Nursing in Contemporary Society
Issues, Trends, and Transition
to Practice

Linda C. Haynes, PhD, RN
Assistant Professor
Baylor University
Louise Herrington School of Nursing
Dallas, Texas

Howard K. Butcher, RN, PhD, APRN, BC
Assistant Professor
University of Iowa College of Nursing
John A. Hartford Foundation
Building Academic Geriatric Nursing Capacity Scholar
Iowa City, Iowa

Teresa A. Boese, MSN, RN
Clinical Assistant Professor
University of Iowa College of Nursing
Iowa City, Iowa

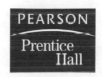
PEARSON
Prentice
Hall

Upper Saddle River, New Jersy 07458

Library of Congress Cataloging-in-Publication Data

Haynes, Linda, (date)
   Nursing in contemporary society : issues, trends, and
transition to practice / by Linda Haynes, Teresa Boese,
Howard Butcher.—1st ed.
      p. cm.
   Includes index.
   ISBN 0-13-094153-0
   1. Nursing. 2. Nursing—Vocational guidance.
   3. Nursing—Social aspects. I. Boese, Teresa. II. Butcher,
Howard, Ph.D. III. Title.
   RT82.H396 2004

   610.73—dc21   2002044572

Publisher: Julie Levin Alexander
Executive Assistant & Supervisor: Regina Bruno
Editor-in-Chief: Maura Connor
Senior Acquisitions Editor: Nancy Anselment
Editorial Assistant: Malgorzata Jaros-White
Director of Manufacturing and Production: Bruce Johnson
Managing Production Editor: Patrick Walsh
Production Liaison: Cathy O'Connell
Production Editor: Linda Begley, Rainbow Graphics
Manufacturing Manager: Ilene Sanford
Manufacturing Buyer: Pat Brown
Design Director: Cheryl Asherman

Senior Design Coordinator: Maria Guglielmo Walsh
Cover Designer: Mary Siener
Senior Marketing Manager: Nicole Benson
Marketing Coordinator: Janet Ryerson
Channel Marketing Manager: Rachele Strober
Media Editor: John Jordan
Media Production Manager: Amy Peltier
Media Project Manager: Stephen Hartner
Composition: Rainbow Graphics
Printer/Binder: Courier/Westford
Cover Printer: Coral Graphics

Pearson Prentice Hall™ is a trademark of Pearson Education, Inc.
Pearson® is a registered trademark of Pearson plc
Prentice Hall® is a registered trademark of Pearson Education, Inc.

Pearson Education LTD.
Pearson Education Australia PTY, Limited
Pearson Education Singapore, Pte. Ltd
Pearson Education North Asia Ltd
Pearson Education, Canada, Ltd
Pearson Educación de Mexico, S.A. de C.V.
Pearson Education–Japan
Pearson Education Malaysia, Pte. Ltd
Pearson Education, Upper Saddle River, NJ

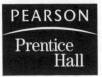

PEARSON
Prentice
Hall

1 0 9 8 7 6 5
0-13-094153-0

Dedication

To the nursing students and nurses who will create the future for nursing

Contents

Unit 6   Challenge of Management   481

Epilogue   Toward the Future   543

Preface

The intent of this textbook is to provide both a comprehensive review of current trends and issues in nursing and a synthesis of practical approaches to facilitate the nursing students' transition from the educational environment to a rewarding career as a professional nurse. Change is occurring at an ever-accelerating pace in health care. As students are prepared to enter professional practice in the Third Millennium, it is essential that they are made aware of the most relevant and current issues and trends affecting professional nursing practice. The content in this textbook is an evidenced-based blend of critical contemporary issues and trends with practical application developed using the framework of *The Essentials of Baccalaureate Education for Professional Nursing Practice*, published by the American Association of Colleges of Nursing (AACN) in 1998. The *Essentials* document provides direction for the educational preparation of professional nurses in the twenty-first century. Using the *Essentials* document, as a guide, *Nursing in Contemporary Society: Issues, Trends and Transition into Practice* combines contemporary approaches to issues, trends, and the transition to practice with a vision for future health care and market place consumer demands. Concepts are illustrated and made relevant by transition into practice–based examples.

The inspiration for writing this book comes from years of teaching issues, trends, professional roles, responsibilities, and critical decision-making as part of the education and preparation of baccalaureate graduate nurses. These experiences have led to the conclusion that a comprehensive, transition into practice–based textbook for baccalaureate graduates is needed which will integrate the importance of accountability, responsibility, and critical decision-making with an understanding of contemporary issues, trends, and transition into practice concerns for future nurses.

The primary goals of *Nursing in Contemporary Society: Issues, Trends, and Transition into Practice* are therefore twofold: to clearly review current trends and issues in nursing and health care and to present a synthesis of practical approaches designed to facilitate the transition into professional practice. This textbook aids in building a foundation for students to become lifelong learners who maintain an ongoing understanding

of contemporary health care concerns. Furthermore, the book will serve as a reference for new graduates and experienced nurses who seek to be informed regarding the most current issues and trends facing the nursing discipline.

We have enhanced the content by assembling a cast of distinguished nurse scholars and leaders who have expertise and are passionate about the specific issues and topics addressed in this book. The content is organized into six major units. Unit 1, Evolution and Context for Professional Nursing Practice, provides an overview of the evolution of the image, education, knowledge, and professional organizations of nurses. Unit 2 focuses on the professional values and core competencies described in AACN's *Essentials* document and includes chapters on professional values in ethical practice, caring, reflective clinical reasoning, technology, and developing and maintaining competence. Unit 3 describes the current trends impacting nursing practice, which include cultural diversity, spiritual care, evidence-based practice, health promotion, and complementary and alternative therapeutic modalities. Major changes occurring in the health care delivery system from an economic, political, and legal perspective are covered in Unit 4. The content in Unit 5 places emphasis on the nursing student's transition into professional nursing practice. Chapters focus on obtaining professional employment, licensure, issues which impact the transition from student to employee, and strategies for coping with employment-related stress. Issues concerning advanced practice preparation and opportunities for employment are also presented in this unit. Unit 6 provides an overview of the challenge of management by including chapters on collaboration, nursing management and leadership, and legal issues for the nurse manager. The book concludes with an Epilogue envisioning future trends and challenges that will face nurses.

A number a features have been incorporated into each chapter to enhance student interest and promote their understanding of current issues, trends, and challenges as they prepare to transition into practice. These features are also designed to assist nurse educators in providing focus for study and discussion.

Learning Objectives appear at the beginning of each chapter to help focus students learning.

Figures appear throughout the text and offer visual interpretations of the underlying content, issues, and trends.

Tables are included as a means to highlight, list, and summarize important information.

Critical Thinking and Reflection boxes are special features found throughout each chapter. These are designed to raise questions and challenge students to think and dialogue about important ideas and content.

Transition into Practice is a unique feature in each chapter that places particular emphasis on how the content and ideas in the chapter are relevant and affect the student's transition from the educational setting into professional nursing practice.

Research Applications are incorporated in each chapter as a means to emphasize the importance of evidence-based thinking as a focus for lifelong learning and professional practice.

Key Points appear near the end of each chapter and are organized in a way to provide a brief summary of the chapter.

Suggested Readings are included at the end of each chapter in addition to the References cited in the text. The readings are included so that the interested student can further explore the information presented in each chapter.

This textbook will facilitate students as they prepare for careers in nursing and the ultimate transition into practice. Today's students are the leaders of tomorrow. If nursing is to be at the forefront of the transformation of health care, then future nurses must be prepared to define and transform the profession to meet ever-changing and emerging health care needs of society. Preparing nurses in this new millennium requires increased emphasis on (a) identifying, articulating, and utilizing nursing's unique body of knowledge to guide nursing practice; (b) changing the image of nursing in the eyes of the public so nursing's contribution to the health and well-being of all is understood, recognized, and rewarded; (c) integrating humanistic values rehumanize the mechanical, corporate, patriarchal, institutional, and bureaucratic practices of our health care system; and (d) incorporating creativity and innovation to improve the delivery of quality nursing care.

Web-based Teaching and Learning Support are also available at a Web site dedicated to *Nursing in*

Contemporary Society: Issues, Trends, and Transition into Practice (http://www.prenhall.com/). This Web site offers learning objectives, key terms with definitions, an overview and outline, and learning activities, which include critical thinking questions, real world projects, and other Web activities for each chapter. In addition to this array of learning activities NCLEX©-type test questions are provided along with Web links, which are continually updated.

Also available on the *Nursing in Contemporary Society: Issues, Trends, and Transition into Practice* (http://www.prenhall.com/) Web site and CD-ROM are resources specifically designed for the instructor. For each chapter, the instructor is also provided an extensive chapter outline with PowerPoint slides that can easily be adapted by the instructor for presentation in the classroom. NCLEX©-type test questions are provided in the Test Bank available on the Web site and CD-ROM. The Web site and CD-ROM also offer the instructor ideas or strategies to stimulate discussion based on critical thinking questions, projects, and Web activities found on the student Web site of *Nursing in Contemporary Society: Issues, Trends, and Transition into Practice.*

Future nurses need to be knowledgeable about issues and trends affecting nursing, including the increasing diversity of health care populations, the movement toward outcome- and evidenced-based practice, complementary health care modalities; and ethical conflicts related to evolving technology. Students require an awareness of the current revolutions in the delivery of health care, including legal, sociopolitical, and economic changes. As a nursing student transitions into professional practice he or she must make career choices, search for employment, function in leadership and management roles, and cope with the stresses of professional practice. The presentation of the topics in this textbook are specifically designed to prepare the next generation of nurse leaders so that nursing can rise to its rightful place in the health care delivery system thus promoting the health and well-being of individuals, communities, and the nation.

Linda C. Haynes, PhD, RN
Howard K. Butcher, RN, PhD, APRN, BC
Teresa A. Boese, MSN, RN

Acknowledgments

Many individuals have contributed to the production of this book particularly the editors of Prentice Hall. We are most grateful to Linda Curran who dedicated her time and skill coordinating, editing, and processing the manuscript. We wish to acknowledge the support of Rita Frantz, PhD, RN, FAAN, without whose contribution our efforts would have been considerably more difficult. We also appreciate the contributions of Kathryn Leonard, Kaye Adams, and Debra Milam for their support, dedication, and tireless effort verifying and researching references. We acknowledge our principal mentors, Melinda Mitchell, MSN, RN; Linda F. Garner, PhD, RN; Melanie McEwen, PhD, RN; Frances Strodtbeck, DSN, RNC, NNP, FAAN; and Pauline Johnson, PhD, RN, who deserve acknowledgment for their unwavering guidance and support. Finally, we wish to thank our families who have inspired and encouraged us. Each of these individuals has been a champion offering a positive attitude while contributing skill, support, and assistance that has made this process enjoyable and rewarding.

Contributors

Joan Carter, PhD, RN
Associate Dean
St. Louis University
School of Nursing
St. Louis, Missouri

Janis C. Childs, PhD, RN, PNP
Associate Professor and Director of the Nursing
    Learning Resource Center
University of Southern Maine
College of Nursing and Health Professions
Portland, Maine

Elizabeth Farren Corbin, PhD, RN, FNP
Professor
Baylor University
Louise Herrington School of Nursing
Dallas, Texas

Patricia Czar, RN
Manager of Clinical Systems
St. Francis Medical Center
Information Services
Pittsburgh, Pennsylvania

M. Patricia Donahue, PhD, RN, FAAN
Executive Associate Dean
The University of Iowa
College of Nursing
Iowa City, Iowa

Melanie C. Dreher, PhD, RN, FAAN
Kelting Dean and Professor
The University of Iowa
College of Nursing
Iowa City, Iowa

Frances Eason, EdD, RNC
Professor
East Carolina University
School of Nursing
Greenville, North Carolina

Jennifer Echols, RN, DSN
Assistant Region Director
Signa Behavioral Health
Tampa, Florida

Debra Franzen, PhD, RN
Professor
Grand View College
Division of Nursing
Des Moines, Iowa

Linda F. Garner, PhD, RN
Associate Professor
Baylor University
Louise Herrington School of Nursing
Dallas, Texas

Deborah R. Garrison, PhD, RN
Chair, Nursing Department
Midwestern State University
Nursing Program
Wichita Falls, Texas

Ginny Wacker Guido, JD, PhD, FAAN
Associate Dean and Director of Graduate Studies
University of North Dakota
College of Nursing
Grand Forks, North Dakota

William Christopher Haynes, JD
Attorney at Law
Erhard and Jennings
Dallas, Texas

Toni Lee Hebda, PhD, RN
Adjunct Professor
Duquesne University
School of Nursing
Pittsburgh, Pennsylvania

Faye Hummel, PhD, RN, CTN
Professor
University of Northern Colorado
School of Nursing
Greeley, Colorado

Debra Woodard Leners, PhD, RN, CPNP
Professor
University of Northern Colorado
School of Nursing
Greeley, Colorado

Jean Logan, PhD, RN
Professor and Head of the Division of Nursing
Grand View College
Division of Nursing
Des Moines, Iowa

Cynthia Mascara, MSN, MBA, RN
Senior Implementation Consultant
Siemens Medical Solutions Health Services
Pittsburgh, Pennsylvania

Merry J. McBryde-Foster, PhD, CCM, RN
Assistant Professor
Baylor University
Louise Herrington School of Nursing
Dallas, Texas

Melanie McEwen, PhD, RN
Associate Professor
Baylor University
Louise Herrington School of Nursing
Dallas, Texas 75246

Jacquelin S. Neatherlin, PhD, RN, CNRN
Associate Professor
Baylor University
Louise Herrington School of Nursing
Dallas, Texas

Carolyn Pauling, MSN, BSN
Assistant Professor
Grand View College
Division of Nursing
Des Moines, Iowa

Daniel J. Pesut, PhD, RN, CS, FAAN
Professor and Department Chair
Indiana University
School of Nursing
IUPUI Campus
Indianapolis, Indiana

Diane Peters, PhD, RN, CTN
Professor
University of Northern Colorado
School of Nursing
Greeley, Colorado

Judith M. Richter, PhD, RN
Professor
University of Northern Colorado
School of Nursing
Greeley, Colorado

Barbara Ritzert, PhD, RN
Thompson, Coe, Cousins & Irons LLP
Dallas, Texas

Lisa Sams, MSN, RNC
President
Clinical Linkages, Inc.
Arlington, Virginia

Leona Stoll, RN, MSN
Consultant
St Louis, Missouri

Frances Strodtbeck, DNS, RNC, NNP, FAAN
Associate Professor
Baylor University
Louise Herrington School of Nursing
Dallas, Texas

Marilyn Terrado, PhD, RN, CS
Assistant Professor
Rush University
College of Nursing
Department of Adult Health Nursing
Chicago, Illinois

Nancy White, PhD, RN
Professor
University of Northern Colorado
School of Nursing
Greeley, Colorado

Reviewers

Margaret W. Bellak, MN, RN
Associate Professor
Indiana University of Pennsylvania
Indiana, Pennsylvania

Joan B. Carlisle, DSN, CRNP-BC
Assistant Professor
University of Alabama at Birmingham, School of
    Nursing
Birmingham, Alabama

Sandra K. Cesario, PhD, RN
Director of Research and Assistant Professor
Texas Woman's University College of Nursing
Houston, Texas

Maureen Cochran, PhD, RN
Adjunct Professor
Suffolk University
Boston, Massachusetts

Peggy Craik, MBA, MS, RN
Associate Professor
University of Mary Hardin-Baylor School of Nursing
Belton, Texas

Vera V. Cull, RN, DSN
Assistant Professor
University of Alabama at Birmingham, School of
    Nursing
Birmingham, Alabama

Cynthia L. Dakin, PhD, RN
Clinical Specialist
Northeastern University, School of Nursing
Boston, Massachusetts

Susan DeSanto-Madeya, RN, DNSc
Assistant Professor
St. Luke's SON at Moravian College
Bethlehem, Pennsylvania

Frances Anne Freitas, MSN, RNC
Assistant Professor
Kent State University—Ashtabula Campus
Ashtabula, Ohio

Tracey C. Gaslin, RN, MSN, CRNI, CPNP
University of Louisville
Louisville, Kentucky

Rebecca Gesler, MSN, RN
St. Catharine College
St. Catharine, Kentucky

Peggy L. Hawkins, PhD, RN
Associate Professor of Nursing
College of Saint Mary
Omaha, Nebraska

Sandra Huddleston, PhD, RN
Associate Professor of Nursing, Foster G. McGaw
    Chair in Nursing
Berea College
Berea, Kentucky

Susan Kardong-Edgren, PhD(c), RN
Director, Baccalaureate School of Nursing Program
University of Texas at Arlington
Arlington, Texas

Nancy Kramer, EdD, CPNP, ARNP
Professor and BSN Program Chair
Allen College
Waterloo, Iowa

Sylvia Kubsch, PhD, RN
Associate Professor of Nursing, Interim Chairperson,
    Professional Program in Nursing
University of Wisconsin Green Bay
Green Bay, Wisconsin

Judith A. Lewis, PhD, RNC, FAAN
Associate Professor and Director of Information
    Technology
Virginia Commonwealth University School of Nursing
Richmond, Virginia

Patrica K. Leary, MS
Allied Health Instructor
MOISD and FSU
Big Rapids, Michigan

Gale E. Manke, MSN, RN
Clinical Associate Professor
University of Arizona, College of Nursing
Tucson, Arizona

Pamela Martin, PhD, RN
Assistant Dean for Nursing Undergraduate Programs
College of Nursing and Health Sciences
Tyler, Texas

Sheila P. Patros, PhD, RN
Chairperson and Associate Professor, Department of
    Nursing
Kentucky State University
Frankfort, Kentucky

Renee S. Schnieder, MSN, RN
Faculty Advisor ADN Program
Southeast Community College
Lincoln, Nebraska

Patricia Spurr, EdD, MSN, RN
Director of Baccalaureate Nursing Program
Spalding University
Louisville, Kentucky

Nancy M. Sweeney, DNSc, RN, PHN
Lecturer
San Diego State University School of Nursing
San Diego, California

Sharon Telban, DEd, RNC
Associate Professor and Director, Masters Program
Wilkes University
Wilkes-Barre, Pennsylvania

Rose Mary Volbrecht, PhD
Professor of Philosophy, Health Care Ethics
    Consultant
Gonzaga University
Spokane, Washington

Carol G. Williams, DNSc, RN
Associate Professor
Central Connecticut State University Department of
    Nursing
New Britain, Connecticut

Janet M. Witucki, PhD, MSN, RN
Assistant Professor
The University of Tennessee College of Nursing
Knoxville, Tennessee

Susan P. Yarbrough, PhD, RN
Assistant Professor and Assistant Dean for Graduate
    Nursing Programs
The University of Texas at Tyler College of Nursing
Tyler, Texas

Unit 1

Evolution and Context for Professional Nursing Practice

1

Turning Points in Nursing History

M. Patricia Donahue

> *My experience of men has never disposed me to think worse of them, nor indisposed me to serve them; nor, in spite of failures which I lament, of errors which I only now see and acknowledge, or of the present aspect of affairs, do I despair of the future. The truth is this: the march of Providence is so slow and our desires so impatient, the work of progress is so immense and our means of aiding it so feeble; the life of humanity is so long, that of the individual so brief, that we often see only the ebb of the advancing wave and are thus discouraged. It is history that teaches us to hope.*
>
> *Robert E. Lee*

LEARNING OBJECTIVES

AT THE COMPLETION OF THIS CHAPTER, THE READER WILL BE ABLE TO:

➤ Identify the great turning points in world progress that represent milestones in nursing's march toward identity.

➤ Discuss the rationale for the study of nursing history.

➤ Compare the achievements of past nursing leaders with leaders of today.

➤ Determine needed strategies to secure nursing's position in health care.

➤ Discuss how visionary nurse inventors formed a set of core ideas consistent with their social context that served to mold the legacy of nursing.

➤ Examine the role of men in nursing.

➤ Explore the relationship between nursing and society.

MediaLink www.prenhall.com/haynes

Additional online resources including NCLEX review questions, critical thinking questions, and real-world activities for this chapter can be found on the Companion Website at www.prenhall.com/haynes.

*S*ome time ago an article entitled "Thank Heavens for Crazy People" appeared in the *American Journal of Nursing*. It contained this advertisement for a job:

> Wanted: People to work long hours with frequent mandatory overtime. Few holidays and weekends off. Must be able to keep massive amounts of paperwork up to date while making split-second, life-or-death decisions. Must be immune to verbal abuse and able to neutralize the occasional physical assault. Must display patience, kindness, understanding, and caring even when personal life is coming apart at the seams. Salary in no way commensurate with training and ability (Mitch, 1991, p. 108).

The author continued: "In case you're thinking no one would ever work at a job like that, you're wrong. Hundreds of people . . . are already working under those conditions. They're called nurses." Some people might indeed contend that those who take on a job such as this are just plain crazy. However, the above environmental conditions under which nurses practice are reflected throughout nursing's history and clearly emphasize that nurses have always possessed a sense of devotion and responsibility to society no matter what the circumstances—two qualities that seem to be nearly extinct in today's world.

The picture that nursing currently presents is complex and impressive. There are hundreds of thousands of nurses in the working world, comprising one of the largest existing bodies of professional women and men. They function in a vast array of settings, so varied, so constantly expanding that it seems almost to defy limitation. Nurses are involved in that vital field of human effort concerned with health care. In addition, the complex mechanism of the modern hospital cannot function without an organized body of nurses. The need for nurses is as great today as it was in the past.

Yet, efforts to stop nursing's march toward identity have been continuous and diligent since Florence Nightingale set modern nursing in motion. Approaches aimed at the control or obliteration of nursing, without concern for social or human welfare, have been designed and attempted. The story of nursing is a great epic involving trials and triumphs, romance and adventure. Its history has been one of frustration, ignorance, and misunderstanding, an epic of an occupational group whose status has always been affected by the prevalent standards of humanity. Great turning points in world progress also represent turning points in nursing. According to Stewart (1929), events that give rise to ". . . higher degrees of consideration for those who are helpless or oppressed, kindliness and sympathy for

the unfortunate and for those who suffer, tolerance for those of differing religion, race, color, etc.—all tend to promote activities like nursing which are primarily humanitarian" (p. 3). At issue in this schema is the fact that nursing must shape and control its own destiny. The power has always been in the hands of nurses to accomplish this, but they have continued to perpetuate the passivity of the past, to behave as an oppressed group and regard themselves as victims. Perhaps nurses need to heed the message in the fable by Styles (1982):

A Biblical Fable on Our Origins

In the beginning, God created nursing.
He (or She) said, I will take a solid, simple,
Significant system of *education* and an
adequate, applicable base of clinical
research, and
On these rocks, will I build My greatest gift
To Mankind—nursing practice.
On the seventh day, He—threw up His hands.
And has left it up to us (p. 154).

The fable certainly does illustrate the fact that nursing is "up to nursing."

Although early philosophy identified nursing strictly with the care of the sick, Florence Nightingale had a different conception of the word, pointing out that there were "nurses of the sick and nurses of health." Nightingale continually spoke of "health" not "illness," described disease as a reparative process, and defined nursing not as the administration of medicines or medical regimens, but as the proper use of air, light, warmth, quiet, cleanliness, and diet—". . . at the least expense of vital power to the patient" (Nightingale, 1860, pp. 1–2). She set forth a clear, concise charge to nurses for a broad definition of nursing—caring for and caring about—not confined to the narrow scope, which limits medicine to the diagnosis and cure of disease. More importantly, she envisioned nursing as the care of the individual: the care of the physical, the mental, and the spiritual.

Nightingale was truly an independent practitioner who viewed herself as the patient's advocate. One need only look at the mortality rates at Scutari for evidence. Prior to her arrival there with 38 nurses, the death rate was over 40% even though physicians and surgeons abounded. Within 6 months, Nightingale and her nurses reduced the death rate to less than 2%. Nightingale proved that *good nursing care made the difference*, since nursing care was the only new variable that had been introduced.

Nightingale also understood the importance of economics, the stratagems of power, and the underlying subtleties of control related to social issues. She used this knowledge to advance nursing in all arenas, including education. She believed that improvements in nursing education would result in improved nursing practice. The entire realm of nursing care based on a holistic concept of man would thus be positively affected. Nightingale was involved in developing a knowledge base for professional practice that went far beyond the simple elements of skill and expertise in the performance of procedures or the manipulation of machines. She was vitally concerned with the very broad responsibilities of nursing and with the role that women, especially nurses, could take in effecting social change. Indeed, Miss Nightingale has been celebrated as one of the most brilliant persons of the nineteenth century, a woman whose ideas and feats of accomplishment stagger the imagination.

Early leaders in nursing, while essentially agreeing with Nightingale's tenets, consistently referred to nursing as an art as well as a science. Art was the essential ingredient in the concept of caring. Art, as such, was a form of inquiry, a qualitative inquiry that stressed the role of intelligence and involved a type of perception that was active, dynamic, and developing. The art of nursing was essentially the creative use of knowledge and a means to create beauty. It was recognized that people could be said to be technically perfect in music and painting, but lacking in soul, mind, or imagination. Thus, a difference did exist between a true artist and a mere technician. It was believed, therefore, that emphasis on the nurse as a true artist was essential to the progression of nursing into something other than a highly skilled trade. Stewart (1929) clearly defined this position:

> The real essence of nursing, as of any fine art, lies not in the mechanical details of execution, nor yet in the dexterity of the performer, but in the creative imagination, the sensitive spirit, and the intelligent understanding lying back of these techniques and skills. Without these, nursing may become a highly skilled trade, but it cannot be a profession or a fine art. All the rituals and ceremonials which our modern worship of efficiency may devise, and all our elaborate scientific equipment will not save us if the intellectual and spiritual elements in our art are subordinated to the mechanical, and if the means come to be regarded as more important than ends (p. 1).

In order to understand nursing and its future, it is necessary to know not only existing conditions, but also influences that have shaped its current status. It is necessary to understand that nursing has been, and always will be, linked to constantly occurring issues generated by changes and/or trends in the medical and human sciences, in technology, in consumers' health care problems and needs, and in health care systems (Donahue, 1998). Professional nursing evolves in response to these trends, as depicted in Figure 1–1. In other words, the profession of nursing continues to be integrally involved in a cyclic process that responds to social change. In addition, economic, political, cultural, social, and ethical considerations provide a contextual background for understanding nursing. The message from the past is clear. Future nurses must continually search for answers in theory, research, and practice, and must be competent in both the art and science of nursing. This competence will not only stimulate the development of new knowledge and contribute to a growing body of nursing science, but will also expand nurses' understanding of humans and their health care needs. In order to achieve this, however, nurses must be empowered by an education with high standards of excellence that adequately prepares them to apply knowledge from every source and be committed to research and scholarship (Donley, 1989).

Why Study Nursing History?

The study of history is not an idle journey into a dead past. It is rather a way to understand and live in the present, since all experience is part of history. What is true of life is also true for nursing. Earlier generations of nurses studied nursing history, recognizing its relevancy to comprehending trends and issues in the discipline. They recognized that without examining their history, they could not understand where nursing had been or where it was going. They recognized that the "past" world was as fascinating as the world in which they were currently living and that the past could provide clues to nursing's future.

Christy (1978) used the phrase "The Hope of History" to refer to the value to be derived from studying nursing history. Everything has a history—families, patients, inventions, cultures, countries, and technology. Contrary to popular belief, history is not only contained in musty materials on library shelves. History is everywhere—even in the mind of every human being. Consider, for example, an individual who has a sudden loss of memory, a loss of all historical knowledge. This loss of memory, diagnosed as amnesia, may be due to a variety of circumstances. Yet, the meaning is clear. The vanished memory has left the individual with a significant void in which life may be viewed as meaningless, with no

Figure 1–1   Sphere of Influence

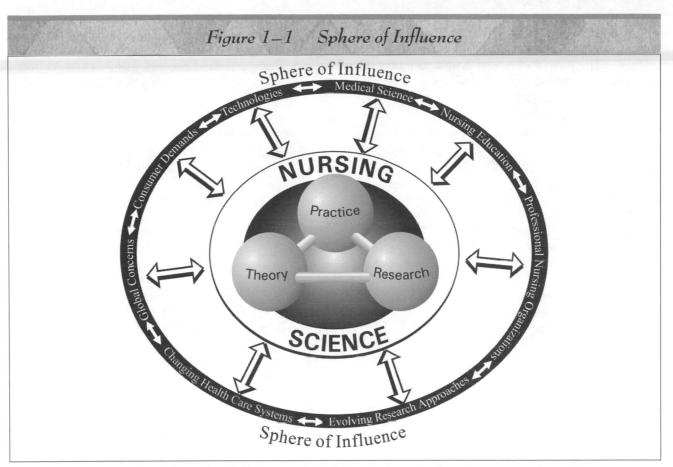

Reprinted from *Issues and trends in nursing*, G. Deloughery (Ed.), The evolution of nursing science and practice, p. 89, Copyright 1998, with permission of Elsevier Science.

reference points to provide guidance (Donahue, 1994). Reflect on this in relation to nursing when nurses are either ignorant of or have no memory of their history. Would it be possible for nurses to make sense of the world around them with no understanding of history? Or would utter helplessness, confusion, and misery abound? Thus, history is a way of thinking about the present in the hope that some sense can be made of complex contemporary events by scrutinizing their origins. History serves to clarify context and provide meaning.

History is not merely a transmitter of tradition or a way to legitimize the status quo. It is also social knowledge concerned with values, meanings, and facts useful for all who deal with human beings in complex situations. Historical thought occurs daily in the professional lives of nurses as they use the nursing process; construct case histories; obtain patient histories; identify nursing diagnoses, interventions, and outcomes; and create research proposals. It stands to reason, then,

that the study of nursing history is not only valuable, but also necessary for understanding the human experience. It is difficult to identify any nursing problem that has not been shaped by history. In Lerner's (1982) analysis, history functions to satisfy a variety of human needs, thereby making history "not a dispensable intellectual luxury" but a social necessity. She further identifies the following historical functions:

- History as memory and as source of personal identity—Generations are linked together; experiences, ideas, and deeds are kept alive; past and future are a source of personal identity.
- History as collective immortality—A sense of immortality is provided through the creation of a structure in the mind.
- History as cultural tradition—Diverse groups are united through a shared body of ideas, values, and experiences that lead to a cultural tradition.

- History as explanation—Historical events become "illustrations" of philosophies and of broader interpretive frameworks through an ordering of the past. The past can become evidence, model, contrast to the present, symbol, or challenge (p. 10).

Finally, the study of nursing history should provide an inspiration. The early leaders such as Isabel Hampton Robb, M. Adelaide Nutting, Lavinia Lloyd Dock, Isabel Maitland Stewart, Lillian D. Wald, Annie Goodrich, and others present a rich heritage that illus-

Research Application

Historical research is the "careful study and analysis of data about past events. The understanding of the importance of the past on present and future events related to the life process" (Brockopp & Hastings-Tolsma, 1995, p. 243). It is more than a collection of data. It is a study of facts, incidents, and themes that have affected the past, continue to impact the present, and may influence the future (Brink & Wood, 1998).

Historical research is undertaken to (a) discover the unknown, (b) answer why something happened, (c) communicate past accomplishments, and (d) look at implications and consequences of relationships. Historical research serves to instill pride in accomplishments. One has only to review the table of contents of the journal *Nursing Historical Review* to experience a small sense of the pride nurses should feel for their profession. Historical research is conducted because most see the past as valuable. This value is conveyed by such common phrases as "We learn from our mistakes" and "What has history taught us?"

All agree that the events of the September 11, 2001, terrorist attacks will be retold for generations to come. The telling of these events will be filtered through the perceptions of historians. This type of filtration depicts one of the major concerns regarding accuracy of historical analysis. Historical researchers must maintain a clear, unbiased quest for answers; otherwise, the data will not accurately portray what took place.

Investigating history is more than reviewing history textbooks. It is complex, as historical investigators have no control over the creation of the data or the environment they study. These historians are at the mercy of those who created and stored the data. Historical research can be costly. It requires researchers to review original data often in the form of diaries, letters, manuscripts, maps, or books. Nurse historians may travel long distances to review primary sources of information in hospitals, archives, or historical societies. Furthermore, access to and viewing of the original sources is restricted by the actions of the controlling agency.

Historical research is complicated as the researcher is attempting to (a) reconstruct events, (b) analyze rationale behind decisions, and (c) trace activities and influences that lead to current events. These researchers may be attempting to trace the scientific origins for procedures. They may be attempting to discover the impetus or the creative thought that led to a sequence of events that culminated in discovery. Further, the job of the historical researcher is difficult as this individual is attempting to analyze the ideas of another person.

We take the facts presented in history books for granted. These textbooks provide a foundation for information, but only nurse historians such as Christy, Lynaugh, Hamilton, Donahue, Bullough, and Fairman provide nurses with greater understanding of the heritage of nursing. Nurses who wish to explore history need not go further than their own nursing school. They need only think about and design a research question. For example, a nurse might ask what led to the idea that resulted in my nursing school? The next step would be to begin gathering information from sources. These sources will initially be secondary sources that will lead to the primary data and the ultimate analysis and synthesis of information to explain the origins of the school of nursing.

History is designed to put into context what has happened in the past to help us understand the present and what lies in the future. For nurses to understand their profession, they need to understand where their profession has come from. Historical research provides a venue for this understanding.

As stated earlier, vanished memories leave individuals with a significant void in which life may be viewed as meaningless, with no reference points to provide guidance (Donahue, 1994). Reflect on this in relation to your own family history—many individuals are either ignorant of or with no memory of their history. Is it possible for individuals to make better sense of the world around them by understanding their history? How does knowledge of your own family history help you make sense or influence your understanding of the world?

trates courage, dedication, standards of excellence, and successes. These leaders did much to shape the course of nursing practice and nursing education. They were involved in the social issues of the times including women's suffrage, child labor laws, public health, and national defense. The insight to be gained by studying these role models is immeasurable.

A Reflection of Social Reality

Changes in response to societal needs lend credence to the fact that nursing is a reflection of social reality. Nursing continually changes, grows, and advances in response to perceived social needs and societal demands for services. In other words, nursing as an occupational group changes in concert with changing needs of society and with advancements in medical science, knowledge, and technology. The impact of these forces, along with shifting public policies, mandates constant fluctuations in nursing roles, functions, and responsibilities. This combination of factors places nursing in a constant state of flux, making the ultimate goal of quality care, at times, more difficult. Perhaps this is why it is extremely difficult to capture the total "essence" of nursing, its true art and its caring spirit. Nursing is abstract yet concrete, complex yet simple. It defies expression! Just when we think we know what nursing is and what it is about, it changes. Paintbrushes, pens, charcoal, pencils, cameras, clay, and any other type of artistic medium are inadequate for capturing the intricacies and complexities of human beings, societies, and cultures, all of which are encompassed in the role of nurses. It is thus apparent that nursing is dynamic, not static, and its definition is continually transformed!

Several significant points have characterized this tight bond between nursing and the societies it serves:

- "The history of nursing is an episode in the history of women." In one sense, the entire history of nursing may be summed up in this statement— "the nurse is the mirror in which is reflected the position of woman through the ages" (Robinson, 1946, p. VII).

- The overall position/status of women within society affects the position/status of nursing within society. In other words, if women are respected in a society or culture and accorded high status, nurses will generally occupy the same position. The reverse is also true. If women are not respected in a society or culture nor accorded high status, nurses will also occupy a low status.

- The care of the sick is always influenced by the nature of the society at any given time and place, the type of civilization, and the ideals that are maintained by the society. For example, nursing among primitive tribes was different than nursing in England during the Renaissance. Nursing is always related to both the social and cultural history of a particular society.

- The status of nursing is always affected by the prevalent standards of humanity. If the society is concerned with humane treatment of individuals, nursing will be promoted. This translates to the idea that when there is a high degree of consideration for those who are helpless or oppressed, or sympathy for the unfortunate and suffering, nursing will be promoted.

- Throughout history, both men and women have served as caregivers within societies. The predominant sex is usually governed by specific world or cultural events (e.g., crusades, Christianity, dark ages).

- Nursing has involved different roles and functions at different eras in history.

- Although caregivers have always been present in society, they have been addressed by a variety of titles. For example, caregivers have been referred to as slaves, servants, attendants, and nurses. In addition, persons such as priests or physicians sometimes assumed the caregiver role.

- Great turning points in world progress are also turning points in nursing. Consider the impact of inventions, technology, and specialization on nursing.
- Wars seriously impact nursing. Nursing has made some of its greatest strides during time of war. Wars harshly illustrate the evils of humankind and create situations where the need for care of the sick and wounded is profound. Wars also create serious ethical dilemmas for nurses who frequently must triage soldiers according to the seriousness of injuries. In addition, they must deal with the knowledge that soldiers returned to health will be sent to battle to face injury and death once again.
- Different types of leaders emerge in nursing depending on the structure of health care, as well as on the social and political forces of the particular era.

Nursing and society have and will continue to occupy a close, indispensable alliance. Nursing's future will continue to be affected by constant change resulting from external and internal forces. It will be up to nursing to develop an understandable road map for dealing with change.

Nature of Nursing—Heritage and Tradition, Values and Virtues

The work of nursing is intimate, involving the "care of strangers." Therein lies its beauty. Throughout nursing history, nurses have cared for individuals they have never known, have never seen. They have cared for individuals in the most intimate way possible—seeing and touching patients' most private parts, as well as listening to their most personal stories, concerns, fears, and secrets. Patients permit this bodily and spiritual intimacy, trusting that nurses will care for them in a way that will retain and maintain their human dignity. The American public loves and trusts nurses. For two years in a row, Gallup's survey on honesty and ethics in professions found that the American public rates nursing as the field with the highest standards of honesty and ethics. "Almost eight in 10 Americans—79%—say nurses have 'very high' or 'high' ethical standards" (Carlson, 2000, p. 1). In the wake of the September 11, 2001, terrorist attacks in the United States, firefighters ranked first in the 2001 poll. Nurses were second with 80% of Americans rating them high or very high on these characteristics (Moore, 2001).

The nursing profession was built on a firm foundation, embodying those traditional values of caring, compassion, commitment, advocacy, and quality of care. Nurses have traditionally valued honesty and engaged in nursing practice based on ethical principals. Although nurses embrace these values, they frequently vacillate in the practice of those values. Issues such as the ongoing struggle for power and authority, the impact of less-than-desirable working conditions, the continuing "entry into practice" debate, and the minimal recognition of nurses' increasing obligations and responsibilities for patient care impede the nurse's ability to place value into practice and serve as a source of dissonance for nurses.

Health care may be changing, but the traditional values of nursing are still relevant. What remains to be done, therefore, is to effectively balance the humanistic, traditional nursing values with a highly technologic, highly specialized delivery system forced to operate under cost containment. Nursing must again move in the direction in which values of individual human dignity, quality caring, and humanitarian concerns are emphasized even while being forced to cut costs. More than ever, the nurse must be the conduit of care, keeping the focus on humane patient care while seamlessly weaving the science of nursing with the art of nursing. This struggle to bridge the gap between science and the humanities in nursing is explicated by Lynaugh (2001):

> Clearly, nurses need intimate understanding of the discipline of nursing and need to grasp the social context in which they function. Nurses need to appreciate the social relevance and value orientations of their field; they need to know how to relate to other disciplines and how our heritage influences our perspective (p. 239).

Perhaps the words of Hamilton (1994) also ring true: ". . . nurses are seeking to reexamine, reframe, and clarify the heritage and tradition of nursing" (p. 25). Such is the challenge for nursing!

Themes in Nursing History

An analysis of nursing history reveals a number of prevalent themes that have directly and/or indirectly affected nursing throughout its evolution. These themes have endured across the ages and continue to impact current nursing practice, education, and research. The themes of politics, power and control, economics, women's work, and education are particularly significant to an understanding of nursing history. In addition, religion, the military, and technology are also significant themes addressed separately as powerful influences on nursing's development.

Politics, Power, and Control

The failure of nursing to emerge as a viable, political force is a result of numerous factors. Chief among these is the reality that women dominate the profession in a society that has constantly regarded women in general and nurses specifically as nonpolitical. Changes are occurring in the political arena with increasing numbers of women and nurses moving into political offices, but the change has been slow. Women and nurses are frequently still underrepresented in political offices and are usually in those positions affording less power. They operate on the fringes of politics, often engaging in menial campaign tasks, rarely seeking positions of power.

Unfortunately, political awareness and political action have not consistently been a vital component of nursing particularly in relation to organized nursing. Yet, there have been nursing role models who have always been involved in politics. Their political strategies involved the written word, the use of statistics, and the enlisting of help from politicians, government officials, and philanthropists in order to advance nursing and its practice. Prominent among these early nursing leaders was Florence Nightingale, an accomplished politician, who was able to initiate and institute considerable reforms. Particularly interesting is the fact that ". . . she was a reformer on a larger scale through the influence which she exercised" (Cook, 1913, p. 214). As such she was both the inspiration and instigator of many achievements completed by others.

Lavinia Lloyd Dock, endowed with one of the keenest and most versatile minds in the profession, completed a careful study of laws under which professional organizations could operate. She contributed important and powerful articles to the *American Journal of Nursing* dealing with the structure and purpose of professional organizations and a variety of social problems. At a time when nurses were novices in legislative matters, Miss Dock wrote a classic and still convincing article, "What We May Expect from the Law" (Dock, 1901). An ardent pacifist, she boycotted World War I as editor of the *Journal*'s "Foreign News." Dock was also a colorful and zealous suffragist and a radical feminist. She was convinced that women would achieve equality with men only through the right to vote. Her many activities against "social evils"

included publishing a book, *Hygiene and Morality* (Dock, 1910), dealing with the then-taboo subject of venereal disease.

Another nurse who looked to legislation to resolve social and health problems was Lillian D. Wald. She was brilliant in her approaches to influential people as she fought to change deplorable conditions of immigrants living in the tenements of New York City's lower east side. With the establishment of the world-famous Henry Street Settlement, she was able to organize the first community nursing services, which expanded to include public health, school, and rural nursing. Lillian Wald's contributions to nursing and society at large were numerous and focused primarily on reforms that would ensure some measure of justice for the "unfortunates." Her initiative and skill in securing support for new ideas and new plans made her one of the most influential health workers of her day. "Throughout her life she had opposed political and social corruption and supported those measures that would improve the health, wealth, and happiness of humanity" (Donahue, 1996, p. 307).

Even the notion that there is "power in numbers" has been elusive in nursing. Although nurses at 2.7 million constitute the largest number of health care providers, these numbers are not reflected in membership in their professional organization, the American Nurses Association (ANA). This is startling since the unity and strength of a powerful organization would be a significant political strategy. But the "free rider" problem continues to plague the professional organization in that nurses who do not belong to the ANA still reap the benefits gained through the organization's initiatives. This is true especially with respect to the political arena. The ANA formed a legislative committee in 1928 that represented nursing throughout the depression and World War II. It was not until 1974, however, that the Nurses' Coalition for Action in Politics (N-CAP) was formed, which became the political arm of the ANA to raise money for political campaigns of aspirants for elective office. Two years later in 1976, the ANA began publicly supporting political candidates for congressional office. Financial support was not always guaranteed due to limited funds. Candidates were endorsed based on their views and actions related to key health issues, funding for nursing and biomedical research, funding for nursing education, and third-party reimbursement for nurses. Endorsement of congressional candidates expanded to include candidates for president and vice president in 1984. In 1986, to promote identification with the ANA, the name N-CAP was changed to ANA/PAC.

Whether or not nurses believe that a professional organization should endorse political candidates, the process is a mechanism for gaining access to persons in high places. It is also a way to make nursing visible at all levels and provide a vehicle through which nursing issues can be heard. The influence of professional organizations as a political force should not be minimized. At this most crucial time in nursing history, nurses need to join, participate, and unite. More importantly, they need to recognize that today's politics mandate the use of power, that many issues currently faced by nursing will undeniably be decided in the political arena, and that a professional organization can't do all the work. Nursing needs the support of all members of the profession.

An interesting dichotomy has existed in nursing related to power and control. The intimate and complex relationships established between nurse and patient permitted nurses to control the relationships. Yet, when nurses functioned outside of these care relationships, their participation in decision-making and negotiation was minimal, at best. Nurses were particularly ineffective when dealing with physicians and hospital administrators (Reverby, 1987). What is perhaps most significant here is an analysis of a lack of power in nursing's history. Although power usually implies more than one person involved in influencing a relationship, power begins with oneself. Frequently, the aspect of risk taking is also involved, a concept not generally embraced by nurses.

Nurses and nursing could exert a powerful influence on the health status of every individual, on the public's health, and on the future of the health care system. Nurses have had a long history of effecting change in health care due to unique experiences and intuition about forces and issues that impact health care delivery. Nurses must continue to be involved with providing strategies for the resolution of these problems. What becomes clear is that power, politics, and risk taking are essential factors for the true attainment of control of nursing practice and the assumption of an influential position in the health care system.

Economics

The history of nursing has been and always will be linked with the issues and trends occurring in economics. Economics is a powerful force that exerts pressures on the health care delivery system. As health care reforms are mandated, economics are a driving force that frequently focus on cost containment and on obtaining the cheapest care from the cheapest provider. These factors are closely correlated with nursing's position in the system. The social and economic utility of nurses in the health field formed the foundations of delivery systems in hospitals, homes, welfare agencies, industries, clinics, and schools—everywhere that nurses practiced. As the economic and managerial value of nurses became obvious to those interested in the development of the health care industry, the social good that nurses did tended to receive less and less public emphasis.

Nursing emerged from interacting social and economic needs related to the care of the ill. Nursing developed from the growth of paternalistic hospitals eager to manipulate females and to profit from nurses' work. Hospital administrators and physicians were not supportive of formal nursing education, the former even believing that requiring one year of high school prior to nursing school placed a hardship on the hospital and the latter in part threatened by their own lack of a college education (Ashley, 1976; Bullough & Bullough, 1964). Student nurses became a source of virtually free labor and provided almost all of patient services under an apprenticeship system. Accompanying this practice were deplorable working conditions that included long hours, hard and demanding work, and low status. Free labor by student nurses enabled hospitals to buy new equipment for use by physicians with money not spent for nursing services. Salaries just above poverty level enabled hospital administrators to improve hospitals. The addition of "old medical techniques" to the work of nurses rarely brought prestige or increased salaries; it just brought more work (Peplau, 1966). Finally, "The availability and persistence of exploitative student labor, a system created and sustained by the problems of

---

Critical Thinking and Reflection

Should nurses and/or nursing organizations endorse political candidates? Why or why not? How could the "free rider" problem in nursing be overcome? How would you describe yourself? Do you take risks? If not, how can you prepare to join that force of nurses dedicated to exerting a powerful influence in health reform?

underfinanced hospitals, corrupted the education of nurses" (Lynaugh, 1991, p. 14).

Deep-rooted traditions have also contributed to the economic plight of nurses. Hospitals have been associated with charitable institutions; nursing has been associated with other forms of Christian service. This altruistic spirit of nursing in which service would be available whenever illness occurred became a barrier to any deliberate consideration of working hours or compensation. In addition, the emphasis on obedience, subservience, and submissiveness required of student nurses added to the undervaluing of nursing contributions. These factors affected the social and economic life of the nurse for a long time and continue to impact such nursing issues as a compressed pay range, minimal additional pay for undesirable shifts, pay unrelated to education, and hiring without consideration of competencies and education.

Inadequate financial support has long been a barrier to nursing education. Isabel Stewart was forceful in her comments that nursing schools needed to be removed from hospitals or there would be no hope for advancements in nursing education. She commented that nursing schools should have independent financial status and the power to develop their own system of education, and be unhampered by the complicated and crushing demands of the hospital. She favored some type of endowment for nursing schools. Otherwise, support should come from state or municipal funds. Stewart (1921) fearlessly stated:

> The plain facts are that nursing schools are being starved and always have been starved for lack of funds to build up any kind of substantial educational structure. As someone has recently said, the nursing school has been literally buried in the hospital, and few people have been aware of its existence. It has fed on the crumbs that fell from the hospital table—a very frugal table, as everyone knows. The educational interests of the school have had no chance whatever against the pressing economic interests of the hospital, and it is probable that even if the hospital recognized its educational obligations, which it has never done, it would find considerable difficulty in meeting them as they should be met (pp. 17–18).

Adelaide Nutting went one step further in declaring "The root of all the main problems in nursing will be found, I believe, if carefully studied, to be economic in nature" (Nutting, 1926, p. vi). She wrote of the economic problems in education, which included (a) the role students played as a source of cheap labor and (b)

the weak economic foundation of training schools for nurses. By 1926, only two large endowments had been made for nursing education. Miss Nightingale gave the first, $200,000, for the founding of the Nightingale School at St. Thomas Hospital in London with an independent financial base. Mrs. Helen Hartley Jenkins for the Department of Nursing and Health at Teachers College, Columbia University in New York gave the second, approximately $150,000. These two endowments were a beginning, but much more work was needed to further growth and progress in nursing education.

Economic issues continue to exist in nursing in both the education and practice settings. However, nursing is no longer a strictly altruistic profession but one that mandates the acquisition of sophisticated knowledge and skills in order to provide quality nursing care. Only by understanding and exploring the relationship between economics and nursing will nurses be prepared to practice effectively in the present and meet complex challenges of the future.

Women's Work

Nursing at its inception was almost exclusively a female profession. Caring for the sick, the helpless, the weak, and anyone in need had long been the task of women. This societal view of nursing as "women's work" often dissuaded men from entering the discipline and functioned as a repressive force for women with "higher aspirations." In general, this "women's work" was devalued. In Ashley's (1976) scrutiny, the progress of nursing and nurses was significantly thwarted by these cultural conventions about women and women's work and further by self-serving male hospital administrators and physicians. Reverby (1987), on the other hand, deduced that nurses were "ordered to care" within a culture in which caring was honored more in discourse than in practice.

Nursing was also hampered by the social misconception that the feminine mind was inherently inferior and that intellectual growth was harmful to women. Women were born to be wives and mothers, and intellectual thought would seriously harm their "reproductive organs," potentially leave them barren, and also affect them psychologically. It was only when this caring function was recognized as significant to hospitals and organizations in the health care field that nursing began to be advertised as an honorable profession for women to enter. The usefulness of nurses was quickly demonstrated to have both social and economic worth. Yet, the utilitarian functions of women in society, a limited exposure to knowledge, and the lack of expectation that women could and would create new knowledge were factors that limited nursing and its education for years thereafter. Ultimately, the ideas of nursing as every woman's work and as a specialized social task mandating a circumscribed education coexisted for approximately 30 years (Lynaugh, 2001). "Designed to provide service in hospitals, the vast majority of nursing schools for nearly a century did not prepare women capable of solving the social problems that impinged on the health of individuals and families within communities" (Ashley & LaBelle, 1976, p. 53).

Education

Throughout nursing's history, one element has consistently been identified as a freeing and powerful agent. That element is education, but more specifically a liberal education upon which the professional component would be built. Liberal education then would serve as the basis for excellence in nursing. But the fact remains—there has always been rhetoric regarding liberal education in nursing, but the translation of words into action has not occurred. According to Russell (1958), liberal education as a base for nursing education was historically a theme highly valued by nurse educators, but actual curricular practices did not reflect the same degree of commitment.

The continued growth of the professions in America has brought with it an extended and deepened interest in the processes of professionalization. Professional schools of law, engineering, medicine, and nursing are critically examining their purposes, substance, method, and organization. The dynamic character of the world of work and the rapidity of change in work situations emphasize the need for evaluating the system within which the professional person is developed, for it is in the professional school that the practitioners' attitudes, values, general orientation, special skills, and knowledge are shaped.

Although critical interest in professional education has always been apparent in nursing, it has been especially so since World War II. The prime emphasis in current reexaminations of nursing programs has been directed toward such questions as what is being taught, what should be taught, and what is effective teaching? In addition, the growth of interest in the process of socialization has contributed strongly to the growth of interest in the field of nursing education.

Schools of nursing are dedicated in part to helping students learn the professional role of the nurse. One of their aims is to teach the skills, attitudes, and norms of the role competency in such a way as to motivate a performance that will be both professionally and socially acceptable. The most obvious acquisition of students going through a nursing program is a store of specialized knowledge. However, acquiring a professional role requires much more than specialized knowledge.

Part of any discussion related to educational programs concerns the following: the inclusion or exclusion of the liberal arts; the emphasis or weight to be given the liberal arts; the emphasis or weight to be given the sciences; the interrelationship between the arts and the sciences; the rationale for including either or both; and, most importantly, the need for a liberal education. This last concern is the most distressing, since the question of the education and status of the nursing profession has been the subject of controversy since the advent of formal nursing programs in America in 1873. This in itself is puzzling, since no one has ever questioned the fact that professions must be "learned." Nor has there ever been serious doubt that for a profession to render its highest form of service, its education must be liberal. Indeed, leading members of the nursing profession have repeatedly made it quite clear that no education can be adequate if it is not liberal. Yet, this issue of a liberal education for nurses is, for all practical purposes, still not resolved.

Arguments for a liberal education in nursing can be found in literature as early as 1893. Many of these are pleas for the incorporation of liberal studies into nursing programs. A classic among them was a speech in 1909 by Richard Olding Beard, who founded the first school of nursing under university control at the University of Minnesota, which was based on the ". . . symmetrical development of the physical, mental, and spiritual possibilities of the individual" (1910, p. 28). Perhaps one of the most distinct passages that described the value of a liberal college education for the nurse was rendered by Isabel Maitland Stewart in 1940:

> We do not expect these nurses will show greater technical skill than the nurses who receive the older type of training, but we believe that they should be better able to think out their problems, to meet the varied and unpredictable demand of society in the future, and to become self-reliant, self-directing, growing, professional women (p. 1033).

In other words, a truly liberally educated nurse must have developed a general intelligence capable of application to a variety of professional tasks.

Others who spoke out included Margaret Bridgman in *Collegiate Education for Nursing*. She asserted that the ". . . essential amalgamating element in the educational process is the application of knowledge from every source to the science and art of nursing" (1953, p. 104). Yet, the best argument delivered by Charles M. Russell appeared in *Nursing Research* in 1958. His article, "Liberal Education and Nursing," clearly documented that "No group which would aspire to the elevated status and position of leadership of a profession can . . . fail to make liberal education its training ground" (p. 124). For it was his belief that: "The liberal ingredient brings knowledge to its humane level, and therefore forms an essential element in the performance of professional service" (p. 116). The key here is the word *humane*, elaborated upon in a more recent quote by Paterson and Zderad (1988):

> When arts and humanities are included in nursing education programs, it is for their humanizing effects. Traditionally they have been recognized as having a civilizing influence. So in nursing they are seen as supporting the elements of humaneness and humanitarianism. Furthermore, they are a necessary antidote for the depersonalization that accompanies scientific technology and mechanization. . . . They stimulate imaginative creativity. They broaden a person's perspective of the human situation, of man in his world (p. 87).

This dialogue very clearly points out the importance and necessity of a balanced education that embraces the arts and humanities as well as the sciences.

Nursing has its roots in the humanities, which address the wholeness of the persons for which care is being delivered. Nursing has been sanctioned by society because nursing care satisfies real human needs. Yet, the liberal arts in nursing's educational programs continue to diminish to accommodate the scientific knowledge also necessary to practice nursing. Forgotten are the struggles of early nursing leaders to incorporate the liberal arts, the humanities, within the mainstream of nursing. The early groundwork for the future identification of the value of liberal education for nurses has not become a reality. Nursing does currently have a strong emphasis and strong programs in nursing research. Yet, something is missing from a historical viewpoint—the aspect of humanitarianism. The original cornerstone of nursing was composed of its historical, philosophical, social, and cultural roots, which have all but disappeared from the curricula of most schools, despite an increased attention to "liberalizing" the education of nurses.

But what does a liberal education mean? Where did the idea come from? How is it defined today? Does it have relevance in today's world of nursing? The idea stems from Greco-Roman times. The word *liberal* comes from the Latin *liber*, meaning "free." This freedom, however, was concerned with the individual's economic and political status in society, a definition quite different from that of more recent centuries. Liberal education then was that education accorded a "freeman," as compared to a slave or an artisan. This freeman, having been released from working for a livelihood, was able to devote his efforts to civic life and the management of the state. As can be imagined, the number of freemen within the ancient society was small. Liberal education became the privilege of the few rather than the many (Brubacher, 1977). Originally, colleges and universities in this country, prior to becoming a vital part of complex contemporary life, also restricted their clientele to the academic elite. In a sense this was logical, since higher education was distinguished by a sophistication that mandated the need for academically "elite" students to handle the content.

Liberal education very quickly became almost synonymous with intellectual excellence in that the intellect would be cultivated. Through reading and study, the mind would be freed. But in addition to acquired knowledge, comprehension and understanding would occur. Consequently, liberal learning, which was transmitted by the university, would exercise a continuous influence on society.

It is interesting to note that four themes on the purposes of a liberal education appeared consistently in the nursing literature between 1893–1952 (Hanson, 1988):

- The development of the individual
- The preparation for citizenship/social reform
- The acquisition of a broad knowledge base
- The development of critical thinking and judgment

These purposes are consistent with those identified in educational philosophy (to provide essential knowledge, to cultivate intellectual skills, to cultivate traits of personality and character). Furthermore, all of the stated purposes reflect the ancient notions regarding the definition and purpose of a liberal education.

The recognized value of a liberal education for nurses does not seem to be at issue here. The translation of that value into the educational program for nurses is the stumbling block. Even more disheartening is the fact that even in some programs professing to have a liberal education base, that base is meager, at best. The liberal education piece has consistently been eroded over time, to make way for a more scientific framework.

There is no doubt that a symbiotic relationship exists among a liberal education, a professional education, and nursing education. One can even go so far as to say that nursing education equals a liberal education base on which the professional component is built. This topic has been the subject for discussion in professional nursing organizational meetings since 1893. It has been examined in major studies of nursing education and practice that have been initiated almost every 5 to 10 years since 1923 (Ashley, 1976; Bridgman, 1953; Brown, 1948; Burgess, 1928; Committee for the Study of Nursing Education, 1923; Committee on the Grading of Nursing Schools, 1934; Department of Health, Education, & Welfare, 1963; Hughes, Hughes, & Deutscher, 1958; Institute of Medicine, 1983; Johns & Pfefferkorn, 1934; National Commission on Nursing, 1983; National League of Nursing Education, 1917, 1927, 1937; West & Hawkins, 1950). The focus of selected landmark nursing studies is presented in Table 1–1. Common elements with regard to nursing education have evolved from these studies: several educational programs leading to entry into the same practice create consumer and employer confusion; the studies have not been conducted by nurses (groups such as government agencies, psychologists, historians, sociologists, allied health organizations, and private foundations became involved); the committees or commissions conducting the studies have not been dominated by nurses; study effects on nursing education and practice were varied; complaints of a shortage of hospital nurses were continual; and nursing experienced considerable difficulty in implementing the recommendations put forth on the education and practice of nursing. Perhaps this lack of followthrough can be attributed to Lynaugh and Brush's (1996) analysis that "Most studies of 'nursing' actually focused on hospital needs for nurses rather than on nursing as a discipline or general public service" (p. xi). These studies did, however, perpetuate the notion that the lack of standardization in educational requirements makes it difficult to entice workers with a strong attachment to the workforce.

Esther Lucile Brown in 1948 minced no words in stating that the only type of education that could prepare nurses adequately to meet the needs of the twentieth century was a professional education on a level with other professions. She made it very clear that nursing should align itself to community and 4-year colleges. Unfortunately, nursing failed to link community colleges with practical and diploma schools and universities with registered nursing. The cliche, "A nurse is a nurse is a nurse," continued intact since nurses from all programs received the same license, were paid the same, and were employed to perform the same hospital/nursing functions. These practices continue today amid numerous efforts for reform.

Primary Influences

It is evident that there have been numerous influences that have shaped nursing's history. Almost every textbook in nursing history makes reference to the origins of organized nursing under religious or monastic orders, the effects of militarism on nursing, and more recently the impact of technology on nursing practice. Nurses are the inheritors of great traditions, which have come from religious organizations and military orders; the influence of religion and militarism on nursing has thus been profound. Roberts (1954) went so far as to say that nursing was ". . . molded by the opposing forces of Christian ideals and war" (p. 32). Leslie (1951) commented on the connection of the profession of nursing with religion as nursing ". . . aptly described as 'Christianity' with its sleeves rolled up" (p. 255). In addition, technological advances have significantly affected the definition of nursing, the role of the nurse, and methods by which care is delivered. Although the old traditions have been slowly disappearing and religious and militaristic restrictions are gradually being eradicated, technology is emerging as a force with, as yet, unimaginable consequences.

Religion

The emergence of a Christian world began the continuous recording of nursing history and resulted in significant differences from previous eras. The first five centuries of the Christian era (1–500 A.D.) witnessed the rise of a religious and social movement, which enabled the systematic development of organized nursing. The principal source of charitable nursing became the Christian church and its chief agent the monastery. Christ's teaching of love and brotherhood transformed not only society at large but also the development of nursing. The organization of nursing was a direct response to these teachings and epitomized the concept of pure **altruism** (disinterested service to humanity done for love of God—devotion to others without hope of any material reward; reward would be realized in the hereafter) initiated by the early Christians. The motive for nursing thus became the marvelous activity of love and mercy embraced by many men and women who responded to the teachings of Christ. Thus, the care of the sick or disabled became a vital component of the Corporal Works of Mercy. These "acts" encompassed basic human needs as well as scientific and humanistic objectives for caring. In addition, a very spiritual meaning became deeply embedded in the care

Table 1-1   Selected Landmark Nursing Studies

Date	Title	Investigator(s)	Funding/ Sponsor	Focus
1912	The Educational Status of Nursing	M. Adelaide Nutting	U.S. Bureau of Education	Revealed appalling educational practices and substandard living and working conditions of students in nursing schools throughout the country. Highlighted need for major reforms.
1923	Nursing & Nursing Education in the United States (The Goldmark Report)	Committee for the Study of Nursing Education C.E.A. Winslow (Chair) Josephine Goldmark (Chief Investigator)	Rockefeller Foundation	Study of American nursing and nursing education. Examined functions of nurses in public health, private duty, and in institutions. Considered the training of nurses in hospital schools, university programs, and postgraduate courses. Dealt with financing of nursing education, licensure, nurse teachers and administrators, and weaknesses of hospital schools.
1928	Nurses, Patients, & Pocketbooks	May Ayres Burgess/ Program Director and Statistician	Committee on the Grading of Nursing Schools/Nurses, Private Foundations, Member Organizations, Interested Layman, Frances Payne Bolton	Inquiry into the supply and demand for nursing service and the problem of shortages of graduate nurses. Demonstrated profound economic problems in nursing. Conclusions consistent with the Goldmark Report.
1934	An Activity Analysis of Nursing	Ethel Johns and Blanche Pfefferkorn	Committee on the Grading of Nursing Schools/Nurses, Private Foundations, Member Organizations, Interested Layman, Frances Payne Bolton	"Job analysis" of what nurses did (analysis of nursing functions) in order to use data to standardize and improve curricula in nursing schools. Two primary questions addressed: What is good nursing and How can it be taught?
1934	Nursing Schools Today & Tomorrow		Committee on the Grading of Nursing Schools/Nurses, Private Foundations, Member Organizations, Interested Layman, Frances Payne Bolton	Final report. Grading (classification) of schools based on factual knowledge about underlying problems in nursing education and service and on needed student qualities to perform required activities.
1917	Standard Curriculum for Schools of Nursing	M. A. Nutting and Isabel M. Stewart/ Education Committee	National League of Nursing Education	Construction of a basic curriculum (a working guide) adaptable to the conditions of particular nursing schools.

(continued)

Table 1–1   (continued)

Date	Title	Investigator(s)	Funding/Sponsor	Focus
				Two primary objectives of the curriculum: serve as a guide for nursing schools; represent an idea to the general public of acceptable training for nursing.
1927	Curriculum for Schools of Nursing	Education Committee	National League of Nursing Education	Revision of the 1917 report. Changes needed to advance standards consistent with newer developments and improvements achieved in more progressive nursing schools. Intent to stimulate thinking rather than dictate requirements.
1937	A Curriculum Guide for Schools of Nursing	Isabel M. Stewart/Education Committee	National League of Nursing Education	Second revision of the 1917 report. Most far-reaching and ambitious effort undertaken in the area of nursing education. Essentially a cooperative research project. Review and reevaluation of existing curricula and traditional philosophies underlying them. Outlined a curriculum for a 2½- to 3-year program to be offered as an educational tool and guide.
1948	Nursing for the Future (The Brown Report)	Esther Lucile Brown	Carnegie Foundation, Russell Sage Foundation, the National Nursing Council	Status of nursing in America. Nursing education and nursing service viewed from the aspect of what was best for society. Oriented to long-range social goals.
1950	Nursing Schools at the Mid-Century	National Committee for the Improvement of Nursing Services	NCINS; Book cost underwritten by six national nursing organizations	Measurable aspects of nursing education. Method for schools of nursing to evaluate their programs. Preparation of an interim classification of nursing schools. Precursor to development of more comprehensive accreditation program.
1958	Twenty Thousand Nurses Tell Their Story	E. Hughes, H. Hughes, and I. Deutscher/authors	American Nurses Association	Total view of the current state of the nursing profession. Report based on numerous studies of nursing functions. Draws attention to situations calling for reform as well as gaps in knowledge.
1959	Community College Education for Nursing	Mildred Montag	Institute of Research & Service in Nursing Education/Teachers College, Columbia University	Findings of 5-year study of eight, 2-year nursing programs. Paved the way for the establishment of additional Associate Degree nursing programs.

Table 1–1   *(continued)*

Date	Title	Investigator(s)	Funding/ Sponsor	Focus
1970	An Abstract for Action	Jerome Lysaught/ National Commission on Nursing & Nursing Education	American Nurses' Foundation, Avalon (Mellon) Foundation, W. K. Kellogg Foundation	Determination of responsibilities and skills required by nurses to render high-quality patient care. Scope of study included an evaluation of present-day changing nursing practice, educational patterns, and potential future requirements in nursing.
1979	The Study of Credentialing in Nursing: A New Approach	Inez G. Hinsvark	American Nurses Association	Investigation of credentialing for nurses. Committee established that advocated a free-standing national nursing credentialing center to coordinate licensure, conduct registration and certification of nurses, and accreditation of nursing services and education for basic and advanced practice.
1982	Magnet Hospitals: Attraction & Retention of Professional Nurses	American Academy of Nursing	American Academy of Nursing/American Nurses Association	National sample of "magnet hospitals," those that retain professional nurses in their employment. Identification of factors that influence nurse job satisfaction and low turnover rates in the hospital setting.
1983	National Institute of Medicine Study	Katherine Bauer	Department of Health and Human Services (DHHS)	Need for continued expenditure of federal money for nursing education.

of the sick and the suffering, which forever had a deep and significant impact on the practice of nursing.

From a chronological point of view, there was a vast difference between nursing in the Christian era and that of the ages that preceded it. Those who understood the best medical and surgical techniques of the times gave a superior type of care. The rich and the powerful that converted to Christianity and engaged in charitable works were socially, culturally, and intellectually endowed. Some were recognized scholars. The educationally prepared included members of the clergy who for several centuries were the only group that was exposed to any type of formal training. Furthermore, a true integration of services was in evidence as medical and nursing care was seldom separated from other forms of charity (Sellew & Nuesse, 1946).

The Christian era is one of the most significant to an understanding of nursing's historical development. Christianity vastly enlarged women's opportunities for useful social service by opening the door to honorable and active careers particularly for the unmarried. Women in organized groups concentrated on social work and nursing, which paved the way for the present role of the public health/community health nurse. At the same time, both men and women were free to engage in humanitarian endeavors, which led to many men entering the field. Nursing activities were thus shared by men and women and at times included the carryover of magic, empirical remedies, and home treatments of the earlier periods of history. With the rapid growth of the monastic movement after the sixth century, large numbers of voluntary celibates, men and women, joined religious orders, and the care of the sick, helpless, and infirm became their permanent vocation.

Gifted nurse leaders emerged and facilitated the development of nursing's roots, purpose, and direction. They founded hostels, hospices, and hospitals. Eventually, names for the various special divisions found in these charitable institutions arose: *Xenodochia*, inns for strangers or travelers; *Nosocomia*, wards or rooms for the sick; *Brephotrophia*; foundling asylums; *Orphanotrophia*, orphan asylums; *Gerontokonia*, homes for the aged; *Cherotrophia*, homes for widows; *Ptochotrophia*, almshouses for the poor. It is interesting to note that nurses with special interests and skills cared for persons with special problems such as the mentally ill, the elderly, and the dying. One wonders how similar these specialists were to our present-day specialists.

Nurses became trusted and respected members of the interdisciplinary team. Many benefits were derived from the influence of religion on nursing. These included a distinctly humanitarian approach to the care of the sick and the poor, the development of organized nursing services, the expansion of nursing services to encompass "all those in need," the entry of many men into the field, and a strong commitment to the nursing work. Eventually, the creation of religious orders of men and women occurred with the primary motivation of nursing the sick. What must be remembered is that character development and purification of the soul were chief aims for the givers and receivers of care during this time period. The essential character trait of a "good nurse" became *obedience* and, more specifically, *unquestioning obedience.*

The beauty of nursing's identification with religion and religious orders cannot be denied at a time in history of plagues, pestilences, the ultimate collapse of Roman power, and the degradation of society. Yet this religious thought also handicapped progress in nursing until well into the second half of the twentieth century. Strict discipline became a way of life.

"In a sense religion forced nurses to make a strong commitment but a commitment at the expense of money, family, and personal freedom. Those engaged in the nursing work were eventually trained in docility, passivity, humility, and total disregard for self. Unquestioning obedience to the decisions of others higher in rank, usually the priest or physician, was promulgated. An individual nurse's accountability, the personal responsibility for decision-making in regard to patient care, was thus bypassed and totally alien in nursing for many years to come" (Donahue, 1996, p. 81).

Military

At the end of the eleventh century, crusaders from many countries responded to a call to the Holy Wars and made their way to Palestine. Here they were faced with multitudes of sick and wounded soldiers and pilgrims with few provisions for their care. Military nursing orders were organized with extreme details dedicated to routines, regulations, and proscribed times for all aspects of their work. They became rescuers of the sick and wounded and introduced great numbers of men into nursing. These military nursing orders combined the attributes of religion and chivalry, as well as militarism and charity, in their dedicated services. Through their endeavors, the military ideal of discipline and order entered nursing.

Great orders were formed, all called by the name *hospitallers*. The Order of St. John of Jerusalem (the name of this order changed as its geographic location shifted to the Knights of Rhodes and then to the Knights of Malta), the Teutonic Knights (der Deutsche Order), and the Knights of St. Lazarus were probably the most well known. So great was their influence on nursing that Nutting and Dock (1907) devoted an entire chapter on their origin and development in the *History of Nursing*, Volume One. They were considered to be benevolent, brave, and charitable. They built magnificent hospitals throughout Europe. Large numbers of women formed a separate chapter of the hospitallers. Unfortunately, these orders began to accumulate vast riches and large land holdings, which proved to be their eventual downfall. At the conclusion of the Holy Wars, the devotion to nursing and works of mercy diminished and aggression against "unbelievers" became their primary focus.

A harsher element entered nursing with the advent of the military orders. Emphasis was now placed on rank, deference to superior officers, uniformity in dress, submergence of the individual, and unquestioning obedience. Many customs and traditions thus arose in nursing that can be traced to military origins. Student nurses were subjected to "inspection" and the use of military insignia to denote class rank and were governed by "doctors' orders." When "on duty," nurses obeyed orders quickly and spontaneously; an order given was an order carried out with no sense of personal accountability. This enormous military influence translated into all aspects of nursing practice including the routinization of medication administration, treatments, and procedures and the development of hospital hierarchies for head nurses and supervisors. All of these profoundly affected the progress of nursing and nursing education for many years to come. Remnants of these influences can still be observed in nursing practice today.

Technology

Unimaginable technological advancements are occurring at a heretofore unprecedented rate, forcing a rethinking of values and assumptions about health care. The impact on nurses and nursing has been and continues to be profound. Throughout nursing's history, new technology served to shape the work of nurses. Although the promise of technology to save time and energy was embraced, in numerous instances it actually increased time and produced labor. Advanced technology also required highly skilled and knowledgeable nurses aware of the impact of technology on patients. The question has now become whether nurses can continue to retain their ability to deal with patients in a humane manner even while using technology? Or will they lose touch with patients? Even in 1977, concerns about the impact of technology on the nurse were being voiced:

> . . . The perspective of history is essential in helping clarify the extent to which the traditional role of the nurse as steadfastly caring and minimally technical, has been a function of the level of technology involved in health care. Without question, the role of the modern nurse encompasses far more knowledge and skill concerning equipment and apparatus than has ever before been the case. Does the advancement of technology in nursing signify a necessary concomitant; a decline in the customary caring which has characterized nursing? Is nursing faced with a decision between preserving its commitment to *caring*, on the one hand, and following the progress of medical science with more technically intricate *curing* (Gadow, 1977, p. 8).

A note of caution is expressed in Gadow's comments. This is understandable since her position is that the nurse is potentially the humanist of health care and that nursing is by definition the most humanistic of the health professions.

The traditional nursing values of caring, compassion, quality of care, commitment, and advocacy are still relevant in nursing. What remains to be seen is the effective balance of these humanistic values with a highly technological, highly specialized health care delivery system. The *challenge* for nursing is to balance *high touch with high tech*! What is particularly disconcerting is the fact that a great deal of the nursing work involves interpersonal relationships, communicating with individuals, families, and communities. Will this significant foundation be continued with what Naisbitt, Naisbitt, and Philips (1999) describe as the dark side of technology and its impact on lives in the twenty-first century? In their book, *High Tech/High Touch*, these authors examine technology's saturation of American society and its devastating effects. "Over time, America has transformed from a technologically comfortable place into a Technologically Intoxicated Zone" in which technology at its best ". . . supports and improves human life, and warning that, at its worst, it alienates, isolates, distorts, and destroys" (pp. 2–3). What is particularly alarming is the devastating impact on relationships that is occurring. Will future nurses know how to communicate, how to maintain a sense of balance, and the essential points of nontechnological connectedness in this constantly evolving high-tech world?

Perhaps the most erudite explication of the nursing–technology relationship is the work by Margarete Sandelowski (2000), *Devices & Desires: Gender, Technology, and American Nursing*. This comprehensive work demonstrates the inexorable link between nursing and technology since formalized training of nurses began in the United States. Sandelowski asserts that nursing has been shaped by technology that has magnified recurring dilemmas in nursing. She also emphasizes the fact that nurses have never wholly succeeded in differentiating themselves from other laywomen or other health-related professionals or workers. She comments on why this difference continues to elude nursing:

> Nursing has been identified—in deed, word, and image, by others and by nurses themselves—both with and against technology and thus, in an ironic way, with and against itself. Early in their history, American nurses identified nursing with technology in order to align themselves with an entity

---

Critical Thinking and Reflection

As technology is emerging at a force with, as yet, unimaginable consequences, the nurse must consider how technology may influence the nurse–patient relationship. How has technology affected or changed your personal and professional life? What strategies can nurses use to balance technology with the humanistic side of nursing? Does the advancement of technology in nursing signify a decline in caring, which has characterized nursing? Identify some benefits resulting from technology in health care. From your perspective, what have been some negative aspects of technology advancements?

Will nurses and nursing be able to attain a balance in which the nursing art and nursing science can mutually not only survive but also thrive in such an environment? Distinguish between the art and science of nursing. How do they influence or complement each other?

associated with science and progress and thus highly valued in Western culture. Physicians identified nursing with technology and thereby appropriated the nurse's body and mind as instruments of medicine. Yet nurses have also positioned nursing against technology to disassociate nursing from an entity that, especially after World War II, was increasingly viewed as dehumanizing patient care. But, in order to separate themselves from technology, nurses realigned their practice with an entity traditionally denigrated in Western culture: feminine caring (p. 178).

The stated points are consistent with all types of literature that stresses the impact of technology on professional roles, responsibilities, and relationships; the implications for patient care; the potential erosion of the essence of nursing as humanistic and caring; and whether technology is a liberating or oppressing force (Ashworth, 1987; Cowan, 1996; Fairman & Lynaugh, 1998; Gadow, 1984; Howell, 1995; Mazlish, 1967; Melosh, 1982; Reverby, 1987; Sandelowski, 1988).

Throughout the twentieth century, nurses not only embraced the latest health care changes but also learned to care in new and different ways by employing increasingly sophisticated technology. Nurses have always used a variety of tools, instruments, appliances, and machines in their practice. Modern technology, however, encompasses a broader meaning that not only incorporates the "past" definition of technology but includes such things as computer and information technology and genetic engineering. This knowledge–technology explosion presents to nursing education, practice, research, and administration an immediate and constantly recurring problem of keeping current in an ever-broadening field while keeping the art of nursing intact. A recent publication by Dinnocenzo and Swegan (2001) explores the issues related to technology that impact society and the workplace and focuses on solutions to problems created. Emphasis is placed on the fact that lives, work, health, and relationships are being compromised, making it difficult to effectively cope in today's "techno" world. No one escapes access overload, information overload, and work overload.

The Fateful Decade (1890–1900)

According to Hamilton (1994), "the society of the 'fateful decade' resonated to an anxious but hopeful rhythm in which ideas of reform, progress, democracy, idealism, good women, and justice harmonized" (p. 12). The United States was in the midst of the Industrial Revolution in which populations in cities soared with people seeking a better life, large numbers of immigrants arrived from Europe, families along with their children toiled in factories 12 to 16 hours a day, and few sanitary laws existed to govern housing, hygiene, or food. The harsh metropolitan realities of exceedingly high illness and death rates and rampant epidemics of cholera, diphtheria, syphilis, tuberculosis, and typhoid demanded reform. Overall, numerous segments of society were depressed and services were needed to counteract the ills of society. A genuine concern for mankind spurred the development of philanthropic and charity aid organizations, a variety of social agencies, and institutions like Jane Addams's Hull House in Chicago and Lillian Wald's Henry Street Settlement in New York (Christy, 1969). The Settlement House Movement became a popular cause.

This 10-year time period was also marked by numerous important events and "fateful decisions" in nursing's history. "Great leaders emerged, schools proliferated, organized nursing was born, and the AJN was started" (Christy, 1975, p. 1163). The impact of these achievements is almost immeasurable. Prior to 1890, there was no official organization of nurses or nurse educators although the first three schools of nursing had opened in 1873. Nursing schools were proliferating at an amazing rate with no established standards for curriculum in place. The first decade of the twentieth century witnessed the development of over 700 nursing schools. This was due to the success of the early schools in improving the care of the sick and hospital environments. All school functions were ultimately placed under the control and general direction of hospital authorities. The biggest problems facing nursing were those dealing with the setting of standards.

The evolution of organized nursing during this decade occurred as a result of serious conditions that jeopardized both the recipients and the providers of nursing care. Farsighted leaders such as Isabel Adams Hampton, Lavinia L. Dock, Louise Darche, Mary E. P. Davis, Sophia Palmer, Anna Maxwell, Annie Goodrich, Irene Sutliffe, Isabel McIsaac, and M. Adelaide Nutting realized that nursing's real power and potential would be achieved through an organized effort of united individuals promoting nursing's interest. The American Society of Superintendents of Training Schools for Nurses (name changed to the National League of Nursing Education [NLNE] in 1912; in 1952 again reorganized under the current National League for Nursing [NLN]) was formed in 1893, an outgrowth of the International Congress of Charities, Corrections and Philanthropy held at the World's Fair in Chicago, which included a subsection of nursing. Following the meeting, a committee was organized by Isabel Adams Hampton to form an association of superintendents whose aim was to develop high educational standards for schools of nursing through established universal admission requirements, sound programs of theory and practice, and improved working conditions. Eventually, the Society formed an education committee to address the question of teacher preparation. In October 1899, a program originally designed to prepare administrators of nursing service and nursing education was launched at Teachers College, Columbia University. This program in hospital economics led to a Department of Nursing Education, a pioneer program for the education of nurses. "The school became known as the 'motherhouse' of collegiate education because it fostered the initial movements toward undergraduate and graduate degrees for nurses" (Donahue, 1996, p. 290).

The Nurses Associated Alumnae of the United States and Canada (renamed the American Nurses Association in 1911) was established in 1896 to unite practitioners of nursing. At its inception, alumnae associations were the mode of entrance to the organization; the development of local and state units would follow. The general needs and common welfare of nurses were the focus of the association along with a primary objective of securing legislation to differentiate between the trained and the untrained nurse. One of the first activities of the association was to consider and investigate the possibility of establishing a professional journal that would be its official means of communication for nurses. The journal would provide a mechanism whereby members could become informed about issues affecting their general welfare as well as those affecting patient care. The original enterprise was financed through shares of stock bought by individual nurses and alumnae associations. The first issue of the *American Journal of Nursing* was published in October of 1900. Sophia Palmer served as editor until her death in 1920, when Mary M. Roberts succeeded her.

During this decade, nurse leaders successfully campaigned for legislation designed to control the practice of nursing in order to both protect the public and standardize or upgrade the preparation of nurses. Through an extensive and ambitious campaign and in the face of strong opposition, the first licensing laws were enacted in 1903 in four states—North Carolina, New Jersey, New York, and Virginia. Within 20 years, all 48 states, Hawaii, and the District of Columbia had enacted laws.

The Nurse Inventors

Visions and challenges are a part of nursing's heritage. These combined with leaders and leadership became the primary components in the search for excellence in nursing. A number of early American leaders were visionaries possessed with unusual discernment or foresight. One of these, M. Adelaide Nutting, was considered by many to be a great visionary of the time. She was said to be an insomniac who might go for days without sleep or with as little as 2 to 3 hours per night. She would frequently write her thoughts and ideas on scraps of paper, which became known as her "midnight musings."

Numerous challenges were faced by leaders who contributed to the growth and development of nursing. These challenges are documented in texts, reports, and studies. Two crucial questions arise when pondering the challenges: Did the visions of early nursing leaders create the challenges, or did the challenges they faced provide the basis for the creation of visions?

According to Stewart, sociologists and psychologists who have studied the nature and conditions of leadership seem to agree that effective leadership depends on three main factors: a situation that calls for leadership (usually a crisis or complicated conditions of affairs); a sufficiently homogeneous group that is responsive to leadership and able to reach an acceptable level of cooperation and understanding; and a leader who possesses traits acceptable to the group and is capable of encountering the specific situation (Stewart, 1940). Whether the situation in nursing's past called for the leaders, for indeed all the factors were present, or the leaders discovered the need and created the movement, need not be of concern here. They would possibly have been leaders in any field, but in nursing and nursing education, they found a congenial cause and ample scope for their unusual abilities.

Numerous individuals have been identified as leaders throughout nursing's history. They have been referred to as nurse leaders, nurse influentials and innovators (Fitzpatrick, 1983), nurse heroines (Christy, 1969), and the developers of nursing's legacy. In addition, Hamilton (1994) refers to a large group of eminent leaders as nurse inventors as she conceptualizes "nurses' thinking," the "thoughts and the thinking patterns of the leaders who designed nursing as a vocation for women" (p. 240). These nurse inventors formed a certain set of core ideas consistent with their social context. These ideas were deliberately chosen, as they were deemed appropriate for nursing practice, for society, and for themselves.

These leaders used their talents in a collaborative effort to shape and develop a viable and much respected nursing art. Each left her mark, not in isolation, but as part of the whole that is nursing's legacy. They truly believed in an educational structure founded on a sound economic base that balanced the art, the science, and the spirit of nursing. Knowledge instead of service should be the driving force of education that would prepare the nurse not only to care for patients but also would prepare the nurse for life in a diverse and complex society.

Important commonalities and differences can be identified among the nursing leaders. The following commonalities can be attributable to most of the leaders, if not all of them:

- Unmarried (Isabel Hampton Robb was the exception.)
- Older, more mature when entering nursing
- Educated in other fields before entering nursing
- Accepted challenges
- Respected and valued one another
- Shared thoughts, ideas, resources
- Risk takers
- Argued, but primarily on an intellectual level
- Compromised when necessary for the good of nursing
- Created networks
- Articulate
- Worked for the good of nursing, not for personal aggrandizement
- Assertive
- Social activists

There is no doubt that their ideas were timely, that they were resolute in their careers, and were able to effect needed change. They had a common concern for patients and were committed to the future development of nursing as a profession. They worked to change the social agenda through public health, education, school and industrial health, and settlement house work. They frequently addressed the interrelationship of thought and action that pervades nursing's history. Annie Goodrich (1932) rendered the most esthetic and inspiring comments on this topic:

> To the nurse, working in the different levels of the social structure, in touch with the fundamentals of human experience, is given a unique opportunity to relate the adventure of thought to the adventure of action,—this to the end that the new social order to which we are committed by our forefathers may be realized. To effectively interpret the truly great role that has been assigned her, neither a liberal education nor a high degree of technical skill will suffice. She must also be master of two tongues, the tongue of science and that of the people (p. 14).

Differences are also apparent among the nurse leaders. These relate particularly to their personal and professional interests, their creativity and innovativeness, and their unique perspectives on issues related to health care and nursing. But differences never interfered with their concerted efforts to move nursing forward. The fulfillment of their visions and dreams, however, would depend on future nursing pioneers. Hopefully, the words of Stewart (1943) will not ring true:

> As I remember some of the older leaders, it seems to me they were a little more ready to stand up for unpopular causes and fight for what they believed in even if they were considered queer or radical by their associates. I realize that times have changed and that causes and crusades are no longer the fashion even among the young. Perhaps they will come in again, and we shall develop more crusaders like Isabel Hampton and Lavinia Dock, Adelaide Nutting, and Annie Goodrich (pp. 144–145). See Table 1–2 for a summary of selected American Nurse Inventors/Leaders.

Struggle for Identity

Modern nursing is still regarded as a women's profession. As such, nurses face special problems indicative of an occupational group constantly struggling for iden-

Table 1–2   Selected American Nurse Inventors/Leaders

Name	Life Span	Primary Focus	Selected Accomplishments
Bunge, Helen Lathrop	1906–1970	Nursing Research	Effective in fostering the development of nursing research Dean at Western Reserve Executive officer of the Institute of Research & Service for Nursing Education at Teachers College (first research institute for nursing in the United States) First voluntary editor of *Nursing Research* Member of the United States Public Health Service's first Nursing Research Study Section
Dock, Lavinia Lloyd	1856–1956	Social Reformer	Pursued equal rights and equal social standing for women Active in the movement for legislation for nursing Ardent suffragist Lobbied for women to have the right to vote Nurse historian Wrote first medication textbook for nurses ever published, *Materia Medica for Nurses*
Goodrich, Annie	1876–1955	Nursing Administration	Superintendent of several nursing schools in New York City Believed that collegiate nursing education was the preferred type of education for all nurses Idea created, developed, and eventually carried through to develop an Army School Established the Vassar Training Program at Vassar College to produce highly trained nurses and the demand for nurses during World War I Dean of the Yale University School of Nursing
Goostray, Stella	1886–1969	Nursing Administration	Dual directorship of nursing school and nursing service at Children's Hospital School of Nursing (Boston) Consultant to the Committee on the Grading of Nursing Schools Chairman of the National Nursing Council for War Service Writer of books and articles on a variety of subjects, including pharmacology and chemistry
Hall, Lydia Williams	1906–1969	Nursing Practice	Earliest of nurse theorists Developed a theory that the direct professional nurse–patient relationship is itself therapeutic Implemented a conceptual system of nursing practice (innovative model of patient care) Established and directed the Loeb Center for Nursing & Rehabilitation at Montefiore Hospital, Bronx, New York Believed professional nurses belonged at the bedside

(continued)

Table 1–2 *(continued)*

Name	Life Span	Primary Focus	Selected Accomplishments
Nutting, Mary Adelaide	1858–1948	Economic Basis for Schools of Nursing	World's first professor of nursing education Nurse historian *Adelaide Nutting Historical Nursing Collection*, housed at Teachers College, dedicated to her memory Educational experimenter and creative thinker Succeeded Isabel Hampton Robb at Johns Hopkins Took charge of Hospital Economics course at Teachers College in 1907 and remained there as head of the department until retirement in 1925
Robb, Isabel Hampton	1860–1910	Nursing Organizations	Achieved important educational reforms at the Illinois Training School Superintendent of Nurses & Principal of the Johns Hopkins Training School of Nurses Initiated establishment of the American Society of Superintendents of Training Schools for Nurses (became NLNE, then NLN) Participated in establishment of and became the first president of the Nurses Associated Alumnae of the United States and Canada (became ANA). Assisted with the development of the *American Journal of Nursing* (AJN)
Roberts, Mary May	1877–1959	Nursing Journalism	Journalist and nurse historian Editor, *American Journal of Nursing* Author: *American Nursing: History & Interpretation* (1954) Charter member of the History of Nursing Source Committee Conceived the notion and creation of a Nursing Information Bureau (NIB)
Palmer, Sophia	1853–1920	Nursing Journalism	First editor of the *American Journal of Nursing* Campaigned for state legislation for nurses Involved in the forefront of professionalism and nursing reform Instrumental in the organization of the New York State Nurses Association Appointed first President of the New York Board of Examiners
Stewart, Isabel Maitland	1878–1963	Nursing Education	"Miss Curriculum" Developed program to train teachers at Teachers College Director of Department of Nursing Education at Teachers College for 22 years Nurse historian Early advocate of nursing research Active in the work that resulted in the three published curriculum guides Credited with idea of an Association of Collegiate Schools of Nursing (ACSN)

Table 1–2 (continued)

Name	Life Span	Primary Focus	Selected Accomplishments
Stimson, Julia Catherine	1881–1948	Army Nurse Corps/Military Nursing	Developed a social service department at Harlem Hospital Became an Army Nurse in 1917 Dean of Army Training School Superintendent of the Army Nurse Corps First woman in the Army to become a major
Wald, Lillian	1867–1940	Public Health Nursing	Accomplished fund raiser Established the Metropolitan Life Insurance Company's nursing service for policyholders Established the Red Cross's Town & Country Nursing Service Organized the first public health nursing service Credited with the development of school nursing Instrumental in the establishment of the United States Children's Bureau Known for work with immigrants in New York's lower east side and the establishment of the Henry Street Settlement Elected first president of the National Organization for Public Health Nursing (NOPHN)

Note: The women listed here represent but a few selected American nurse inventors/leaders. Their identified accomplishments reflect only a mere portion of those that could be listed. In addition, although a primary focus is identified, all of the leaders were participants in nursing educational, organizational, and practice endeavors that contributed to nursing's growth and development.

tity. Many problems faced by nurses and nursing are problems referred to by Muff (1988) as those of "socialization, sexism, and stereotyping." She identifies the problems of nurses as the problems of women; she argues that sexism is the root of the problem and that while men and women are equal they are definitely not the same. These issues profoundly affect the work of nursing since the health care system has long been male-dominated. Paternalism flourished in the apprenticeship model for training nurses. The economic division of labor between male and female jobs still continues, and society continues to devalue nurses and discriminate against them. This is reflected in nursing's constant attempts to distance itself from anything having to do with the medical model and the fact that nurses have typically been characterized along with women as passive, dependent, and emotional. Those factors that keep nurses subservient, overworked, and underpaid endure today. Finally, nursing has not been valued intellectually or monetarily primarily due to its emphasis on altruism, caring, and nurturing.

The Subordinate Sex

In the nineteenth century and at the turn of the twentieth century, tradition and law carefully defined women's activities. Essentially, women had no legal existence except through a father or husband. Women had no legal control over person, property, or children and were not permitted to vote. Education except for elementary levels was reserved for men. Women were even informed through "prescriptive literature" that they should "embody four critical qualities: piety, purity, submissiveness, and domesticity" (Kalisch & Kalisch, 1987, p. 10). If they did not personify these virtues, they should strive to attain them. Nurses, predominantly female during this time period, became a metaphor for all women. The issues that plagued women were embraced in the environments where nurses practiced. The ideas articulated by Passau-Buck (1988) reinforce this relationship:

- The roles of woman, nurse, and mother are viewed by society as similar if not synonymous.

- The hospital family consists of mothers (nurses), fathers (physicians), and children (patients) and is based on the patriarchal family system of Western society.
- The subordinate position of nursing is reinforced by the care/cure myth that values caring, the traditionally female nursing role, less than curing, the male medical role.
- This dichotomy is further emphasized by monetary rewards: physicians are well paid for curing, but not so nurses for caring (p. 204).

Although male dominance is a problem for women in society as a whole, nurses have had special problems in this respect. This is vividly illustrated by the fact that physicians and hospital administrators have remained in positions of dominance and control over nursing and health care since the first decade of the twentieth century (Ashley, 1975, 1976). They have consistently opposed any reforms by nurses that would improve nursing education, improve the status of nursing, set nursing on the path toward professional status, and place nursing in the hands of nurses. Unfortunately, nurses have contributed to this phenomenon by cooperating with the very men who prevented such reforms. As second-class citizens, nurses were subjected to male authority and accepted the situation in relative silence. Organized medicine and the hospital's constant fight for control over nursing was a deliberate strategy to have their own interests served. Establishing a nursing school resulted in improved hospital conditions and reduced the cost of running the hospital since this cost became absorbed as a portion of nurses' training. At the same time, nurses were prevented from achieving equal status with men in the health care field and as professionals. Certainly, a lack of social and personal support for women with careers also entered the equation.

On the other hand, nursing offered women a supportive, caring, and nurturing role that permitted control over their lives and the ability to remain "feminine." This control came after completion of their training program. They would enter private-duty nursing since students were the primary hospital caregivers until the late 1930s and early 1940s. This combination of factors was not provided to the same extent in other women's occupations. Nursing heroines such as Florence Nightingale, Dorothea Dix, Mother Bickerdyke, Clara Barton, Lillian Wald, and others emerged and became excellent role models for nursing as an honorable and respected service to humankind. "No other occupation open to women could match its [nursing's] glamour, its image of dedication, its service, even its freedom" (Bullough & Bullough, 1984, p. 23).

Men in Nursing

The fact that men have been nurses and caregivers in all cultures and throughout the history of humankind is well documented by history and tradition (Figure 1–2). Men are not new to nursing. Men have been a part of the practice and profession of nursing from its inception. A glimpse into the past reveals that ". . . in the early Christian period, and for centuries thereafter, men of the priestly class, or belonging to military or religious orders, have been responsible for at least one half of the nursing service through mediaeval times up to a very recent period" (Nutting & Dock, 1907, p. 101). Nursing was considered as much a male profession as a female one prior to the late nineteenth century. And yet, traditional sex roles continue to permeate society's identification of nurses as females. Cultural conditioning, stereotypes, and the continued depiction of the "female" image of nurses in literature and in the media contribute significantly to the perpetuation of this social perception.

Male nurses face the same type of sex stereotyping and cultural pressures that define nursing as a woman's profession. Men in nursing are constantly plagued by social stereotypes and are often viewed as unable to get into medical school, as being effeminate or homosexual, and as unable to handle or perform well in societal defined jobs for *real men*. This is reflected in unsuccessful attempts to recruit increased numbers of men into nursing. The percentage of nurses who are men in the United States has never been great; numbers vacillate but remain low. The percentage decreased from 7.6% in 1910 to 3.8% in 1920. In 1989, only 3.1% of nurses were men (Miller, 1989). In 1992, the percentage had risen to 4.3% (ANA, 1994). According to Spratley, Johnson, Sochalski, Fritz, and Spencer (2000), this percentage had risen to 5.4%. Various organizations have even questioned the title of *nurse* as a deterrent to men entering nursing and studies have been conducted to determine the opinion of nurses about changing the title. Is the title sexist and is it such a barrier? Some nurses believe yes; other nurses believe no. Perhaps a starting point would be to eliminate the word *male* in all references to men in nursing and call them "nurses." Women in nursing are not called "female" nurses. Nurses themselves thus perpetuate the sex stereotype through the use of the title "male nurse."

Male nurses have been harassed and discriminated against and have suffered minority status. The excellent nursing care given by early generations of men, although documented, has all but been forgotten and/or ignored. Military and other male nursing orders have left their mark on nursing and at times carried the chief burden of nursing.

Figure 1–2   A Brief History of Men in Nursing

500 B.C.	In *Ayur-Veda*, the books from ancient India that discuss the prevention and cure of disease, the "Nurses" mentioned are always male.
	In the New Testament, the Good Samaritan paid the male innkeeper to provide care for an injured man. This story turned particular attention toward the sick poor, and by so doing also affected nursing, medicine, and charity.
A.D.	The first five centuries of the Christian era (1–500) witnessed the rise of a religious and social movement that enabled the systematic development of organized nursing.
300	Men risked their lives to provide nursing care in every plague that swept Europe. The Parabolani was initiated in 300 A.D. during the Black Plague epidemic.
	When western Europe succumbed to Barbarism (500–1000 A.D.), the care of sick men was assigned to monks.
500	The order of Benedictines, established in the sixth century by St. Benedict of Nursia, decreed nursing the sick would be a chief function and duty of community life.
1000	Military nursing orders known as Knights Hospitallers surfaced in the 1100s. They nursed the sick and defended the Holy Land during the Crusades.
	The Order of the Santo Spirito or Holy Ghost, established in 1070, was identified with the development of general hospitals within city walls.
	An order of men established in 1095, the Antonines (Hospital Brothers of St. Anthony), devoted themselves to sufferers of "St. Anthony's Fire," probably the ergotism that caused hallucinations.
1200	St. Dominic also founded orders to take nursing out among the people (Dominican order founded 1206).
	St. Francis of Assisi (1182–1226) established three religious nursing orders including the Gray Friars, distinguished by gray robes with a rope girdle. This order chose to identify itself with the care of lepers and contributed to a public health movement (Franciscan order founded 1211).
	St. Louis IX was another saint whose endeavors with lepers were well known. Louis personally tended to the sick and devoted his life to humane treatment for all individuals (inherits throne of France 1226).
	The brotherhood of Misericordia was started in Florence in 1244. Founded primarily as a volunteer ambulance society, they became known as the "Masked Brotherhood." This name arose from the members' belief that their contributions would gain spiritual reward only if they prevented themselves from being recognized by others.
1300	The Alexian Brothers were organized in the 1300s to provide nursing care for the victims of bubonic plague in the Netherlands.
1500	The Brothers of Mercy (also known as the Brothers of St. John of God or the order of the Fatebene-Fratelli) was founded in Spain in 1538 by John Ciudad. They were mendicants who devoted themselves to nursing, hospital work, the distribution of medicines, the tender care of the mentally ill and abandoned children, and the visitation of the sick at home.
	In the sixteenth century, St. Camillus founded the Nursing Order of Ministers of the Sick who pledged themselves to the work of nursing, doing hospital work and caring for those stricken with the plague in Rome in 1590.
1860	Large numbers of men and women volunteered as nurses during the American Civil War. Walt Whitman served as a volunteer Civil War nurse in Washington, D.C. He described his experiences in a collection of poems.

(continued)

Figure 1–2 (*continued*)

1886–1888	In 1886, the School for Male Nurses was established in connection with the New York City Training School for Nurses on Blackwell's (Welfare) Island. In 1888, the Mills College of Nursing was established in Bellevue Hospital in New York, the first nursing college for men.
1898–1928	The Congregation of the Alexian Brothers established two schools for men nurses in their hospitals in Chicago (1898) and St. Louis (1928), which provided all types of care for men and boys.
1940	According to the U.S. Census, the number of men in nursing in 1940 was approximately 2% of the total number of graduate and student nurses.
	Although the U.S. government badly needed nurses during World War II, they refused to allow males to receive equal opportunity in the military. Although female nurses received full commission rank in U.S. military service in 1947, the first men were not commissioned as nurses until 1955.
1960	Philip E. Day became the first male to be elected president of a state nurses' association in 1960.
1966	A congressional bill authorizing appointment of male nurses to the regular forces of the Air Force, Army, and Navy Nurse Corps was signed by President Lyndon Johnson in 1966. Men constituted 22% of the Army's total nursing population.
1974	Male nurses face the sex stereotyping and cultural pressures that define nursing as a woman's profession.
	The American Assembly for Men in Nursing was established in 1974.

Reprinted with permission: College of Nursing (2001). *Men in nursing* (p. 3). Iowa City, IA: College of Nursing, The University of Iowa. Copyright 2001 M. Patricia Donahue, Professor and Associate Dean for Academic Affairs, College of Nursing, The University of Iowa.

Along with the Knights Hospitallers, the Benedictines, the Order of the Santo Spirito, the Antonines, the brotherhood of Misericordia, the Alexian Brothers, and numerous other orders of men distinguished themselves as caring and competent nurses. Men risked their lives to provide nursing care in every plague that swept Europe. Individual men also markedly contributed to the progress of nursing throughout different periods in history. St. Francis of Assisi and St. Dominic founded orders to take nursing out among the people. Large numbers of men volunteered as nurses during the American Civil War, including the poet Walt Whitman. Whitman attended the wounded in military hospitals in Washington, D.C. His poem "The Wound Dresser" remains one of the most moving examples from a nurse's viewpoint of the experience of nursing in time of war (Fiedler, 1988).

In an effort to overcome some of the gender barriers preventing men from becoming nurses, several nursing schools for men were established in the United States, one of the earliest being the School for Male Nurses (1886) in conjunction with the New York City Training School for Nurses on Blackwell's (Welfare) Island. In 1940, there were four accredited schools of nursing that admitted only men; 63 schools were coeducational (Kalisch & Kalisch, 1995, p. 402). Unfortunately, the educational barrier was not the only one that prevented men from contributing to the work of nursing. Men who volunteered for the military faced not only the horrors and dangers of war but other types of conflicts and frustrations as well. Men who were nurses were barred from the Army Nurse Corps since its original title was the "Army Nurse Corps, Female." The Navy Nurse Corps followed suit in 1908. The view held by society and nurses alike was that a man's place in wartime was on the battlefield, not doing nursing care. The first men were actually not commissioned as nurses until 1955; full commissioned rank for "female" nurses in the military services was permanently established in 1947.

Discriminatory practices against men in nursing may be easing, but some men continue to relate stories about unfair treatment both in the educational and practice settings. Absolute change will not occur, however, until men in nursing are free to develop their full potential as nurses and until both society and nurses no longer view nursing totally as a women's occupation.

Creating New Patterns— The Future

The key to nursing's future is predicated on the need for the incorporation of an evolutionary spirit into the discipline. This evolutionary spirit may be painful but is needed to provide nursing with growth, achievement, and great satisfaction. It is necessary in order that nursing not only survive, but also thrive in a new era and emerge as the creator of new knowledge about human behavior, health, human reactions to illness, and the management of care. Challenges and controversy must be met with thoughtful action. New ideas, exploration, innovation, and experimentation must be the focus of nursing education, practice, and research. Horizons must be broadened and identification made, through careful deliberation, of those things that can be changed versus those that cannot. Whatever changes are agreed upon to take the profession to a new pinnacle must be chosen to ensure quality patient care.

Nurses, now more than ever, will need to be risk takers to take up the challenge of nursing's future—to be the leaders in the movement to balance the humanistic and traditional values of nursing with the highly technological, specialized care delivery system in which they practice. They will need to be visionaries, dreamers, innovators, and creators of new patterns in order to have a pivotal role in determining the health care system of the future. Nurses will need to be politically involved to steer American health policy toward greater social harmony, to alleviate those social dilemmas created by competing or changing sets of values. Nurses can have an impact on institutional and political forces that control health care and its development. In other words, nurses must be the creators of new "turning points in nursing history."

Each and every nurse has a significant role to play in this movement toward new spheres of action. The excuse that "I'm only one person" is unacceptable. One human being can indeed make a difference in the determination of life's pathways and create a new page in history. Numerous examples of such happenings are available if one but searches for them. Several years ago

an article appeared in an Iowa newspaper entitled, "Refuge Named for Eagle-Watcher." It was the story of Elton Fawks from East Moline, Illinois, who waged a one-man campaign, which environmentalists say helped to save the bald eagle from extinction. He took up bird watching after childhood polio kept him from more active pursuits; bald eagles became his passion. With a pair of binoculars and a keen curiosity in nature, he noticed in the 1950s a marked decrease in the number of immature bald eagles that nested around the river's locks and dams. He took it upon himself to confer with Charles Broley, an ornithologist who was among the first to determine that DDT damages the eagle's eggshells. Fawks then began a lobbying campaign for tough state laws to control pesticides. In the 1960s, the Illinois general assembly adopted measures based on his proposals, DDT was banned nationwide in the 1970s. What started as the effort of one human being escalated into nationwide involvement, the result being the removal of the bald eagle from the endangered species' list. Visions and challenges are a part of Fawks's story just as they have been and are a part of nursing's heritage.

A semantic jungle has historically existed in nursing: New categories of nurses have developed; new titles have been manufactured; definitions lack precision; labels have proliferated; and ambiguous, vague, and unclear terms are used. According to Montag (1975), terms must be defined not in esoteric but in operable ways. Unless the language of nursing becomes precise, nursing will continue to find itself in the situation of Humpty Dumpty, when he said to Alice in *Through the Looking Glass*, "When I use a word," Humpty Dumpty said in a scornful tone, "it means just what I choose it to mean—neither more nor less." "The question is," said Alice, "whether you can make words mean so many different things." A mere glimpse into nursing's history reveals that terms have been consistently unclear, undefined, or used to mean many different things. Currently, a standardized language and classification system is being developed in nursing, which should contribute to a clearer understanding of nursing activities.

The early nursing leaders were sufficiently liberated to successfully undertake the challenges of revolutionizing nursing education and practice. They are a source of inspiration for contemporary nurses to continue the work these leaders began. Their stories provide motivation for newly emerging nursing leaders to be proactive in meeting current and future challenges. Will today's emerging leaders be as visionary as M. Adelaide Nutting, as eloquent and diplomatic as Isabel Maitland Stewart, as humanitarian as Lillian Wald, as charismatic as Isabel Hampton Robb, and as feisty as Lavinia Dock? Will they question whether the current reality of nursing is the way it should be? Will they use their collaborative efforts to shape and develop a viable nursing for the future? Will they be the master of two tongues—the tongue of science and that of the people? Will they set standards of excellence that will serve to influence and "convert" physicians, administrators, and the public?

In the final analysis, nursing needs members who are willing to face uncharted territory even when faced with dragons!

> When a cartographer ran out of known world before he ran out of parchment, he inscribed the words "Here be dragons" at the edge of the ominously blank terra incognita, a signal to the voyager that he entered the unknown region at his peril (Lewis, 1977, p. 21).

TRANSITION INTO PRACTICE

Technology has made communication almost instantaneous across many regions of the world. The growth of electronic modes of communication has been remarkable; many remain unsure of the full potential for information storage and retrieval. Because computers bought today will be relatively obsolete within a few years, data retrieval could be problematic. With the technological evolution, applications become outmoded, cast off, and replaced by new and improved hardware and software programs. Data retrieval can be impossible as a result of incompatibilities between old and new systems. Consider retrieval of information from videotape. When a facility moves to an all-CD format, how is the video data retrieved? Agencies and decision makers have to consider the impact of possible lost data when the format for information storage is changed.

If nursing history is to be saved, nurses along with nurse historians need to be involved in decisions regarding information storage. Nursing history involves not only the history of nurses but also the involvement of nurses in the social, economic, political, and cultural setting of their time. Nursing history also involves documentation of patient care. Nurses are far too uninvolved in saving the legacy of their profession. Nurse historians have assumed the lead in rescuing historical data in a manner that allows it to be saved and accessed by future nurses. If accurate data of desirable quality, which reflects the history of nursing, is not stored, then the legacy of the profession will be distorted.

Hewitt and Donahue (2001) suggest that nurse historians be more proactive and assume greater leadership roles in the selection and storage of electronic data. Simply placing information on a disc is not an adequate method of preserving the past. With technologic advances, vast volumes of information are stored electronically; there are few who use electronic storage who have not felt the pain of lost data when a disc or hard drive "crashes." Nurses, and specifically nurse historians, should take a role in the management of information to ensure preservation of data.

Hewitt and Donahue (2001) suggest that nurse historians also take a greater role in cultivating historical interests of other nurses. Nurse historians can serve as leaders in the need to store and manage historical data, but they need every nurse to recognize the value of historical documents and artifacts. While many nurses show a distinct disinterest in the past and in archival documents, scholars are able to demonstrate the clear value these records provide to better understand how events of the past impact the present and future. The past provides knowledge for nurses to navigate the future.

Hewitt and Donahue (2001) further suggest that nurse historians need to take the lead in determining the quality and quantity of databases that are conserved and preserved. They add that historical nursing research needs to be guided by policy and information management issues. As part of this involvement, these historians need to engage in communal dialogue with the community of electronic users as policy for information storage is developed.

While all the information presented here clearly challenges the nurse historian to preserve the history of nursing, it is also incumbent on all nurses, novice and veteran, to aid these leaders in the collection and preservation of data. Proactive protection of information ensures a legacy for the future.

1. The need for nurses is as great today as it was in the past. Yet, efforts to stop nursing's march toward identity have been continuous and diligent since Florence Nightingale set modern nursing in motion. Approaches aimed at the control or obliteration of nursing, without concern for social or human welfare, have been designed and attempted.

2. The history of nursing has been one of frustration, ignorance, and misunderstanding, an epic of an occupational group whose status has always been affected by the prevalent standards of humanity.

3. The power to shape the destiny of nursing has always been in the hands of nurses to accomplish, but they have continued to perpetuate the passivity of the past, to behave as an oppressed group and regard themselves as victims.

4. Nightingale proved that <u>good nursing care made the difference</u>. She and other early leaders in nursing consistently referred to nursing as an art as well as a science.

5. History is a way of thinking about the present in the hope that some sense can be made of complex contemporary events by scrutinizing their roots. History serves to clarify context and meaning.

6. An analysis of nursing history reveals a number of prevalent themes that have directly and/or indirectly affected nursing throughout its evolution. The themes of politics, power and control, economics, women's work, and education are particularly significant to an understanding of nursing history. Additionally, religion, the military, and technology are also significant themes with a powerful influence on nursing's development.

7. Nurses are the inheritors of great traditions, which have come from religious organizations and military orders; the influence of religion and militarism on nursing has thus been profound. The impact of technology on nursing practice is likely to be no less profound.

8. The evolution of organized nursing that took place during the fateful decade occurred as a result of serious conditions that jeopardized both the recipients and the providers of nursing care.

9. Although male dominance is a problem for women in society as a whole, nurses have had special problems in this respect. Physicians and hospital administrators, both predominantly male, have remained in positions of dominance and control over nursing. They have consistently opposed reforms that would place nursing in the hands of nurses; unfortunately, nurses have contributed to this phenomenon by cooperating with the very men who prevented nurses from achieving professional status. Nurses must unite for each and every voice to be heard.

10. Male nurses face the same type of sex stereotyping and cultural pressures that define nursing as a woman's profession. Men in nursing are constantly plagued by social stereotypes.

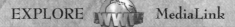

EXPLORE   MediaLink

Critical thinking questions, essay questions, key terms, web links, activities, NCLEX review questions, and more interactive resources can be found on the Companion Website at www.prenhall.com/haynes. Click on Chapter 1 to select activities for this chapter.

REFERENCES

American Nurses Association. (1994). *Today's registered nurse—numbers and demographics*. Washington, DC: ANA Publications, Pub. No. PR-17.

Ashley, J. A. (1975). Nursing and early feminism. *American Journal of Nursing, 75*(9), 1465–1467.

Ashley, J. A. (1976). *Hospitals, paternalism, and the role of the nurse*. New York: Teachers College Press.

Ashley, J. A., & LaBelle, B. M. (1976). Education for freeing minds. In J. A. Williamson (Ed.), *Current perspectives in nursing education: The changing scene* (pp. 50–65). St. Louis, MO: Mosby.

Ashworth, P. (1987). Technology and machines: Bad masters but good servants. *Intensive Care Nursing, 3*(1), 1–2.

Beard, R. O. (1910). The university education of the nurse. In the *Fifteenth Annual Report of the American Society of Superintendents of Training Schools for Nurses, Including Report of the Second Meeting of the American Federation of Nurses*.

Bridgman, M. (1953). *Collegiate education for nursing*. New York: Russell Sage Foundation.

Brink, P. J., & Wood, M. J. (1998). *Advanced design in nursing research* (2nd ed.). Thousand Oaks, CA: Sage Publication.

Brockopp, D. Y., & Hastings-Tolsma, M. T. (1995). *Fundamentals of nursing research* (2nd ed.). Boston: Jones and Bartlett Publication.

Brown, E. L. (1948). *Nursing for the future.* New York: Russell Sage Foundation.

Brubacher, J. S. (1977). *On the philosophy of higher education.* San Francisco: Jossey-Bass Publishers.

Bullough, V. L., & Bullough, B. (1984). *History, trends, and politics of nursing.* Norwalk, CT: Appleton-Century-Crofts.

Bullough, V., & Bullough, B. (1964). Nursing and history. *Nursing Outlook, 12,* 27–29.

Burgess, M. A. (1928). *Nurses, patients, and pocketbooks.* New York: Committee on the Grading of Nursing Schools.

Carlson, D. K. (2000, November). Nurses remain at top of honesty and ethics poll. Princeton, NJ: *Gallup News Service,* 1–4.

Christy, T. E. (1969). *Cornerstone for nursing education. A history of the Division of Nursing Education of Teachers College, Columbia University, 1899–1947.* New York: Teachers College Press.

Christy, T. E. (1975). The fateful decade, 1890–1900. *American Journal of Nursing, 75*(7), 1163–1165.

Christy, T. E. (1978). The hope of history. In M. L. Fitzpatrick (Ed.), *Historical studies in nursing.* New York: Teachers College Press.

Committee for the Study of Nursing Education. (1923). *Nursing and nursing education in the United States.* New York: Macmillan.

Committee on the Grading of Nursing Schools. (1934). *Nursing schools—Today and tomorrow.* New York: National League of Nursing Education.

Cook, E. (1913). *The life of Florence Nightingale.* London: Macmillan and Co., Limited.

Cowan, R. S. (1996). Technology is to science as female is to male: Musings on the history and character of our discipline. *Technology and Culture, 37*(3), 572–582.

Department of Health, Education, and Welfare. (1963). *Toward quality in nursing. Report of the Surgeon General's consultant group on nursing.* Washington, DC: Author.

Dinnocenzo, D. A., & Swegan, R. B. (2001). *Dot calm: The search for sanity in a wired world.* San Francisco: Berrett-Koehler Publishers, Inc.

Dock, L. L. (1901). What we may expect from the law. *American Journal of Nursing, 1,* 8.

Dock, L. L. (1910). *Hygiene and morality.* New York: G. P. Putnam's Sons.

Donahue, M. P. (1994). Developing a sound philosophy of nursing: Is historical nursing knowledge necessary? In J. F. Kikuchi & H. Simmons (Eds.), *Developing a philosophy of nursing.* Thousand Oaks, CA: Sage Publications.

Donahue, M. P. (1996). *Nursing the finest art: An illustrated history* (2nd ed.). St. Louis, MO: Mosby.

Donahue, M. P. (1998). The evolution of nursing: Science and practice. In G. Deloughery (Ed.), *Issues and trends in nursing* (3rd ed.) (pp. 57–104). St. Louis, MO: Mosby.

Donley, Sr. R. (1989, Winter). A coming home. *Reflections, 15*(4), 10.

Fairman, J., & Lynaugh, J. (1998). *Critical care nursing: A history.* Philadelphia, PA: University of Pennsylvania Press.

Fiedler, L. A. (1988). Images of the nurse in fiction and popular culture. In A. H. Jones (Ed.), *Images of nurses: Perspectives from history, art, and literature* (pp. 100–112). Philadelphia, PA: University of Pennsylvania Press.

Fitzpatrick, M. L. (1983). *Prologue to professionalism.* Bowie, MD: Robert J. Brady Co.

Gadow, S. (1977). Humanistic issues at the interface of nursing and the community. Unpublished manuscript from paper delivered at the Conference of Humanists and Nursing. Hartford, Connecticut, March 4.

Gadow, S. (1984). Touch and technology: Two paradigms of patient care. *Journal of Religion and Health, 23*(1), 63–69.

Goodrich, A. W. (1932). *The social and ethical significance of nursing.* New York: Macmillan.

Hamilton, D. (1994). Constructing the mind of nursing. *Nursing History Review, 2,* 3–28.

Hanson, K. S. (1988). A historical analysis of the liberal education theme in nursing education: 1893–1952. Unpublished dissertation, The University of Iowa, Iowa City, Iowa.

Hewitt, H., & Donahue, M. P. (2001). Passing on more than a blank disc: A task for nursing historians. *Nursing History Review, 9,* 207–215.

Howell, J. D. (1995). *Technology in the hospital: Transforming patient care in the early twentieth century.* Baltimore, MD: Johns Hopkins University Press.

Hughes, E. C., Hughes, H. M., & Deutscher, I. (1958). *Twenty thousand nurses tell their story.* Philadelphia, PA: J. B. Lippincott.

Institute of Medicine (IOM). (1983). *Nursing and nursing education: Public policies and private actions.* Washington, DC: National Academy Press.

Johns, E., & Pfefferkorn, B. (1934). *An activity analysis of nursing.* New York: Committee on the Grading of Nursing Schools.

Kalisch, P. A., & Kalisch, B. J. (1987). *The changing image of the nurse.* Redwood City, CA: Addison-Wesley.

Kalisch, P. A., & Kalisch, B. J. (1995). *The advance of American nursing* (3rd ed.). Philadelphia, PA: J. B. Lippincott.

Lerner, G. (1982). The necessity of history and the professional historian. *Journal of American History, 69*(1), 7–20.

Leslie, R. R. C. (1951). Religion and the mentally ill. *American Journal of Nursing, 51*(4), 255.

Lewis, E. (1977). Editorial: Heroines and dragons. *Nursing Outlook, 25*(1), 21.

Lynaugh, J. E. (1991). Nursing's history: Looking backward and seeing forward. In L. Aiken & C. Fagin (Eds.), *Charting nursing's future* (pp. 435–447). Philadelphia, PA: J. B. Lippincott.

Lynaugh, J. E. (2001). Introduction. In E. D. Baer, P. D'Antonio, S. Rinker, & J. E. Lynaugh (Eds.), *Enduring issues in American nursing* (pp. 237–239). New York: Springer Publishing Company.

Lynaugh, J. E., & Brush, B. L. (1996). *American nursing: From hospitals to health systems.* Cambridge, MA: Blackwell Publishers.

Mazlish, B. (1967). The fourth discontinuity. *Technology and Culture, 8*(1), 1–15.

Melosh, B. (1982). *The physician's hand: Work culture and conflict in American nursing.* Philadelphia, PA: Temple University Press.

Miller, T. (1989). Men in nursing. *California Nursing Review, 11,* 2, 11.

Mitch, C. (1991). Thank heavens for crazy people. *American Journal of Nursing, 91*(1), 108.

Montag, M. L. (1975). *Where is nursing going?* New York: National League for Nursing, Pub. No. 23-1585.

Moore, D. W. (2001, December 5). Firefighters top Gallup's "honesty and ethics" list. Princeton, NJ: *Gallup News Service,* 1–4.

Muff, J. (Ed.). (1988). *Socialization, sexism, and stereotyping: Women's issues in nursing.* Prospect Heights, IL: Waveland Press, Inc.

Naisbitt, J., Naisbitt, N., & Philips, D. (1999). *High tech/High touch: Technology and our search for meaning.* New York: Broadway Books.

National Commission on Nursing. (1983). *Summary report and recommendations.* Chicago, IL: Hospital Research and Educational Trust.

National League of Nursing Education. (1917). *Standard curriculum for schools of nursing.* New York: Author.

National League of Nursing Education. (1927). *Curriculum for schools of nursing.* New York: Author.

National League of Nursing Education. (1937). *A curriculum guide for schools of nursing.* New York: Author.

Nightingale, F. (1860). *Notes on nursing: What it is and what it is not.* New York: D. Appleton and Company.

Nutting, M. A. (1926). *A sound economic basis for schools of nursing and other addresses.* New York: G. P. Putnam's Sons.

Nutting, M. A., & Dock, L. L. (1907). *A history of nursing* (Vol. I). New York: G. P. Putnam's Sons.

Passau-Buck, S. (1988). Caring vs. curing. In J. Muff (Ed.), *Socialization, sexism, and stereotyping* (pp. 203–209). Prospect Heights, IL: Waveland Press, Inc.

Paterson, J., & Zderad, L. (1988). *Humanistic nursing.* New York: National League for Nursing.

Peplau, H. E. (1966). Nurse–doctor relationships. *Nursing Forum, 5*(1), 60–75.

Reverby, S. M. (1987). *Ordered to care: The dilemma of American nursing, 1850–1945.* New York: Cambridge University Press.

Roberts, M. M. (1954). *American nursing: History and interpretation.* New York: Macmillan.

Robinson, V. (1946). *White caps: The story of nursing.* Philadelphia, PA: J. B. Lippincott.

Russell, C. H. (1958). Liberal education and nursing. *Nursing Research, 7*(3), 116–126.

Sandelowski, M. (1988). A case of conflicting paradigms: Nursing and reproductive technology. *Advances in Nursing Science, 10*(3), 35–45.

Sandelowski, M. (2000). *Devices & desires: Gender, technology, and American nursing.* Chapel Hill: University of North Carolina Press.

Sellew, G., & Nuesse, C. J. (1946). *A history of nursing.* St. Louis, MO: Mosby.

Spratley, H., Johnson, A., Sochalski, J., Fritz, M., & Spencer, W. (2000). *The registered nurse population. Findings from the National Sample Survey of Registered Nurses.* Washington, DC: U.S. Department of Health and Human Services.

Stewart, I. M. (1921). Developments in nursing education since 1918. *U.S. Bureau of Education Bulletin, 20,* 6.

Stewart, I. M. (1929, Winter). The science and art in nursing. *The Nursing Education Bulletin, 2*(1), 1–3.

Stewart, I. M. (1940, September). The philosophy of the collegiate school of nursing. *American Journal of Nursing, 40,* 1033.

Stewart, I. M. (1943). Forty-ninth Annual NLNE Convention. New York: National League of Nursing Education.

Styles, M. M. (1982). *On nursing: Toward a new endowment.* St. Louis, MO: Mosby.

West, M., & Hawkins, C. (1950). *Nursing schools at the mid-century.* New York: National Committee for the Improvement of Nursing Services.

SUGGESTED READINGS

Brown, E. L. (1970). *Nursing reconsidered, a study of change.* Philadelphia, PA: J. B. Lippincott.

Bush, B. L. (2001). Caring for life: Nursing during the holocaust. *Nursing History Review, 110,* 60–81.

Cramer, S. (1992). The nature of history: Mediations on Cleo's craft. *Nursing Research, 41*(1), 4–7.

Dock, L. L., & Stewart, I. M. (1925). *A short history of nursing* (2nd ed.). New York: G. P. Putnam's Sons.

Dossey, B. M. (2000). *Florence Nightingale: Mystic, visionary, healer.* Springhouse, PA: Springhouse Publications.

Hamilton, D. (1992). Research and reform: Community nursing and the Framingham Tuberculosis Program, 1914–1923. *Nursing Research, 41*(1), 8–13.

Hanson, K. S., & Donahue, M. P. (1996). Doing the work of history. The diary of historical evidence: The case of Sarah Gallop Greg. *Nursing History Review, 4,* 169–186.

Kalisch, P. A., & Kalisch, B. J. (1976). Nurses under fire: World War II experiences of nurse on Bataan and Corregidor. *Nursing Research, 25*(6), 409–425.

King, M. G. (1989) Nursing shortage, Circa 1915. *Image: Journal of Nursing Scholarship, 21*, 124–127.

Pokorny, M. E. (1992). A historical perspective of Confederate nursing during the Civil War, 1891–1865. *Nursing Research, 41*(1), 28–32.

Mitch, C. (1991). Thank heavens for crazy people. *American Journal of Nursing, 91*(1), 108.

Spratley, E., Johnson, A., Sochalski, J., Fritz, M., & Spencer, W. (2000). *The registered nurse population. Findings from the National Sample Survey of Registered Nurses.* Washington, DC: U.S. Department of Health and Human Services.

Stuart, M. (1992). Half a loaf is better than no bread: Public health nurses and physicians in Ontario 1920–1925. *Nursing Research, 41*(1), 21–27.

Winderquest, J. G. (1992). The spirituality of Florence Nightingale. *Nursing Research, 41*(1), 49–55.

2

The Evolution of Nursing Education

MELANIE DREHER

> *There are two classes of people in the world—those who take the best and enjoy it and those who wish for something better and try to create it. The world needs the appreciation of the first and the discontent of the second.*
>
> *Florence Nightingale*

LEARNING OBJECTIVES

AT THE COMPLETION OF THIS CHAPTER, THE READER WILL BE ABLE TO:

- Trace the evolution of professional nursing education in the United States.
- Identify the powerful obstacles that proponents of collegiate-based nursing education confronted throughout the twentieth century.
- Explain why it is important for professional nursing education to be located in universities and 4-year colleges.
- Link curriculum with professional roles by comparing contemporary nursing education with earlier decades.
- Review graduate education in nursing and its impact on academic nursing.

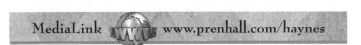

MediaLink   www.prenhall.com/haynes

Additional online resources including NCLEX review questions, critical thinking questions, and real-world activities for this chapter can be found on the Companion Website at www.prenhall.com/haynes.

Two momentous developments, occurring on separate continents almost a century apart, were turning points in the evolution of nursing education. The first, of course, occurred in 1860 when Florence Nightingale established the first formal program of nursing education and nursing came into being as a distinguished, secular profession. Although located at St. Thomas Hospital, Nightingale's school was an independent educational program in which the preparation of nurses was the primary goal. The second momentous development, which spanned nearly a century, was the movement of nursing education from hospitals to universities and 4-year colleges. Unlike the singular, transforming event at St. Thomas Hospital, the transition from hospitals to universities, which began in the first decade of the twentieth century, assumed the greatest momentum in the last half of the twentieth century and to this day remains incomplete. Drawing from the most famous history of nursing education by preeminent educator Isabel Maitland Stewart, *The Education of Nurses* (1953), this chapter summarizes the consistent themes that characterize the evolution of nursing education during the first half of the twentieth century. While the evolution of nursing education is an agonizingly long chapter in the history of nursing, it is one of the most fascinating and unique social movements of the century. The evolution of nursing education over the past century and a half truly is a testimony to the brilliance, creativity, dedication, and tenacity of nursing leaders against powerful odds.

In 1869, the American Medical Association acknowledged the need to have well-prepared nurses to assist them and recommended that every hospital operate a school of nursing in which nurses would be "trained" for both hospital practice and home care. The importance of formal education for nurses had been confirmed by the Civil War experience of women from both the North and the South who courageously volunteered to care for the wounded. They were, however, ill prepared for the overwhelming battlefield responsibilities they encountered. It was about the same time that the work of Florence Nightingale in the Crimean War was becoming known in the United States. Four years later, the first American schools of nursing, based on the principles promoted by Florence Nightingale, were founded at the Connecticut Training School, the Boston Training School, and the Bellevue Training School in New York City (Stewart, 1953).

By 1880, there were 15 training schools for nurses, and by 1909, the number had grown to 35, with 1,552 students (Stewart, 1953, p. 128). Training schools continued to proliferate, and by 1919 there were almost 1,100 hospital-based schools throughout the United States offering a diploma in nursing. Unfortunately, the guidelines promoted by Florence Nightingale, with a few exceptions, had all but disappeared. In most cases, the service needs of the hospital were not distinguished from the needs of the school.

Being largely philanthropic in purpose, these schools did not discriminate clearly between the aim of supplying a good nursing service for the hospital and that of developing a good educational system—indeed they considered these more or less identical. Economic pressure, even in the independent schools, tended to push the educational aim in the background and to merge the school more and more in the nursing service of the hospital. The hospitals, at first opposed to the new type of nurses, discovered in them forces of incalculable value—practical and moral. It soon became an accepted principle that a school of nursing was indispensable in running a hospital and most hospitals set up their own schools or took over schools that had been organized on an independent basis. This change in the control of nursing education undoubtedly helped in the rapid expansion of hospitals and nursing schools, but it only covered up and did not solve the fundamental conflicts which had existed before, between the economical servicing of the hospital and the proper education of nurses (Stewart, 1953, p. 131).

In these hospitals, students were required to work long hours with no compensation other than room and board. They had insufficient time even for meals and sleep, much less learning. Many were required to do private duty in homes and then return their earnings to the hospital. Hospitals were not required to follow any formal curriculum or standards and often manipulated admission criteria to assure that they would have sufficient quantity, if not quality, of staff. Thus it was commonplace for students to have met neither the minimum age nor the high school completion requirements. Many hospitals were small and offered narrow clinical experience, typically focusing on operating room and surgical services. Students essentially staffed the hospitals with "duties" that included scrubbing the beds and mopping the floors as well as attending to the care of patients.

Why did women take these positions? Mainly because of the opportunity to engage in "private duty" home care at the end of their training at wages that were significantly higher than other occupations open to working-class women at that time. While women were beginning to succeed in being admitted to 4-year colleges and universities, there was little interest in transitioning hospital training programs into 4-year colleges and universities. In 1899, Teachers College at Columbia University offered the first course for nurses in the United States, and in 1909, the University of Minnesota established the first baccalaureate program in nursing. Unfortunately, the latter did not differ substantially from hospital diploma programs, and even though nursing students had to meet the same admission standards as other university requirements, they continued to work long hours in the hospital and received a diploma instead of a degree.

Over the ensuing decades, concerned nursing leaders continued to spearhead attempts to set standards for nursing education and promote curricula that would include (a) the sciences as a basis for practice, (b) content that focused on health care, and (c) comprehensive experiential opportunities to provide patient care. At the end of World War I, the United States faced a serious shortage of nurses, attributable mainly to the widely acknowledged exploitation of nursing students who literally ran the hospitals. Many studies were commissioned to study the "nursing problem," the most famous of which was the Goldmark Report. Published in 1923, the report advocated for the setting of educational standards and a liberal education for nurses in 4-year colleges. Although the report did not have a significant impact on nursing education, it did result in the establishment of the Yale University School of Nursing and the Case Western Reserve School of Nursing, both of which were administratively and fiscally independent from their hospitals (Stewart, 1953).

By 1928, the year before the stock market crash, there was an oversupply of nurses, accompanied by low educational standards, poor working conditions, and dangerously unsatisfactory levels of care. When the depression officially hit, there were over 2,200 diploma programs, but as the economy worsened, there were fewer opportunities for private duty employment after graduation. Several hospitals closed their training programs and began to hire graduate nurses at a minimum wage to staff their hospitals. By 1936, the number of hospital diploma schools had been reduced to less than 1,500. In the meantime, almost 70 collegiate programs had been established, but even there, scientific theory represented only a small percentage of the nursing education curriculum, which was restricted primarily to physical and medical sciences (Stewart, 1953).

The poor quality of nursing education continued through and after World War II. Diploma schools, where the majority of nurses were educated, frequently had inadequately prepared teachers who also directed the nursing services of the hospital. Hospitals continued to depend on nursing students to provide the bulk of nursing services. Two decades after the Goldmark Report, a report by anthropologist Esther Lucile Brown lamented the lack of progress since the earlier study and once again recommended that professional nursing education be located in 4-year colleges and universities. Throughout the many decades that followed the establishment of the first Nightingale-based schools in the United States, three persistent themes motivated generations of nursing leaders who aspired to promote college-based education for professional nursing practice.

- Increasing recognition within the nursing leadership of the complexity of nursing care and its emerging theoretical and scientific base, independent of medicine
- Increasing significance of public health as a venue for nursing practice, requiring theory and practice experience that could not be provided in a hospital curriculum
- The quest for professional self-determination, consistent with other professions such as medicine, law, education, and social work

Report after report cited the value of a liberal education, including the arts and humanities, as well as the sciences, as the foundation for professional nursing. Even early studies acknowledged that hospital apprentice training, in most cases, simply was not sufficient preparation for the increasingly complex role nurses played in health care—particularly in public health content, such as disease prevention and child health and development. Largely focused on the care of the sick, under the direction of physicians, nursing students were required to spend time in each of the medical specialty areas (e.g., surgery, orthopedics, etc.). The need for nurses to have knowledge of social and behavioral sciences emerged largely from the experiences of public health nurses. This knowledge provided the framework for the development of nursing theory and science. Yet, despite its expanding role and growing body of knowledge, nursing remained the only profession in which educational standards were controlled by another industry—specifically hospitals. Medicine, law, education, dentistry, and later social work and public health all were responsible for setting their own standards for professional education and practice, while nursing education remained under the control of the parent institution—namely hospitals.

Fortunately, the 1950 report, *Nursing Schools at Mid-Century*, resulted in the establishment of accreditation procedures in nursing. This was very important not only because it put the process of determining and requiring educational standards under the control of nursing, but also because it became a vehicle for enhancing good programs and closing inferior ones. It was at this time that professional nursing education truly began to shift, still incrementally but incontrovertibly, to colleges and universities. In the fall of 2001, the Enrollment and Graduation Report 2001–2002 (American Association of Colleges of Nursing, 2002, p. 9) showed there were 663 baccalaureate nursing educational programs in the United States and its territories. From the enduring university program at Minnesota in 1909 and then the Goldmark Report in 1923, it still took over half a century for the majority of professional nursing education programs to be housed in universities and 4-year colleges and even to this day, hospital diploma programs continue to exist, primarily in the northeastern states.

Why has the transition to collegiate-based education been so long in coming? It is clear that from the beginning, powerful opposition from the hospital and medical communities served as a major obstacle to the advancement of nursing as a profession. Although hospitals complained about the cost of "training," they were reluctant to give up their control over the supply and demand of nurses. Physician organizations championed the value of skilled nurses but regarded them mostly as able assistants. Both the hospital industry and medical associations used every opportunity to oppose collegiate programs, accreditation standards, and even professional licensure. The first nursing licensure laws were passed in 1903 as a means of protecting the public by assuring minimal competency, but hospital and medical associations paid little attention to them, asserting that patient care would be seriously compromised by the resulting shortage of nurses. Physicians and other members of the hospital industry sought to reframe their patently economic motives by addressing quality of care concerns. The clinical skill of "overtrained" nurses, who would have too much knowledge and not enough practical experience, was brought into question. Technical skills, industry, and obedience to the physicians were seen as the most desirable attributes for nurses. These self-serving policies of hospital and physician organizations surfaced again and again throughout the century, including opposition to an 8-hour day for nurses (instead of the usual 12 hours). Sadly, many nurses, powerless and manipulated by hospitals and physi-

cians, also saw little value in collegiate education (Friss, 1994).

Nursing Education Curriculum

As early as 1917, the National League of Nursing Education, which eventually became the National League for Nursing, published the *Standard Curriculum for Schools of Nursing*, with the intent to improve nursing education by establishing and publishing standards of quality. In 1929, responding to the expansion of nurses into the field of public health, the League revised this curriculum to include an emphasis on health as well as illness, instituting educational content that Nightingale believed should be integral to nursing education. In spite of these efforts, the quality of nursing education continued to vary widely, and in 1934, the National League of Nursing Education undertook preparation of its third and perhaps most comprehensive curriculum. When it was published in 1937, the vast majority of nurses still were educated in hospitals. *A Curriculum Guide for Schools of Nursing* (National League of Nursing Education, 1937) (Box 2–1) represented the most progressive thinking in basic nursing education at the time and was used for several decades.

Although referred to as a "guide," the curriculum was highly prescriptive, including requirements for the number of hours and placement of each element, as well as the content itself. While it may appear rigid by today's standards, *The Guide* evolved in a context of great variability among hospitals, where there was often more concern with getting the work done than establishing and maintaining the quality of nursing education. It was, in many respects, a "how to" for establishing a professional nursing education program, and despite its hospital orientation, *The Guide* continued to influence nursing education for decades. It was grounded clearly in Nightingale's principles of professional nursing education based in the sciences while embracing the concept of health as well as illness.

The most recent curriculum guidelines of national significance can be found in the 1998 revision of the *Essentials of Baccalaureate Education for Professional Nursing Practice* advanced by the American Association of Colleges of Nursing (AACN). Although it might be considered the contemporary equivalent of *The Guide*, it reflects, without question, the transition of professional nursing education to the collegiate setting (Box 2–2).

Box 2–1   1937 Curriculum

Table 3. A schematic outline of theory and practice in nursing arts and clinical courses showing one of many possible arrangements. This plan may be varied to suit different student groups, different classifications of clinical experience, and minimum as well as maximum periods in the different clinical divisions.

	FIRST TERM	SECOND TERM	THIRD TERM	

FIRST TERM	Introduction to Nursing Arts
	45 hours theory
	16 weeks clinical practice
	6–9 hours per week
		Introduction to Nursing Arts
		90 hours theory
		16 weeks clinical practice
		18–21 hours per week
			Medical and Surgical Nursing
			80 hours theory
			16 weeks clinical practice
			  8 weeks Medical Nursing (general)
			  8 weeks Surgical Nursing (general)
			33–36 hours per week	

	Varied Services–mainly Medical and Surgical	Varied Services–mainly Medical and Surgical	M M M M S S S S M M M M S S S S	

SECOND TERM	Medical and Surgical Nursing
	80 hours theory
	16 weeks clinical practice
	  4 weeks Diet Kitchen
	  6 weeks Operating Room
	  4 weeks Eye, Ear, Nose, and Throat
	  2 weeks Orthopedic
	38–42 hours per week
		Medical and Surgical Nursing
		80 hours theory
		16 weeks clinical practice
		  2 weeks Orthopedic
		  6 weeks Communicable Disease
		  4 weeks Tuberculosis
		  4 weeks Gynecological
		38–42 hours per week
			Obstetric Nursing
			60–80 hours theory
			16 weeks clinical practice
			38–42 hours per week	

	D D D D OR OR OR OR OR OR E E E E O O	O O CD CD CD CD CD CD Tb Tb Tb Tb G G G G	Ob Ob Ob Ob Ob Ob Ob Ob Ob Ob Ob Ob Ob Ob Ob Ob	
THIRD TERM	Nursing of Children 60–80 hours theory 16 weeks clinical practice 38–42 hours per week	Psyciatric Nursing 60–80 hours theory 16 weeks clinical practice 38–42 hours per week	Nursing and Health Service in Family 30–40 hours theory 8 weeks practice 38–42 hours per week	Advanced Nursing and Electives 30–40 hours theory 8 weeks clinical practice 38–42 hours per week
	C C C C C C C C C C C C C C C C	P P P P P P P P P P P P P P P P	F F F F F F F F	A A A A A A A A

Total Length of Course	Key—Assignment to Clinical Practice
3 years—144 weeks—9 terms of 16 weeks each, exclusive of 12 weeks' vacation, 4 weeks per year.	(Each letter above indicates one clinical week.)

Total period of organized instruction
1200–1300 hours approximately.

Total period of clinical practice
4400–5000 hours approximately.

Key—Assignment to Clinical Practice
(Each letter above indicates one clinical week.)

M—Medical (general)   Tb—Tuberculosis
S—Surgical (general)   G—Gynecological
D—Diet Kitchen   Ob—Obstetric
OR—Operating Room   C—Nursing of Children
E—Eye, Ear, Nose, Throat   P—Psychiatric
O—Orthopedic   F—Nursing and Health Service
CD—Communicable Disease   in the Family
   A—Advanced Nursing and Electives

Reprinted with permission: National League of Nursing Education. (1937). *A curriculum guide for schools of nursing*. New York: National League of Nursing Education. Copyright National League for Nursing.

As can be seen in the outline above, the 1998 curriculum looks very different from the one that preceded it by just over 60 years. Its comparative flexibility may be its most obvious feature. Rather than a rigid sequence of courses and content, it is a distillation of the three major components of a baccalaureate curriculum for the practice of professional nursing—*role, knowledge,* and *practice.*

Role

The *Essentials* document begins quite logically with the end (or outcomes), identifying three broad roles of professional nursing: (1) provider of care, (2) designer/manager/coordinator of care, and (3) member of a profession. Understanding the roles of professional nursing in contemporary society thus guides the knowledge and clinical practice that students will need to prepare for those roles. Some might argue that various components of the roles identified in the AACN document represent a vision of the potential of professional nursing rather than the current realities, which is exactly what is expected when nursing education moves from hospital to collegiate setting. The responsibility of institutions of higher education is not simply to prepare

The Discipline and Role

Nurses are providers of care.

Nurses are designers, managers, and coordinators of care.

Nurses are members of a profession.

Core Knowledge

Health promotion, risk reduction, and disease prevention

Illness and disease management

Information and health care technologies

Ethics

Human diversity

Global health care

Health systems and policy

Core Competencies

Critical thinking

Communication

Assessment

Technical skills

These essentials are based on a liberal education as a foundation for nursing and on professional values, including:

Altruism

Autonomy

Human dignity

Integrity

Social justice

---

nurses for existing jobs, as hospitals did, but to *prepare nurses who will create new positions and new roles to address the changing and emerging health needs of society.* One of the most daunting challenges faced by educators is to prepare graduates to practice in a world that is as yet unimagined. This preparation requires foresight, flexibility, creativity, and a broader definition of nursing than ever has existed in the past.

Knowledge

The second dimension of the AACN *Essentials* document consists of the fundamental areas of knowledge required to prepare students for careers in professional nursing. When the role of nursing was limited to care of the sick in hospitals and homes, the required knowledge base also was more limited and focused primarily on anatomy, physiology, chemistry, biology, and what were referred to as medical sciences, such as pathophysiology and pharmacology. Nurses who entered the field of public health became cognizant of the social, cultural, and economic influences on health. Later, anthropology, economics, and political science, along with biostatistics and epidemiology, emerged as additional disciplines from which professional nursing takes nourishment. Knowledge of health promotion, risk reduction, and disease prevention; illness and disease management; information and health care technologies; ethics; human diversity; and global health care, along with health care systems and policy formulation, is grist for the contemporary nursing education mill. In addition, better under-

standing of the relationship between physiological and behavioral processes mandated that nurses have an equally sound grounding in behavioral sciences. Finally, leadership and political activism have become as essential as direct care if nurses are to be successful advocates for patients, as well as the nursing profession.

Practice

Since nursing is a practice discipline, nursing education is not only about acquiring knowledge but also about learning how to apply it. Referred to as "Core Competencies" in the AACN *Essentials* document, this part of the curriculum addresses the question of how nurses use knowledge to achieve goals. Rather than attending to the minutiae of clinical practice, the AACN has elegantly identified *assessment, communication,* and *critical thinking* as the three main components of practice in any context.

The most elemental component of practice is the ability to establish therapeutic relationships with patients. A therapeutic relationship is not just any relationship, but rather a relationship that *makes a difference.* Examples of therapeutic relationships include the effective management of pain, a drug prevention program in schools, helping to keep a child with asthma out of the hospital, teaching an individual how to manage anticoagulant therapy, or changing a national policy to improve the health of elders. A therapeutic relationship is an advocacy relationship, helping patients, whether they are individuals, a family, a group, a community, or a whole nation, to stay well, to manage illness, and to create order out of the chaos that comes with sickness and vulnerability.

Assessment is fundamental to everything that a professional nurse does. Nurses cannot engage patients, families, or communities in therapeutic partnerships unless they can communicate with them, and they cannot communicate with them effectively unless they assess them, their illness, and the context in which health and illness are manifested. Nurses have many vehicles of communication—they communicate through observation and touch, as well as verbal, written, telephonic, electronic, and public media. Communication and assessment are not linear but interwoven and mutually enhancing; better assessment will enhance communication, which, in turn, will result in a more comprehensive and richer assessment.

Clinical reasoning (or *critical thinking* in the *Essentials*) is the third leg of the practice enterprise. It weds *knowledge* about human responses, health, illness, and treatment to *information* derived from assessments of *specific* patients, families, and communities to generate a plan for the clinical management of our patients. The evolution of nursing education is perhaps most obvious in the clinical reasoning component of practice, where the nursing model emerges, based in the social and behavioral as well as the physical sciences, and distinct from that of medicine. Through research and scholarship, the university-based intellectual community in nursing ultimately exposed the limitations in the medical model that had been deeply unsatisfying for nurses in both practice and academia for some time. Thus, clinical management in nursing is different from clinical management in medicine. In nursing, it is the process of individualizing treatment to meet the specific needs of patients, families, and communities. Physicians,

on the other hand, are less concerned with the individualization of care and more concerned with the treatment of the disease or infirmity. They start with the disease or health problem, which just happens to be located in a specific patient, and look for a cure or treatment. Nurses start with the specific patient or client, who just happens to have a health problem, and search for contextual explanations. For example, a physician is likely to treat frequent headaches by prescribing vasodilators, while the nurse will explore dimensions of the patient's home and work life, tracing the incidence of headaches and looking for contextual factors that may both explain their presence and suggest ways to prevent them. Both approaches are very important and useful and even complement one another, but they are not the same. The unique contribution that nursing brings to interdisciplinary clinical management of patients can and should, at the very least, be a reliable and comprehensive knowledge of the patient—whether that be an individual, family, community, or group.

The differences between nurses educated in the hospital and those educated in universities are far from superficial, as some members of the hospital and medical communities would like to think. When the emphasis shifted from skills to concepts, nursing education resolutely and manifestly required that care move from process to outcomes. Rather than learning *how* to do something, nurses learn to identify the desired outcomes of patient care and let those desired outcomes determine *what* care is provided. Nursing practice has gone from ritualistic to evidence-based. Critical thinking mandates that nurses constantly challenge existing practices and theories and question not only whether care is being provided most effectively and most efficiently, but also whether the action needs to done at all.

Research Application

To better understand employer expectations of the entry-level nurse, the National Council of State Boards of Nursing (NCSBN) conducts job analysis studies every 3 years (Hertz, Yocom, & Gawel, 1999). The NCSBN formulated a list of descriptors expected of newly licensed registered nurses based on past job analysis studies. The studies were initiated to identify changes over time in the work environment, employment characteristics, and activities of newly licensed nurses. Data from these studies are analyzed in relation to the frequency of performance, impact on maintaining patient safety, criticality of nursing activities performed, and the various settings where nursing activities were performed.

While these studies provide valuable data regarding employer expectations of new graduates, it is important to recognize that the studies do not dictate the framework or guidelines for baccalaureate nursing education. Using AACN guidelines, Daggett and others (2002) offer an organizing

(continued)

framework for nursing education. This framework provides new graduates with a broader understanding of those skills needed for successful practice in the twenty-first century than does the NCLEX job analysis survey, which simply outlines those skills nurses do today.

According to Daggett et al. (2002, p. 35), "successful nursing practice will require nurse to:

- Use resources in a more socially appropriate manner and design ways to offer services that will maintain or improve quality and lower costs.
- Improve access to care.
- Create less resource-intensive health care but more fulfilling lives for people as they age.
- Master information technologies.
- Develop practice protocols for new technologies that balance costs and benefits.

- Welcome the discipline of continuous improvement of quality.
- Understand the empowered role of the health care consumer and develop skills to change individual attitudes.
- Move organizations, systems, and policies toward strategies that improve equity of resourse distribution.
- Incorporate a more holistic perspective into care delivery."

The job analysis survey tells us what nurses do today. Baccalaureate education should prepare the professional not only for today but also for the future. How does your education rank with regard to preparation for the above tasks? Do you feel capable of taking on these responsibilities?

Old Habits

In spite of the enormous progress that has occurred in nursing education, there continue to be remnants of hospital-based learning that are so inherent that they are almost unrecognizable. One, for example, is the emphasis on specific time periods, often phrased in "hours," required for the successful completion of a component of the curriculum. In 1937, it was necessary to designate specific hour requirements to ensure that students have a broad and comprehensive clinical practicum and not spend all their time in the operating room assisting surgeons. There also has been a tendency among nurses to correlate mastery with time spent (i.e., if twice as much time is spent in labor and delivery, then the nurse will be twice as good). Today, educators understand that students learn at different rates and that mastery is correlated not only with time but also with the challenge and comprehensiveness of the experience. But even now, some schools and some State Boards of Nursing have continued to have specific "hour" requirements for different aspects of clinical nursing (e.g., care of child, psychiatric–mental health, etc.). This practice, unfortunately, is not only misguided, it reinforces a "job" mentality of the nursing culture in which professional nurses are viewed and paid as *hourly* workers rather than *salaried* professionals.

Another example of a diploma school dinosaur is the continued allegiance to the acquisition of technical proficiency as the fundamental component of nursing education. Even the *Essentials* document could not escape reference to specific technical skill competency (vital signs, pulse oximetry, three-lead electrocardiogram, etc.). There is no doubt that in the process of learning to nurse, students will be required to master certain aspects of current technology, to support the fundamental components of practice, assessment, communication, clinical reasoning, and therapeutic intervention. But unlike the enduring aspects of nursing practice, nursing technology changes more swiftly each day. Since the publication of the *Essentials*, nurses already are beginning to use a technology that can ascertain heart functioning without using a three-lead electrocardiogram. Today's curriculum prepares knowledgeable workers, not just "doers" who carry out the orders of others, but also professional nurses who are able to make clinical decisions themselves. Rather than an endless list of technical skills (spirometry, proper use of tubes and drains, suture and staple removal) that, given the rate of technological advancement, will never capture all the procedures nurses do, a more useful list of accomplishments might include things like:

- Support a patient and family at end of life.
- Manage a chronically ill, co-morbid adult patient across settings.
- Establish a community partnership to reduce health disparities.
- Provide guidance and support to healthy, first-time childbearing parents.
- Develop a project to promote healthy lifestyles in middle-aged persons.

Are there "diploma dinosaurs" in your nursing program? How could they be eliminated? What have we learned from our educational past, the diploma framework of education?

- Provide therapeutic intervention to a woman and her children who have been victims of domestic violence.
- Manage the immediate postoperative care of a patient undergoing cardiac surgery.

Ironically, despite the obvious differences between 1937 and 1998, both curricula are grounded in the lasting values of professional nursing, advanced by Nightingale. The contemporary role of the professional nurse not only as caregiver, but also as the manager and coordinator of care and as member of a profession, fulfills Nightingale's assertion that nursing is not just a matter of carrying out a doctor's instructions, but nursing is also a matter of relating as a colleague. That role is extended to collaboration with all health professions (e.g., physical therapy, social work, pharmacists, etc.), to which nurses bring a set of independent decisions and activities.

The separation of professional nursing education from hospitals was a painful but necessary step in the evolution of nursing education. Unlike medicine, in which medical school faculties and students have continued to provide patient care in their hospitals and clinics, the shift of nursing education from hospital to university resulted in two separate trajectories—education and practice—between which there has been an almost palpable tension. Despite the tension, both Deans and Chief Nursing Officers in hospitals are concluding that to move the profession of nursing forward, nursing education and practice should be reunited—to the detriment of neither and the benefit of both. In fact, the roles of clinicians and faculty members are becoming increasingly less distinguishable. Clinicians have taken on teaching and research responsibilities while faculty members are finding ways to engage in practice. The capacity of nursing students to function as clinical scholars is embedded in the remarriage of practice and academia.

The Associate Degree in Nursing and the Debate on Entry into Practice

In 1951, Dr. Mildred Montag proposed the training of "technical nurses" in 2-year colleges, who could provide high-quality assistance to the professional nurse and build cost-effective nursing teams. To protect the safety of the public and secure the confidence of the professional nurses who would supervise them, these technical nurses are required to pass the Registered Nurse licensing exam. The associate degree in nursing (ADN) was not the first experiment in abbreviated educational programs for producing a cadre of nursing staff prepared to function at a safe level of practice. The Cadet Nursing Corps of World War II, in which nurses were instructed in an abbreviated and intensive program of study to meet the urgent demands of wartime, was another example. The postwar nursing shortage and the success of the Cadet Nursing Corps provided both the impetus and feasibility for the preparation of nurses at the associate degree level.

Unfortunately, but not surprisingly, the hospital industry, anxious to meet staffing needs while keeping costs low, used the fact that associate degree graduates sit for the Registered Nurse licensing exam (NCLEX) as justification for deploying associate degree and bachelor's degree nurses interchangeably. Conveniently endorsing licensure, rather than education, as the entry into professional practice, hospitals have justified conferring the same title, assigning the same responsibilities, and providing the same orientation and compensation to 2-year graduates as to 4-year graduates. The tragedy of this is not that associate degree nurses are assuming responsibilities for which they are not qualified, but rather that bachelor's degree nurses are *not* fulfilling the role of professional nurse for which they are qualified—clinical leadership and delegation, outcomes management, evidence-based practice, policy evaluation, interdisciplinary practice, fiscal responsibilities—all of which would improve both the practice environment and the quality of care. A 2-year technical education simply does not prepare nurses for the daunting responsibilities of high-level clinical management, patient advocacy, and health care leadership. By treating BSN graduates as if they were associate degree graduates, hospitals are losing the value added by BSN competency.

For reasons that are less clear (but likely linked to the earlier competition between diploma and collegiate programs), the nursing profession also has chosen, perhaps inadvertently, perhaps by default, to endorse licensure rather than education as the entry into practice, thus confusing *professional practice* with *minimum safe practice*. As a result, the issue of entry into practice literally has consumed the nursing profession, generating endless debate and studies dedicated to proving and justifying the clinical superiority of nurses graduating with a bachelor's degree. Interestingly, nursing is singular in this respect. Medicine, dentistry, and physical therapy, for example, feel no compulsion to demonstrate that they are more qualified than physician's assistants, dental assistants, and physical therapy assistants, respectively. Nor do lawyers waste time proving that they are better prepared than paralegals. Nursing seems to be the only profession that feels the need to prove, rather than assume, that there is a correlation between education and performance.

Nurses have allowed the entry into practice issue to become a profession-wide obsession and, in turn, have chosen to view themselves as victims of an unenlightened hospital industry, yet they remain co-conspirators in this confusion. Nurses express resentment about being used interchangeably in hospitals, yet they accept positions in those institutions that fail to distinguish between the two types of graduates. Nurses insist on the importance of well-prepared leaders but do not insist that hospital-accrediting bodies set educational standards for nursing leadership. Professional nurses continue to join nursing organizations in which the membership consists of both levels of practice and then are dismayed by the ascendancy of associate degree majority control. They complain about the fact that associate degree graduates are required to sit for the same licensing exam but voluntarily permit them to sit for advanced certification exams. And in spite of nursing's insistence that the bachelor's degree should be the minimum entry into professional nursing practice, professional nurses persist in treating associate degree nurses as their equals rather than as capable, licensed assistants to whom selected aspects of patient care are delegated. It is unlikely that nursing's medical colleagues would take a position in which they function as physician's assistants or that they would report to a physician's assistant, or that they would include physician's assistants in the decision-making of their professional organizations that affect the future practice of medicine, or that they regard them as equally meritorious colleagues, entitled to the same rewards and having the same responsibilities.

It is time to reframe the entry into practice issue in a way that more accurately reflects contemporary realities. The complexity of patient care management in today's health care system simply requires nurses who have *at least* a 4-year college education in nursing. Graduates of associate degree programs have a useful and important role to play as direct caregivers under the guidance and direction of bachelor's-prepared professional nurses. Just because associate degree nurses (ADNs) sit for the same licensing exam as bachelor's degree graduates does not make them equal. Licensure as a registered nurse simply protects the public in both instances.

The confusion between licensure and education as the criterion for entry into practice does not have to exist. The U.S. military services provide an excellent example of an employer that has used the educational degree, rather than the license, as the basis for professional practice, requiring a bachelor's degree in nursing to be a commissioned officer, while nurses with less preparation are hired as enlisted persons. Using the military example, the baccalaureate nurse must stop worrying about competing with ADNs as the preferred level for entry into practice and simply endorse the bachelor's degree as the level for entry into *professional* nursing practice.

There are elements of nursing care that are accomplished quite effectively by nurses with less education. These elements are primarily procedural in nature (e.g., taking vital signs, changing a dressing, catheterizing patients, starting an IV, or even patient teaching). But who performs a particular nursing procedure—bachelor of science nurse (BSN), ADN, licensed practical nurse (LPN), nursing assistant, a family member, or even the patient—is not the basis for determining professional competence. Nor is it an automatic designation (e.g., ADNs can change dressings but only BSNs can start an IV). Who performs what responsibilities in the care of a patient is a clinical decision that should be based on clinical reasoning by a professional nurse with sufficient education, knowledge, and expertise to assign nursing procedures responsibly, according to circumstances. Thus, it may be fine for an ADN to teach some patients how to manage insulin therapy while other patients may require a more complex approach for the same task.

Associate degree graduates are thus capable, licensed assistants to whom nurses delegate selected aspects of care for selected patients. Two-year programs provide opportunities for men and women to have satisfying midlevel careers in health care. Although 4-year colleges have responded aggressively to requests for streamlined professional advancement opportunities with accessible and affordable RN–BSN programs, only 14% of ADNs, nationally, continue their education by seeking a bachelor's degree in nursing (AACN, 2002).

This suggests that the vast majority of ADNs are quite contented with where they are and what they are doing. While it is true that some of these nurses perform at a very high level, it is not a sufficient reason to forsake education as the minimal entry into professional practice or to assume that they are equal to the bachelor's-prepared nurses. Likewise, nurses may be able to point to specific physician's assistants who function at a level that is comparable to many physicians. Without the MD after their name, however, they are viewed simply and solely as well-prepared individuals who can extend the practice and expertise of the physician. The best advice that professional nurses can give to those extraordinary ADNs is to complete a bachelor's degree so that they can reap the rewards commensurate with their performance. In the meantime, professional nurses have the advantage of being assisted by well-prepared technical nurses who have demonstrated, by exam, that they can practice at a level that is at least minimally safe.

The debate on entry into practice is not only fruitless and distracting, it is unnecessary. As intended by Montag, the introduction of the associate degree in nursing was neither a bad nor confusing idea. Nurses should always be looking for more efficient and less costly ways of doing things in any field, and there are many aspects of nursing practice that can be performed by persons less prepared than professional nurses, just as there are aspects of medical and dental practice that can be performed by physician's assistants and dental assistants. Most would agree that the work of professional nurses should *not* be encumbered with having to do procedures that someone with less education can do. Advances in health care technology have made it possible for ADNs to do things that at one time only nurses from 4-year colleges could do, just as nurses can now do what once only physicians did.

The associate degree in nursing has proven to be adequate for passing the RN licensure exam. That being the case, the question has been called; it is the responsibility of bachelor's degree nurses to clearly define what distinguishes professional nursing practice from technical practice. One thing that is clear is that the distinction lies

not in the performance of nursing procedures, but rather in the integration of theoretical knowledge and information and its application in the construction of therapeutic relationships and clinical management.

Prelicensure Professional Degrees

In a bold attempt to establish nursing as equal in stature to medicine and other health professions, Case Western Reserve initiated the ND (Doctor of Nursing) program for college graduates in 1979. As the nursing equivalent of medicine and dentistry and other professional doctorates, it was intended to build on a liberal undergraduate education and to be offered in academic health science centers where clinical scholarship and research flourish. Like the baccalaureate degree, it is a prelicensure program, although most ND students sit for the NCLEX during their educational program rather than at the end. This professional doctorate is not a substitute for the PhD, which is a research degree. Just as the MD who desires a career in research must go on to acquire a PhD, the ND who wishes to pursue a career in research and university education must do the same.

The ND was a logical idea for bringing nursing to the interdisciplinary professional table at the same level as our colleagues in other health science disciplines. Unfortunately, it was an idea ahead of its time, and today there are only four ND programs in the country. While post-bachelor's education terminating in a *professional* master's degree has been the dominant model in physical therapy (MPT), occupational therapy (MOT), social work (MSW), and others, nursing generally has not taken that route. There are a number of "direct entry" master's degree programs in nursing, but they generally lead to advanced practice certification in which students frequently complete a BSN in the process. For the vast majority of the applicants who already have degrees in other fields, prelicensure programs are limited to second bachelor's degrees. In the *Essentials* document, the American Association of

Critical Thinking and Reflection

The failure of hospitals to differentiate bachelor's degree graduates from associate degree graduates is understandable, given the obvious economic motives, but why do you think that bachelor's pre- pared nurses have elected to treat associate degree nurses as their equals? Do you think this practice should continue? If not, what would you do to change it?

Why is nursing the only health profession that prepares prelicensure professional students below the master's level? What would happen if all existing bachelor's programs became professional master's program (master of nursing practice or MNP), comparable to social work or physical therapy? How would you accommodate currently practicing nurses who have a bachelor's degree? What impact would such a change have on our relationships with other health professions?

Colleges of Nursing (1998) addresses the impending debate on the post-bachelor's route to professional nursing education.

> Increasingly, we see the development of programs that prepare entry-level nursing professionals with graduate degrees (e.g., the nursing doctorate and the generic master's program). These programs are able to build on a broad base of education already acquired by students and then focus on several years of professional nursing education. These innovative models provide us with a variety of graduate education approaches for professional entry, and they need to be carefully examined and evaluated. The decisions we make or fail to make regarding nursing education today will determine whether those who come after us will be able to continue the tradition of professional nursing within the context of 21st century health care delivery (p. 20).

There is no doubt that it has become increasingly difficult within a 4-year program to fulfill the promises of the liberal education advocated by enlightened educators since the inception of professional nursing. In addition to a liberal education, contemporary nursing leaders have argued the importance of having a professional designation that is commensurate with the length and complexity of nursing education and comparable to the graduates of other health professions (e.g., MSW, MPT, MOT, DDS, PharmD, MD, etc.).

Graduate Education and Preparing the New Professoriate

Master's Education

The first graduate programs in nursing were established at Teachers College, Columbia University. The purpose of the early graduate programs was to prepare teachers and administrators of nursing who would assume the leadership roles required for advancing the profession—namely faculty members and nurse executives. Until clinical specialist roles appeared on the nursing practice horizon, these "functional" roles dominated graduate education in nursing. Within the past two decades, however, the emphasis in graduate nursing education has shifted away from teaching and administration to programs in *clinical* leadership and advanced practice nursing—generally referring to four roles: clinical specialists, nurse practitioners, nurse-midwives, and nurse anesthetists. In the 2001 Enrollment and Graduation Report 2001–2002, there were 388 nursing education programs that offered master's degrees, of which 327 offered nurse practitioner programs (AACN, 2002, p. 3). By far the most popular of the advanced practice roles, nurse practitioners accounted for 67% of the graduates from master's programs. The rest were divided among clinical nurse specialists (12%), nurse anesthetists (5%), nurse-midwives (4%), and teaching or administration (11%).

Of the four categories of advanced practice nurses, the roles of the nurse-midwife and nurse anesthetist are most clearly defined. While nurse practitioners and clinical specialists generally are distinguished by their emphasis on primary care or institution-based clinical leadership, respectively, there are many nurse practitioners functioning as clinical leaders in institutions and clinical specialists who have taken community-based positions on primary care teams. While the legal authority of nurse practitioners to prescribe medication is commonly considered a distinguishing factor, prescriptive authority varies from state to state. In some states, all advanced practice nurses have prescriptive authority.

Doctoral Education

Like the master's programs, the early doctoral programs in nursing were located in schools of education—Teachers College of Columbia University and the School of Education at New York University, both of which offered an EdD (Doctor of Education) for successful completion of doctoral work in nursing. Currently, there are 79 programs nationally that offer a PhD or DNS. The academic doctorate, usually a PhD (Doctor of Philosophy), is a research degree. It is focused on scientific discovery and research in which doctoral candidates demonstrate their proficiency by writing a dissertation. Thus, the PhD prepares the student for a career in university teaching and research. Recent studies by the AACN indicate that both the PhD and DNS degree are research focused and virtually indistinguishable in their purpose, which is "to prepare students to pursue intellectual inquiry and conduct independent research for the purpose of extending knowledge" (AACN, 1998, p. 10).

The most rapid growth of doctoral programs occurred in the 1980s and 1990s, during which 52 institutions initiated programs of doctoral study in nursing. The proliferation of programs, however, has not resulted in a proliferation of graduates. In 1998, there were only 200 more graduates than there were in 1989, and the average number of graduations each year is less than six per program. Since these doctoral programs prepare the next generation of faculty members, the failure to produce more PhD or DNS graduates poses a serious problem for nursing education.

Unlike medicine, dentistry and other professions in which students who have an interest in science, research, and teaching at the university level move quickly on for their PhD, nursing faculty members have tended to spend much more time in practice, often pursuing advanced degrees part time after several years of practice. A common pattern for faculty preparation would include graduation from a bachelor's degree program, practice for 2 or 3 years, return part time for an advanced practice master's program, complete the program in 4 to 5 years, practice again, and then return for a doctorate in another 5 to 10 years. Thus, it is not uncommon for nurses to be middle-aged by the time they acquire their doctorate and take an assistant professor faculty position, compared to other disciplines in which new doctorates are in their late twenties and early thirties.

Recently, some schools and colleges of nursing have developed programs for undergraduate students who have a particular interest in science and knowledge development to move directly into a PhD program, similar to other disciplines. In almost all nursing education programs, there is an eagerness to identify such students and encourage them to move quickly into graduate work. While it is true that nursing is a practice discipline and requires opportunities for clinical practice within the graduate plan of study, it also is an intellectual and scientific endeavor. Just like public health, medicine, biology, or anthropology, nursing is charged with the responsibility for developing knowledge and theories that will improve nursing practice to achieve better patient outcomes and producing the next generation of researchers and educators.

Nursing Faculty

Within nursing schools, there are various kinds of faculty roles, leading to two fundamental kinds of faculty appointments—*clinical track* and *tenure track*. Members of the clinical track faculty generally are focused on practice and clinical teaching. Some members of the clinical track may have a PhD or DNS, but frequently their highest degree is a master's in one or more areas of nursing clinical specialization and leadership. Clinical track faculty members often are the instructors who guide clinical theory and practice instruction, working with colleagues in hospitals and other nursing institutions to prepare students for practice as professional nurses. Members of the clinical faculty are expected to be up to date on the practice innovations and clinical research in their fields, including the most recent technology and its application. In contrast, academic or tenure track faculty have the additional responsibility of conducting research and/or other forms of scholarship, disseminating their results and contributing to the body of science that guides nursing practice. In most nursing programs, appointment to a tenure track position requires an academic earned doctorate (most commonly a PhD) in nursing or a related field, and a commitment to research and scholarship as well as teaching. Both types of faculty members are expected to provide service to the profession (e.g., leadership in professional organizations, writing questions for certification exams, serving on editorial boards of nursing journals, conducting accreditation site visits, etc.).

When students enter a nursing program, becoming a faculty member usually is not the first thing they think of as a career option. Often, this realization comes after a number of years of clinical practice and having the opportunity to precept a student or mentor a new graduate. Teaching novice members of the profession is both a role and a responsibility of professional practice, particularly if employed in a teaching hospital or other kind of teaching facility. Typically, nurses have thought of teaching hospitals only as

Faculty members have many responsibilities in addition to teaching. What is the impact of those many roles on students? What should the relationship between students and faculty be like? What are the advantages and disadvantages of a career in academic nursing?

those that have medical students and residents, but there is no reason why that same designation should not be applied to hospitals in which nurses are taught. Being a faculty member in a college of nursing is both a challenging and gratifying role and another career option for nurses who enjoy teaching others. It provides an opportunity to be part of an intellectual community that shapes the direction of the profession by influencing literally hundreds of nurses throughout a lifetime.

Nursing Shortages and the Future of Nursing Education

The standard response to a nursing shortage is to educate more nurses. At first blush, this response appears intuitively correct and, as discussed in this chapter, is exactly what hospitals did when they controlled the education and thus the supply of nurses. But before simply increasing the volume of nurses, it is useful to consider why there is a nursing shortage and where the nursing shortage is most acute. The current crisis in nursing is not just a contemporary problem, rather it is a chronic condition that has plagued nursing for over 100 years.

It was the shortage of qualified nurses in the Civil War that spurred the establishment of schools of nursing in the United States. Subsequent shortages—both national and local—were powerful incentives for hospitals throughout the country to establish their own schools. On the other hand, the poor working conditions in hospital-based programs were powerful disincentives, overcome only by necessity (i.e., women from working-class backgrounds for whom the option of private duty wages on completion of the program made it worth enduring). Through its control of nursing education, the hospital industry was able to prevent the market forces that had worked so well for other professions to increase status and compensation from having any impact on the nursing profession. In medicine, for example, when the demand for physicians was greater than the supply, physicians were able to command higher fees and higher social standing. In nursing, however, when the demand was greater than the supply, hospitals simply trained more nurses, precluding any increase in either salaries or status.

Unfortunately, this did not change when nursing education moved to universities and 4-year colleges. Although most hospitals no longer have direct control over the supply of nurses through education, they have developed alternative strategies to achieve the same objectives; for example, employing less qualified nursing staff to replace professional nurses and then extinguishing any differentiating symbols such as name tag identification, or violating immigration laws to recruit foreign nurse graduates. Furthermore, in the past, it was typical for new graduate nurses, most of whom were young women, to work for 3 to 5 years until they married and began to have children. Since few stayed in the profession—particularly in hospital nursing—hospitals used this 3- to 5-year turnover as an economic strategy that resulted in the "glass ceilings" that characterize nursing compensation today. But today's young people—women as well as men—are seeking a lifelong career that is both intellectually and emotionally satisfying and that offers monetary rewards and leadership opportunities in nursing that are comparable to those of other professions.

Why are recruitment incentives such as "sign-on bonuses" (trips to Hawaii, discounts on cars, etc.) not a good idea? Give examples of what you would do to address the nursing shortage.

The fact that the shortage is worst in hospitals, where the rewards and leadership opportunities for clinical nursing practice have been least attainable, is unsurprising and has resulted in superficial, short-term, ineffective, and even offensive recruitment strategies, including everything from "sign-on bonuses" to spa memberships and trips to Hawaii. Some hospital leaders have gone so far as to explore the idea of reinstituting diploma programs to ensure a supply of nurses sufficient to meet their needs. In their desperation for a "quick fix," hospitals have focused all of their attention on *recruitment* when the real problem is *retention*, which can be addressed only by long-term, fundamental, organizational changes required for improving the practice environment and creating career, rather than job, incentives.

At the same time, the nursing education community also must agree to let market forces play out and not be tempted by hospital promises of faculty support to increase enrollment and thus produce an oversupply of professional nurses. It is becoming increasingly urgent for nurse educators to come together and formulate a plan for sizing and shaping the future nursing workforce and to assist the hospital community to develop more stringent educational requirements for their nursing leadership and improve the practice environment.

Perhaps the greatest challenge for nursing educators today is not only to prepare nurses for a world that does not yet exist, but also to be the architects of that future. The good news is that professional nursing is particularly well equipped for that role. One has only to look at the dominant health issues of the future—prevention of disease and health promotion, chronicity, aging, and the problems and illnesses that result from socioeconomic dislocations and global migration—to see that each is grist for the nursing mill. The advancement of medical science and technology has changed the landscape of health and illness. Not only are people living much longer, they are living with chronic illnesses that would have been fatal 20 years ago. This is true not only in adults but also in children, resulting in the need for providers who can manage the ongoing health needs of such children and their families at home and in schools. The necessity for practitioners who focus on the promotion of health and wellness and the prevention of disease has emerged as not only a good and wholesome thing to do in our society but also as a means of addressing escalating medical costs. Finally, global migration and social and economic disparities have resulted in problems that are most effectively addressed in partnerships with communities. Whether we are working with elders, children, refugees, ethnic minorities, persons with chronic illness, or whole communities, the predominant theme is the promotion and maintenance of *health*, Florence Nightingale's legacy to the nursing profession.

The Essentials of Baccalaureate Education for Professional Nursing Practice captures the role and significance of professional nursing in the future. The promise lies in the extent to which nursing acknowledges that creativity will be even more important than knowledge, that risk taking must replace conservatism, and that we must move from a position that has been insular and monolithic to interdisciplinary and multicultural. If ever there was a time in which educators should not just tolerate but also actively solicit dissension and debate, encourage venture, and promote a liberal education as the foundation for nursing practice, this is it.

TRANSITION INTO PRACTICE

As you read this book and this chapter, think about where nursing education is heading in the next 10 years. How has your education prepared you for the direction health care is taking? Were most of your clinical experiences based primarily in a hospital setting or a community setting? How did you learn to be a beginning nurse?

For many years, faculty have assigned students a certain number of patients for which they develop a plan of care and then provide care for that patient based on that plan. Faculty supervise students as they provide care. Students learn by doing, and then absorb whatever other information they can during the time they are in the clinical area. Furthermore, students attend classes, take notes, and study for and take exams designed to test their knowledge.

Tanner (2002) states that clinical education must be changed. Because of technology advances and availability of information, the ways of teaching need to adapt. She notes that educational principles should be altered to match how students learn. Thus, broad ranges of learning activities should be developed from which students can choose. Students also need to be taught to think and then function like nurses.

In addition, technology advances need to be incorporated as part of, or instead of, classroom lectures. Faculty should be increasing the use of online education to enhance the classroom time, if not replace meeting altogether.

Finally, within the next 10 years, many faculty members will be retiring. If you've never given any thought to teaching, do so. You will need a graduate degree. Plan on how to further your education. Get involved in teaching other nurses where you will work. Serve as a preceptor for students. Talk to nursing faculty after you graduate. An insufficient number of nurses prepared to teach will perpetuate the nursing shortage.

KEY POINTS

1. The most significant turning points in the evolution of nursing education included (a) the first formal program of nursing education established in 1860 by Florence Nightingale and (b) the U.S. movement of nursing education from hospitals to universities and 4-year colleges.

2. The 1950 report, *Nursing Schools at Mid-Century*, resulted in the establishment of accreditation procedures in nursing. These procedures placed the process of determining and requiring educational standards under the control of nursing and thus became a vehicle for enhancing good programs and closing inferior ones.

3. Hospitals and the medical community served as a major obstacle to the advancement of nursing as a profession and used every opportunity to oppose collegiate programs, accreditation standards, and even professional licensure.

4. The earliest standards of quality designed to improve nursing education were established and published by the National League for Nursing. In 1998, the American Association of Colleges of Nursing outlined curriculum guidelines in *The Essentials of Baccalaureate Education for Professional Nursing Practice*, which, without question, places professional nursing education in the collegiate setting. The curriculum offers flexibility and is a distillation of three major components—role, knowledge, and practice.

5. The differences between nurses educated in hospitals and those educated in universities are far from superficial. When the emphasis shifted from skills to concepts, nursing education resolutely and manifestly required that care move from process to outcomes.

6. Sadly, hospitals and the nursing profession endorse licensure, rather than education, as the entry into professional practice, conferring the same title, assigning the same responsibilities, and providing the same orientation and compensation to 2-year graduates as to 4-year graduates.

7. Contemporary nursing leaders have argued for the importance of having a professional designation that is commensurate with the length and complexity of nursing education and comparable to the graduates of other health professions.

8. Early graduate programs sought to prepare teachers and administrators; contemporary programs have shifted to clinical leadership and advanced practice.

9. The academic doctorate is a research degree; nurses are charged with the responsibility for developing knowledge and theories that will improve nursing practice to achieve better patient outcomes and produce the next generation of researchers and educators.

10. The standard response to a nursing shortage is to educate more nurses rather than to carefully analyze why we have a nursing shortage; the focus instead should be on retention of both currently prepared nurses as well as new nurses entering the profession.

Critical thinking questions, essay questions, key terms, web links, activities, NCLEX review questions, and more interactive resources can be found on the Companion Website at www.prenhall.com/haynes. Click on Chapter 2 to select activities for this chapter.

REFERENCES

American Association of Colleges of Nursing. (1998). *The essentials of baccalaureate education for professional nursing practice.* Washington, DC: Author.

American Association of Colleges of Nursing. (2002). *Enrollment and graduations in baccalaureate and graduate programs in nursing, 2001–2002.* Washington, DC: Author.

Daggett, L. M., Butts, J. B., & Smith, K. K. (2002). The development of an organizing framework to implement AACN guidelines for nursing education. *Journal of Nursing Education, 41*(1), 34–37.

Friss, L. (1994). Nursing studies laid end to end form a circle. *Journal of Health, Politics, Policy and Law, 19,* 597–631.

Hertz, J. E., Yocom, C. J., & Gawel, S. H. (2000). Linking the NCLEX-RN National Licensure Examination to Practice: 1999 Practice Analysis of Newly Licensed Registered Nurses in the U.S. National Council of State Boards of Nursing: Chicago.

Montag, M. (1951). *The education of nursing technicians.* New York: John Wiley & Sons, Inc.

National League of Nursing Education. (1937). *A curriculum guide for schools of nursing.* New York: National League of Nursing Education.

Stewart, I. M. (1953). *The education of nurses.* New York: Macmillan.

Tanner, C. A. (2002). Clinical education, circa 2010. *Journal of Nursing Education, 41,* 51–52.

SUGGESTED READINGS

Anderson, C. A. (2000). The time is now. *Nursing Outlook, 48,* 257–258.

Bellack, J. P., & O'Neil, E. H. (2000). Recreating nursing practice for a new century: Recommendations and implications of the Pew Health Professions Commission's final report. *Nursing and Health Care Perspectives, 21*(1), 14–21.

Boyce, C. A., Brow, M. B., Cote, K. C., DeSisto, M. C., Evans, D. A., Gorman, D., et al. (2001). End the debate: Entry level into practice should be the master's degree. *Journal of Nursing Administration, 31*(4), 166–168.

Porter-O'Grady, T. (2001). Profound change: 21st century nursing. *Nursing Outlook, 49*(4), 187–192.

3

Achieving Professionhood Through Participation in Professional Organizations

JEAN LOGAN
DEBRA FRANZEN
CAROLYN PAULING
HOWARD K. BUTCHER

"The professionalism of nursing will be achieved only through the professionhood of its members."

Margretta M. Styles, 1982

LEARNING OBJECTIVES

AT THE COMPLETION OF THIS CHAPTER, THE READER WILL BE ABLE TO:

> Describe the requisites of a profession.

> Describe how participation in professional organizations enhances the development of professionhood.

> Analyze the responsibilities inherent to membership in professional nursing practice.

> Explore the relationship of social responsibility to nursing practice.

> Recognize the role the National Student Nurses' Association plays in developing a lifelong connection with professional organizations.

> Discuss the purpose and function of the American Nurses Association and Sigma Theta Tau, International.

> Describe how participation in professional organizations empowers nurses to influence health care.

MediaLink   www.prenhall.com/haynes

Additional online resources including NCLEX review questions, critical thinking questions, and real-world activities for this chapter can be found on the Companion Website at www.prenhall.com/haynes.

*I*n laying the foundations for nursing, Nightingale (1893) declared, "no system can endure that does not march" (p. 198). Nursing has endured; yet, the long *march* toward professionalism remains unfulfilled. Without professional status, nursing will lack the power, prestige, and recognition necessary to fulfill the social contract to enhance human health and the betterment of all. A major catalyst in the movement of an occupation toward achieving professional status is the collective participation of its members in professional organizations. This chapter (a) explores the progress nurses have made in moving nursing from a mere occupation to a recognized profession, (b) addresses the need for nurses to participate in professional organizations as a practice arena for learning the values and culture of nursing, and (c) recognizes the role professional organizations have to influence change in today's rapidly evolving health care system.

▨ Professionalism and Professional Practice

Qualities of a Profession

Few beginning nursing students are able to articulate what professional nursing practice is . . . for that matter, few practicing nurses would be able to succinctly define nursing. Yet, a clear understanding of professional practice is key to the role development of baccalaureate-prepared nurses. Rogers (1964) pointed out that "the loose usage of the prestigious word 'professional' must give way to a more precise definition" (p. 10). Although the terms *occupation* and *profession* are often used interchangeably, it is important to understand critical differences between the two. All professions are occupations, but not all occupations are professions. An occupation can be either a career or a job. The training period of an occupation may be extensive or may occur on the job. In some occupations, workers are supervised and accountability rests with the employer, while in others workers are autonomous and responsible for their own actions. Only in occupations that are defined as professional does training include the values, beliefs, and ethics of the occupation as a prominent feature. Professionals are generally committed to their occupation and rarely leave their occupation (Beletz, 1990). Choosing nursing as a profession entails a commitment to a *career*. For a nurse, this career represents a path or journey.

In general, as an occupational category, professions are highly esteemed and are at the pinnacle of power, income, and prestige. Professions provide society with an essential social service that affects the lives and safety of people. In *The Oxford Dictionary* (1989), a profession is defined as

> "the occupation which one professes to be skilled in and to follow . . . a vocation in which a professed knowledge of some department of learning or science is used in its application to the affairs of others or in the practice of an art founded upon it . . . The body of persons engaged in a calling" (p. 354).

Some may consider use of the term *calling* rather provocative in that it may infer divine influence, with a strong emphasis on altruistic impulses. However, a **calling** is also a deep internal desire to choose a profession that the person is devoted to and experiences as valuable. Individuals who are called to a profession strive to act according to the profession's highest principles (Raatikainen, 1997). For some, the calling and life vision of a career emerges with great clarity. For others, career callings take shape gradually as personal and professional passions, preferences, interests, and strengths are identified and developed. One chooses to answer the call by choosing to devote oneself to the profession and strive to act according to the highest principles of that profession. Responding to the call requires commitment to a set of values that imbue the chosen profession and often involves walking a particular path that requires courage, boldness, creativity, and a strong will (Raatikainen, 1997).

A number of individuals have established criteria for defining a profession (Begun & Lippincott, 1993;

Critical Thinking and Reflection

Recall what motivated you to first choose nursing as a career. How did you first become aware of nursing as a possible choice for a career? What were the aspects or features about nursing that attracted you to choose nursing?

Bixler & Bixler, 1959; Flexner, 1910; Goode, 1960; Greenwood, 1957; Houle, 1980). Based on a synthesis of the literature, Styles (1982) identified five commonly cited requisites or qualities that an occupation must have in order to denote professional status:

- An extensive university education
- A unique body of knowledge
- An orientation of service to others
- Autonomy, self-regulation, Code of Ethics
- A professional society

Thus, a **profession** is a prestigious, autonomous, self-regulating occupation providing an essential service to society. A profession requires a lengthy and rigorous education, which is grounded in a unique body of knowledge taught in an institution of higher learning. The members are called to the profession, actively participate in its professional societies, and are guided by the profession's Code of Ethics. **Professionalism** is the process by which an occupation strives for and achieves professional status.

Quality 1—Extensive University Education

Few would refute that the practice of nursing requires specialized education, and yet there remain multiple educational entries for individuals into nursing practice. Only just over one third of all practicing nurses have been educated in an institution of higher learning. In 2000, 122,000 nursing students were enrolled in 2-year associate degree programs in community colleges, 12,500 in 3-year hospital-based diploma programs, and 102,000 in university-based baccalaureate programs (National League for Nursing, 2000). North Dakota is the only state that requires a baccalaureate degree in nursing for licensure as a registered nurse. However, in 2005, all nurses seeking first-time registration in Ontario, Canada, must hold a minimum of a baccalaureate degree.

Each year, nearly twice as many nurses graduate with an associate degree than those who graduate with a bachelor's degree. Since as far back as 1923, with the publication of the Goldmark Report, many committees, reports, and organizations have repeatedly called for enhanced nursing education placed within university settings. In 2000, the American Nurses Association (ANA) reaffirmed their 1965 resolution that a bachelor's degree in nursing be the standard for new licensees in the United States.

The multiple educational entries for nursing practice have led to confusion regarding the specialized nature of the educational foundation for the practice of nursing. There is a lack of clarity regarding the role that nurses of differing educational backgrounds play in the health care delivery system. The confusion over what nurses do is fostered by the misrepresentation of nursing in the practice arena; many institutions and agencies ignore the distinction that baccalaureate education brings to the practice setting. Nursing roles have been created that do not distinguish or appreciate the differences in role preparation and outcome expectation.

Quality 2—Unique Body of Knowledge

Nurses require knowledge from other disciplines, including psychological, sociological, and biological sciences. However, the nursing discipline has a unique body of knowledge comprised of existing nursing conceptual frameworks, nursing practice models and theories, and nursing classifications systems. Nursing theories are designed to guide nursing practice, education, research, and administration. Nursing practice models derived from specific nursing theories, nursing diagnosis, nursing intervention classification, and nursing outcome classification all contribute to distinguishing the unique focus of nursing.

Unfortunately, despite the vast amount of literature demonstrating the utility of nursing theories and classification systems, few nurses base their practice on them. Furthermore, few practice settings have implemented nursing theories as a way of organizing nursing care. Without understanding the knowledge specific to nursing, many nurses have difficulty articulating and practicing nursing that is distinct from the biomedical model. If nursing is to achieve full professional status, the body of knowledge unique to nursing must be at the core of nursing education, practice, and research.

Quality 3—An Orientation of Service to Others

Professions provide society an essential service. The notion that nurses provide a human service, which in most cases is provided for people during vulnerable times of their life, seems to support the requisite of a service orientation. Nursing's service orientation is an unrelenting dedication and unselfish attention to improving the health and well-being of all. Work is central to the profession, and any sharp demarcation between work and leisure almost disappears. Intrinsic to the service commitment in professionalism is the commitment to a calling, the service ideal, and altruism

(Beletz, 1990). The service orientation encompasses (a) a commitment to the standards of practice and lifelong learning, (b) a commitment to the community of nurses that share common goals, and (c) a commitment to civility (nurse-to-nurse) despite individual differences. Professional values of service guide collegial relationships, which are expected to be cooperative, egalitarian, and supportive.

Quality 4—Autonomy, Self-Regulation, Code of Ethics

Autonomy refers to independence. According to Gross (1962), **autonomy** in professions involves control of practice, control of entry into the profession, and the ability to determine the qualifications needed for entry into the profession. Autonomy allows the profession to control services, deal with competition, and influence state and federal policy makers. Licensure does not guarantee autonomy and has little relation with professionalism. Governments grant licenses to practice when the nature of the work is viewed as sufficiently complex to require a minimum amount of knowledge in order to protect the public from unqualified practitioners. Professional autonomy is granted only when society is convinced the occupation has a unique and valuable knowledge base to exert self-control over its education and practice (Goode, 1960).

Oermann (1997) rightly points out that **autonomy in nursing** refers to the freedom to make decisions and clinical judgments within the scope of nursing practice. Lack of autonomy has often been cited as a major shortcoming in nursing practice. Other professional groups threaten the autonomy of nursing (e.g., organized medicine and health services administration) through well-organized, effective lobbyist actions that attempt to control nursing.

Emerging employment opportunities for nurse entrepreneurs (e.g., nurse-owned and -managed nursing centers, nurse practitioner primary care, and private practice) will provide additional opportunities for nurses to experience autonomous practice. In addition, as more nurses become educated at the graduate level and are prepared as advanced practice nurses, their ability to function in independent roles will increase.

Recognized professions have promulgated a Code of Ethics. A Code of Ethics is a mechanism by which professions establish Standards of Practice for self-regulation. The ANA has established both a Code of Ethics for Nurses and Standards of Practice. Nursing has long been viewed as one of the most honest and ethical "professions." While nursing dropped to second place in 2001 in the annual CNN/USA Today/Gallup poll ranking for honesty and integrity, the percentage of individuals rating nursing as high or very high actually increased from 79% to 84%. In the wake of the widely praised heroic efforts of fire and rescuer workers during the September 11, 2001, terrorists attacks in the United States, only firefighters ranked higher (90%) than nurses in the CNN/USA Today/Gallup poll ranking for honesty and integrity (Honesty and Ethics Poll, 2001).

The public's expression of trust does not necessarily imply recognition of nurses' knowledge, competence, and expertise. Buresh and Gordon (2000) point out that the public generally does not understand what nurses contribute to health care, and that the high regard for nursing is based on a sentimentalized image of nursing.

Both the Standards of Practice and Code of Ethics for Nurses provide a framework for professional nursing practice. When one violates either, strong sanctions by state boards of nursing can lead to loss of licensure. Licensure through independent state boards of nursing provides the predominant mode for self-regulation. Other means of self-regulation in nursing include registration and certification.

Quality 5—Professional Society

The structural embodiment of a professional community is a professional society or association. A voluntary association is a major catalyst in the movement of an occupation toward professional status. Freidson (1986) points out that the professional association is the major "formal means by which the interests of its members are pressed collectively and focused politically" (p. 185). Professional organizations provide the vehicles that serve to create a collective identity, political entity, and a voice for the profession (Beletz, 1990). A major deterrent in nursing's march toward actualizing full professional status is the low participation of nurses in their primary professional organization, the American Nurses Association (ANA). Despite all its activities and accomplishments, the ANA has yet to reach its full potential as nursing's primary professional organization. Only about 6% of all RNs are members of the ANA. To *march* means to "proceed directly and purposely . . . to walk steadily and rhythmically forward in step with others" (*American Heritage Dictionary*, 2000, p. 1068). Through collective actions of the organization's members, the profession can impact the status of nurses and increase their power in relation to

Styles (1982) lists five requisites or qualities of a profession. As you consider each of the five criteria, what meaning do they have for you as you think about nursing as a profession? Reflect on an experience you had with someone you considered to be a professional. What was it about that person that caused you to consider them to be a professional? Who or what influenced you to become a nurse? How does this influence relate to professionalism?

other occupations and professions. The only limit to the force of collective action is the number of members working together to effect change.

Achieving Professionhood

Styles (1982) takes a different approach to professionalization by proposing that instead of applying the five external criteria to determine nursing's professional status, nurses should focus on the characteristics of each individual member of the profession. Therefore, the seeds of professional reformation actually lie within the individual nurse as that nurse achieves **professionhood**. Styles (1982) differentiates professionhood from professionalism. "Professionhood focuses on the characteristics of the individual as a member of a profession. Professionalism emphasizes the composite character of the profession" (p. 8). The characteristics of professionhood include a belief in the social significance of nursing, a personal commitment to doing one's best work, and a commitment to collegiality and collectivity. A commitment to the social significance of nursing is achieved through each nurse's *desire and confidence* to make a significant social contribution.

Being committed to doing one's best work means having a career orientation and plan rather than a job orientation. **Collegiality** refers to our shared responsibility at the micro or practice level of nursing while collectivity refers to each nurse's participation in professional organizations that shape the profession's agenda. Only when all nurses embrace the values of professionhood and work collectively in professional organizations will nursing achieve full recognition as a profession.

Essential Professional Role Development

The process of achieving professionhood begins as nursing students are socialized. They learn the responsibilities inherent to their membership in professional nursing practice, which includes a commitment to lifelong learning. Lifelong pursuit of knowledge and knowledge development is an ongoing process and not a terminal outcome. Nurses must have opportunities to develop leadership skills. Membership in the profession requires effective interpersonal skills, which includes written and verbal communication. Professional socialization creates an awareness of the need for lifelong interpersonal skill development.

Nurses must also come to value the power that emerges from collaboration and engaging in caring relationships with colleagues. This colleagueship includes a commitment to mentorship. Vance and Olson (1998) describe the mentor connection as a developmental, empowering, and nurturing relationship extending over time where professional growth occurs in an atmosphere of respect, collegiality, and affirmation. Participation in professional organizations provides opportunities to live the experience of being mentored, be socialized to expect mentorship from colleagues, and in turn be committed to mentoring others. This generational effect, or the idea that those who have been mentored will mentor others, has been well documented. Mentoring relationships have important implications for leadership development and the advancement of professional nursing practice (Giese, 1986; Larson, 1986; Rawl & Peterson, 1992).

Nurses must learn to be politically astute and come to value the importance of political activity in professional nursing practice that includes agenda setting and creation of policy. **Policy** has been defined as "the principles that govern action directed towards given ends" (Titmus, 1974, p. 23), "a consciously chosen course of action (or inaction) directed toward some end" (Kalisch & Kalisch, 1982, p. 61), and "broad guidelines that reflect the values of the individuals making the statement" (Skaggs & DeVries, 1998, p. 538). Cohen et al. (1996) examined nursing's political development and concluded that the values of

Reflect on the values you bring to nursing. Identify several practice issues you have become aware of and the impact of those issues on society and well-being. Now consider a range of policy possibilities that would have implications for this practice issue. How might professional nursing practice make a difference with each of the issues you have considered?

nursing can serve to transform political processes and public policy. Among the strategies identified to promote an agenda-setting political identity, nurses must integrate health policy and politics into nursing practice. This strategy would enable nurses to see connections between health, nursing, practice, policy, and political activism, as well as the connection to the broader social issues of the times. Nurses need to be socialized to view politics as a process that exerts control over nursing and health care, and view politics as a way to influence the thinking of others.

Social Responsibility and Nurses

Enabling nurses to see connections between health, policy, and the broader social issues of the times is vitally linked to active, real involvement in issues. Nurturing social responsibility in nurses is a developmental process. Beginning students discover what it means to value social responsibility within the context of professional nursing practice and promotion of health and well-being. Nursing students draw on their knowledge and past experiences to establish a foundation on which to build social responsibility.

Establishing this foundation is an essential step that serves as a reference point from which nurses may consider new possibilities related to health care delivery and professional nursing practice. This discovery will be most meaningful for the beginning nursing student or novice nurse if it is grounded in real experience with an issue that has personal relevance (e.g., consideration of campus health concerns or current community issues).

Ultimately, the social responsibility goal associated with transition into professional nursing practice is that graduates will be confident with the dynamic process for effecting change that impacts themselves, health care, and society. Students preparing for transition into practice must examine the importance of colleagueship and coalition building in a broader context, appreciating their role and responsibility as professional nurses in relation to issues impacting the health care delivery system and society as a whole.

Professional Organizations in Nursing Education and Practice

Nursing students need opportunities to experience colleagueship, research utilization, policy development, political activity, and advocacy. Professional organizations enhance the development of professionhood and give student nurses a forum where a collective voice on health care issues can be heard and policy can be created in the shape of resolutions, main motions, statements of action priorities, legislative platforms, and position papers. At the beginning of a nurse's career, the National Student Nurses' Association offers the nursing student a place to develop social responsibility, professional values, and value-based behavior.

The National Student Nurses' Association

For nursing students, the primary professional organization is the National Student Nurses' Association (NSNA), founded in 1952. The mission of NSNA is as follows:

- Organize, represent, and mentor students preparing for initial licensure as registered nurses, as well as those nurses enrolled in baccalaureate completion programs.
- Promote development of the skills that students will need as responsible and accountable members of the nursing profession.
- Advocate for high quality health care (*Getting the Pieces to Fit*, 2002, p. 2).

Purposes and functions of the NSNA mirror the essentials of professional role development advocated by the American Association of Colleges of Nursing (AACN). The purposes and functions of NSNA are located in Table 3–1.

In 1999, the House of Delegates of NSNA adopted the Code of Professional Conduct, which describes a high standard of behavior guided by ideals

Table 3–1   Purposes and Functions of NSNA

Purposes

To assume responsibility for contributing to nursing education in order to provide for the highest-quality health care.

To provide programs representative of fundamental and current professional interests and concerns.

To aid in the development of the whole person, his or her professional role, and his or her responsibility for health care of people in all walks of life (*Getting the Pieces to Fit*, 2002, p. 11).

Functions

To have direct input into standards of nursing education and influence the educational process.

To influence health care, nursing education, and practice through legislative activities as appropriate.

To promote and encourage participation in community affairs and activities toward improved health care and the resolution of related social issues.

To represent nursing students to the consumer, institutions, and other organizations.

To promote and encourage students' participation in interdisciplinary activities.

To promote and encourage recruitment efforts, participation in students' activities, and educational opportunities regardless of a person's race, color, creed, sex, age, lifestyle, national origin, or economic status.

To promote and encourage collaborative relationships with the American Nurses Association, the National League for Nursing, the International Council of Nurses, as well as the other nursing and related health organizations (*Getting the Pieces to Fit*, 2002, p. 11).

Reprinted with permission: National Student Nurses' Association. (2002). *Getting the pieces to fit 2002–2003* (p. 11). Copyright National Student Nurses' Association.

and values that are expected of students who participate in NSNA activities. In 2001, the House of Delegates approved the Code for Academic and Clinical Professional Conduct (*Getting the Pieces to Fit*, 2002, p. 9). The two documents comprise the NSNA Code of Ethics, which, when coupled with the NSNA Student Bill of Rights and Responsibilities for Students of Nursing, sets the tone for professional development.

Nursing students actively involved in the NSNA learn a wide array of the culture and values of the nursing profession including leadership skills (Logan, 1994). Thus, the NSNA could be viewed as a professional clinical arena. Dr. Diane Mancino, executive director of the NSNA, calls NSNA the training ground, the "boot camp" for learning the lessons of leadership (Mancino, 1999, p. 2). Based on this practice arena concept, the 1998–1999 NSNA Board of Directors initiated the NSNA Leadership U—a self-governing body of students studying and practicing leadership and management skills (Mancino, 1999, p. 2). The purposes of the NSNA Leadership U are to:

- Link service-learning activities to professional values development and socialization into the nursing profession.

- Develop competencies that future leaders and managers need to successfully provide for the health care needs of society.
- Validate that learning has taken place.
- Provide formal recognition to NSNA members who demonstrate leadership and management skill development.
- Assist students to develop a professional portfolio.
- Create opportunities for mentor–protégé relationships and peer networks to develop and grow.

The Leadership U Web site offers an Admissions Office where students register for NSNA Leadership U offerings. It also includes a Leadership Library where leadership opportunities can be explored. Nursing programs, which serve as models for other schools, are found in this area of the Web site. Each of these programs offers nursing curriculum opportunities for participation within NSNA, whether at the local chapter or state or national level. A Student Leadership Union offers a chat room to discuss topics with fellow nursing students and access the latest health care news. The Faculty Lounge facilitates discussion among faculty peers and the Mentor Lounge is a place where student leaders meet. Finally, the International Lounge facili-

A recent qualitative study with a case study approach investigated learning and changes experienced by members of a chapter of critical care nurses as they moved from being new members to becoming board members and officers (Stein, 2001). The 20 members learned through mentoring, coaching, and experience. There were observable changes such as attainment of high-level interpersonal skills and the ability to apply these skills in other settings. Life changes occurred as a result of involvement for most members. These changes included members changing career paths, achieving certification in the specialty, attaining new career positions and promotions, and earning a higher degree. As a result of their involvement, chapter leaders described an increase in confidence. They also were able to see more possibilities for themselves and developed a broader understanding of the world.

In another qualitative study, Logan (1994) studied how student experiences within the National Student Nurses' Association relate to internalizing the culture and values of the nursing profession. Six nursing students actively involved in two local NSNA chapters were individually interviewed and eight nursing faculty from the same two universities were interviewed in focus group sessions. Results suggest that students actively involved are learning a wide array of the culture and values of the nursing profession. Findings indicated three main routes through which students learn in NSNA: experience, involvement, and connections to others. It was concluded that viewing NSNA as a "professional clinical" arena is a useful way to understand its meaning for nursing students.

tates students and faculty meeting and interacting with people around the world.

Total School Membership, a NSNA plan that includes membership fees in student activity or tuition bills, facilitates having all students actively involved in a professional organization. This membership commitment also provides an opportunity to merge NSNA experiences directly with the nursing curriculum. By participating in NSNA activities, students can incorporate NSNA experiences throughout their educational preparation as they journey from novice to expert in leadership skill acquisition.

Leadership Within Constituency NSNA Chapters

Many opportunities exist in beginning nursing courses for nursing students to immerse themselves in leadership development. Participation in their school NSNA chapter provides additional opportunities to develop leadership skills. For example, students can form leadership teams with each team member assuming one of several leadership roles such as (a) Mentor Committee Member, (b) NSA Delegate, (c) Resolution Writer, (d) Community Service Committee Member, and (e) Free Clinic Volunteer. Engagement in these roles allows students to value these aspects of their nursing career and make meaning of class concepts related to professional-

ism. Concepts such as decision-making, research utilization in practice, leadership, colleagueship, policy, the health care delivery system, and legal and ethical aspects of professional nursing practice become real as students engage in their leadership roles over time (Logan & Franzen, 2001).

Students can discover the interaction of professional service and community service within these roles as they engage in team dialogues. Through team dialogue, students are challenged to identify a service need and respond to this need in the form of "giving back" to society. The outcome of each team's efforts includes the discovery of an issue related to health care and nursing and the implementation of a project to effect change including the development of a resolution.

Resolutions are indications of an organization's position on key issues. These resolution outcomes are not seen as the end of the semester-long project, but as the beginning of the student's professional organization connection on a new level. At this point, the team is creating direction for policy. Creating and presenting these resolutions engages students in the process of developing an understanding of the power of collective voice in the issues raised and the opportunity to effect change. As a result, teams broaden their perspective from a narrow provincial view of nursing responsibility in the workplace to a broader view of societal responsibility (Logan & Franzen, 2001). Along this journey, students can develop leadership skills and learn to embrace the professional values of altruism, autonomy, human dignity, integrity, and social justice that they will carry with them throughout the rest of the nursing curriculum and into their professional practice as baccalaureate-prepared nurses (AACN, 1998).

The Power of Social Responsibility

The following scenarios depict examples of nursing students engaged in social responsibility at different levels. These students were challenged to identify and pursue an issue of interest to them. Students chose a variety of issues from pain management to antibiotic resistance (see Table 3–2). As the following examples are read, consider how the experience contributes to an understanding of the nurse as a professional. Reflect on how the experience will enable a new nurse to incorporate professionalism into practice and come to identify with the values of the profession.

Antibiotic Resistance: Awareness and Action

Sophomore students Tysheka, Curt, Abby, and Sara were challenged to pursue a health care issue that they could impact. Drawing on their collective experiences from personal situations as well as coursework in microbiology, they decided to tackle the issue of antibiotic resistance. As they examined the literature, gathered anecdotal information, and dialogued about their discoveries in class, they began to see the social impact this issue had and the implications for professional nursing practice. They were challenged to collaborate as a team to develop and implement a project that would address social responsibility related to the antibiotic resistance issue. Most importantly, the team was directed to funnel their efforts through their local nursing student professional organization, the Nursing Student Association (NSA). It was through this organization that the students were mentored in the process and came to realize the importance of collective voice and collaboration. There were several outcomes of this experience, including:

- An antibiotic resistance education booth at the campus wellness week activities
- Student-designed materials that were distributed on campus and at clinics to generate greater community awareness of the issue
- Collaboration with a newly created statewide task force working on the antibiotic resistance issue

Perhaps the greatest influence these students created was the resolution that they wrote, which was passed within their local chapter NSA and taken to the state convention the following fall term (see Box 3–1). The State House of Delegates adopted the resolution, and it was taken to the national convention. Collaboration with another state constituent resulted in a resolution that was adopted by the NSNA House of Delegates. These students, mentored by the NSA and faculty at the local, state, and national levels, were thus supported in their role development as a "member of a profession" that is advocated by AACN's *Essentials of Baccalaureate Education* (AACN, 1998).

Table 3–2   Workplace, Community/State, and National Issues Students Have Impacted

Workplace Issues	Community/State Issues	National Issues
• Pain management	• Sexual abuse	• Rotavirus
• Hospital/patient safety	• Women's health in prison	• Antibiotic resistance
• Family presence in the emergency department	• School nurse staffing	• Head lice in schools
• Restraints in the mental health unit	• Attention deficit–hyperactivity disorder (ADHD) assessment in schools	• Nursing shortage
• Staff satisfaction and retention	• RN pronouncing of death	• Nursing retention and recruitment
• Latex allergy	• Mental health in long-term care	• Meningitis in college-age population
• Nurses' back injuries	• Education in schools	• Contraception
• Radiology safety	• Tobacco settlement monies	
• Needless devices		

Box 3–1   *Antibiotic Resistance Education Resolution*

In Support of Education on the Prevention and the Consequences of Antibiotic Resistance
Submitted by: Grand View College, Des Moines, Iowa; Texas Nursing Students' Association

WHEREAS, in the United States alone, an estimated 100 million unnecessary antibiotic prescriptions are written annually and in 1 year 13,300 hospital patients died from bacterial infections that were resistant to antibiotic treatment; and WHEREAS, consequences of antibiotic resistance include the following:

Decreased ability to cure the infection; increased morbidity and mortality; greater health costs through expensive isolation procedures; longer hospital stays; more drug investigations; and utilization of new, expensive, toxic, and more complicated antibiotics; and

WHEREAS, strains of at least three bacterial species capable of causing life-threatening illnesses (*Enterococcus faecalis, Mycobacterium tuberculosis,* and *Pseudomonas aeruginosa*) already evade every available antibiotic; and

WHEREAS, in 1941 all strains of *Staphylococcus aureus (S. aureus)* were susceptible to penicillin. Today, 90% of all *S. aureus* strains are penicillin resistant; and

WHEREAS, a variety of preventable human practices have contributed to the rise of antibiotic resistance: the overprescription of antibiotics, patient demand for antibiotics to treat viral infections, the failure of patients to follow prescribed treatment, the use of antibiotics by immunosuppressed patients to prevent infections, and the treatment of acne with long-term, low-dose antibiotics; and

WHEREAS, the control of antibiotic use can decrease the number of antibiotics distributed per admission, decrease the number of antibiotic-resistant nosocomial infections, and decrease antimicrobial expenditures; and

WHEREAS, antimicrobial compounds mixed with soaps, lotions, and other common household products destroy the skin's natural flora and ultimately promote the growth of resistant bacteria; and

WHEREAS, A MAJOR SEGMENT OF THE GENERAL POPULATION IS UNAWARE OF THE HARMFUL EFFECTS OF MISUSING ANTIBIOTICS AND USING ANTIMICROBIALS; THEREFORE BE IT

RESOLVED, that Iowa Nurses' Association (NSNA) encourage health care facilities and local NSNA chapters to support implementation of antibiotic resistance education for nursing students, other health care professionals, and the general public; and be it further

RESOLVED, that the NSNA encourage its constituents to participate in community service projects related to this issue; and be it further

RESOLVED, that the NSNA send copies of this resolution to the American Nurses' Association, the American Association of Colleges of Nursing, the American Hospital Association, the National League for Nursing, and to any other organization deemed appropriate by the NSNA board of directors.

Differentiated Practice: Rediscovery of an Issue

Sanna and Donna had become aware of differences in the educational preparation of nurses working in units and agencies where they had their student clinical experiences. They were interested in the lack of difference in practice expectations by most employers despite significant differences in educational preparation and nursing program outcomes. The students approached the practice issue systematically and gathered data from as many different sources as possible considering the many and varied stakeholders involved. They discovered this differentiated practice issue was not a new issue but one that has existed as long as entry into nursing practice has been questioned. They quickly discovered the multifaceted nature of the issue and were intrigued and overwhelmed as they explored the many interrelated elements, including work environment concerns, job satisfaction, patient care, and the nursing shortage. They gathered data from a variety of sources, including the literature, interviews of local nursing staff in a variety of practice settings, Internet sources and e-mail contacts of individuals working on the issue in other states, and contacts from local and national coalitions for differentiated nursing practice. They explored nursing and related research and discovered a need for more information. Sanna and Donna came to identify that their social responsibility was to help others develop a clearer understanding of this issue. Based on their past participation in the NSNA, they were aware of the visibility a resolution can have and the power it has to raise awareness. With this in mind, Sanna and Donna developed a resolution on differentiated practice that they presented to their chapter NSNA (see Box 3–2). Their presentation of this resolution was the first step in educating others. Subsequently, it has been accepted as one of the resolutions that will go to the state convention in the fall, and it is anticipated the study and debate on the resolution will create the intended effect—to raise awareness and to educate their peers and the public on this issue.

Differentiated Practice: Affirming Commitment

Senior students Kate and Angie had also become aware of differences in the educational preparation of nurses working in units and agencies where they had their student clinical experiences. They noted that one hospital unit functioned from a unique paradigm—one that respected and valued the different preparation and skills team members brought to their nursing practice. Here they discovered job satisfaction, low turnover, and quality of patient care.

These students utilized the NSA resolution on Differentiated Nursing Practice as a basis for their work. This effort focused on promoting a demonstration unit and affirming the need for data collection to assist in the discovery process and identify connections to job satisfaction, staff turnover, the nursing shortage, and quality patient care.

The process that Kate and Angie were engaged in was more important than the outcome that they eventually developed. As these students proceeded with their verbal and written contacts, they were able to strengthen their communication abilities and gain confidence in being included in leadership networks such as attending planning meetings for examining job satisfaction issues and the development of demonstration units. They also engaged in collaboration and colleagueship with nurse managers, care coordinators, and

---

Box 3–2   Differentiated Practice Resolution

In Support of Education of Nurses and Nursing Students on Differentiated Nursing Practice
Submitted by: Sanna K. Henzi and Donna Keizer
WHEREAS, the current system of nursing education and licensure, which fails to differentiate competencies of each type of nurse, has confused the public and the employer, and created fragmentation within nursing (Koerner, 1992); and
WHEREAS, licensure rather than an education credential has defined the entry level into practice (Fosbinder, Ashton, & Koerner, 1997); and
WHEREAS, differentiated practice is a plan that implements nursing practice according to education experience and competence (Fosbinder, Ashton, & Koerner, 1997); and
WHEREAS, the implementation of differentiated practice has provided an environment for patient satisfaction due to the increase in staff satisfaction (Barra & Johnson, 1998); and
WHEREAS, differentiated nursing practice further demonstrates the need for integration to avoid further fragmentation (Baker et al., 1997); and
WHEREAS, collegial and collaborative partnership can emerge only when the varied nursing roles are understood and valued mutually (Koerner, 1992); therefore be it further
RESOLVED, that the GVCNSA and Grand View College Nursing Faculty support the education of differentiated nursing practice to but not limited to nursing students, professional nurses, and nurse educators throughout the state of Iowa; and therefore be it further
RESOLVED, that the GVCNSA send this resolution along with the provided fact sheet to stakeholders within but not limited to the state of Iowa; and therefore be it further
RESOLVED, that the GVCNSA send a copy of this resolution to the GVC Faculty, Iowa Association of Nursing Students, Iowa Nurses' Association, Iowa Workforce Development, Iowa Nursing Colleges and Universities, Hospitals of Iowa, and any other organization deemed appropriate by the GVCNSA board of directors.

administrative personnel. There grew out of these meetings a reciprocal respect of all involved. In addition, the result of this work has led to discussion and planning to conduct qualitative research to address the need for data collection.

Kate and Angie presented their policy proposal to the nurse manager and two care coordinators for the unit. Their proposal contributed to the affirmation of a differentiated practice demonstration unit with continued work toward the development of additional units. Kate and Angie's work caused them to discover a new awareness of the political implications of the nursing shortage, job satisfaction, colleagueship, and the different roles involved in patient care delivery. Most importantly, they came to a new understanding of ethical considerations for how units conduct the business of managing patient care with staff turnover issues impacting not only quality patient care but also the integrity of care providers. Most importantly, they were viewed as valued colleagues and equipped with essential skills for their transition to professional practice.

Mental Health Parity: Emergence of Practice Passion

Julie had been a practicing registered nurse for a number of years. She had chosen to return to school on a part-time basis to complete a baccalaureate degree in nursing but continued to work full time in a mental health unit in a local hospital. Julie's coursework challenged her to consider relevant issues with policy implications from this practice arena.

Early in her BSN program of study, Julie was empowered to participate in resolution writing with fellow nurses of the Iowa Nurses' Association. The RN to BSN student has the opportunity to join either the NSNA or ANA and its state constituent organization. Julie had not belonged to a professional organization prior to returning to school. As a result of this opportunity, Julie chose to join her state nursing association and thereby ANA. As a result of this membership she co-authored a resolution on Mental Health Parity, which was presented at the state nurses association fall convention (see Box 3–3). This experience proved to

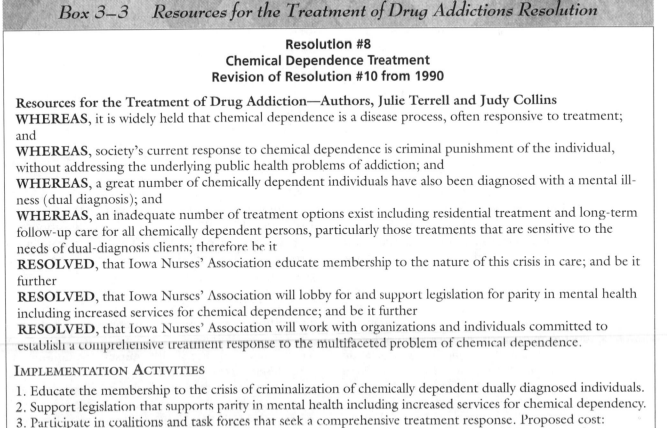

Box 3–3   Resources for the Treatment of Drug Addictions Resolution

Resolution #8
Chemical Dependence Treatment
Revision of Resolution #10 from 1990

Resources for the Treatment of Drug Addiction—Authors, Julie Terrell and Judy Collins

WHEREAS, it is widely held that chemical dependence is a disease process, often responsive to treatment; and

WHEREAS, society's current response to chemical dependence is criminal punishment of the individual, without addressing the underlying public health problems of addiction; and

WHEREAS, a great number of chemically dependent individuals have also been diagnosed with a mental illness (dual diagnosis); and

WHEREAS, an inadequate number of treatment options exist including residential treatment and long-term follow-up care for all chemically dependent persons, particularly those treatments that are sensitive to the needs of dual-diagnosis clients; therefore be it

RESOLVED, that Iowa Nurses' Association educate membership to the nature of this crisis in care; and be it further

RESOLVED, that Iowa Nurses' Association will lobby for and support legislation for parity in mental health including increased services for chemical dependence; and be it further

RESOLVED, that Iowa Nurses' Association will work with organizations and individuals committed to establish a comprehensive treatment response to the multifaceted problem of chemical dependence.

IMPLEMENTATION ACTIVITIES

1. Educate the membership to the crisis of criminalization of chemically dependent dually diagnosed individuals.
2. Support legislation that supports parity in mental health including increased services for chemical dependency.
3. Participate in coalitions and task forces that seek a comprehensive treatment response. Proposed cost: $1,500. Proposed priority: 5 (highest)

be very empowering for Julie. When asked to describe this collegial experience, Julie stated that she believed it helped her to identify an issue that put passion back into her nursing practice.

She further stated, "I thought that the faculty was crazy, making me participate in an organization where I had to pay for membership. Ultimately, I discovered how important membership and active participation in one's professional organization could be. I was able to collaborate with seasoned members of the local district organization and co-author a resolution on mental health parity. Seeing this resolution pass the INA House of Delegates, actually sitting in the room, was something I can barely describe. I felt that I could make a difference. I was powerful, even as a student."

American Nurses Association

Active involvement in the workings of the NSNA prepares students for transition to membership in professional nursing organizations, specifically the ANA. The purpose and functions of the NSNA mirror the purpose and functions of the ANA. Both organizations have state and national conventions with a House of Delegates, resolution hearings and debates to influence health care policy, and codes of ethics governing the conduct of their members. The ANA has served as the forum in which the nation's critical health issues have been discussed throughout the last century. Like the NSNA, which has represented nursing students' voice for 50 years, the ANA serves as a collective voice for registered nurses and a vehicle for influencing health care policy in local, state, and national arenas.

Founded in 1897 as the Nurses' Associated Alumnae of the United States and Canada, the ANA was originally created to establish and maintain a code of ethics, to elevate the standard of nursing education, to promote the profession's usefulness, and to honor the financial and other interests of nursing. Today, the ANA continues to focus on the advancement of the nursing profession by (a) fostering high standards of nursing practice, (b) promoting the economic and general welfare of nurses in the workplace, (c) projecting a positive and realistic view of nursing, and (d) lobbying Congress and the regulatory agencies on health care issues affecting nurses and the public. The organization is composed of 53 constituent state members, 3 related entities, and 13 organizational affiliate members. It is the only full-service professional organization representing the nation's 2.7 million registered nurses. There are currently 180,000 members, which is approximately 6% of the potential membership.

There is debate as to why nurses fail to join the ANA. Some nurses disagree with the ANA's economic and general welfare policies, and others are opposed to the 1965 position the ANA took on the baccalaureate degree as the entry level for professional nursing practice. Still others are opposed to position statements on women's reproductive rights or believe that the ANA does not represent their specific practice concerns. As a result of differing agendas, over the last century, the number of organizations for which nurses can hold membership has proliferated. Most of these organizations are specialty interest groups that exist to develop and maintain expertise in a given field and provide support for clinical practice. Some nurses have argued that they cannot afford to belong to several organizations, and their support must go to their special interest groups. Multiple organizations have splintered nursing as a profession and have diluted the power of the collective voice.

In an attempt to bring all groups together, in 1989, the ANA established the Nursing Organization Liaison Forum (NOLF), which comprises more than 70 national nursing organizations including the NSNA (see Table 3–3) and serves as a platform for addressing important issues that affect nursing and health care in general. Each participating organization sends one registered nurse representative to an annual forum hosted by the ANA. The ANA gathers agenda items from each participating organization. At the forum, recommendations emerge and are forwarded for consideration to the ANA board of directors and the board of directors of each participating organization.

In addition to NOLF and the affiliated organizations identified in Table 3–3, there are four ANA-related entities: (1) the American Nurses' Foundation (ANF), (2) the American Nurses' Credentialing Center (ANCC), (3) United American Nurses (UAN), and (4) the American Academy of Nursing (AAN). The ANF was founded in 1955 as the research education and charitable affiliate of the ANA. It is the national philanthropic organization that promotes the continued growth and development of nurses and services to advance the work of the nursing profession.

The ANCC was established in 1973 to provide recognition of professional achievement in a defined functional or clinical area of nursing. Since 1991, it has certified more than 150,000 nurses throughout the United States. The ANCC also provides the following services: (a) accreditation of education providers and approvers, (b) recognition of excellence in nursing services through the Magnet Recognition Program, and (c) education of the public regarding the value of professional nursing credentialing.

Table 3–3 Professional Nursing Organizations

Academy of Medical Surgical Nursing	Air and Surface Transport Nurses
American Academy of Ambulatory Care Nurses[a]	American Assembly for Men in Nursing
American Association for Continuity of Care	American Association of Critical Care Nurses[a]
American Association of Legal Nurse Consultants	American Association of Neuroscience Nurses
American Association of Nurse Anesthetists[a]	American Association of Nurse Attorneys
American Association of Occupational Health Nurses	American Association of Spinal Cord Injury Nurses
American College of Nurse Practitioners	American Heart Association Council on Cardiovascular Nursing
American Holistic Nurses Association[a]	American Medical Informatics Association
American Nephrology Nurses Association	American Psychiatric Nurses Association[a]
American Public Health Association	American Radiological Nurses Association
American Society for Parenteral and Enteral Nutrition	American Society of Ophthalmologic Registered Nurses, Inc.
American Society of Plastic and Reconstructive Surgical Nurses, Inc.	American Society of PeriAnesthesia Nurses (ASPAN)[a]
American Thoracic Society	Association for Child & Adolescent Psychiatric Nurses, Inc.
Association of Black Nursing Faculty in Higher Education, Inc.	Association of Community Health Nursing Educators
Association of Occupational Health Professionals	Association of Nurses in AIDS Care
Association of PeriOperative Registered Nurses, Inc.[a]	Association of Pediatric Oncology Nurses
Association of Rehabilitation Nurses[a]	Association of State and Territorial Directors of Nurses
Association of Women's Health, Obstetric & Neonatal Nurses[a]	Chi Eta Phi Sorority
Consolidated Association of Nurses in Substance Abuse International	Council on Graduate Education for Administration in Nursing
Dermatology Nurses Association	Developmental Disabilities Nurses Association
Drug & Alcohol Nursing Association, Inc.	Emergency Nurses Association[a]
Hospice Nurses Association	International Society of Psychiatric Mental Health Nurses
International Society of Nurses in Genetics	Intravenous Nurses Society[a]
National Association of Clinical Nurse Specialists	National Association of Directors of Nursing Administrator in Long Term Care
National Association of Hispanic Nurses	National Association of Neonatal Nurses
National Association of Nurse Massage Therapists	National Association of Nurse Practitioners in Reproductive Health
National Association of Orthopaedic Nurses[a]	National Association of Pediatric Nurse Associates & Practitioners
National Association of School Nurses, Inc.[a]	National Association of State School Nurse Consultants, Inc.
National Gerontological Nursing Association	National League for Nursing
National Nurses Society on Addictions	National Nursing Staff Development Organization
National Organization of Nurse Practitioner Faculties	National Student Nurses' Association
North American Nursing Diagnosis Association	Nurses Organization of Veterans Affairs

Table 3-3   (continued)

Oncology Nursing Society[a]	Philippine Nurses Association of America, Inc.
Respiratory Nursing Society	Sigma Theta Tau, International, Inc.
Society for Vascular Nursing	Society of Gastroenterology Nurses & Associates, Inc.
Society of Otorhinolaryngology & Head–Neck Nurses, Inc.[a]	Society of Pediatric Nurses
Society of Urologic Nurses & Associates, Inc.	Wound, Ostomy & Continence Nurses Society
National Black Nurses Association	National Assembly of Men in Nursing

[a]Also an ANA organizational affiliate member.

The UAN, formally established in 2000, is the largest and most effective labor union for registered nurses in the country. Because of its association with the ANA, the UAN has instant credibility, resources, and a voice in state legislatures, governors' offices, the U.S. Congress, and the White House.

The AAN was established in 1973 and consists of an organization of leaders in nursing that are recognized nationally and internationally in education, management, practice, and research. Currently there are 1,300 Fellows of the academy. The mission of the Academy is to potentiate the contributions of nursing leaders in transforming the health care system to optimize public well-being. The AAN is a member of the Nursing Practice and Education Consortium (N-PEC), which is a collaborative group of many nursing organizations focused on the future of nursing. Led by Sigma Theta Tau, International, the consortium of 10 organizations has created a strategic plan, "Vision 2020 for Nursing: A Strategic Plan to Transform Nursing Practice and Education." The Academy is also a supporting member for Research America, an organization that focuses on providing information to the public about health research and various research agendas.

Sigma Theta Tau, International

Sigma Theta Tau, International (STTI), identified as one of the NOLF organizations, is a unique nursing organization in that it is an honor society. Founded by six nursing students at Indiana University in 1922, these women recognized the value of scholarship and the importance of excellence in practice. Their vision helped bring recognition of nursing as a science. Membership is by invitation only to baccalaureate and graduate nursing students who demonstrate excellence in scholarship and to community leaders who have shown exceptional achievement in nursing. Baccalaureate students must be in the upper one third of their graduation class to be considered for membership. Membership criteria create an exclusive honor society that is highly regarded worldwide.

STTI has a vision to create a global community of nurses who lead in using scholarship, knowledge, and technology to improve the health of the world's people. The STTI mission is to provide leadership and scholarship in practice, education, and research to enhance the health of all people, and supports the learning and professional development of members who strive to improve nursing care worldwide.

Education and research initiatives are strong priorities for STTI. The society publishes a scholarly journal and many other publications that disseminate nursing knowledge. In addition, the International Center for Nursing Scholarship, located in Indianapolis, Indiana, houses the society's headquarters and its electronic library, the Virginia Henderson International Library. Leadership development opportunities exist through the International Leadership Institute, which helps nurses across the globe develop abilities to improve the health and welfare of people in their communities. The Mentor–Fellow program offers opportunities for local chapters to nurture and develop members focusing on preparing the next generation for leadership roles. STTI also offers a Directory of Nurse Experts to provide accurate information on nursing and health care to the media and the public.

There are 120,000 active STTI members, which makes it the second largest nursing organization in the world. Sixty percent of active members hold a master's degree and/or doctoral degree. The power of this collective voice of nursing worldwide is important to the profession as well as international health care. For most of its history, STTI claimed to be an apolitical organization; however, at its biennial convention in the mid-1990s, the House of Delegates took on a political presence. The organization has since formed coalitions such as "Nurses for a Healthier Tomorrow," which is a politically active consortium focused on providing the public with a strong, exciting image of what it means to be a nurse.

The past President Pat Thompson's vision for STTI included both leadership development and political activism. Thompson identified the need to create an organization of collegial learning networks in which opportunities exist for members to affect the health status of local communities—an organization in which the collective talents and scholarship of members are fostered and disseminated. This powerful synergy is expected to influence the health of people worldwide.

Involvement in professional nursing organizations contributes to ongoing professional role development, which includes commitment to lifelong learning, enhancement of the repertoire of leadership skills, and caring collegial relationships, including mentoring. As students begin their professional practice, participation in professional organization activities provides the framework to engage in coalitions, which support agendas that enhance high-quality, cost-effective health care, and the advancement of the profession. Ultimately, it is our imperative to accept social responsibility and act as catalysts in influencing health care policy.

TRANSITION INTO PRACTICE

Preparation for Collective Action

Involvement in political activity is a hallmark of professional nursing practice. Nurses must give consideration to strategies that prepare them for political activity. To facilitate transition to professional nursing practice and support skill acquisition, the environment for learning strategies to support political action must closely resemble the real experience. A mock convention supports the development of confidence in the political arena and prepares nursing students and nurses for future political activity. The event sets the stage for mentorship, provides a forum for resolution writing, and prepares students for the colleagueship and coalition-building opportunities that meetings and conventions provide.

The following stories reflect actual beginning students' perspectives on their development through leadership experiences and preparation for political activity:

Kirsten

The mock convention was actually kind of intimidating. I think we have awesome role models and leaders to look to for mentoring, but it still seems intimidating. It's hard to believe that the board is only one year ahead of us (in their nursing education). They seem to know so much. I guess it's probably because some of them have had so much experience with NSNA. I think that by watching and hearing about the past conventions, we are becoming prepared to be leaders ourselves. We have excellent mentors who seem to be more than willing to help any time needed. They also encourage us to be leaders and be heard as well.

Jamie

I feel as a nursing student it is important to become involved in the nursing student organization. I have become active in the Grand View College Nursing Student Association (GVCNSA) community service committee. I felt the need for a community service committee, so I wrote a letter supporting such a committee and had other students sign it. I then presented this letter to GVCNSA. As a result of this letter, the executive committee proposed a change to the organization bylaws. This change was passed and we now have a formal committee for community service.

As the result of successful membership and influence at the local level, Jamie has since gone on to become an elected member of the National Student Nurses' Association as a regional member of the Nominations and Elections committee.

I also feel that by being active in the student organization I am trying to allow my classmates and me to have a voice in our education. What we do may not affect us, but maybe it will help the next class of nursing students.

The following reflections depict students' lived experiences related to the state and national conventions. These students' voices emphasize the value of real experiences and the empowerment that results.

Megan

Serving as a delegate was one of the best experiences I have ever had. I was already excited about going into nursing, but after attending convention, I was nothing short of ecstatic. By seeing what nursing students were capable of when they pooled their resources and talents was completely amazing. Through the team experience and attending convention, students get to see a side of nursing which the bulk of nursing students may not even be aware. These experiences are, I believe, what sets professional nurses apart from the masses. Convention encourages nursing students to care about their chosen profession and try to make a difference in policies that currently affect them and will affect future students.

We all plan to serve our fellow humans by becoming an integral part of the health care delivery system. What sets us apart from other nursing students, however, is our desire to become further involved in our chosen vocation. This convention is designed so that nursing students are given opportunities to develop many of the skills necessary to become caring, professional nurses. This is a forum for learning.

Laura and Michelle
We started thinking about attending the National Convention after hearing the stories of people who had gone before us. We were excited that we would be part of our school group and contribute to a strong representation of our school at the national level. Not only that, but a resolution from our school had been selected to go before the House of Delegates and we wanted to be able to support our peers in person. The president of the American Nurses Association gave a speech, and one of the most exciting events from the convention was getting to meet her and interview her for the video we brought back to campus. There was relationship building between our school group and we were able to meet and interact with delegates from other schools in our state. Most importantly, we met people from all over the country and saw how we are all connected through our shared interest in the education of professional nurses. We found that through this process we truly have a voice and it will be heard.

Through experiences within professional organizations, nursing students learn to form an essential covenant with society. These experiences both challenge the student with the realities of the contemporary health care delivery system and the economic, legal, and political factors that influence it, and support their empowerment by engaging them in opportunities to influence health care policy on behalf of patients or the profession.

KEY POINTS

1. A profession is a prestigious, autonomous, self-regulating occupation providing an essential service to society requiring a lengthy and rigorous education grounded in a unique body of knowledge taught in institutions of higher learning. The members are called to the profession, actively participate in its professional societies, and are guided by the profession's Code of Ethics.
2. Full professional status is achieved through the actualization of the qualities and values of professionhood and the collective action of all nurses in professional organizations.
3. Nursing students must be socialized to the responsibilities inherent to their membership in professional nursing practice.
4. Lifelong pursuit of knowledge and knowledge development is an ongoing process and not a terminal outcome.
5. Nurses must be empowered to approach practice issues systematically by using professional literature and an evidence-based approach to clinical management of patients.

6. Membership in the profession requires effective interpersonal skills, including written and verbal communication.
7. The values of the nursing profession can serve to transform political process and public policy.
8. Enabling students to see the connections between health, policy, and the broader social issues of the times is vitally linked to active, real involvement in these issues.
9. Professional organizations give nurses forums where a collective voice on health care issues can be heard and policy created.
10. Participation in the National Student Nurses' Association represents the beginning of a lifelong connection to professional organizations.
11. Experiences with professional organizations contribute to the development of professionhood, challenge the student with realities of the contem-

porary health care delivery system, and support their empowerment by engaging them in opportunities to influence health care policy on behalf of patients or the profession.

12. The future of nursing is dependent on the achievement of professionalization through the actualization of professionhood and the empowerment of students to influence health care.

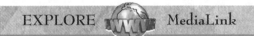

EXPLORE MediaLink

Critical thinking questions, essay questions, key terms, web links, activities, NCLEX review questions, and more interactive resources can be found on the Companion Website at www.prenhall.com/haynes. Click on Chapter 3 to select activities for this chapter.

REFERENCES

American Association of Colleges of Nursing (AACN). (1998). *The essentials of baccalaureate education for professional nursing practice.* Washington, DC: Author.

American Heritage Dictionary (2000). Fourth Edition. Boston: Houghton Mifflin.

Baker, C. M., Lamm, G. M., Winter, A. R., Robbeloth, V. B., Ransom, C. A., Conly, F., Carpenter, K. C., & McCoy, L. E. (1997). Differentiated nursing practice: Assessing the state-of-the-science. *Nursing Economics, 15*(5), 253–261.

Barra, J., & Johnson, V. V. (1998). The healing web: Implementation for education. *Journal of Nursing Education, 37*(7), 329–331.

Begun, J. W., & Lippincott, R. C. (1993). *Strategic adaptation in health profession.* San Francisco: Jossey-Bass.

Beletz, E. (1990). Professionalization—A license is not enough. In N. Chaska (Ed.), *The nursing profession: Turning points.* St. Louis, MO: Mosby.

Bixler, G. K., & Bixler, R. W. (1959). The professional status of nursing. *American Journal of Nursing, 59,* 1142–1147.

Buresh, B., & Gordon, S. (2000). *From silence to voice: What nurses know and must communicate to the public.* Ottawa: Canadian Nurses Association.

Cohen, S. S., Mason, D. J., Kovner, C., Leavitt, J. K., Pulcini, J., & Sochalski, J. (1996). Stages of nursing's political development: Where we've been and where we ought to go. *Nursing Outlook, 44*(6), 259–266.

Flexner, A. (1910). *Medical education in the United States and Canada.* New York: Carnegie Foundation for the Advancement of Teaching.

Fosbinder, D., Ashton, C. A., & Koerner, J. G. (1997). The national healing web partnership: An innovative model to improve health. *Journal of Nursing Administration, 27*(4), 37–41.

Freidson, E. (1986). *Professional powers: A study of the institutionalization of formal knowledge.* Chicago: Chicago University Press.

Giese, J. (1986). *A study to explore the differences in job satisfaction between leaders in hospital settings who have had mentor relationships and those who have not.* Unpublished master's thesis, University of Washington, Seattle.

Goldmark, J., & The Committee for the Study of Nursing Education. (1923). *Nursing and nursing education in the United States.* New York: Macmillan.

Goode, W. J. (1960). The profession: Reports and opinion. *American Sociological Review, 25,* 902–914.

Greenwood, E. (1957). Attributes of a profession. *Social Work, 2*(3), 45–54.

Gross, E. (1962). When occupations meet: Professions in trouble. *Hospital Administration, 7,* 40–59.

Honesty and Ethics Poll. (2001). Gallup Organization. Princeton, NJ: Princeton.

Houle, C. O. (1980). *Continued learning in the professions.* San Francisco: Jossey-Bass.

Kalisch, B. J., & Kalisch, P. A. (1982). *Politics of nursing.* Philadelphia, PA: Lippincott.

Koerner, J. (1992). Differentiated practice: The evolution of professional nursing. *Journal of Professional Nursing, 8*(6), 335–341.

Larson, B. A. (1986). Job satisfaction of nursing leaders with mentor relationships. *Nursing Administration Quarterly, 11*(1), 53–60.

Logan, J., & Franzen, D. (2001). Leadership and empowerment: The value of the National Student Nurses' Association for beginning students. *Nurse Educator, 26*(4), 198–200.

Logan, J. E. (1994). *The National Student Nurses' Association: A "professional" clinical arena for learning the culture and values of the nursing profession.* Unpublished dissertation.

Mancino, D. J. (1999). The NSNA Leadership U—Giving credit where credit is due. *Dean's Notes, 21*(1), 1–4.

National League for Nursing. (2000). *National League for Nursing official guide to undergraduate and graduate nursing school.* New York: National League for Nursing Press.

National Student Nurses' Association. (2002). *Getting the peices to fit, 2002–2003.* Brooklyn, NY: National Student Nurses' Association.

Nightingale, F. (1893). Sick-nursing and health nursing. In B. B. Coutts (Ed.), *Woman's mission.* London: Sampson, Low, Martson.

Oermann, M. H. (1997). *Professional nursing practice.* Stamford, CT: Appleton & Lange.

Oxford English Dictionary. (1989). Second Edition. Oxford: Oxford University Press.

Raatikainen, R. (1997). Nursing care as a calling. *Journal of Advanced Nursing, 25,* 1111–1115.

Rawl, S. M., & Peterson, L. M. (1992). Nursing education administrators: Level of career development and mentoring. *Journal of Professional Nursing, 8*(3), 161–169.

Rogers, M. E. (1964). *Revelle in nursing.* Philadelphia, PA: F. A. Davis.

Skaggs, B. J., & DeVries, C. M. (1998). You and your professional organization. In D. J. Mason & J. K. Leavitt (Eds.), *Policy and politics in nursing and health care* (pp. 535–545). Philadelphia, PA: W. B. Saunders.

Stein, A. S. (2001). Learning and change among leaders of a professional nursing association. *Holistic Nursing Practice, 16*(1), 5–15.

Styles, M. M. (1982). *On nursing: Toward a new endowment.* St. Louis, MO: Mosby.

Titmus, R. M. (1974). *Social policy: An introduction.* New York: Pantheon Books.

Vance, C., & Olson, R. K. (Eds.). (1998). *The mentor connection in nursing.* New York: Springer.

SUGGESTED READINGS

Anderson, C. F. (1999). *Nursing student to nursing leader: The critical path to leadership development.* New York: Delmar.

Buresh, B., & Gordon, S. (2000). *From silence to voice: What nurses know and must communicate to the public.* Ottawa: Canadian Nurses Association.

Diekelmann, N. (1988). Curriculum revolution: A theoretical and philosophical mandate for change. In *Curriculum revolution: Mandate for change* (pp. 137–157). New York: National League for Nursing.

Diekelmann, N. (1990). Nursing education: Caring, dialogue and practice. *Nursing Education,* 300–305.

Leavitt, J. K., & Pinsky, J. B. (1998). Coalitions for action. In D. J. Mason & J. K. Leavitt (Eds.), *Policy and politics in nursing and health care* (pp. 180–190). Philadelphia, PA: W. B. Saunders.

National League for Nursing Center for Research in Nursing Education. (1997). *Nursing data review (1997).* Publication No. 19-7327. New York: National League for Nursing Press.

Pew Health Professions Commission. (1995). *Critical challenges: Revitalizing the health professions for the twenty-first century.* San Francisco: University of California Center for the Health Professions.

Styles, M. M. (1982). *On nursing: Toward a new endowment.* St. Louis, MO: Mosby.

Tracy, J., Samarel, N., & DeYoung, S. (1995). Professional role development in baccalaureate nursing education. *Journal of Nursing Education, 34,* 180–182.

4

Nursing's Distinctive Knowledge

HOWARD K. BUTCHER

"If we want to ensure the survival of our discipline, all of us must fall in love with nursing [knowledge] now and develop a passion for the destiny of the discipline of nursing.

Jacqueline Fawcett, 1999"

LEARNING OBJECTIVES

AT THE COMPLETION OF THIS CHAPTER, THE READER WILL BE ABLE TO:

➤ Identify three major philosophies of science that have influenced nursing knowledge development.

➤ Explain how each of Carper's fundamental patterns of knowing are present in every nursing practice encounter.

➤ Identify the relationships of the major concepts that make up nursing's distinctive knowledge.

➤ Describe how conceptual frameworks and theories are used to guide nursing practice.

➤ Define concepts used by various nursing theorists.

➤ Explain the importance of theory-based nursing practice for the advancement of the nursing profession and promotion of excellence in practice.

MediaLink www.prenhall.com/haynes

Additional online resources including NCLEX review questions, critical thinking questions, and real-world activities for this chapter can be found on the Companion Website at www.prenhall.com/haynes.

$\mathcal{C}$linical practice is central to nursing and is built on nursing knowledge, theory, and research. While the knowledge used to guide nursing practice is derived from a wide array of other disciplines and fields, the *Essentials of Baccalaureate Education for Professional Nursing Practice* (American Association of Colleges of Nursing, 1998) cogently points out "in the senior college and university setting, every academic discipline is based on a discrete scientific body of knowledge with unique and distinctive applications" (p. 4). Most scholars agree that *a unique body of knowledge is an essential quality of a profession* (Styles, 1982). A unique body of knowledge is a foundation for attaining the respect, recognition, and power granted by society to a fully developed profession and scientific discipline. Furthermore, the autonomy of a profession rests most firmly on the uniqueness, recognition, and recognized validity of the discipline's theoretical knowledge.

Undergraduate nursing students expect to become knowledgeable, competent, ethical, and caring professionals who provide nursing care for promoting health and well-being. To meet this goal, it is essential that they acquire the knowledge, skills, values, meanings, and experience that are specific to nursing. The use of nursing knowledge is a *hallmark* of clinical practice (Fawcett & Carino, 1989). This knowledge represents nursing's unique contribution to the health care system and thus distinguishes nursing as an autonomous health profession (Parse, 1995). Nursing's distinctive knowledge base is expressed in the concepts, philosophy, patterns of knowing, conceptual frameworks, theories, classification systems, and practice models specific to nursing.

A number of nursing scholars (Cody, 1997; Fawcett, 1999; Levine, 1995; Mitchell, 1997; Rawnsley, 1999; Reed, 1998) have noted the decreased emphasis on the application of unique nursing knowledge in nursing education and clinical practice. Recently, DeKeyser and Medoff-Copper (2002) commented that "over the decade of the 90s nursing theory seemed to take an increasingly smaller role in the content of schools of nursing" (p. 330) and "practicing nurses are continuing with their daily routines and are often unaware that the world of nursing theory is changing" (p. 329). The vast majority of published nursing research continues to be conceptualized from theories borrowed from other disciplines. More importantly, few practicing nurses use a nursing conceptual framework or theory as the foundation for guiding clinical practice. The continued advancement and very survival of nursing as an emerging profession and academic practice discipline rests on the ability of all nurses to understand, express, and use nursing's distinctive knowledge base to guide nursing practice, research, and education.

Some undergraduate programs include "nursing theory" as part of the curriculum. There are a number of current textbooks (Alligood & Marriner-Tomey, 2002; Fawcett, 2000; George, 2002; Johnson & Webber, 2001; Marriner-Tomey & Alligood, 2002; McEwen & Wills, 2002; Parker, 2001) that describe the relevance and application of nursing's unique knowledge base in practice. Lutjens Johnson and Horan (1992) point out that it is not sufficient to isolate nursing theory in one course. Furthermore, confining nursing theory to graduate studies, which is the custom in many schools of nursing, conveys the false notion that theory is too esoteric. This custom underestimates the intelligence and capabilities of undergraduate students to learn how to engage in theory-guided practice. Lutjens Johnson and Horan (1992) assert that baccalaureate nurses, on completion of their education, be able to:

- Understand the concepts of differing nursing conceptual models
- Conceptualize nursing as nursing theory–guided practice
- Utilize theoretical thinking grounded in nursing conceptual frameworks in applying the nursing process
- Articulate the practice–theory–research cycle
- Use theoretical thinking grounded in nursing models to conceptualize components of the research process
- Identify the goal of research as theory building or theory testing

Critical Thinking and Reflection

What organizing framework currently guides your thinking about nursing? Is your image of nursing your own private image or is it based on a specific nursing conceptual framework? What conceptual framework organizes the nursing knowledge in your nursing program? How would you clearly and succinctly describe and explain the nature of nursing to a patient, the public, or another health care professional?

More than a decade ago Schlotfeldt (1989) asserted that "there can be little doubt that one of the highest priorities for creating an appropriate future for nursing is that of identifying, structuring, and continuously advancing the knowledge that underlies the practices of professionals in the field" (p. 35). The organization and structure of nursing's unique philosophical and scientific knowledge offered in this chapter is a new and unique synthesis of the vast amount of literature on nursing theory.

The purpose of this chapter is not to summarize or repeat the content presented in popular nursing theory textbooks, but rather to: (a) demonstrate essential need for using nursing's unique body of knowledge to advance the discipline of nursing; (b) offer a structure or way of organizing nursing's unique and distinctive knowledge base; (c) describe the essence of nursing's distinctive body of knowledge; and (d) illustrate the relevance of nursing theory in guiding nursing practice.

A format for organizing and structuring nursing's unique knowledge base is presented in Figure 4–1. This template places the knowledge base specific to nursing at the core of nursing education, research, and practice. The structure of nursing's distinctive body of knowledge as depicted in Figure 4–1 serves to organize the content in this chapter. (Not all nursing conceptual frameworks and theories are included in Figure 4–1 due to space limitations.)

It is important to note that in addition to Orem's Self-Care Deficit Nursing Theory, The Roy Adaptation Model, and King's Interaction Systems and Theory of Goal Attainment, the totality paradigm also includes: Peplau's Theory of Interpersonal Relations, Levine's Conservation Model, Johnson's Behavioral Systems Model, The Newman Systems Model, Leininger's Theory of Cultural Care Diversity and Universality, and Boykin and Schoenhofer's Nursing as Caring. Table 4–1 lists the primary resources for the conceptual framework of leading nurse theorists.

The Nature of Scientific Disciplines

Disciplines are branches of knowledge and are identified by distinct conceptualizations of the phenomena of concern. Disciplines are branches of knowledge organized by concepts/paradigms, or what Kuhn (1970) later referred to as disciplinary matrices. The fourth edition of the *American Heritage Dictionary* (2000) defines a discipline as a branch of instruction or learning. The idea of a "branch" suggests that there are dis-

tinctions among branches or disciplines. The uniqueness of a discipline stems from its belief systems articulated in its major paradigms, theoretical structures, and conceptualizations. As a science and academic discipline, nursing has a unique and distinct content or knowledge base. Like all professional fields, nursing also has roots or "linkages" to basic sciences, social science, humanities, and the arts.

Having a unique body of knowledge is the very essence of a discipline. Donaldson and Crowley (1978) pointed out in their classic article, "a discipline is not global; it is characterized by a unique perspective, a distinct way of viewing all phenomena, which ultimately defines the limits and nature of its inquiry" (p. 113). Similarly, Meleis (1997a) pointed out that "a discipline provides a unique way of considering the phenomena that are of interest to its members" (p. 42). Nursing practice is the application of nursing knowledge for the promotion of health, quality of life, and betterment of all humans.

Science exists within all disciplines. Nursing is a science and an intellectual discipline. The goal of the discipline is to expand knowledge relevant to nursing practice through research and creative conceptualization. Knowledge generated through scientific inquiry provides a scientific base for nursing practice. As early as 1959, Johnson (1959) referred to nursing as a science, noting that each science emerged from the study of different phenomena using a unique perspective of observation and interpretation. Nursing science has developed as the result of creative thinking by nurse philosophers, theorists, and scientists. The result of this creative thinking is a matrix of knowledge that cements together disciplinary perspectives that serve as a guide for nursing education, practice, and research. Fawcett (2000) explains the status conferred by being a member of the professional discipline of nursing. Unlike an occupation or a trade, professional membership carries with it responsibility to develop, disseminate, and use knowledge specific and unique to nursing.

Nursing's Metaparadigm

Toulmin (1972) explained that the core of a discipline is its domain, or the territory for practice and investigation. Similarly, Meleis (1997a) asserted that a domain of knowledge is the crux of a discipline. The domain is made up of central concepts, central concerns, and focal areas of investigation. Thus, the domain is the territory that shapes both the discipline's theoretical and practical boundaries. The central concepts of a disci-

Figure 4–1   The Structure of Nursing's Distinctive Body of Knowledge

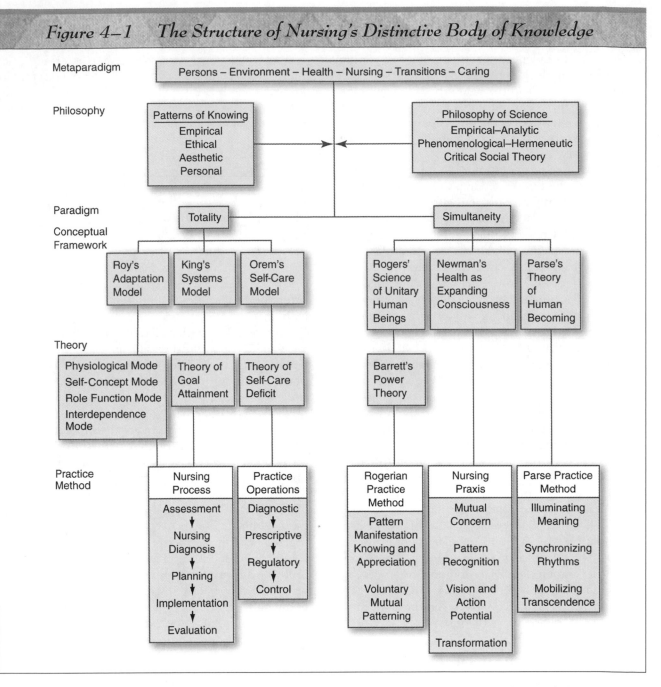

pline are comprised of metaparadigm, and the discipline's central concern evolves from its metaparadigm concepts.

All nurses have some awareness of nursing's metaparadigm by virtue of being educated as nurses. However, they may not be as familiar with the term *metaparadigm*. A metaparadigm represents the "broadest consensus within a discipline. It provides the general parameters of the field and gives scientists [and clinicians] a broad orientation from which to work"

(Hardy, 1978, p. 38). Thus, the **metaparadigm** of any discipline comprises of the most global and abstract central concepts that identify the phenomena of interest to the members of the discipline and includes global propositions that state relationships among those central concepts (Kuhn, 1970).

Fawcett (1996, 2000) specified four characteristics for the metaparadigm of a discipline. First, the central concepts specified by the metaparadigm are distinctive from the central concepts of other disciplines; second,

Table 4–1 Resources for the Conceptual Framework of Leading Nurse Theorists

Theorist	Conceptual Framework	Most Current Comprehensive Reference
Florence Nightingale	Environmental Model of Health	Nightingale, F. (1860/1992). *Notes on nursing: What it is, and what it is not.* Commemorative Edition. Philadelphia, PA: Lippincott.
Hildegard Peplau	Theory of Interpersonal Relations	Peplau, H. (1952). *Interpersonal relations in nursing: A conceptual framework of reference for psychodynamic nursing.* New York: Springer.
Myra E. Levine	Conservation Model	Levine, M. E. (1991). The conservation principles: A model for health. In K. Schaefer & J. Pond (Eds.), *Levine's conservation model: A framework for nursing practice* (pp. 1–11). Philadelphia, PA: F. A. Davis.
Dorothy Johnson	Behavioral Systems Model	Johnson, D. E. (1990). The behavioral systems model for nursing. In M. Parker (Ed.), *Nursing theories in practice.* (pp. 23–32). New York: National League for Nursing.
Martha Rogers	The Science of Unitary Human Beings	Rogers, M. E. (1992). Nursing science and the space age. *Nursing Science Quarterly, 5,* 27–34.
Dorthea E. Orem	Self-Care Deficit Nursing Theory	Orem, D. E. (2001). *Nursing: Concepts of practice* (6th ed.). St. Louis, MO: Mosby.
Imogene M. King	Interaction Systems and Theory of Goal Attainment	King, I. M. (1995). A systems framework for nursing. In M. Frey & C. Sieloff (Eds.), *Advancing King's systems framework and theory of goal attainment* (pp. 14–22). Thousand Oaks, CA: Sage.
Betty Neuman	The Neuman Systems Model	Neuman, B. (2001). *The Neuman systems model* (4th ed.). Upper Saddle River, NJ: Prentice Hall.
Callista Roy	The Roy Adaptation Model	Roy, S. C., & Andrews, H. A. (1999). *The Roy adaptation model* (2nd ed.). Stamford, CT: Appleton & Lange.
Margaret A. Newman	Health as Expanding Consciousness	Newman, M. A. (1994). *Health as expanding consciousness* (2nd ed.). New York: National League for Nursing.
Madeleine Leininger	The Theory of Cultural Care Diversity and Universality	Leininger, M. (2002). *Transcultural nursing: Concepts, theories, research, & practice* (3rd ed.). New York: McGraw-Hill.
Jean Watson	Theory of Human Caring	Watson, J. (1999). *Postmodern nursing and beyond.* London: Churchill Livingstone.
Rosemary Parse	The Theory of Human Becoming	Parse, R. R. (1998). *The human becoming school of thought: A perspective for nurses and other health care professionals.* Thousand Oaks, CA: Sage.
Anne Boykin and Savina Schoenhofer	Nursing as Caring	Boykin, A., & Schoenhofer, S. (1993/2001). *Nursing as caring: A model for transforming nursing practice.* New York: National League for Nursing.

the metaparadigm must encompass all phenomena of interest to the discipline in a parsimonious manner; third, the metaparadigm must be perspective neutral, meaning that the concepts do not represent a particular paradigm or theoretical perspective; and finally, the metaparadigm must be international in scope and substance, and not reflect particular national, cultural, or ethnic beliefs and values. While there continues to be some debate as to what concepts identify nursing's metaparadigm, there is increasing consensus around Fawcett's (1984) original proposal that person, environment, health, and nursing are the four metaparadigm concepts that identify nursing's distinctive domain of knowledge. *Person* refers to the recipient of nursing and includes individuals, families, groups, and communities. The *environment* includes the person and significant others' physical surroundings as well as the setting in which nursing occurs, which may range from the person's home, where he or she seeks nursing care, to society as a whole. The *environment* also refers to all local, regional, national, and international cultural, social, political, and economic conditions that are associated with the person's health. *Health* is the person's condition of well-being, which ranges from high-level wellness to terminal illness. The metaparadigm concept of nursing refers to the definition of nursing, the actions taken by nurses on behalf of or in conjunction with the person, and the goals or outcomes of nursing actions (Fawcett, 1997, 2000).

Fawcett (2000) writes that her version of nursing's metaparadigm should not be regarded as a premature closure on the central phenomena or concern of the discipline and anticipates that modifications to the metaparadigm will be offered as nursing continues to evolve. The metaparadigm for nursing proposed in this chapter includes Fawcett's four concepts and proposes two additional concepts central to nursing—caring and transitions.

Caring

Caring is central to nursing. **Caring** is to be concerned, to be interested in, or to give close attention to another and provide needed assistance (*American Heritage Dictionary*, 2000). Caring designates the nature of nursing practice. Leininger (1991) has long maintained that caring is the essence of nursing and the central, dominant, and unifying focus of nursing. Watson (1990) also advocated that human caring needs to be explicitly incorporated into nursing's metaparadigm. Both the *Nursing's Social Policy Statement* (American Nurses Association, 1995) and *The Essentials of Baccalaureate Education for Professional Nursing Practice* (American Association of Colleges of Nursing, 1998) recognize caring as a central domain in nursing. Clearly, all conceptualizations of nursing and all aspects of nursing practice involve the process of caring.

Transition

Schumacher and Meleis (1994) convincingly argued that the concept of *transition* is a central concept of knowledge in nursing. All health–illness situations can be viewed as a change or transition. Nurses interact with persons who are experiencing some sort of transi-

tion or are anticipating a transition (Meleis, 1997b). A **transition** denotes a change in health status, in role relations, in expectations, or in abilities. Transition also refers to changes in needs of all human systems and requires the person to incorporate new knowledge and alter behavior (Meleis, 1997b). Schumacher and Meleis (1994) described four types of transitions relevant to nursing: developmental, situational, health–illness, and organizational. Nursing care gives attention to the processes and consequences of transitions in the lives of patients. The notion of transition or changing is present in all nursing conceptual frameworks and theories. Nursing care may be viewed as creating conditions that assist patients in making healthful transitions.

Focus of the Discipline

Since Nightingale, a number of nurse scholars have offered definitions of nursing. Some of the most significant and enduring definitions of nursing are highlighted in Table 4–2. Schlotfeldt (1987) remarked that, ideally, a definition of any field of professional endeavor gives guidance concerning the practice domain. A definition identifies the goal and focus of the practitioners' concerns, endeavors, and work. Metaparadigm concepts can be linked together to form a single statement, which serves as the definition and focal statement of a discipline. Using the six metaparadigm concepts in nursing offered in this chapter, the focal definition of the discipline is:

> *Nursing is the study of caring for persons experiencing human–environment–health transitions.*

The strength of a clear and concise statement describing the focus of nursing is that it enables all nurses to clearly understand the focus of nursing and communicate to other disciplines and the public nursing's purpose. This statement expands on Newman, Sime, and Corcoran-Perry's (1991) focal statement of nursing as the study of caring in the human health experience. Like Newman et al.'s (1991) definition, the definition offered here incorporates caring, while expanding their definition by explicitly incorporating the domain of environment, and adds the domain of transitions. Defining nursing as the "study of" recognizes that nursing is an academic and learned profession with a body of unique knowledge. The knowledge generated from "study" and research is used in practice to promote health, well-being, and human betterment. The inclusion of the term *experiencing* emphasizes the

Table 4–2   Definitions of Key Theory Terms

Metaparadigm	A metaparadigm represents the most global perspective of a discipline and consists of the central concepts with which the discipline is concerned. There is some consensus that the metaparadigm concepts of nursing are: nursing, persons, environment, and health. Caring and transitions are two additional concepts that a number of nurse scholars have suggested should be included in nursing's metaparadigm.
Philosophy	Philosophy is the love and pursuit of wisdom by intellectual means and moral self-discipline. A philosophy comprises statements of enduring values and beliefs held by members of a discipline. The branches of philosophy addressed most commonly in nursing include: ethics, aesthetics, epistemology (theory of knowledge), and ontology (theory of reality, existence, and being). Philosophical statements are practical guides for examining issues and clarifying priorities of the discipline.
Paradigm	A worldview or ideology. A paradigm implies standards or criteria for assigning value or worth to both processes and the products of a discipline, as well as for the methods of knowledge development within a discipline. A paradigm contains conceptual frameworks consistent with the paradigm's particular worldview.
Conceptual Framework (Model)	A logical grouping of related concepts or theories, usually created to draw together several different aspects that are relevant to a complex situation such as a practice situation or an educational program. Nursing conceptual frameworks (grand theories) convey a mental image and symbolically represent the field of nursing by identifying and describing concepts and their relationships of central concern to nurses.
Theory	A creative and rigorous structuring of ideas that project a tentative, purposeful, and systematic view of a phenomenon. A theory consists of a logical set of interrelated concepts, statements, propositions, and definitions that have been derived from philosophical beliefs and scientific data from which questions or hypotheses can be deducted, tested, and verified.
Practice Method	A practice methodology is derived from the concepts and propositions of a particular nursing theory. Therefore, the steps or processes of the practice method are congruent with the particular nursing theory's concepts and propositions.

Sources: Adapted from Chinn and Kramer (1999); Fawcett (2000); McEwen and Wills (2002); Meleis (1997a); and Parker (2001).

nurse's focus on the patient's thoughts, emotions, behaviors, knowledge, and skills when considering their health situation. The dashes between human, environment, and health signify the nursing discipline's holistic philosophical perspective, which views persons as being integral or in interaction with the environment and health as emerging from or a result of person–environment interactions. While each of the major nursing theorists has defined nursing, the definition offered does not reflect any particular paradigmatic or theoretical perspective (Table 4–3).

Science and Patterns of Knowing

Nursing knowledge development does not occur in a vacuum. Particular philosophical perspectives about the nature of science have influenced the development of knowledge via particular "pathways" or "patterns of

knowing." Knowing here refers to ways of perceiving and understanding self and the world. The ways in which knowledge and knowing are developed in nursing reveal how nurses come to know and acquire the shared knowledge in the discipline.

Philosophical Traditions Influencing Nursing Knowledge Development

Within any discipline, both students and scholars should be aware of the philosophical orientations that provide the basis for developing theory and advancing knowledge (DiBartolo, 1998). Increasingly, basic undergraduate textbooks in nursing theory and research are introducing students to the concepts and language of nursing philosophy and science. **Philosophy** is a form of rigorous inquiry for the purposes of discerning general characteristics and statements of enduring beliefs about the nature of reality and principles of value (Chinn & Kramer, 1999). It is essential to understand the way in which nursing knowledge develops in

Table 4–3 Classic Definitions of Nursing

The function of nursing is "to put the patient in the best condition for nature to act upon him" (Nightingale, 1860, p. 75).

"The unique function of the nurse is to assist the individual, sick or well, in performance of those activities contributing to health or its recovery (or to a peaceful death) that he would perform unaided if he had the necessary strength, will, or knowledge. And to do this in such a way as to help him gain independence as rapidly as possible" (Henderson, 1960, p. 3).

"Nursing is the diagnosis and treatment of human responses to actual and potential health problems" (ANA, 1980, p. 9).

"Nursing is the appraisal and the enhancement of the health status, health assets, and health potentials of human beings" (Schlotfeldt, 1987, p. 67).

"Nursing is the study of caring in the human health experience." (Newman, Sime, & Corcoran-Perry, 1991, p. 4).

"The focus of nursing . . . is person as living in caring and growing in caring." (Boykin & Schoenhofer, 2001, p. 393)

"The core focus of nursing, the metaparadigm, is the human–universe–health process" (Parse, 1997, p. 74).

order to determine the quality, relevance, and legitimacy of knowledge gained. Three major philosophical schools describing the nature of knowledge have influenced nursing knowledge development: empirical–analytic, phenomenological–hermeneutic, and critical social theory. Each of these major schools of philosophy has led to unique and distinctive forms of knowledge that guides nursing practice.

EMPIRICAL–ANALYTIC PHILOSOPHY OF SCIENCE

The empirical–analytic schools of thought dominate the broader scientific community, especially in the North American philosophy of science. This approach to knowledge development in nursing is the one most familiar to nursing students. Often, empirical–analytic methods of knowledge development are presented as if these methods are the only way for developing "scientific" knowledge. Most undergraduate nursing research courses place great emphasis on understanding the steps of the "scientific research process," which typically involves quantitative research designs with tight controls over context. In this view of science, the scientist tests measurable hypotheses that can be generalized, reproduced, and verified to produce evidence-based knowledge.

An important assumption of the empirical–analytic view of science is that the world is structured by law-like regularities that can be identified and manipulated. The world is viewed as ordered and can be broken down into a system of independent and dependent variables. Many of the central features of this view of science are its emphasis on theory, the centrality of observation and measurement, the ideal of experimental designs, objectiv-

ity, prediction, and control (Allen, Benner, & Diekelman, 1986). Among health care disciplines, the empirical–analytic perspective of science is most common in the culture of biomedicine and its associated biomedical model.

Historically, in seeking to be recognized as a science, nursing has placed great emphasis on the scientific method as the legitimate way of developing nursing knowledge. In the 1950s, the shift toward science was a welcome change from the traditional focus of nursing on technically competent performance of delegated medical tasks, blind duty, and womanly virtue (Chinn & Kramer, 1999). Initially, nursing research focused primarily on nursing education; however, through the 1960s and 1970s, nursing research increasingly focused on nursing practice. By the 1980s, more nurses were being educated at the doctoral level, and many master's programs required a thesis for degree completion. Increasing attention was given to research questions asked, research methods, the linking of research to theory, and the utilization of research findings in practice. One of the most pivotal events in the rise of the empirical–analytic scientific perspective was the establishment of the National Center for Nursing Research (NCNR) at the National Institutes of Health (NIH). In 1993, the NCNR was promoted to full institute status within NIH and today is known as the National Institute of Nursing Research (NINR). The persistent dominance of the empirical–analytic approach to knowledge development can be attributed in part to the need of academic nurses to gain legitimacy in university communities and to the need of nurses to achieve political and personal legitimacy within medicine and society in general (Chinn & Kramer, 1999).

PHENOMENOLOGICAL–HERMENEUTIC PHILOSOPHY OF SCIENCE

A second thread of influence in nursing is grounded within a phenomenological–hermeneutic perspective of knowledge development. The phenomenological–hermeneutic view of science has also been referred to as the interpretive, naturalistic, or constructivist philosophy of science (Lincoln & Guba, 2000). This scientific tradition views truth as a matter of perspective. In other words, truth is relative and there is no objective reality.

Central to the phenomenological–hermeneutic view is the term *human science*, which can be traced back to the philosopher Wilhelm Dilthey (1833–1911). Dilthey proposed that the human sciences require concepts, methods, and theories that are fundamentally different from those of the physical and biological sciences. Dilthey proposed, "human sciences study meanings, values, and relationships to enhance understanding of experiences as humanly lived" (Parse, 2002, p. 3). Rather than to seek to control and manipulate the phenomenon of investigation using the "scientific method," the human scientist's approach to knowledge development recognizes the inseparability of human beings from their environment, context, history, and background (Cody & Mitchell, 2002; Mitchell & Cody, 1992). The research is done without control or manipulation of variables, but rather is conducted in natural settings with the goal to produce (a) narratives, rather than statistical descriptions and (b) interpretations, to help understand the nature of human experiences. In nursing, the works of Patterson and Zderad (1988), Parse (1998), Boykin and Schoenhofer (1993, 2001), Benner and Wrubel (1989), Watson (1999), and Newman (1997) are most closely associated with the phenomenological–hermeneutic perspective of science and knowledge development. These authors view nursing as a *human science*, concerned with understanding a person's meanings, relations, values, patterns, and themes in relation to their health–illness experience.

CRITICAL SOCIAL THEORY

Critical social theory is part of a tradition of scientific theory that stands in sharp contrast to the empirical–analytic. The roots of critical social theory can be traced to the Institute of Social Research founded in Frankfurt, Germany, in 1923. The goal of the Frankfurt School was to revise Marxism and the objectivist interpretation of historical materialism. It was a response to the domination of technological knowledge developed through logical positivist science and its consequent contribution to the oppression of working classes. Critical social scientists seek to expose social inequalities that keep people from reaching their full potential and inspire others to seek instrumental or communicative action for social change through the promotion of justice and freedom. Approaches to critical social theory endeavor to understand how oppression operates within society and how human perception shapes the social world (Boutain, 1999).

From a critical social theory perspective, oppression is understood as unequal power relations embedded in the basic structures and functions of society (Stevens, 1989). A growing number of nursing scholars, including Allen (1985), Campbell and Bunting (1991), Chinn and Wheeler (1985), Stevens (1989), Taylor (1999), and Thompson (1987), have used a critical social theory perspective to bring about awareness of oppression (e.g., racism, sexism, and classism) that is embedded in nursing and health care and contributes to health care disparities. The research methods used by critical social theorists may include the interpretive critical analysis of text, narratives, diaries, and/or statistical analyses. The aim of critical inquiry is to critique and reveal the nature of inequities as a means to empower others to transform the social, political, cultural, economic, ethnic, and gender structures that exploit humankind. Confrontation, conflict, advocacy, empowerment, emancipation, and action are key concepts of critical social theory.

Each of these scientific traditions are present in nursing and have contributed to the development of nursing knowledge relevant to understanding the health experiences of patients, establishing a scientific base for nursing practice, and illuminating the social processes that limit patients from achieving their full health potentials. Neither of the three scientific approaches to nursing knowledge development has a final grasp on truth. From a disciplinary perspective, all three approaches should be equally valued in nursing.

Patterns of Knowing Influencing Nursing Knowledge Development

Disciplines are not only identified by domain concepts and sources influencing knowledge development, but are also identified by ways in which knowledge is characterized and developed (Meleis, 1997b). How nurses come to know and understand the kinds of knowledge that are of most value in the discipline of nursing is critical to developing a full understanding of the development of knowledge used to guide nursing practice.

Carper (1978) examined early nursing literature and uncovered four fundamental patterns of knowing that nurses value and use in practice: aesthetic, ethical, empirical, and personal. While other authors have proposed viable additions and adaptations to Carper's original work, the four fundamental patterns have endured as an essential feature to understanding the nature of nursing knowledge. Chinn and Kramer (1999), extending Carper's original work, explain that the fundamental patterns remain valuable because they conceptualize the broad scope of knowing that accounts for nursing's holistic perspective. While empirical knowing has been the prevailing approach to knowledge development, Carper's work draws particular attention to other equally valuable personal, aesthetic, and ethical ways of knowing that are often neglected in nursing education, research, and practice.

AESTHETIC KNOWING

Aesthetics is a branch of philosophy that focuses on the critical analysis of art and beauty. *Aesthetic knowing* involves the art of nursing. Nursing has long been recognized as an art as well as a science. Nightingale (1860) described nursing as one of the "finest of the fine arts" (p. 362), and Stewart (1929) proclaimed the "real essence of nursing, as any fine art, lies not in the mechanical details of execution, nor in the dexterity of the performer, but in the creative imagination, the sensitive spirit, and the intelligent understanding lying back of those techniques and skills" (p. 1). More recently, Rogers (1988) defined the art of nursing as "the creative use of the body of abstract knowledge in human service" (p. 100). The art of nursing is expressed through the nurse's empathy, caring, skillfulness, and compassion. "Nursing aesthetics in nursing is that aspect of knowing that connects with the deep meanings of a situation and calls forth inner creative resources that transform experience into what is not yet real, but possible" (Chinn & Kramer, 1999, p. 183). Aesthetic knowing makes it possible to move beyond the surface toward a deeper meaning of the moment and to connect with the depths of human experience in health, sickness, suffering, recovery, birth, and death. The nurse's coordinated balance, finesse, style, timing, and synchrony with the patient are all representative of the nurse's artistic skillfulness in practice. Aesthetic knowing allows the nurse to act at once, without protracted deliberation, and it permits the nurse to see what is most important in a given situation.

ETHICAL KNOWING

Ethics is the branch of philosophy that focuses on matters of obligation and morality. *Ethical knowing*, Carper (1978) explains, is that ethical component of nursing that is concerned with matters of obligation or what ought to be done. In nursing, ethical knowing arises from both experiential knowledge, from which ethical reasoning arises, and knowledge from formal principles, ethical codes, and discipline-specific theories and ethical theories. However, ethical knowing goes beyond the knowledge of norms, ethical codes for nursing, and obligation and encompasses the judging of moral values related to motives, intention, and character. Like each of the patterns of knowing, ethical knowing is expressed through nursing actions. Ethical knowing involves making moment-to-moment decisions about what ought to be done, what is good and right, and what is responsible and guides and "directs how nurses conduct their practice, what they select as important, where loyalties are placed, and what priorities demand advocacy" (Chinn & Kramer, 1999, p. 5). Clearly, nursing is a discipline that requires the use of ethical knowing in every nursing situation. For example, *every* nursing situation involves the preserving of human dignity by protecting confidentiality and privacy; enacting justice by treating patients equally and fairly; cultivating fidelity and veracity by keeping the commitments made with the patient and being truthful about information; engendering beneficence by doing "good" for patients; and fostering the patient's autonomy and personal freedom in making decisions concerning their own care.

EMPIRICAL KNOWING

Empirical knowing is most closely associated with science and theory. "Science seeks to understand the real world. Theory is the product of science: research its tool" (Stainton, 1982, p. 24). *Empirical knowing* draws on the assumption that what is known is accessible through the five senses and is based on knowledge that is considered objective, abstract, often quantifiable, and publicly verifiable. Empirical knowledge can be verified by other observers through repeated testing and over time can be formulated into scientific generalizations, scientific laws, statements of what is considered fact, theories, and principles that describe, explain, and predict phenomena of concern to the discipline of nursing (Carper, 1978).

Empirical knowledge has been considered the foundation of nursing practice ever since Nightingale first established formal education as a requirement to

Consider the patient you last cared for. How did the patterns of knowing guide your nursing care? For example, what empirical or theoretical knowledge helped you understand the patient's condition? What personal knowledge did you bring into the situation and how did your personal knowledge help you understand the patient's experience? What ethical principles were present in the situation? How did you use aesthetic knowledge in your care of the patient?

practice as a nurse. Nightingale also emphasized the importance of accurate observation and careful record keeping (Chinn & Kramer, 1999). Principles and facts gleaned from observation were the basis of early procedural guides nurses used for providing routine hygienic care to patients and for performing delegated medical tasks. Nursing's emergence as a scientific discipline placed great emphasis on empirical knowing as a way of building a scientific body of nursing knowledge.

PERSONAL KNOWING

Carper's (1978) fourth fundamental pattern of knowing is concerned with the nurse's inner experience of becoming whole, aware, and genuine. *Personal knowing* encompasses knowing one's own self and the self of others and is fundamental to nursing practice since interpersonal processes are inherent to nursing practice (Chinn & Kramer, 1999). Full awareness of oneself, the moment, and the context of the interaction with patients make possible meaningful, shared human experiences. The idea of the therapeutic use of self in nursing practice would not be possible without using personal knowing. Carper (1978) believes personal knowing is the pattern most essential to understanding the meaning of health in terms of individual well-being. Personal knowing is not limited to personal observations and perceptions, but also includes spiritual and mystical forms of knowing. The personal aspect of spiritual knowing is not necessarily linked with any particular religious tradition but can be a set of values, attitudes, hopes, and beliefs that can inspire one to confront life-challenging issues and provide meaning while caring for others who are suffering and in despair.

Moch (1990) described personal knowing as including three overlapping components: experiential knowing, interpersonal knowing, and intuitive knowing. Experience comes from the nurse's everyday participation in the events of daily living and is deepened by attending to the experiences, studying the process of experiences, and connecting an experience to previous experiences. Interpersonal knowing is increased awareness through intense interactions with others or being with another. Interpersonal knowing emerges when one is open to sharing of feelings with another. Intuitive knowing is the immediate knowing of something without conscious use of reason (Chinn & Kramer, 1999). Benner (1984) notes that expert nurses are characterized as having an intuitive grasp of situations and being able to rapidly identify problems without wasting consideration on a wide range of alternative diagnoses and solutions.

Personal knowing is discovered by reflection, synthesis of perceptions, and connecting with what is known (Moch, 1990) and can be cultivated in the nurse by private journaling, meditation exercises, and focusing or centering practices. Personal knowing is essential to healing relationships because it expands what is accessible to the self in the experience with another and enables the experiencing of a deeper level of meaning shared in the interaction (Chinn & Kramer, 1999).

▓ Evolution of Nursing Theory Development

Theories from other disciplines, including medicine, psychology, sociology, and education, were borrowed and applied to nursing practice. Borrowed theories that have been useful to nursing include: general systems theory, symbolic interactionism, role theory, feminist theory, psychodynamic and behavioral theories, developmental theories, stress and coping theories, theories of disease causation, theories of infection and immune function, genetic theories, pain management theories, leadership theories, and learning theories.

While borrowed theory influenced nursing education, research, and practice, as early as the mid-1950s, there was a flourish of activity at Columbia University Teachers College focusing on the development of empirical theories specific to nursing. Hildegarde Peplau, Virginia Henderson, Lydia Hall, and Faye Abdellah were a few of the early nursing scholars at Teachers College who published the first conceptualizations or theories of nursing. In 1965, the American Nurses Association (ANA) position paper identified theory development as significant to the development of the profession (ANA, 1965). The availability of federal dollars to support doctoral education led to an increasing focus on theory development, the formulation of a definition of nursing theory, and the development of theory to guide nursing curricula. By the early 1970s, a number of nursing theorists published the first editions of their conceptual frameworks. The works by Rogers (1970), Roy (1970), King (1971), Orem (1971), and Neuman (1974) were evidence of the new emphasis on nursing theory development. Throughout the 1980s, nurses witnessed phenomenal growth of nursing science and theory. In the early to mid-1980s, books published by Fawcett (1984), Chinn and Jacobs (1983), Riehl and Roy (1980), Fitzpatrick and Whall (1983), Meleis (1985), Walker and Avant (1983), and Stevens (1979) describing and critiquing theories specific to nursing were common texts in many graduate programs in nursing, and these programs offered specific courses in nursing theory and theory development.

Throughout the 1990s, nurse theorists continued to develop, expand, and test their conceptualizations of nursing. Nurse theorists, scholars, and students, especially graduate students, published a mass of research and practice articles demonstrating the usefulness of nursing theories in guiding practice, education, research, and administration. Paradoxically, the 1990s were also marked by decreasing emphasis on nursing theory, particularly nursing conceptual frameworks. Typically, nursing theory was not integrated throughout the curriculum as theory is in the education of students in other disciplines. Few nurses actually use nursing theory in their practice settings upon graduation, as few practice settings implement nursing. In addition, professional nursing organizations failed to explicitly make nursing theory a standard for nursing education and practice. Rather, empirical knowing in nursing today continues to be dominated by borrowed theory from other disciplines and by an emphasis on mid-range theory development. The continued dominance of borrowed theories from outside of nursing and mid-range theories not linked to extant nursing theories in nursing education, research, and practice fails to distinguish nursing science from other disciplines and does not add to the development of nursing as a scientific discipline.

Nursing's Scientific Paradigms

Scientific disciplines are characterized by paradigms (Meleis, 1997b). A **paradigm** is a broad organizing framework or worldview that represents a particular philosophical stance about the phenomenon of concern. A paradigm is developed by a community of scholars who share commitment, a constellation of values, norms, beliefs, views, goals, attributes, and methods (Meleis, 1997b). Paradigms house the various conceptual frameworks or schools of thought within a discipline. The conceptual frameworks within a particular paradigm are each distinct but share a common worldview or set of values, norms, beliefs, views, goals, attributes, and methods. Each paradigm holds particular assumptions and beliefs about the discipline.

Every discipline has more than one paradigm. However, often one paradigm may be more dominant. A **"paradigm shift"** occurs when the new or emerging paradigm begins to explain observed anomalies that were not explained by a more dominant and older paradigm. A **"paradigm revolution"** occurs when the emerging paradigm replaces the older paradigm.

Parse (1987) was among the first to identify paradigms in nursing. Her work remains an influential force in the literature describing nursing paradigms (Cody, 2000). She identified two major paradigms in nursing: totality paradigm and simultaneity paradigm.

Totality Paradigm

Within the totality paradigm (see Table 4–4), human beings are defined as holistic, a total or summative organism, made up of biological, psychological, sociological, spiritual, and cultural components. The environment consists of internal and external stimuli surrounding the person. Human beings interact with and adapt to environmental stimuli to maintain balance and achieve goals. Nursing research and practice based on this paradigm focus on preventing disease and promoting health. Johnson's Behavioral Systems Model, King's Interaction Systems Framework, Levine's Conservation Model, Neuman's Systems Model, Orem's Self-Care Deficit Theory, Roy's Adaptation Model, Leininger's Theory of Culture Care Diversity and Universality, and Peplau's Theory of Interpersonal Relations are all conceptual frameworks or theories that are consistent with the general values, norms, beliefs, views, goals, attributes, and methods of the totality paradigm. Furthermore, the nursing process and nursing

Table 4–4   Characteristics of the Totality and Simultaneity Paradigms

Totality Paradigm	Simultaneity Paradigm
Humans are the sum of bio-psycho-social-cultural-spiritual parts	Humans are unitary wholes who are more than and different from the sum of parts
Human beings adapt to an ever-changing environment	Humans are in a rhythmical process of becoming ever co-evolving with the universe toward patterns of increasing diversity, innovation, and complexity
Humans are in interaction with the environment	Humans are in simultaneous mutual process with the environment
Humans can be reduced into parts	Humans are irreducible and have no parts
Humans react to stimuli and causal relationships can be identified	Everything is interconnected, therefore causality cannot be determined
Change is causal and predictable	Change is acausal and unpredictable
Health and illness are defined by societal norms	Health is defined by the person
Health is a state of biological, psychological, sociological, and spiritual well-being	Health is a continuous changing process of changing value priorities
Nurses diagnose and treat human responses to actual and potential health problems	Nurses focus on experiences, perceptions, and expressions as manifestations of the human–environmental field mutual process
Nursing focuses on preventing disease, maintaining and promoting health according to social norms	Nursing focuses on pattern recognition, health experiences as they are lived, and quality of life

Modified and expanded based on Parse's 1987 original work and her 1998 expanded work. Reprinted with permission Dr. Rosemarie Rizzo Parse.

classification systems including North American Nursing Diagnosis Association (NANDA), Nursing Interventions Classification (NIC), and Nursing Outcomes Classification (NOC) are most consistent with the totality paradigm.

Simultaneity Paradigm

In contrast, the simultaneity paradigm represents a radically different view of nursing. Rogers (1970) founded the simultaneity paradigm when she posited human beings as *more and different than the sum of parts*. If persons are more than and different than the sum of their parts, then the sum of biological, psychological, sociological, spiritual, and cultural parts does not explain the nature of human beings. Within the simultaneity paradigm, human beings are viewed as "unitary" or irreducible wholes that cannot be understood by reducing them into bio-psycho-social-spiritual-cultural parts. Ultimately, there are no parts. Human beings are integral and inseparable from their environment. Therefore, human beings do not respond to stimuli, interact, or adapt to the environment, but rather the human being and the environment simultaneously co-evolve together. Health is a process of changing values, and the focus of nursing is on patterns, well-being, lived experiences, and quality of life.

Nursing Conceptual Frameworks and Theories

The terms *conceptual framework*, *conceptual model*, *conceptual system*, *grand theory*, *theoretical framework*, and *theory* have been used interchangeably in the nursing literature and refer to a set of concepts that are defined and linked by broad generalizations. The development of conceptual frameworks of nursing emerged during the 1960s and early 1970s when there was a major interest in defining and describing the functions and roles of nurses. Conceptual models of nursing are explicit and formal presentations of an image of nursing. Since conceptual frameworks provide a description of nursing and identify the purpose and scope of nursing, they are not only useful in nursing practice, but are also useful in helping nurses describe the nature of nursing to other health care professionals and the general public.

Popper (1965) explained that a conceptual model provides a distinctive frame of reference and a coherent, internally unified way of thinking about events and processes. Conceptual frameworks are more specific in scope than the paradigm but are more abstract than theories. Conceptual frameworks provide broad perspectives for defining and organizing major concepts in nursing and provide global viewpoints for guiding nursing practice, research, education, and administration. Each conceptual model, then, presents a unique focus that guides how to observe, interpret, and understand the phenomenon of interest to the discipline.

Conceptual frameworks have existed ever since humans first began to think about themselves and their environment. Conceptual frameworks exist in all areas of life and disciplines. Everything a person experiences, sees, hears, and reads is interpreted or filtered through a cognitive lens representing a conceptual frame of reference (Fawcett, 2000). Fawcett (2000) explains that conceptual models evolve from the empirical observations and intuitive insights of scholars or are derived by creatively combining knowledge from other fields of study.

While there is considerable confusion in the nursing literature concerning the differences between paradigms, conceptual frameworks, and theories, for the purpose of clarity, theories are viewed in this chapter as being more specific and less abstract than conceptual frameworks. Theories are derived from conceptual frameworks and therefore are less abstract or narrower in scope than their parent conceptual model.

Based on a synthesis of the nursing theory literature, Chinn and Kramer (1999) defined **theory** as an expression of the empiric pattern of knowing and "a creative and rigorous structuring of ideas that projects a tentative, purposeful, and systematic view of a phenomenon" (p. 51). The ideas are structured as concepts represented by word symbols. In addition to concepts, theories contain definitions of each concept and propositions that explain the nature of the relationships between specific concepts. In general, a conceptual framework cannot be tested directly because its concepts and propositions are too broad to be empirically measurable. Conversely, theories are

Research Application

There is a vast quantity of research literature on nursing theory. When conducting research, there is nothing wrong with conceptualizing the research problem within a theory from another discipline. However, research conceptualized using non-nursing theories or borrowed theories from other disciplines does not advance nursing science nor does it advance the development of a unique body of disciplinary knowledge (Parse, 1994). Nursing science, as defined in this chapter, consists of conceptual frameworks and theories designed by nurse theorists for the specific purpose of guiding nursing research, practice, education, and administration.

Rather than present one particular research study conceptualized within a specific nursing theory, it may be more useful for students to be aware of the quantity of published nursing theory literature. A computer search using Cumulative Index to Nursing and Allied Health Literature (CINAHL) 1982–June 2003, revealed the following number of citations for each of the nursing conceptual frameworks addressed in this chapter: Nightingale (13 citations specific to her model); Orem's Self-Care Deficit Theory (758 citations); Rogers' Science of Unitary Human Beings (509 citations); Roy's Adaptation Model (430 citations); Johnson's Behavioral Systems Model (45 citations); Watson's Theory of Caring (204 citations); Parse's Theory of Human Becoming (353 citations); Newman's Theory of Health as Expanding Consciousness (121 citations); Leininger's Theory of Cultural Care Diversity and Universality (261 citations); King's Interaction Systems Framework (165 citations); and Boykin and Schoenhofer's Nursing as Caring Theory (10 citations) (Table 4–5). In addition, there are many book chapters in edited books, master's theses, and dissertations focusing on a particular nursing theory not included among the CINAHL referencing system. Students who desire to learn more about a particular nursing theory would be well served by conducting a search of publications based on the particular nursing conceptual model or theory demonstrating the theory's application in specific nursing situations.

Table 4–5 Chronology of Evolution of Selected Major Conceptual Frameworks in Nursing

Theorist/Author	Year	Title of Theoretical Writings
Florence Nightingale	1860	*Notes on Nursing*
Hildegard Peplau	1952	*Interpersonal Relations in Nursing*
	1997	*Peplau's Theory of Interpersonal Relations*
Myra E. Levine	1967	*The Four Conservation Principles of Nursing*
	1973	*Introduction to Clinical Nursing*
	1989	*The Conservation Principles: Twenty Years Later*
	1991	*The Conservation Principles: A Model for Health*
	1996	*The Conservation Principles: A Retrospective*
Martha Rogers	1970	*An Introduction to the Theoretical Basis of Nursing*
	1980	*Nursing: A Science of Unitary Man*
	1983	*Science of Unitary Human Being: A Paradigm for Nursing*
	1988	*Nursing Science and Art: A Prospective*
	1989	*Nursing: A Science of Unitary Human Beings*
	1992	*Nursing and the Space Age*
	1994	*Martha E. Rogers: Her Life and Her Work* (Barrett and Malinski)
Madeleine Leininger	1970	*Nursing and Anthropology: Two Worlds to Blend*
	1978	*Transcultural Nursing: Theory, Concepts, Research, & Practice*
	1988	*Leininger's Theory of Nursing: Cultural Care Diversity and Universality*
	1995	*Transcultural Nursing: Theory, Concepts, Research, & Practice*, 2nd edition
	2001	*Madeleine M. Leininger Theory of Nursing: Cultural Care Diversity and Universality*
	2002	*Transcultural Nursing: Theory, Concepts, Research, & Practice*, 3rd edition
Dorothy Orem	1971	*Nursing: Concepts of Practice*
	1980	*Nursing: Concepts of Practice*, 2nd edition
	1985	*Nursing: Concepts of Practice*, 3rd edition
	1991	*Nursing: Concepts of Practice*, 4th edition
	1995	*Nursing: Concepts of Practice*, 5th edition
	2001	*Nursing: Concepts of Practice*, 6th edition
Imogene M. King	1971	*Toward a Theory for Nursing: General Concepts of Human Behavior*
	1981	*A Theory for Nursing: Systems, Concepts, Process*
	1989	*King's General Systems Framework and Theory*
	1995	*A Systems Framework for Nursing*
	1997	*King's Theory of Goal Attainment in Research and Practice*
	2001	*Imogene M. King Theory of Goal Attainment*
Betty Neuman	1974	*The Betty Neuman Health-Care Systems Model: A Total Person Approach to Patient Problems*
	1982	*The Neuman Systems Model*
	1989	*The Neuman Systems Model*, 2nd edition
	1995	*The Neuman Systems Model*, 3rd edition
	2001	*The Neuman Systems Model*, 4th edition
Dorothy Johnson	1976	*Behavioral Systems and Nursing* (Auger)
	1980	*The Behavioral System Model for Nursing*
	1990	*The Behavioral System Model for Nursing*
	1984	*Introduction to Nursing: An Adaptation Model*, 2nd edition
	1989	*The Roy Adaptation Model*
	1999	*The Roy Adaptation Model*, 2nd edition

(continued)

Table 4–5   (continued)

Theorist/Author	Year	Title of Theoretical Writings
Jean Watson	1979	*Nursing: The Philosophy and Science of Caring*
	1985	*Nursing: Human Science and Human Care*
	1999	*Postmodern Nursing and Beyond*
	2001	*Jean Watson Theory of Human Caring*
Rosemary Parse	1981	*Man–Living–Health: A Theory for Nursing*
	1985	*Man–Living–Health: A Man–Environment Simultaneity Paradigm*
	1987	*Nursing Science: Major Paradigms, Theories, Critiques*
	1989	*Man–Living–Health: A Theory of Nursing*
	1998	*The Human Becoming School of Thought*
	2001	*The Human Becoming School of Thought*
Margaret A. Newman	1983	*Newman's Health Theory*
	1986	*Health as Expanding Consciousness*
	1994	*Health as Expanding Consciousness*, 2nd edition
Anne Boykin and	1993	*Nursing as Caring: A Model for Transforming Practice*
Savina Schoenhofer	2001	*Nursing as Caring*

Note: The table contains the major, most current, and primary sources for the works of these theorists.

derived from a conceptual framework and contain concepts, propositions, and hypotheses that can be empirically tested.

The Purpose of Nursing Conceptual Frameworks and Theories

In addition to identifying the unique focus of nursing, nursing conceptual frameworks and theories describe, explain, and/or predict phenomena of concern to nurses. Conceptual frameworks and theories provide a way of organizing a multitude of facts and ideas into a meaningful whole and provide a common theoretical basis for understanding relationships for communication within the discipline of nursing. Conceptual frameworks and theories function like a map of a particular territory. Maps cannot and do not display the full terrain as an aerial photograph; however, maps do show the important features of the territory. The map's aim is to guide travelers by using symbols to describe the terrain. Nursing conceptual frameworks and theories use concepts as symbols to describe the terrain of nursing. Visintainer (1986) used the map analogy in explaining conceptual frameworks:

> The maps of a discipline operate in a way similar to that of maps of a geographic region. They pro-

vide a framework for selecting and organizing information from the environment. In studying a discipline, one learns the maps and through mastery of the maps learns what to ask about, what to observe, what to focus on, and what to think about (p. 33).

Each nursing conceptual framework provides a definition of nursing, identifies the major concepts of nursing's concern, and describes the purpose and goal of nursing care. More specifically, theories derived from conceptual framework are designed to guide all aspects of nursing care. A nursing theory gives direction to the focus of assessment by identifying the phenomenon of concern; providing a scientific basis for understanding the nature of patient problems; and providing the specifics for guiding all aspects of planning, implementing, and evaluating nursing care (Fawcett, 2000; Meleis, 1997b). Nursing theories are designed to (a) provide a perspective for understanding the person the nurse is caring for, (b) direct the approach to be taken to deliver care, and (c) structure critical thinking, reasoning, and decision-making in practice (Alligood, 2002). Nursing conceptual frameworks and theories are also designed to: (a) guide all aspects of nursing research; and (b) provide a general outline for organizing nursing knowledge (Fawcett, 2000).

The Language of Nursing Science

Few words conjure up more anxiety and dread among nursing students than the terms *theory* and *research*. Often, the difficulty revolves around the terminology used to describe and define concepts in particular nursing conceptual frameworks and theories. The terminology is often viewed as too abstract, as esoteric, or as "jargon." Students may wonder, "Why don't nurse theorists use common language or 'speak English'?" The use of common language terms is a sign of the early stages of a developing science. Nursing's disciplinary language can no longer be considered to be in early phases of development. Nursing disciplinary language has been evolving for 30 years. As Levine (1995) beautifully states:

> Theory is the poetry of science. The poet's words are familiar, each standing alone, but brought together they sing, they astonish, they teach. The theorist offers a fresh vision, familiar concepts brought together in bold, new designs. . . . A lovely poem will wait forever to be discovered, but a theory caught in the intellectual exercises of the academy becomes alive only when it is made a true instrument of persuasion (p. 14).

The nature of theory requires concepts and a specific language in order to provide clarity of meaning. The terminology in nursing conceptual frameworks and theories only sounds "bizarre" or difficult to one who has not studied or learned the theory. As a science matures, a more precise terminology is used to communicate abstract formulations in a clear and unambiguous way. The language of psychoanalytic theory (i.e., ego, superego, transference, counter transference) sounds equally meaningless and cumbersome when one first learns psychoanalytic theory. The terminology of nursing theory pales in comparison to the complex medical language of pathophysiology and pharmacology that all nurses learn. Nurses first exposed to medical terminology often require a "medical dictionary." Once familiar with the terminology, the meaning of these abstract concepts is so clear that most anyone understands their meaning. Clarity of meaning enhances communication and understanding of the theory. As Cody (1994a) points out, "nurses who read in other disciplines take it upon themselves to learn the language . . . shouldn't they be expected to do the same with regard to their own discipline" (p. 99)?

All disciplines are characterized by the language embedded in their conceptual frameworks and theories. Classification systems organizing the knowledge of a discipline contribute to the discipline's distinctive language (Stark & Lattuca, 1997). Every discipline educates its future practitioners by immersing them in a knowledge and language base unique to that discipline. Nursing conceptual frameworks, theories, and classification systems provide the language of nursing.

Watson (1995) has pointed out that if you don't have a language, you don't exist. "In a fundamental way, one is one's language" and "is a way of being" (Allen, 1995, p. 177). Throughout nursing history, nursing has adopted or adapted other disciplines' language to explain nursing phenomena. Not surprisingly, when nursing adopts the language of medicine, nursing is seen as an extension of medicine rather than a separate and unique discipline.

Some nurses have suggested that since nurses will need to work more within a multidisciplinary perspective, nursing theory language limits interdisciplinary communication and collaboration and prevents the formation of interdisciplinary partnerships. However, collaboration depends on the ability of each discipline to clearly communicate their professional focus and the nature and extent of their contribution to the common shared goal. If the nurse is using only knowledge derived from other disciplines such as medicine or psychology, the nurse would have little to contribute to the care of the patient distinct from what physicians and psychologists contribute. If nurses use a nursing theory to guide assessment, the nurse would have information distinct from any other member of the team and therefore contribute to a new understanding of the patient's situation that likely is not otherwise addressed. There are also nurses who argue that we should abandon nursing theory because other health care professionals do not understand it and argue that all health care professionals should speak the same language. Such statements really translate into "we all need to speak the language of medicine." Why should the nurses relinquish their valued knowledge base? Other health care professionals, such as psychologists and social workers, do not abandon their theoretical heritage when working with the multidisciplinary team. Rather, other professionals translate abstract theoretical concepts in a manner that those unfamiliar with the theory can understand.

Another concern expressed about the nature of theoretical language is the idea that "patients do not understand nursing theory jargon." Theoretical language or the language of nursing theory is not what is communicated to patients or to other health care professionals in practical situations. The concepts and terminology embedded within nursing theories guide conceptualization of nursing phenomena. Theory is a conceptual road map that organizes nursing knowledge.

Theorizing is a way of *thinking* and *being* in nursing situations. Some critics of nursing theory believe basing nursing practice on nursing theory is too narrow and that nursing is more than what is articulated in nursing theories. It is the use of non-nursing theory that limits nursing, not the use of nursing theory. Practicing from a non-nursing theory base potentially limits the full extent of a nurse's contribution to promoting the health in persons needing nursing care. All nursing theories extend beyond any borrowed biomedical, psychological, sociological, or even critical theories. Because nursing theories are consistent with nursing's metaparadigm (persons, health, environment, nursing, caring, transitions) and are holistic in nature, they provide a base for a practice more expansive than any particular sociological, psychological, biological, cultural, or spiritual theory (Table 4–6). Most nursing theories are inclusive of all these components while at the same time organizing them all into a coherent, systematic, logical, and scientific whole. Conceptualizing and understanding nursing through the lens of a nursing theory opens up new possibilities. Nurses who base their practice on an explicit nursing conceptual framework are assured that they "follow in Nightingale's footsteps and articulate what nursing is and what it is not" (Fawcett & Bourbonniere, 2001, p. 312).

Table 4–6 Selected Major Contemporary Nursing Conceptual Frameworks and Metaparadigm Concepts		
Conceptual Framework	**Metaparadigm Concepts**	**Definitions/Descriptions**
Peplau's Theory of Interpersonal Relations	Person	Man is an organism in an unstable environment. Human beings are reducible, one way or another. All behavior is purposeful and goal seeking. Humans act on the basis of the meaning of events (Peplau, 1952).
	Environment	Existing interpersonal forces outside the organism and in the context of culture from which mores, customs, and beliefs are acquired (Peplau, 1952).
	Health	Forward movement of personality and other ongoing human processes in the direction of creative, constructive, productive, personal, and community living (Peplau, 1952).
	Nursing	A significant, therapeutic, interpersonal process. Nursing is an educative instrument, a maturing force that functions cooperatively with other human processes that make health possible for individuals in communities (Peplau, 1952).
	Caring	The nurse–patient relationship is the primary human contact that is central in a fundamental way to providing nursing care (Peplau, 1997). Reframing empathic linkages occurs when the ability of the nurse, the patient, or both feel in the self the emotions experienced by the other in the same situation (Peplau, 1952).
	Transitions	The nurse–patient relationship is an interpersonal process, which moves through three phases: orientation, working, and termination phase. Termination occurs when the patient becomes self-reliant (Peplau, 1997).

Table 4–6 (continued)

Conceptual Framework	Metaparadigm Concepts	Definitions/Descriptions
Levine's Conservation Model	Person	A holistic being; wholeness is integrity. Integrity means that the person has freedom of choice and movement (Levine, 1991). Persons experience life as change through adaptation with the goal of conservation (Levine, 1989).
	Environment	The context in which we live our lives. The person cannot be described apart from their environment. We are active participants in the environment in that the person explores, seeks, and tests understanding of the world in which they inhabit. The nurse is an essential factor in the patient's environment. The interface between the individual and the environment is an orderly, sometimes predictable, but always a limited process (Levine, 1989, 1991)
	Health	The goal of conservation is health. Conservation is a product of adaptation. Homeostasis is a state of conservation (Levine, 1989).
	Nursing	The goal of nursing is to promote adaptation and maintain wholeness and involves nursing actions designed to conserve the patient's energy, structural integrity, personal identity, and social integrity (Levine, 1973).
	Caring	Nursing practice is a cascading repertoire of skill, knowledge, and compassion (Levine, 1989).
	Transitions	Nursing care must allow for progress and change and project into the future the patient's response to treatment (Levine, 1989). In the illness process, the daily flux of events causes a continuing pattern of change requiring revision of nursing care. Interventions must be designed so that they foster successful adaptation (Levine, 1973).
Johnson's Behavioral Systems Model	Person	The person is a behavioral system with patterned, repetitive, and purposeful ways of behaving that link the person to the environment (Johnson, 1980).
	Environment	All factors that are not part of the individual's behavioral system, but influence the system, some of which can be manipulated by the nurse to achieve the goal of health for the person (Johnson, 1980, 1990).
	Health	An elusive, dynamic state influenced by biological, psychological, and social factors. Health is reflected by the organization, interaction, interdependence, and integration of the subsystems of the behavioral system (Johnson, 1980, 1990).
	Nursing	An external force acting to preserve the organization of the patient's behavior by means of imposing regulatory mechanisms or providing resources while the patient is under stress (Johnson, 1980, 1990).
	Caring	If the person is unable to provide adequate protection, nurturance, and stimulation to his or her subsystem functions, those requirements must be supplied by other individuals or institutions (Johnson, 1990).

(continued)

Table 4–6   (continued)

Conceptual Framework	Metaparadigm Concepts	Definitions/Descriptions
	Transitions	Persons are active beings who adjust to their environment. Change occurs only when necessary of survival (Johnson, 1990).
Rogers' Science of Unitary Human Beings	Person	An irreducible, indivisible, pandimensional energy field identified by pattern and manifesting characteristics that are specific to the whole (Rogers, 1992).
	Environment	An irreducible, pandimensional energy field identified by pattern manifesting characteristics different from those of parts (Rogers, 1992).
	Health	Well-being is a value; it is not absolute and is an expression of the life process (Rogers, 1988, 1992).
	Nursing	A learned profession that is both a science and an art. Professional practice in nursing seeks to promote a symphonic mutual process in the patterning of human–environmental fields; facilitates knowing participation in change; strengthens the integrity of the human field; and promotes human well-being and betterment for all (Rogers, 1970, 1992).
	Caring	Nursing is a humanistic science and a compassionate concern for human beings (Rogers, 1970).
	Transitions	Change is continuous, innovative, unpredictable, rhythmical, mutual, and ever evolving toward increasing diversity of human and environmental field patterning (Rogers, 1988, 1992).
Orem's Self-Care Deficit Nursing Theory	Person	Persons in need of nursing care are unable to continuously maintain self-care in sustaining life and health, in recovering from disease or injury, or in coping with their effects. Patients are characterized by their therapeutic self-care demands, self-care agency, and basic conditioning factors (Orem, 2001).
	Environment	The environment encompasses physical, chemical, biologic features; socioeconomic features; and community features (Orem, 2001).
	Health	The ability to meet self-care demands that contribute to the maintenance and promotion of soundness or wholeness of developing human structures and bodily and mental functioning (Orem, 2001).
	Nursing	Nursing is indicated when patients have a self-care deficit. Nursing is attending to and serving others; providing close care of others unable to care for themselves; and helping such persons become sound in health and self-sufficient. The goal of nursing is to help the patient accomplish therapeutic self-care (Orem, 2001).
	Caring	Nursing is a form of care. Nurses are producers of care when they *do for* others. Care and concern for others is an element of human love, mature love. The active character of love is giving and always includes care, responsibility, respect, and knowledge. Caring occurs through the exercise of nursing agency by doing for, guiding, teaching, providing physical and psychological support, and creating an environment that supports development (Orem, 2001).

Table 4–6   (continued)

Conceptual Framework	Metaparadigm Concepts	Definitions/Descriptions
	Transitions	Persons are viewed developmentally as dynamic, ever changing and moving toward maturation and achievement of their potential. Nursing helps persons move toward responsible self-care by increasing independence in self-care actions and helping persons adjust to interruptions in self-care abilities (Orem, 2001).
King's Interaction Systems and Theory of Goal Attainment	Person	Human beings are social, sentient, rational, reacting, perceiving, spiritual, holistic, controlling, purposeful, action-orientated, and time-orientated (King, 1981; Sieloff, 2002).
	Environment	There are internal, external, health care, and social environments. The external environment is any social system in society. Social systems are dynamic forces that influence social interaction, perception, and health (King, 1981). Environment is a function of balance between internal and external interactions, in particular, the performance of activities of daily living depends on one's internal and external environments working in some sort of harmony and balance (King, 1990).
	Health	A dynamic life experience that implies continuous adjustment to stressors in the internal and external environment through optimum use of one's resources to achieve maximum potential for daily living (King, 1989).
	Nursing	Nursing is a helping profession that provides a service to meet a social need. The domains of nursing include the promotion of health, maintenance and restoration of health, care of the sick and injured, and care of the dying. Nursing is an interpersonal process of action, reaction, interaction, and transactions (King, 1981).
	Caring	Caring occurs in the process of perception, judgment, action, reaction, interaction, and transaction to attain mutual goals.
	Transitions	Change is constant and ongoing. Nursing functions to help persons, families, groups, and communities attain, maintain, and restore health so that they can function in their respective roles (King, 1981).
The Neuman Systems Model	Person	An open system that interacts with both internal and external environmental forces or stressors. Persons consist of a central core, lines of defense, and lines of resistance. Physiological, developmental, psychological, sociocultural, and spiritual variables make up the central core (Neuman, 2001).
	Environment	A vital arena that is germane to the system and its function: it includes internal, external, and the created environment. The environment may be viewed as all factors that affect and are affected by the system (Neuman, 2001).
	Health	Health is optimum system stability or the optimal state of wellness at a given time (Neuman, 2001).

(continued)

Table 4–6 *(continued)*

Conceptual Framework	Metaparadigm Concepts	Definitions/Descriptions
	Nursing	The major concern of nursing is to help the patient system attain, maintain, or retain stability between and among patient system variables and environmental stressors through primary, secondary, and tertiary prevention (Neuman, 2001).
	Caring	Caring is prevention as intervention and includes primary, secondary, and tertiary prevention (Neuman, 2001).
	Transitions	Humans are in constant change, moving toward a dynamic state of system stability or toward illness of varying degrees. The goal of the nurse is to guide the patient in conserving energy and to use energy as a force to move beyond the present in a way that preserves or enhances the patient's wellness level (Neuman, 2001).
The Roy Adaptation Model	Person	Humans are holistic, adaptive systems with internal processes (regulator and cognator) acting to maintain adaptation within for adaptive modes: physiological, self-concept, role function, and interdependence (Roy & Andrews, 1999).
	Environment	All conditions, circumstances, and influences surrounding and affecting development and behavior of persons or groups. Factors in the environment that affect persons are categorized as focal, contextual, and residual stimuli (Roy & Andrews, 1999).
	Health	Health is a state and process of being and becoming an integrated and whole person. Health ensues as humans continually adapt to stimuli (Roy & Andrews, 1999).
	Nursing	A health care profession that focuses on human life processes and patterns and emphasizes promotion of health for individuals, families, groups, and society as a whole. Nursing judgments are based on the assessment of stimuli and behaviors in each of the four adaptive modes, and interventions are planned and implemented to manage stimuli for promoting adaptation (Roy & Andrews, 1999).
	Caring	Persons have mutual relationships with the world and God. The nurse takes a values-based stance focusing on awareness, enlightenment, and faith. Nursing's concern is for the person as a total being. Caring occurs in the context of promoting adaptation for individuals and groups (Roy & Andrews, 1999).
	Transitions	Humans are in the process of constant change. Expanding the person's adaptive abilities facilitates person and environment transformation. Person and environment transformations are created in human consciousness (Roy & Andrews, 1999).
Parse's Human Becoming Theory	Person	The human being is in a continuous process of becoming inseparable from health and the universe. The person: is an open system in mutual process with the universe co-creating patterns of relating with others; lives at multidimensional realms of the universe all at once, freely choosing ways of becoming as meaning is given in situations (Parse, 1992, 1998).

Table 4–6 *(continued)*

Conceptual Framework	Metaparadigm Concepts	Definitions/Descriptions
Parse's Human Becoming Theory (*continued*)	Environment	The environment is the universe, which is multidimensional, and co-evolves in mutual process with human beings (Parse, 1992, 1998).
	Health	Health is structuring meaning, co-creating rhythmical patterns of relating, and co-transcending with the possibles. Health is a personal commitment, a process of becoming, a continuously changing process of choosing and living one's valued priorities (Parse, 1992, 1998).
	Nursing	Nursing is a basic science whose processes include illuminating meaning through explicating, synchronizing rhythms through dwelling, and mobilizing transcendence through moving beyond (Parse, 1992, 1998).
	Caring	True presence is a special way of "being with" in which the nurse is attentive to moment-to-moment changes in meaning as she or he bears witness to the person's or group's own living of value priorities. Bearing witness as an interpersonal art, "an intentional reflective love" and a free-flowing attentiveness. The nurse offers presence in the patient's universe unconditionally, is open to the reality the patient lives, and is available to bear witness without judging or labeling (Parse, 1998).
	Transitions	Change is continuous. Persons are in a continuous process of becoming. Mobilizing transcendence is moving beyond the meaning moment with what is not yet. Moving beyond is propelling with envisioned possibles of transforming (Parse, 1998).

Practice Methods

Methods provide a means or systematic way of accomplishing something. Typically, methods have processes, techniques, and orderly components that are characteristic to a discipline (*American Heritage Dictionary*, 2000). Mature disciplines are characterized by research and practice methods that are unique, specific, and distinct (Butcher, 2001; Parse, 2001). In nursing, there are specific research and practice methods that have been derived from particular nursing conceptual frameworks. While the conceptual framework frames the nurse's thinking about phenomena by identifying the focus, purpose, critical thinking, decision-making, and organizing information, the practice method is designed to guide all aspects of nursing practice.

The practice method most familiar to nursing students is the nursing process. The nursing process is a systematic problem-solving approach to practice that was first identified in 1955 by Lydia Hall. The term also appeared in Orlando's 1961 text, *The Dynamic Nurse–Patient Relationship*. It is important to note that the nursing process is not unique to nursing. It is identical to any problem-solving method; however, the nursing process has different terminology identifying each step of the process. The nursing process is not a theory or conceptual framework. Rather, conceptual frameworks and theories provide the scientific rationale and understanding for guiding each step in the nursing process. Unfortunately, most students learn the nursing process in isolation of a nursing conceptual framework and come to believe that pathophysiology or other borrowed theories from medicine, psychology, and sociology provide the theoretical underpinning for guiding most aspects of the nursing process. The nursing process is most consistent with the philosophical beliefs and worldview of the totality paradigm but is not consistent with the beliefs articulated in the simultaneity paradigm. Therefore, conceptual frameworks and theories within the simultaneity paradigm have their own distinct practice methods.

Nursing Process Practice Method: Totality Paradigm

In 1967, Yura and Walsh wrote the first comprehensive book describing the components of the nursing process. In 1973, the American Nurses Association adopted and legitimized the nursing process in the *Standards of Nursing Practice*. The manual of the Joint Commission on Accreditation of Healthcare Organizations requires documentation according to the nursing process. Furthermore, since 1975, the state board NCLEX exams test knowledge of all five major components of the nursing process.

Nursing educators originally developed the nursing process as a teaching guide to assist students to learn critical thinking skills essential for making appropriate clinical judgments concerning patient care. The nursing process consists of five components, each with several phases that are interactive and sequential (Kenney, 1995). **Assessment** "is a continuous process of collecting relevant data about the patient's human responses, health status, strengths, and concerns" (Kenney, 1995, p. 10). Gordon's (1994) eclectic multifocal model for guiding nursing assessment based on 11 functional health patterns offers nurses a way of assessing patients, families, groups, or communities from a unique nursing perspective that can also be applied to many of the nursing conceptual frameworks and theories in the totality paradigm. The functional health patterns identified by Gordon (1994) are: (a) health perception–health management; (b) nutritional–metabolic; (c) elimination; (d) activity–exercise; (e) cognitive–perceptual; (f) sleep–rest; (g) self-perception–self-concept; (h) sexuality–reproductive; (i) coping–stress tolerance; and (j) value belief pattern. In her work, Gordon defines each pattern and provides questions and direction to guide assessment and patient examination according to each of the 11 patterns. Assessment data are then interpreted within the selected nursing conceptual framework.

Nursing diagnosis is the analysis and synthesis of data to identify patterns and compare them to norms and conceptual frameworks as a means to recognize abnormal patterns, make inferences, or assign meaning to the problem (Kenney, 1995). Since 1973, NANDA (North American Nursing Diagnosis Association) has guided the process of identifying and naming the phenomena that nurses diagnose and treat as a means for creating a common language identifying the focus of nursing care, thereby differentiating nursing from medicine. NANDA defines nursing diagnosis as "a clinical judgment about individual, family, or community responses to actual or potential health problems/life processes. Nursing diagnoses provide the basis for selection of nursing interventions to achieve outcomes for which the nurse is accountable" (NANDA, 2001, p. 245). NANDA's latest work, *Nursing Diagnoses: Definitions and Classifications, 2001–2002*, features 155 nursing diagnoses, their definitions, defining characteristics, and related-to factors. The new edition also features "Taxonomy II," and new multiaxial health patterns framework that organizes the diagnoses into domains according to Gordon's Functional Health Patterns (NANDA, 2001).

Planning, the third step in the nursing process, occurs when the patient and the nurse identify the expected outcomes and actions to correct the nursing diagnosis (Kenney, 1995). Planning includes prioritizing the patient's concerns, determining desired health outcomes, selecting appropriate nursing interventions, and designing a plan of care based on scientific knowledge both from nursing and theories from other disciplines relevant to nursing care.

Since 1991, a research team at the University of Iowa has been developing a classification of nursing outcomes. In the second edition of *Nursing Outcomes Classification (NOC)* published in 2000, 260 "nurse-sensitive" outcomes have been identified and defined. A "nursing-sensitive patient outcome" is defined "as a variable patient or family caregiver state, behavior, or perception that is responsive to nursing interventions" (Johnson, Maas, & Moorehead, 2000, p. 25). Each of the 260 outcomes have a label name, a definition, a list of indicators to evaluate patient status in relation to the outcome, and a five-point scale to measure patient status (Johnson, Maas, & Moorehead, 2000). All NOC outcomes have been linked to NANDA nursing diagnoses, making the NOC classification system a powerful and useful tool for identifying appropriate nursing outcomes when planning nursing care.

Implementation is performing the nursing actions designated in the plan by the patient, nurse, and others. Yura and Walsh (1988) defined implementation, the fourth phase of the nursing process, as "the initiation and completion of actions necessary to accomplish the defined goal of optimal wellness for the patient" (p. 154). The implementation phase for the nursing process relies heavily on intellectual, interpersonal, critical thinking, and technical skills of the nurse. Nursing interventions are first identified in the planning phase but are carried out in practice during the implementation phase.

Since 1987, research to develop a vocabulary and nursing intervention classification system (NIC) has been conducted at the University of Iowa by a team led by Joanne McCloskey and Gloria Bulechek. A nursing intervention is "any treatment, based on clinical judgment and knowledge, that a nurse performs to enhance patient/patient outcomes" (Iowa Intervention Project, 2000, p. xix). The implementation phase of the nursing process is enhanced by the use of NIC since the NIC offers a comprehensive, standardized classification of 486 interventions that are linked to both NANDA nursing diagnoses and NOC nursing outcomes (Johnson, Bulechek, McCloskey Dochterman, Maas, & Moorhead, 2001). Each NIC intervention consists of a label name, a definition, and a set of activities that indicate the actions needed for delivering the intervention.

The final phase of the nursing process, **evaluation**, is the process of comparing the patient's current health status with the patient's expected outcomes and determining the patient's progress or lack of progress toward achievement of the outcomes (Kenney, 1995). The use of NOC outcomes allows the nurse to measure the outcome status at any point on a continuum from most negative to most positive, as well as identify changes in the patient's status at different points of time (McCloskey & Bulechek, 2000). The use of criterion-based tools such as the NOC facilitates the determination of the degree of the patient's progress toward desired health outcomes and provides direction to revising the plan of care.

Nursing Classification Systems and the Nursing Process

As early as 1989, Fawcett and Carino (1989) recognized classification systems or standardized vocabularies and nomenclatures as a hallmark of success in nursing practice. Collaboration in patient care requires the sharing of each discipline's unique perspective and is characterized by mutual trust and respect for the contribution of each discipline (Iowa Outcomes Project, 2000).

Today, nursing has a number of classification systems, the most prominent being NANDA, NIC, and NOC. There are indications that NIC and NOC are becoming the standard for nursing practice much in the way NANDA has become the standard for nursing diagnoses. Classification systems are increasingly being implemented into clinical practice settings, used in nursing curriculums, and presented in nursing textbooks. Vendors that develop computer information systems for health care systems and hospitals are increasingly including NANDA–NIC–NOC as part of the nursing documentation system. NANDA–NIC–NOC provides the content focus for the nursing process and therefore serves to identify and communicate the unique function of nursing consistent with the values and beliefs of the totality paradigm. Along with nursing conceptual frameworks and theories, nursing classification systems are the language of the nursing discipline.

The professional languages of nursing classification systems contribute to identifying the disciplinary boundaries of nursing. They supply the vocabulary for communicating nursing diagnoses, interventions, and expected outcomes. Standardized languages help clarify nursing's role to other health care professionals, patients, and to the public. Johnson et al. (2001) point out that NANDA, NIC, and NOC: (a) allows for the collection and analysis of information documenting nursing's contribution to patient care; (b) facilitates the evaluation of patient care; (c) fosters the development of nursing knowledge; (d) facilitates teaching decision-making to nursing students; (e) allows for the development of electronic clinical information systems and the electronic patient record; and (f) provides information for the formation of organizational and public health policy concerning health and nursing care.

It is important to understand that nursing classification systems are consistent with the perspective of the totality paradigm, but by nature, the nursing process and classifications systems are not theoretical. How one conceptualizes the nursing diagnoses, interventions, and outcomes will be specific to each nursing conceptual framework and theory. The traditional nursing process is most consistent with Roy's Adaptation Model, King's Interaction Systems, and Johnson's Behavioral Systems Model, while other nursing conceptual frameworks and theories within the totality paradigm have developed practice models similar to the nursing process. For example, within Roy's Adaptation Model, all steps of the nursing process are conceptualized by Roy's concepts of stimuli, behavior, and four adaptive modes. The goal of nursing is to promote adaptation within each of the four adaptive modes. Initially, the nurse assesses behaviors that may be observable or nonobservable action or reaction to a stimulus. Assessment of behaviors focuses on the four adaptive modes: physiological, self-concept/group identity, interdependence, and role function modes. Once behaviors are identified that are not supportive of adaptation, the second phase of assessment focuses on identifying focal, contextual, and residual stimuli in each of the four modes that arise for the internal and external environment that are causing or contributing to the ineffective behavior (Roy & Andrews, 1999). The NANDA nursing diagnosis statement is an actual or potential problem related to adaptation and specifies the behaviors that led to the diagnosis by relating the stimuli (related-to factors) to the adaptive problem (human response). The goals focusing on promoting adaptation and outcome statement (NOC) are conceptualized behaviors that can be changed through interventions (NIC) that are designed to change the stimuli or strengthen the adaptive process. Finally, evaluation determines how well the person has moved toward adaptation (Roy & Andrews, 1999).

Nursing Practice Methods: Simultaneity Paradigm

New world views require new ways of thinking, sciencing, languaging, and practicing. It is important to note that the nursing process practice method and classification systems are not consistent with the assumptions and beliefs articulated in the simultaneity paradigm (Butcher, 2001). In early writings, Rogers (1970) did refer to nursing process and nursing diagnosis. However, in later years, she asserted that nursing diagnoses were not consistent with her scientific system. Rogers (quoted in Smith, 1988) stated:

> Nursing diagnosis is a static term that is quite inappropriate for a dynamic system . . . it [nursing diagnosis] is an outdated part of an old world view, and I think by the turn of the century, there is going to be new ways of organizing knowledge (p. 83).

Nursing diagnoses are normative, particularistic, and reductionistic labels describing cause-and-effect (i.e., "related-to") relationships inconsistent with the view of a person as an irreducible whole more than and different from the sum of parts. Nursing diagnoses are judgments based on societal norms for what is considered healthy and what is a deviation from health. Within the simultaneity paradigm, health is a value that reflects the choices that each person makes. The nursing process is a stepwise sequential process inconsistent with this nonlinear or a causal view of reality.

The term *intervention* is not consistent with practice within conceptual frameworks in the simultaneity paradigm. Intervention means to "come, appear, or lie between two things" (*American Heritage Dictionary*, 2000, p. 916). From a simultaneity perspective, persons and their environment are integral and mutually

related. No in between exists; human and environmental fields are inseparable. The nurse and the patient are inseparable and interconnected. The idea of outcomes infers predictability. Therefore, outcomes are inconsistent with the simultaneity paradigm's notion that the universe is characterized by unpredictability (Butcher, 1997). As a way to contrast how radically different nursing practice is when practiced from the perspective of conceptual frameworks in the simultaneity paradigm, two practice methods are briefly described.

HUMAN BECOMING PRACTICE METHODOLOGY

Each practice method derived from a conceptual framework in the simultaneity paradigm is consistent with that frameworks assumptions, concepts, and principles. For example, within the Human Becoming School of Thought, the goal of practice is quality of life from the person's perspective (Parse, 1998). Mitchell (2002) explains that the essence of practice is to make a commitment to be truly present with others and to bear witness and participate with another's unique process of becoming. The nurse respects each individual's or families' view of quality and does not attempt to change that view to be consistent with their own perspective. The nurse practices "true presence" by being with the person to explore the depth of ideas, events, and issues.

According to Parse (1998), nursing practice consists of the following dimensions and processes: illuminating meaning, synchronizing rhythms, and mobilizing transcendence (pp. 69–70). The dimensions and processes are not sequential steps, but rather happen all at once. Nurses have opportunities to be truly present with the person, family, or group and to participate with them during times of change, struggle, upset, uncertainty, recovery, and hope (Mitchell, 2002). Rather than making a nursing diagnosis, the nurse writes and documents a Personal Health Pattern Description, which conveys the person's patterns of becoming related to his or her health situation. The nurse accepts what the person or family says or does as the meaning of the situation and moves with the person or family without judging, labeling, or specifying a nurse-generated change. Nursing actions would flow from the person's areas of concern and interest. The effectiveness of nursing practice is evaluated by asking the person about his or her satisfaction with care (Mitchell, 2002). While the nurse may be engaged in some traditional aspects of nursing practice by virtue of the "job description," these traditional medically orientated functions are not unique or specific to nursing.

Nurses report that nursing practice guided by the Human Becoming Theory does not take more time; however, the way the nurse spends time with patients changes dramatically. Nurses who practice Human Becoming Theory work in the same hospitals and with all the same pressures regarding performance and efficiency as nurses who practice in the traditional way (Mitchell, 2002).

SCIENCE OF UNITARY HUMAN BEINGS PRACTICE METHODOLOGY

The focus of nursing care guided by Rogers' (1970, 1988, 1992) Science of Unitary Human Beings is (a) recognizing *pattern manifestation knowing and appreciation* and (b) *voluntary mutual patterning*. Both processes are designed to facilitate the patient's ability to participate knowingly in change, harmonize the person–environment relationship, and promote the actualization of healing potentials (Butcher, 2001).

Pattern is the distinguishing feature of the human–environmental field. All experiences, perceived and expressed, are manifestations of patterning. During the process of pattern manifestation knowing and appreciation, the nurse and patient are equal participants. Patients may be persons, families, and/or communities. Intentionality is expressed by approaching nursing situations with the intent to facilitate human betterment. It is important to create an atmosphere of openness and freedom so patients can participate. Approaching the care situation with an appreciation of the uniqueness of each person, unconditional love, compassion, and empathy can help create an atmosphere of openness and healing (Butcher, 2001).

Throughout pattern manifestation knowing and appreciation processes, the nurse is open to and uses multiple forms of knowing, including intuition, meditative insights, and tacit knowing. Since all information about the patient–environment–health situation is relevant, various health assessment tools such as the comprehensive holistic assessment tool developed by Dossey, Keegan, Guzzetta, and Kolkmeirer (1995) may also be useful. However, all information must be interpreted within a unitary context, which refers to all information being interconnected and inseparable from the environmental context, unfolding rhythmically, acausally, and reflecting the whole. Data are not divided into physical, psychological, social, spiritual, or cultural categories. The focus on experiences, perceptions, and expressions is a synthesis, which is more than, and different from, the sum of the parts.

More importantly, this unitary perspective of nursing practice leads to an appreciation of new information that may not be considered, using other conceptual approaches to nursing practice. For example, pattern information concerning time perception, sense of rhythm or movement, sense of connectedness with the environment, ideas of oneself, and sense of integrity are relevant indicators of human–environment–health potentialities (Madrid & Winstead-Fry, 1986). A person's hopes and dreams, communication patterns, sleep–rest rhythms, comfort–discomfort, waking–beyond waking experiences, and degree of knowing participation in change provide important information regarding thoughts and feelings concerning a health situation.

The nurse synthesizes all pattern information into a meaningful pattern profile. Usually, the profile is a narrative that describes the properties, features, and qualities of the human–environment–health situation. It reflects the essence of the patient's experiences, perceptions, and expressions. The pattern profile may also include diagrams, poems, listings, phrases, and/or metaphors (Cowling, 1997). Interpretations of any measurement tools also may be incorporated into the pattern profile.

Voluntary mutual patterning is an ongoing process in which both the nurse and patients are changed with each encounter. The process is voluntary and intentional in that the nurse approaches each nursing situation with the *intention* to promote well-being and human betterment (Barrett, 1998). Rogers (1988, 1992) placed great emphasis on what is traditionally viewed as holistic noninvasive modalities. Therapeutic touch, guided imagery, humor, dialogue, affirmations, music, massage, journaling, exercise, nutrition, reminiscence, aroma, artwork, meditation, storytelling, literature, poetry, movement, and dance are examples of voluntary mutual patterning strategies. Sharing knowledge through health education also has the potential to enhance knowing participation in change. Regardless of which combination of voluntary patterning strategies is used, the intention is for patients to actualize their potential related to human well-being and betterment.

Embracing the Unique Nature of Nursing

Whether conscious or unconscious, all nurses practice from a conceptual frame of reference. Unfortunately, the practicing nurse's conceptual frame often is grounded in an untested and unscientific implicit personal model of nursing or a perspective grounded in

Nursing theory–based practice is a hallmark of excellence in nursing practice. Some of the barriers that have been identified that may limit the implementation of nursing theory–based practice include: not being taught nursing theory and its value to the profession and significance in guiding practice; devaluing the work of women and nurse theorists; anti-intellectualism among nurses; the unfamiliar language embedded within nursing theories; and the false belief nursing theories are not specific enough to guide research or practice. What additional barriers do you believe limit nurses' ability to base their practice on a nursing theory? For each barrier, identify two strategies that can be employed to overcome the barriers limiting the realization of nursing theory–based practice.

another discipline such as medicine. The realization of theory-guided practice begins with a choice each practicing nurse must make. Nurses can choose to base their practice within the biomedical model, thereby reducing nursing to the traditional domain of medical practice and function as junior doctors (Meleis, 1993), mini-doctors (Barnum, 1998), or physician extenders (Sandelowski, 1999) engaging in pseudomedicine (Kendrick, 1997) and nursing qua medicine (Watson, 1996), or nurses can choose to embrace the knowledge generated by nurse theorists.

It's time for nursing to end its romance with non-nursing models as guides for nursing practice (Fawcett, 1999). Nursing conceptual frameworks and theories collectively identify the focus of the discipline and provide a holistic "discipline-specific lens for viewing clinical situations" (Fawcett, 2002, p. 468). Theory gives meaning to knowledge to improve practice by describing, explaining, and predicting phenomena of concern. Kuhn (1970) asserted that conceptual frameworks and "paradigms of a scientific discipline primarily prepare students for practice as members of that professional community" (p. 11). Students studying to enter a professional discipline are introduced to the conceptual frameworks and theories as an orientation to the approaches used in the practice of the discipline. After students are introduced to a variety of theoretical approaches to nursing practice, they must begin to learn how the nursing conceptual frameworks and models are used to guide all aspects of nursing practice, for it is "by studying them and practicing with them, the members of their corresponding community learn their trade" (Kuhn, 1970, p. 43). If a discipline's content and contribution to the betterment of society is not distinguishable from other disciplines, then the discipline's continued existence may be questioned.

Nursing theory–guided practice is a hallmark of excellence in professional nursing practice (Fawcett, 1999, 2002). "Nursing theory–guided practice is based on theory that is specific to the discipline of nursing, explicitly rooted in a philosophy of nursing, and intended solely to guide nursing practice and research" (Cody, 1994b, p. 145). Using nursing theory to guide nursing practice distinguishes nursing from a trade (Anderson, 1995), and grounding nursing practice in the distinctive knowledge base as articulated in nursing conceptual frameworks and theories ensures that our care is based on a solid scientific foundation. More importantly, nursing theory–guided practice distinguishes nursing as an autonomous health profession and distinguishes nursing's contribution to the health of society from other health care professionals (Parse, 1995). "If we want to ensure the survival of our discipline, all of us must fall in love with nursing [knowledge] *now* [italic added] and develop a passion for the destiny of the discipline of nursing" (Fawcett, 1999, p. 12). If not *now*, when?

TRANSITION INTO PRACTICE

Transitioning to Nursing Theory–Based Practice

The first step in choosing a nursing theory as one's disciplinary lens is to have the courage to make the decision to embrace nursing's distinctive and unique body of knowledge. Exploring a variety of nursing conceptual frameworks enables one to select a conceptual framework that is most congruent with their values and perspective of nursing. Secondly, nurses need to recognize that the adoption of a conceptual model of nursing means an adjustment in thinking about nursing and clinical situations. Essentially, the switch from one conceptual frame of reference to another involves a switch from one meaning perspective or frame of reference to another. Basing one's practice on a nursing conceptual framework requires an initial investment of learning new theory to complete the shift from one frame of reference to another. When one makes a commitment to adopt a specific conceptual framework, effort must be directed toward immersing oneself in the literature describing and demonstrating the frameworks application to specific practice situations.

In selecting a particular conceptual framework, one should consider their personal values and beliefs about nursing. It would be helpful to write out your beliefs about each of the metaparadigm concepts, and after reviewing a variety of conceptual frameworks, select two or three that best fit with your own values about the nature of nursing. Based on her experience of implementing nursing conceptual frameworks in a number of practice settings in Toronto, Canadian nurse Martha Rogers (1992) identified nine phases one can expect when experiencing a transformation from one conceptual frame of reference to another: stability, dissonance, confusion, dwelling with uncertainty, saturation, synthesis, resolution, reconceptualization, and return to stability. The initial period of *stability* is disrupted when the notion of nursing theory–based practice or changing from one nursing conceptual framework to another is first introduced. *Dissonance* arises when the nurse examines and compares his or her current image of nursing to a new vision of nursing as articulated within the new conceptual model or theory. Often, a phase of *confusion* follows as the nurse initially struggles to learn more about the theory and understand its implications for chang-

ing his or her view of practicing nursing. Nurses may experience anger, anxiousness, and feeling overwhelmed with trying to understand the new perspective, while at the same time realizing their previous way of understanding nursing makes sense. The phase of confusion is usually followed by a dwelling with uncertainty as the nurse realizes that the confusion is not due to personal inadequacy, but a normal part of the process when changing from one theoretical perspective to another. *Saturation* occurs as the nurse focuses on understanding the new framework while feeling a need to distance oneself from the process of transformation. As the fog of confusion lifts, *synthesis* occurs through flashes of insight into understanding the new frameworks, which leads to a new sense of understanding and clarity. The moment of clarity moves one toward a deeper and more coherent understanding of the theory. Reading various applications of the theory in various practice situations facilitates synthesis. Reviewing applications in various nursing practice situations highlights the flexibility of the framework as you see its utility in these areas (Alligood, 2002). *Resolution* is characterized by feeling comfortable with the new conceptual framework as feelings of dissonance, discontent, and anxiety dissipate. Often nurses in this phase feel changed, enlightened, and empowered by practicing within a new conceptual frame of reference. Finally, *reconceptualization* occurs as the nurse consciously reconceptualizes nursing practice using the new nursing theory leading to a return to a new phase of *stability* characterized by professional nursing theory–based practice.

KEY POINTS

1. The explicit use of nursing knowledge is a *hallmark* of nursing practice that distinguishes nursing as an autonomous health profession and represents nursing's unique contribution to the health care system.

2. Upon completion of their education, baccalaureate nurses should be able to: (a) understand how differing nursing conceptual models view the metaparadigm concepts; (b) conceptualize nursing as nursing theory–based practice; (c) utilize theoretical thinking grounded in nursing conceptual frameworks in applying nursing the process; (d) articulate the practice–theory–research cycle; (e) use theoretical thinking grounded in nursing models to conceptualize components of the research process; and (f) identify the goal of research as theory building or theory testing.

3. The definition of nursing as the study of caring for persons experiencing human–environment–health transitions links six metaparadigm concepts identified in this chapter.

4. Three major philosophical schools have influenced nursing knowledge development: empirical-analytic, phenomenological-hermeneutic, and critical social theory. Each of these major schools of philosophy has led to unique and distinctive forms of knowledge that informs nursing practice.

5. Nurses use empirical, ethical, aesthetic, and personal knowing in every nursing situation.

6. Nursing has two major paradigms in nursing: totality paradigm and the simultaneity paradigm.

7. Conceptual models of nursing are explicit and formal presentations of an image of nursing that are designed to guide all aspects of nursing practice, research, and education.

8. The nursing process is the dominant nursing practice model in the totality paradigm.

9. The professional languages of nursing classification systems contribute to identifying the disciplinary boundaries of nursing and supply the vocabulary for communicating nursing diagnoses, interventions, and expected outcomes.

10. If a discipline's content and contribution to the betterment of society is not distinguishable from other disciplines, then the discipline's continued existence may be questioned.

11. Nursing theory–based practice is a hallmark of excellence in professional nursing practice.

EXPLORE MediaLink

Critical thinking questions, essay questions, key terms, web links, activities, NCLEX review questions, and more interactive resources can be found on the Companion Website at www.prenhall.com/haynes. Click on Chapter 4 to select activities for this chapter.

REFERENCES

Allen, D. (1985). Nursing research and social control: Alternative models of science that emphasize understanding and emancipation. *Image: The Journal of Nursing Scholarship, 17*, 59–64.

Allen, D. G. (1995). Hermeneutics: Philosophical traditions and nursing practice research. *Nursing Science Quarterly, 8*, 174–182.

Allen, D. G., Benner, P., & Diekelman, N. K. (1986). Three paradigms for nursing research: Methodological implications. In P. Chinn (Ed.), *Nursing research methodology: Issues and implications.* Rockville, MD: Aspen Systems.

Alligood, M. R. (2002). Philosophies, models, and theories: Critical thinking structures. In M. R. Alligood & A. Marriner-Tomey (Eds.), *Nursing theory: Utilization & application* (pp. 41–61). St. Louis, MO: Mosby.

Alligood, M. R., & Marriner-Tomey, A. (2002). *Nursing theory: Utilization & application.* St. Louis, MO: Mosby.

American Association of Colleges of Nursing. (1998). *The essentials of baccalaureate education for professional nursing practice.* Washington, DC: Author.

American Heritage Dictionary (2000). Fourth Edition. Boston: Houghton Mifflin.

American Nurses Association. (1965). Educational preparation for nurse practitioners and assistants of nurses. *American Journal of Nursing, 65*(12), 106–111.

American Nurses Association. (1980). *Nursing's social policy statement.* Washington, DC: Author.

American Nurses Association. (1995). *Nursing's social policy statement.* Washington, DC: Author.

Anderson, C. A. (1995). Scholarship: How important is it? *Nursing Outlook, 43*, 247–248.

Auger, J. R. (1976). *Behavioral systems and nursing.* Englewood Cliffs, NJ: Prentice Hall.

Barnum, B. S. (1998). The advanced nurse practitioner: Struggling toward a conceptual framework. *Nursing Leadership Forum, 3*, 14–17.

Barrett, E. A. M. (1998). A Rogerian practice methodology for health patterning. *Nursing Science Quarterly, 11*, 136–138.

Benner, P. (1984). *From novice to expert: Excellence and power in clinical nursing practice.* Menlo Park, CA: Addison-Wesley.

Benner, P., & Wrubel, J. (1989). *The primacy of caring: Stress and coping in health and illness.* Reading, MA: Addison-Wesley.

Boutain, D. M. (1999). Critical nursing scholarship: Exploring critical social theory with African American studies. *Advances in Nursing Science, 21*(4), 37–47.

Boykin, A., & Schoenhofer, S. (1993). *Nursing as caring: A model for transforming practice.* New York: National League for Nursing Press.

Boykin, A., & Schoenhofer, S. (2001). Nursing as caring. In M. Parker (Ed.), *Nursing theories and nursing practice* (pp. 391–402). Philadelphia, PA: F. A. Davis.

Butcher, H. K. (1997). Energy field disturbance. In G. K. McFarland & E. A. McFarlane (Eds.), *Nursing diagnosis & intervention* (3rd ed.) (pp. 22–33). St. Louis, MO: Mosby.

Butcher, H. K. (2001). Nursing science in the new millennium: Practice and research within Roger's science of unitary human beings. In M. Parker (Ed.), *Nursing theories in research and practice* (pp. 205–226). Philadelphia, PA: F. A. Davis.

Campbell, J., & Bunting, S. (1991). Voices and paradigms: Perspectives on critical and feminist theory in nursing. *Advances in Nursing Science, 13*(3), 1–15.

Carper, B. (1978). Fundamental patterns of knowing. *Advances in Nursing Science, 1*(1), 13–23.

Chinn, P. L., & Jacobs, M. (1983). *Theory & nursing: A systematic approach.* St. Louis, MO: Mosby.

Chinn, P. L., & Kramer, M. K. (1999). *Theory and nursing: Integrated knowledge development* (5th ed.). St. Louis, MO: Mosby.

Chinn, P. L., & Wheeler, C. (1985). Feminism and nursing. *Nursing Outlook, 33*(2), 74–77.

Cody, W. K. (1994a). The language of nursing science: If not now, when? *Nursing Science Quarterly, 7,* 98–99.

Cody, W. K. (1994b) Nursing theory-guided practice: What it is and what it is not. *Nursing Science Quarterly, 7,* 144–145.

Cody, W. K. (1997). Of tombstones, milestones, and gemstones: A retrospective and prospective on nursing theory c. 1997. *Nursing Science Quarterly, 10*(1), 3–5.

Cody, W. K. (2000). Paradigm shift or paradigm drift? A meditation on commitment and transcendence. *Nursing Science Quarterly, 13,* 93–102.

Cody, W. K., & Mitchell, G. J. (2002). Nursing knowledge and human science revisited: Practical and political considerations. *Nursing Science Quarterly, 15,* 4–13.

Cowling, W. R. (1997). Pattern appreciation: The unitary science/practice of reaching essence. In M. Madrid (Ed.), *Patterns of Rogerian knowing* (pp. 129–142). New York: National League for Nursing.

DeKeyser, F. G., & Medoff-Cooper, B. (2002). A non-theorist's perspective on nursing theory: Issues in the 1990s. *Scholarly Inquiry for Nursing Practice: An International Journal, 15,* 329–341.

DiBartolo, M. C. (1998). Philosophy of science in doctoral education revisited. *Journal of Professional Nursing, 14*(6), 350–360.

Donaldson, S. K., & Crowley, D. (1978). The discipline of nursing: *Nursing Outlook, 26,* 113–120.

Dossey, B., Keegan, L., Guzzetta, C., & Kolkmeirer, L. (1995). *Holistic nursing: A handbook for practice.* Gaithersberg, MD: Aspen.

Fawcett, J. (1984). *Analysis and evaluation of conceptual models of nursing.* Philadelphia, PA: F. A. Davis.

Fawcett, J. (1996). On requirements for a metaparadigm: An invitation to dialogue. *Nursing Science Quarterly, 9,* 94–97.

Fawcett, J. (1997). The structural hierarchy of nursing knowledge: Components and their definitions. In I. King & J. Fawcett (Eds.), *The language of nursing theory and metatheory* (pp. 11–17). Indianapolis, IN: Sigma Theta Tau, International.

Fawcett, J. (1999). The state of nursing science: Hallmarks of the 20th and 21st centuries. *Nursing Science Quarterly, 12,* 311–315.

Fawcett, J. (2000). *Analysis and evaluation of contemporary nursing knowledge: Nursing models and theories.* Philadelphia, PA: F. A. Davis.

Fawcett, J. (2002). Conceptual models of nursing, nursing theories, and nursing practice: Future directions. In M. R. Alligood & A. Marriner-Tomey (Eds.), *Nursing theory: Utilization & application* (2nd ed.) (pp. 465–481). St. Louis, MO: Mosby.

Fawcett, J., & Bourbonniere, M. G. (2001). Utilization of nursing knowledge and the future of the discipline. In N. L. Chaska (Ed.), *The nursing profession: Tomorrow and beyond.* Thousand Oaks, CA: Sage.

Fawcett, J., & Carino, C. (1989). Hallmarks of success in nursing practice. *Advances in Nursing Science, 11*(4), 1–8.

Fitzpatrick, J., & Whall, A. (1983). *Conceptual models of nursing: Analysis and application.* Bowie, MD: Brady.

George, J. B. (2002). *Nursing theories: The base for professional nursing practice.* Upper Saddle River, NJ: Prentice Hall.

Gordon, M. (1994). *Nursing diagnosis: Process and application* (3rd ed.). St. Louis, MO: Mosby.

Hardy, M. E. (1978). Perspectives on nursing theory. *Advances in Nursing Science, 1*(1), 37–48.

Henderson, V., (1960). *Basic principles of nursing care* (pamphlet prepared for the International Council of Nurses). Geneva, Switzerland: International Council of Nurses.

Johnson, B. M., & Webber, P. B. (2001). *An introduction to theory and reasoning in nursing.* Philadelphia, PA: Lippincott.

Johnson, D. E. (1959). A philosophy of nursing. *Nursing Outlook, 7*(4), 198–200.

Johnson, D. E. (1980). The behavioral system model for nursing. In J. Riehl and C. Roy (Eds.), *Conceptual models for nursing practice* (2nd ed.) (pp. 23–32). New York: Appleton-Century-Crofts.

Johnson, D. E. (1990). The behavioral systems model for nursing. In M. Parker (Ed.), *Nursing theories in practice* (pp. 23–32). New York: National League for Nursing.

Johnson, M., Bulechek, G., McCloskey Dochterman, J., Maas, M., & Moorhead, S. (2001). *Nursing diagnoses, outcomes, & interventions: NANDA, NOC, and NIC linkages.* St. Louis, MO: Mosby.

Johnson, M,. Maas, M,. & Moorhead, S., (Eds.). (2000). *Nursing outcomes classification (NOC)* (2nd ed.). St. Louis, MO: Mosby.

McCloskey, J. C., & Bulechek, G. M., (Eds.). (2000). *Nursing intervention classification (NIC)* (3rd ed.). St. Louis, MO: Mosby.

Kendrick, K. (1997). What is advanced nursing? *Professional Nurse, 12*(10), 689.

Kenney, J. (1995). Relevance of theory-based nursing practice. In P. J. Christensen & J. W. Kenney (Eds.), *Nursing process: Application of conceptual models* (4th ed.) (pp. 3–23). St. Louis, MO: Mosby.

King, I. M. (1971). *Toward a theory for nursing.* New York: Wiley.

King, I. M. (1981). *A theory for nursing: Systems, concepts, processes.* New York: Wiley.

King, I. M. (1989). King's general systems framework and theory. In J. Riehl (Ed.), *Conceptual models for nursing practice* (3rd ed.) (pp. 149–158). New York: Appleton-Century-Crofts.

King, I. M. (1990). Health as the goal for nursing. *Nursing Science Quarterly, 3,* 123–128.

Kuhn, T. S. (1970). *The structure of scientific revolutions* (2nd ed.). Chicago, IL: Chicago University Press.

Leininger, M. (1991). *Culture care diversity and universality: A theory of nursing.* New York: National League for Nursing.

Levine, M. E. (1973). *Introduction to clinical nursing* (2nd ed.). Philadelphia, PA: F. A. Davis.

Levine, M. E, (1989). The four conservation principles: 20 years later. In J. Riehl (Ed.), *Conceptual models for nursing practice* (3rd ed.) (pp. 325–337). New York: Appleton-Century-Crofts.

Levine, M. E. (1991). The conservation principles: A model for health. In K. Schaefer & J. Pond (Eds.), *Levine's conservation model: A framework for nursing practice* (pp. 1–11). Philadelphia, PA: F. A. Davis.

Levine, M. E. (1995). The rhetoric of nursing theory. *Image: Journal of Nursing Scholarship, 27,* 11–14.

Lincoln, Y. S., & Guba, E. G. (2000). Paradigmatic controversies, contradictions, and emerging confluences. In N. K. Denzin & Y. S. Lincoln (Eds.), *Handbook of qualitative research* (2nd ed.) (pp. 163–188). Thousand Oaks, CA: Sage.

Lutjens Johnson, L. R., & Horan, M. J. (1992). Nursing theory in nursing education: An educational imperative. *Journal of Professional Nursing, 8,* 276–281.

Madrid, M., & Winstead-Fry, P. (1986). Rogers' conceptual model. In P. Winstead-Fry (Ed.), *Case studies in nursing theory* (pp. 73–102). New York: National League for Nursing.

Marriner-Tomey, A., & Alligood, M. R. (2002). *Nurse theorists and their work* (5th ed.). St. Louis, MO: Mosby.

McEwen, M., & Wills, E. M. (2002). *Theoretical basis for nursing.* Philadelphia, PA: Lippincott, Williams & Wilkins.

Meleis, A. I. (1985). *Theoretical nursing: Development & progress.* Philadelphia, PA: Lippincott.

Meleis, A. I. (1993, April). Nursing research and the Neuman model: Directions for the future. Panel discussion with B. Newman, A. I. Meleis, J. Fawcett, L. Lowery, M. C. Smith, & A. Edgil, conducted at the Fourth Biennial International Neuman Systems Model Symposium, Rochester, New York.

Meleis, A. I. (1997a). Theoretical nursing: Definitions and interpretations. In I. King & J. Fawcett (Eds.), *The language of nursing theory and metatheory* (pp. 41–50). Indianapolis, IN: Sigma Theta Tau, International.

Meleis, A. I. (1997b). *Theoretical nursing: Development & progress* (3rd ed.). Philadelphia, PA: Lippincott.

Mitchell, G. J. (1997). Have disciplines fallen? *Nursing Science Quarterly, 10,* 110–111.

Mitchell, G. J. (2002). Parse's theory of human becoming in nursing practice. In M. R. Alligood & A. Marriner-Tomey (Eds.), *Nursing theory: Utilization & application* (2nd ed.) (pp. 403–428). St. Louis, MO: Mosby.

Mitchell, G. J., & Cody, W. K. (1992). Nursing knowledge and human science: Ontological and epistemological considerations. *Nursing Science Quarterly, 5,* 54–61.

Moch, S. D. (1990). Personal knowing: Evolving research and practice. *Scholarly Inquiry in Nursing Practice: An International Journal, 4,* 155–170.

Neuman, B. M. (1974). The Betty Neuman Health-Care Systems Model: A total person-approach to patient problems. In J. P. Riehl & C. Roy (Eds.), *Conceptual models for nursing practice.* New York: Appleton-Century-Crofts.

Neuman, B. (2001). *The Neuman systems model* (4th ed.). Upper Saddle River, NJ: Prentice Hall.

Newman, M. A. (1997). Evolution of the theory of health as expanding consciousness. *Nursing Science Quarterly, 10,* 22–25.

Newman, M. A., Sime, A. M., & Corcoran-Perry, S. A. (1991). The focus of the discipline of nursing. *Advances in Nursing Science, 14*(1), 1–6.

Nightingale, F. (1860). *Notes on nursing.* London: Harrison and Sons.

North American Nursing Diagnosis Association. (2001). *Nursing diagnosis: Definitions & classification 2001–2002.* Philadelphia, PA: NANDA.

Orem, D. E. (1971). *Nursing: Concepts of practice.* New York: McGraw-Hill.

Orem, D. E. (2001). *Nursing: Concepts of practice* (6th ed.). St. Louis, MO: Mosby.

Parker, M. (2001). *Nursing theories and nursing practice.* Philadelphia, PA: F. A. Davis.

Parse, R. R. (1987). *Nursing science: Major paradigms, theories, and critiques.* Philadelphia, PA: Saunders.

Parse, R. R. (1992). Human becoming: Parse's theory of nursing. *Nursing Science Quarterly, 5,* 35–42.

Parse, R. R. (1994). Editorial: Scholarship: Three essential processes. *Nursing Science Quarterly, 7,* 143.

Parse, R. R. (1995). Commentary. Parse's theory of human becoming: An interactive guide to nursing practice for pediatric oncology nurses. *Journal of Pediatric Oncology Nursing, 12,* 128.

Parse, R. R. (1997). The language of nursing knowledge: Saying what we mean. In I. King & J. Fawcett (Eds.), *The language of nursing theory and metatheory* (pp. 73–77). Indianapolis, IN: Sigma Theta Tau, International.

Parse, R. R. (1998). *The human becoming school of thought: A perspective for nurses and other health care professionals.* Thousand Oaks, CA: Sage.

Parse, P. R. (2001). *Qualitative inquiry: The path of sciencing.* New York: NLN Press.

Parse, R. R. (2002). 15th Anniversary Celebration. Editorial. *Nursing Science Quarterly, 15,* 3.

Patterson, J. G., & Zderad, L. T. (1988). *Humanistic nursing.* New York: National League for Nursing.

Peplau, H. E. (1952). *Interpersonal relations in nursing.* New York: Putnam.

Peplau, H. E. (1997). Peplau's theory of interpersonal relations. *Nursing Science Quarterly, 10,* 162–167.

Popper, K. R. (1965). *Conjectures and refutations: The growth of scientific knowledge.* New York: Harper Torchbooks.

Rawnsley, M. M. (1999). Polarities in nursing science: The plight of the emerging nurse scholar. *Nursing Science Quarterly, 12,* 277–282.

Reed, P. G. (1998). Breaking through a breakdown in nursing logic. *Nursing Science Quarterly, 11,* 146–148.

Riehl, J. P., & Roy, C. (1980). *Conceptual models for nursing practice* (2nd ed.). New York: Appleton-Century-Crofts.

Rogers, M. E. (1970). *An introduction to the theoretical basis of nursing*. Philadelphia, PA: F. A. Davis.

Rogers, M. E. (1988). Nursing science and art: A prospective. *Nursing Science Quarterly, 1*, 99–102.

Rogers, M. E. (1992). Nursing science and the space age. *Nursing Science Quarterly, 5*, 27–34.

Roy, C. (1970). Adaptation: A conceptual framework for nursing. *Nursing Outlook, 18*(3), 42–45.

Roy, S. C. & Andrews, H. A. (1999). *The Roy adaptation model* (2nd ed.). Stamford, CT: Appleton & Lange.

Sandelowski, M. (1999). Venous-envy: The post World War II over IV nursing. *Advances in Nursing Science, 22*(1), 52–62.

Schlotfeldt, R. M. (1987). Defining nursing: A historical controversy. *Nursing Research, 36*, 64–67.

Schlotfeldt, R. M. (1989). Structuring nursing knowledge: A priority for creating nursing's future. *Nursing Science Quarterly, 1*, 35–38.

Schumacher, K. L., & Meleis, A. I. (1994). Transitions: A central concept in nursing. *Image: Journal of Nursing Scholarship, 26*, 119–127.

Sieloff, C. L. (2002). Imogene King: Interacting systems framework and theory of goal attainment. In A. M. Tomey and M. R. Alligood (Eds.), *Nursing theorists and their work* (5th ed.) (pp. 336–360). St. Louis, MO: Mosby.

Smith, M. J. (1988). Perspectives on nursing science. *Nursing Science Quarterly, 1*, 80–85.

Stainton, M. C. (1982). The birth of nursing science. *The Canadian Nurse, 78*(10), 24–28.

Stark, J. S., & Lattuca, L. R. (1997). *Shaping the college curriculum: Academic plans in action*. Boston, MA: Allyn and Bacon.

Stevens, B. J. (1979). *Nursing theory: Analysis, application, and evaluation*. Philadelphia, PA: Lippincott.

Stevens, P. (1989). A critical social reconceptualization of environment: Implications for methodology. *Advances in Nursing Science, 11*(4), 56–68.

Stewart, I. (1929). The science and art of nursing (Editorial). *Nursing Education Review, 2*, 1.

Styles, M. M. (1982). *On nursing: Toward a new endowment*. St. Louis, MO: Mosby.

Taylor, J. Y. (1999). Colonizing images and diagnostic labels: Oppressive mechanisms for African American woman's health. *Advances in Nursing Science, 21*(3), 32–45.

Thompson, J. L. (1987). Critical scholarship: The critique of domination in nursing. *Advances in Nursing Science, 10*(1), 27–38.

Toulmin, S. (1972). *Human understanding: The collective use and evaluation of concepts*. Princeton, NJ: Princeton University Press.

Visintainer, M. A. (1986). The nature of knowledge and theory in nursing. *Image: The Journal of Nursing Scholarship, 18*, 32–38.

Walker, L. O., & Avant, K. C. (1983). *Strategies for theory construction in nursing*. Norwalk, CT: Appleton & Lange.

Watson, J. (1990). Caring knowledge and informed passion. *Advances in Nursing Science, 13*(1), 15–24.

Watson, J. (1995). Postmodernism and knowledge development in nursing. *Nursing Science Quarterly, 8*, 60–64.

Watson, J. (1996). The theory of human caring: Retrospective and prospective. *Nursing Science Quarterly, 10*, 49–52.

Watson, J. (1999). *Postmodern nursing and beyond*. London: Churchill Livingstone.

Yura, H., & Walsh, M. (1988). *The nursing process, assessing, planning, implementing, and evaluating*. Norwalk, CT: Appleton & Lange.

SUGGESTED READINGS

Alligood, M. R., & Marriner-Tomey, A. (2002). *Nursing theory: Utilization & application*. St. Louis, MO: Mosby.

Chinn, P. L., & Kramer, M. K. (1999). *Theory and nursing: Integrated knowledge development* (5th ed.). St. Louis, MO: Mosby.

Fawcett, J. (2000). *Analysis and evaluation of contemporary nursing knowledge: Nursing models and theories*. Philadelphia, PA: F. A. Davis.

George, J. B. (2002). *Nursing theories: The base for professional nursing practice*. Upper Saddle River, NJ: Prentice Hall.

Johnson, B. M., & Webber, P. B. (2001). *An introduction to theory and reasoning in nursing*. Philadelphia, PA: Lippincott.

Marriner-Tomey, A., & Alligood, M. R. (2002). *Nurse theorists and their work* (5th ed.). St. Louis, MO: Mosby.

McEwen, M., & Wills, E. M. (2002). *Theoretical basis for nursing*. Philadelphia: Lippincott, Williams & Wilkins.

Nursing Science Quarterly (1988–Current). Thousand Oaks: CA: Sage. *Note*: All issues of this quarterly journal have relevant and key articles on nursing theory and its application to practice and research.

Parker, M. (2001). *Nursing theories and nursing practice*. Philadelphia, PA: F. A. Davis.

Young, A., Taylor, S. G., & McLaughlin-Renpenning, K. (2001). *Connections: Nursing research, theory, and practice*. St. Louis, MO: Mosby.

Unit 2

Professional Values and Core Competencies

5

Professional Values and Ethical Practice

LINDA C. HAYNES
DEBRA WOODARD LENERS

Ethics, a dynamic process of conversation and action, is sensitive to the constantly changing context of health care.

Volbrecht, 2002

LEARNING OBJECTIVES

AT THE COMPLETION OF THIS CHAPTER, THE READER WILL BE ABLE TO:

➤ Discuss the evolution of ethics in health care.

➤ Define selected ethical concepts.

➤ Explain moral development, ethical decision-making, and values clarification.

➤ Apply ethical principles.

➤ Examine theoretical perspectives of ethical decision-making.

➤ Demonstrate understanding of a written Code of Ethics for Nurses.

MediaLink www.prenhall.com/haynes

Additional online resources including NCLEX review questions, critical thinking questions, and real-world activities for this chapter can be found on the Companion Website at www.prenhall.com/haynes

Technological advances, financial considerations, and changes in health care delivery have had far-reaching effects on nursing. Moreover, health care faces a crisis marked by a serious shortage of nurses. The summative effect of changing boundaries, priorities, and methods of health care delivery has led to a restructuring of health care in the United States that raises many ethical questions.

To adequately address changes in health care delivery and the resulting ethical concerns, nurses, other health care providers, and consumers must engage in dialogue to discern the values that will guide the ethical restructuring of health care delivery. Governmental, educational, commercial, and social institutions should be heavily involved in this dialogue for change (Volbrecht, 2002).

Nurses must also choose to have an active role in the dialogue. They offer a unique perspective as patient educators, advocates, and providers of bedside care. Nurses are trusted by the general public and are often asked to address consumer needs for health care. Given the active role nurses can expect to play in promoting change in the current health care delivery system, it is important for them to be able to frame decision-making within an ethical context.

This chapter will review the evolution of ethics in health care, moral development, ethical decision-making, and values clarification. Ethical principles will be defined and applied to ethical decision-making.

Evolution of Ethics in Health Care

Burkhardt and Nathaniel (2002) write, "Moral action is the historical basis for the genesis, evolution, and practice of nursing" (p. 3). The following review of the evolution of ethics in health care will reflect on (a) the subordinate role women have historically assumed as caretakers, (b) societal needs, and (c) spiritual influences that have impacted the moral and ethical foundation of nursing. Nurses can use their knowledge of these influences to mold an ethical practice, which respects individual differences of the patients served.

Since ancient times the role of the "healer" has been influenced by spiritual and religious practices. These practices or customs have impacted not only the activities of healers, but also the gender, importance, and legitimacy of the healer within the society. The value of individuals and the meaning of life, death, and health have been strongly influenced by cultural beliefs, which historically were often defined by spiritual and religious leaders.

The nature of the god(s) worshiped has dictated healing practices. Healing was thought to involve an individual's spirit, which could be restored to health through sacred elements within the environment. Healers were believed to possess "special spiritual gifts" and represented "the embodiment of the cultures' god(s) on earth" (Burkhardt & Nathaniel, 2002, p. 7). Often, religious doctrine mandated health care activities necessary for health promotion and maintenance.

Ancient care providers believed the health and well-being of the patient were a reflection of the individual's moral behavior. Sickness was associated with the presence of evil or sin in a person's life. Priests and religious leaders disagreed with the scholar, physician Hippocrates (460–377 B.C.), who suggested a clinical rather than spiritual approach to treat illness. Hippocrates's work marked the beginning of clinical medicine, which sought to implement treatment based on observation.

Early Christianity had a profound effect on health care practices and beliefs of Western civilization. Biblical interpretations stressed the importance of caring for others as a means to achieve spiritual blessing and a heavenly reward after death. Christianity placed great emphasis on the individual value of all people—including women. Wealthy widows and women rejected by mainstream society were attracted to Christian-based altruistic works of charity. Women from upper social classes dedicated space in their homes in order to meet the health care needs of the sick.

The Middle Ages brought war, famine, and pestilence, which led to social disorder and chaos. Religious groups provided much of the health care offered during this time. Early nursing nuns and monks took vows of poverty, chastity, and obedience—obedience to church doctrine, not principles of health and healing. Many care providers believed they were "called" to care for the sick in much the same way Jesus cared for people from all walks of life. The care provided was deemed a "life's ministry." Through service, the health care provider sought to achieve salvation by works of self-sacrifice. These care providers donated their possessions to the church and dedicated their lives to serving others.

The religious fervor of the Middle Ages was anti-empirical in nature, thus hindering scientific advancement. There was no motivation for scientific exploration. God was believed to be responsible for health; religious interventions were the primary source of treatment. Little attention was paid to hygiene or physical health; unsanitary lifestyles and disease were widespread.

During the Crusades, as Christians sought to liberate the Holy Land from Islam, greater numbers of health care providers were needed. Men were attracted into nursing through the military. The Crusades brought tremendous wealth and, thus, power to the Catholic Church, which continued to monitor and establish standards of practice for health care. Despite the attempt by the church to control and manage health care, treatment practices varied widely. Some military nursing orders were renowned for high-quality care; individuals would feign illness for admittance to these hospitals. In other settings, patients were not only poorly treated, but, in some instances, punished for the sins attributed to mental or physical illness.

The fourteenth century marked the beginning of the Renaissance, which was highlighted by a quest for knowledge, the birth of the scientific era, and advances in healing practices. There was a renewed appreciation for mathematics and the sciences. Rene Descartes proposed a philosophical theory that separated the mind from the physical body. This philosophical theory served as the basis for a model of health care, which would begin to separate the concepts of "caring" and "curing." Health care was henceforth no longer regarded as a religious-based discipline that provided a service within a sacred realm. While the Renaissance served to elevate science and those who offered a "cure," the status of nurses, whose role was to "care," was not valued in the new social paradigm.

Widespread corruption in the Catholic Church led to the sixteenth-century Reformation. The religious doctrine of the time was rejected and modified, establishing a variety of protestant denominations. Health care for the "downtrodden and the weak" (Donahue, 1996, p. 193) was minimized following the social upheavals of the Reformation. Religious nursing orders were disbanded. Hospital care was relegated to disreputable groups of prostitutes, drunkards, and criminals. Nursing entered a dark age lasting from 1550–1850.

The abysmal state of health care strongly influenced the impact Florence Nightingale would have on nursing. Though a strongly spiritual woman, Nightingale sought to associate nursing directly with education and scientific knowledge. Her care of the ill and education of nurses emphasized "caring for the mind *and* the body" (Achterberg, 1990). Nineteenth-century nursing leaders followed in the Nightingale tradition as they advocated for a university-based education for nurses that focused on holistic caring. One nursing leader, Lavima Dock's struggles for social justice within health care during the late nineteenth and early twentieth centuries led to the publication of *Hygiene & Morality*, the first nursing text devoted to ethics and health care issues.

Early in the twentieth century there was little dialogue regarding health care ethics, as the goal of health care as directed by physicians was the physical well-being of patients. The two World Wars, the Korean War, and the Vietnam War led to advancements in technology and the development of autonomous nursing roles. The tremendous "high-tech" approach to cure, exclusive focus on quantity of life over quality, and a resurgent interest in spirituality have raised a variety of ethical issues in health care (Farley, 2001).

Moral Development

Moral development refers to human values that develop within a sociocultural context and therefore are culturally relative (Gostin, 1995). It is useful to think of moral development using theoretical models. As moral development is dependent on cognitive development, Piaget's (1963) four stages of cognitive development will be reviewed along with prominent theories of moral development outlined by Kohlberg (1981) and Gilligan (1982).

Piaget's Stages of Cognitive Development

Piaget (1963) sought to explain how intellectual capabilities developed from birth to 15 years of age. Piaget believed that although individuals are capable of acquiring new knowledge, cognitive development ceased in adolescence with no further quantifiable maturity after the age of 15. In Piaget's first stage, sensorimotor (birth to 2 years), development is dominated by motor activity and reflex. Examples of these activities include the reflexive behavior of sucking or developmental motor activity (e.g., learning to sit, stand, and ultimately walk). The second stage, preoperational thought (age 2 to 7 years), included two substages—preconceptual and intuitive. During this stage the child develops and learns to use symbolic representations such as language. Stage three, concrete operations (age 7 to 12 years), is marked by the child's ability to apply logical thought to concrete situations (e.g., touching a hot stove causes pain). In the final stage, formal operations (age 12 to 15), the adolescent begins to apply logical thought to abstract situations (e.g., lying to a friend will result in loss of a trusting relationship). Table 5–1 summarizes Piaget's stages of cognitive development.

Table 5–1 Piaget's Stages of Cognitive Development

Stage	Behavior	Clinical Application
Stage 1—Sensorimotor (birth to 2 years)	Motor reflexes present at birth are developed so that activity can be generalized to multiple situations; motor activities become increasingly coordinated to include chains of behavior (e.g., learning to sit, stand, and ultimately walk).	Sequential changes in development are a result of continual interaction between the infant and the environment: Infants repeat behavior that previously led to a novel response; eventually, the infant initiates the same behaviors to purposely elicit the desired response (e.g., moving from a social smile to cooing to vocalizations to repetition of specific sounds).
Stage 2—Preoperational Thought (2 to 6–7 years)	Representational skills and mental imagery are acquired, language develops, and the individual is highly egocentric and views the world only from his or her own perspective.	Hallmark behavior in this stage is the ability to function symbolically using language. Words, as symbols, mentally provide an image of something. Verbal requests and sentences are meaningful and understood: The meaning of "on," "in," and "under" becomes meaningful.
Stage 3—Concrete Operations (6–7 to 11–12 years)	Individuals learn to consider the point of view of others; problem solving remains concrete rather than abstract, and at this stage the individual lacks the capacity to understand all logical outcomes of a problem.	Children can project themselves into other people's situations and realize their own way of thinking isn't the "only" way. This age group can sort and organize facts; they understand that changing the shape of a substance does not change its volume (conservation principle).
Stage 4—Formal Operations (11–12 to 15 years)	Once this level of development has been attained, the individual can think logically and abstractly; knowledge continues to be acquired (e.g., lying to a friend will result in loss of a trusting relationship).	Putting across ideas and listening to ideas of others leads to a constant interest in conversations with friends, argumentation, or use of a scientific approach to solve problems. The individual is able to solve complex problems using abstract reasoning.

Kohlberg's Theory of Moral Development

In the Piagetian tradition, Kohlberg (1963) presented a theory of moral development. To Kohlberg (1976), "the most essential structure of morality" was the principle of justice, and the "core of justice is the distribution of rights and duties regulated by concepts of equality and reciprocity" (p. 4). His approach was similar to Piaget's in that (a) his was a general organismic orientation and (b) he was in opposition to psychoanalytic and teaching–learning perspectives that suggest morality is learned through education.

Kohlberg (1969) believed that as an individual matures, so too does his or her moral understanding. He believed that moral development was based on moral reasoning. The theory, which Kohlberg espoused, is based on 20 years of interviews with children, adolescents, and adults using the Moral Judgment Interview, a series of stories depicting varying moral dilemmas. These stories were presented to subjects who were then asked questions about each dilemma. Based on the responses to the various moral dilemmas, Kohlberg identified six stages of moral reasoning, which are presented in Table 5–2. Kohlberg proposed that each of the six stages form a universally invariant sequence. These six stages are then conceptualized into three different levels of moral development.

At the first level, the preconventional level, individuals demonstrate no internalization of moral values. Rather, one responds to either punishment (stage one) or rewards (stage two), both of which are a consequence of behavior. At the second level, the conven-

Table 5–2   Kohlberg's Theory of Moral Development

Level	Stage	Basis for Decision-Making	Clinical Application
Level 1—Preconventional	Stage 1 Punishment/ Obedience Orientation	Behavior is determined by possible consequences.	Avoid breaking rules to avoid punishment; the child desires pleasure; conformity is demontrated to avoid punishment or "bad" things happening.
	Stage 2 Personal Reward Orientation	Behavior is determined by what is right or wrong.	Egocentric focus; decisions about behavior are usually based on what provides satisfaction out of concern for self: "I'll do something if I get something for it or because it pleases you and then you owe me something later."
Level 2—Conventional	Stage 3 Good Boy/Nice Girl Orientation	Behavior is determined by what pleases others.	Need to see self as "good"; "I'll behave this way so you will approve of me or because it is expected of good people."
	Stage 4 Law and Order Orientation	Behavior is determined by the desire to maintain social order.	Black and white rules of behavior; obey the rules because those are the rules and it is a good person's duty to respect and obey the rules.
Level 3—Postconventional	Stage 5 Social Contract Orientation	Good behavior is determined by a socially agreed upon standard of human rights; the U.S. Constitution is based on this type of orientation.	Right actions are defined in terms of higher moral principles such as equality, justice, or due process. The individual is aware that a variety of values exist, but the way to make change in law/rules is through a designated process (right actions may not be popular, but it is good for the greatest number).
	Stage 6 Universal Ethical Principle Orientation	Good and right are matters of individual conscience and involve abstract concepts of justice, human dignity, and equality.	"I choose this behavior because it is morally, ethically, and spiritually right, even if it is illegal in the eyes of the law." Unjust laws may be broken if there is conflict with higher principles.

tional level, the individual has an intermediate internalization of moral values. One selectively abides by either the standards of other people, parents (stage three), or the rules of society (stage four). At the conventional level, it is important to note the individual is selective in the internalization of standards by which he or she chooses to abide. At the third level, the post-conventional level, moral values are completely internalized and not dependent on the standards of others. The individual recognizes a variety of moral options and develops a moral code of his or her own. This code may be the same as that generally accepted by the commu-

nity (stage five) or it may be more individualized (stage six). Table 5–2 summarizes Kohlberg's theory of moral development.

While Kohlberg's theory increased our understanding of moral development, various aspects of his theory have been criticized. First, his view has been described as placing too much emphasis on moral thought and too little emphasis on what should be done from a moral point of view (Gibbs & Schnell, 1985). Gibbs and Schnell (1985) stress that one's actions should be considered as well as one's ability to reason through a moral dilemma. Simpson (1976) has suggested Kohlberg's view is too cognitive, disregarding emotion.

A second common criticism of Kohlberg's research focuses on the manner in which data were gathered. Actions of individuals in real life situations were not studied. Kohlberg used stories to investigate moral development. These stories focused on issues of justice and fairness related to competition, property rights, right to life, and obligations.

Garbarino and Bronferbrenner (1976) further criticized Kohlberg, who assumed a universal application of moral development theory. These researchers suggested that Kohlberg's levels of moral development may be more tied to culture than Kohlberg originally suggested.

A fourth criticism of Kohlberg's theory was raised by one of Kohlberg's students, Carol Gilligan (1982), who suggested that Kohlberg's theory and research relied predominantly on a longitudinal sample of males. Gilligan argued that females contribute unique concerns and perspectives to moral development. She believed that Kohlberg grossly underestimated the role of interpersonal relationships and caring in the development of moral reasoning.

Gilligan's Ethic of Caring

Studying under Kohlberg, Carol Gilligan (1982, 1987) challenged traditional theories of moral development by suggesting that gender plays a role in moral decision-making. She believed the moral development of women is distinctly different from that of men. Gilligan wrote that moral reasoning in men reflects a "justice perspective" based on the virtues, rights, and formal reasoning. From "the justice perspective, an autonomous moral agent discovers and applies a set of fundamental rules through the use of universal and abstract reason" (Davis, Aroskar, Liaschenko, & Drought, 1997, p. 39). When applying justice to health care, one assumes obligation to be "fair." Fairness implies all individuals are entitled to the same level of health care. Rules are followed to treat illness and promote health regardless of situational variance. From a justice standpoint, the central focus for decision-making is to follow established guidelines rather than consider contextual or relational concerns specific to a situation. Justice-based ethics assumes that people are the same with regard to basic needs, freedoms, and goals. Distributing a "fair share" of health care may mean lowering standards of care when scarce or limited resources are distributed too thinly.

In contrast, Gilligan (1982) believed that the moral development of women is based on a morality of care and responsibility. From "the care perspective, the central preoccupation is a responsiveness to others that dictates providing care, preventing harm, and maintaining relationships" (Davis et al., 1997, p. 39). Rights and justice are not sufficient by themselves; they need to be based on caring and responsibility. To care and feel cared for promotes personal and social health. From the caring perspective, the central focus for decision-making is concern for the patient. Decisions about health care resources are made by asking questions that determine (a) the patient's goals for his or her health, (b) whether quality of life is of higher value than longevity, and (c) what kind of family support is available to lessen economic or social burdens that technology can create.

Similar to Kohlberg, Gilligan proposed that moral development progresses through a series of phases. With each successive stage, the individual has progressively greater understanding of the relationship of him- or herself with others. Moral development progresses from stage one, an initial selfish concern for survival, to stage two, a more responsible focus on goodness, and ultimately to stage three, an understanding that caring for another is intimately related to care for self; caring and responsibility provide an adequate guide for resolving moral conflict. Table 5–3 summarizes Gilligan's ethic of caring.

Basic Ethical Concepts

Nurses are committed to caring for patients, families, and communities. Care of an individual patient may involve long hours with the patient and their family during periods of intense physical and psychosocial vulnerability. The nurse–patient relationship involves professional intimacy and a trusting relationship. The nursing care provided to an individual often extends to the family and even to the community in which the patient and/or the nurse lives. The intimate, trusting relationship that exists between a nurse and patient serves as the core for ethical decision-making.

According to Volbrecht (2002), "**Ethics**, a process of reflecting consciously on our moral beliefs, consists of an ongoing dialogue about what communities value and what they should do in light of these values" (p. 1). **Ethical inquiry** is a method for answering questions regarding what "ought" to be done in a given situation. The study of ethics offers neither blanket rules for decision-making nor precise answers for difficult questions. However, using an ethical decision-making

Table 5–3 Gilligan's Ethic of Caring—Developmental Progression of Moral Thinking

Phase	Concern/Focus	Clinical Application
Phase 1	**Concern for Survival** Focus on what is best for self; selfish dependence on others.	Morality is behavior that submits to authority/acceptance of sanctions imposed by society.
Phase 2	**Focusing on Goodness** As the individual transitions to the second phase, there is an appreciation of connectedness with others; there is a recognition of the value of self-sacrifice; accepting responsibility for others; the individual maintains a narcissistic, manipulative concern for how others will appreciate the individual's effort.	Personal desires are set aside to meet others' needs; very aware of connectedness with others. Indirect efforts to control others' behavior may turn into manipulation through use of guilt.
Phase 3	**Imperative of Care** There is greater honesty for self-sacrifice; a deeper appreciation of connectedness and responsibility for self and others; predicted consequences and personal intention motivate behavior.	Behavior is based on the desire to be good to others, but also responsible to personal needs. Hurt no one, including self—attempt to understand and resolve conflict between selfish and selfless actions. Less concerned with "how others will view me" and more concerned with consequences of action for all, including self.

model affords the nurse an approach for examining and resolving ethical dilemmas.

Ethical decision-making involves communal dialogue between involved groups. Nurses are well suited to facilitate health-related ethical dialogue with patients, families or caregivers, professional groups, health care agencies, organizations, and society at large. Nurses who understand ethical concepts, decision-making models, and the various theoretical perspectives that shape the communal dialogue will be better prepared to resolve ethical dilemmas. An understanding of basic ethical principles is necessary to the nurse's participation in ethical dialogue.

Ethical Principles

When examining ethical issues, moral or ethical principles serve to guide reflection and action. "**Principles** are the most fundamental guiding precepts of action from which more specific rules may be derived" (Volbrecht, 2002, p. 2). Moral or **ethical principles** are basic philosophical concepts and statements that provide a foundation for guiding behavior—in the words of one author, "basic and obvious moral truths" (Burkhardt & Nathaniel, 2002, p. 41). **Ethical dilemmas** are situations that require a choice between equally favorable or unfavorable alternatives. By the very nature of an ethical dilemma there is no one good

solution, and decisions are upheld by adherence to one or more ethical principles. Beneficence, nonmaleficence, fidelity, veracity, confidentiality, and accountability are the principles that guide ethical decision-making. These ethical principles are summarized in Table 5–4.

BENEFICENCE

In its simplest form, **beneficence** is defined as helping others. Nurses have a strong desire to help others and do good deeds. The nurse's commitment to behave in a beneficent manner guides decision-making when his or her actions cause adverse consequences that threaten the patient's well-being or dignity. In some situations, "doing good" does not always mean avoiding harm. For example, immunizations have long-term benefits for promoting health; however, they are not without complications, the injection is often uncomfortable, the patient can experience transient side effects, and in some rare instances serious adverse effects can occur. Generally, it has been asserted that the long-term benefits of health promotion and disease prevention for both the individual and society far outweigh the possible harm associated with immunization.

Recognizing that many health care treatment modalities have potential adverse consequences, the nurse is obligated to respect the patient's autonomy by ensuring that informed consent is obtained. Before an

Table 5–4   Nursing Values and Ethical Principles

Ethical Principle	Definition	Sample Behavior
Beneficence	Promoting good and actively seeking benefits	• Promotes good while recognizing patient autonomy by ensuring informed consent. • Prevents harm while differentiating between the patient's rights to self-determination and noncompliance. • Removes harm though avoids paternalistic decision-making based on benevolence, protection, leadership, or discipline.
Nonmaleficence	Behaving in a manner that actively seeks to do no harm	• Analyzes each intervention to determine the risk for harm to the patient. • Bases nursing action on evidence-based knowledge and critical judgment.
Fidelity	Faithfulness and an attempt to keep promises	• Recognizes that the nurse–patient agreement to provide care is a promise. • Act to keep promises. • Monitor the patient status to ensure the promise was kept. • Develop and employ alternative strategies when initial efforts are unsuccessful.
Veracity	Telling the truth	• Values truth over deception. • Role model truth rather than deception to patient and family.
Confidentiality	Respect for the privacy of others	• Ensures all patient data, personal experiences, choices, and outcomes are kept private and confidential at all times.
Accountability	Acceptance of responsibility for one's own actions	• The nurse is responsible for his or her professional actions; assures high standards of care are provided and the patient is protected from harm. The nurse is ethically responsible to practice in a legally accountable way, to the standard of the "prudent" nurse.

immunization is administered, the patient is provided with information regarding benefits, but information regarding possible adverse consequences must also be provided. It is then the patient's decision whether to accept or reject treatment. When a patient rejects treatment health care providers deem beneficial, the patient is often labeled "noncompliant." In accordance with the principle of beneficence, nurses must recognize the patient's rights to self-determination as an alternative perspective from that of noncompliance. When explaining the benefits of treatment, it is important for nurses to avoid paternalistic decision-making behavior based on a desire to control or be protective of the patient. Beneficence must be tempered with a patient's right to self-determination in health care decisions.

NONMALEFICENCE

As defined previously, beneficence involves positive actions that help others; however, beneficence can be defined on a broader continuum, as doing no harm, or **nonmaleficence**. In cases in which beneficence and nonmaleficence come into conflict, the duty to avoid harm may override the desire to do good. Health care professionals try to balance the risks and benefits of a plan of care while striving to do no harm. For example, many medications are known to have toxic effects. Less toxic drugs are used when possible; however, with more resistant organisms, drugs with potentially harmful side effects are prescribed. To avoid harming the patient, serum drug levels are assessed, body functions are monitored, and the impact of treatment on the infecting organism is evaluated. As long as the medication is presumed to be effective, treatment is continued. When harm is detected, the health care team members act to prevent injury (e.g., the nurse notifies the physician and the physician adjusts the treatment protocol).

A more complicated example of nonmaleficence involves end-of-life decisions. Health care providers struggle with these decisions daily. Some may perceive the use of costly technology such as ventilator support as a source of good in a terminally ill patient. Others may view technology as cruel treatment, which simply postpones inevitable death. When decisions regarding potential patient harm are considered, the health care provider determines if the potential for harm outweighs the potential to promote good.

FIDELITY

Fidelity refers to being faithful to promises and commitments made to patients. Though rarely stated as such, nurses regularly make promises to patients that impact whether or not a nurse is trustworthy. When the nurse states, "I'll be right back" or "I will bring your pain medication right away," a commitment has been made. When a nurse accepts his or her patient assignment, that nurse is committing to provide prescribed care to a patient. Failure to provide that care is unethical and may constitute abandonment, neglect, or malpractice. A nurse who agrees to address a patient's pain has established an agreement with that patient to (a) implement a pain relief strategy, (b) assess the effectiveness of the strategy, and (c) employ alternative strategies if pain relief is not at a level acceptable to the patient. In order to maintain the principle of fidelity, the nurse will seek to directly resolve patient pain by exploring all options, not simply wait until the next dose of narcotic can be administered.

CONFIDENTIALITY

Maintaining **confidentiality** requires that the nurse protect the private records or personal information with which he or she has been entrusted. Patient confidentiality enjoys widespread legal protection in the United States. Confidentiality is clearly addressed in the American Nurses Association (ANA) Code of Ethics for Nurses and the International Council of Nursing (ICN) Code of Ethics and legally in federal and state statutes. The practice of confidentiality extends to include a protection of the patient's right to privacy from family members and friends. Maintaining confidentiality is more complicated in the care of dependent patients (young children, adolescents, and the elderly). While parents have a right to all information regarding the care of their children, it is prudent to preserve the relationship established with the pediatric patient by avoiding an unnecessary exchange of information. For example, when a teenager discusses concerns over pregnancy or drug use, the adolescent may simply be seeking information from a trusted health care provider. When there is no concern regarding safety of the child or others, the nurse should carefully consider the need or motivation to share such a conversation with the parent.

Confidentiality has been challenged by today's technologically advanced world. With the advent of computer-based medical records, health care institutions are required to take added measures to ensure security and privacy of patient data.

VERACITY

Veracity relates to the practice of conforming to or telling the truth. From early childhood, society exhorts telling the truth and avoidance of lying. Dilemmas arise when the question becomes: Do you tell the truth when you believe the truth will cause harm to an individual? Often, nurses may be uncomfortable giving patients "bad news" and would prefer to avoid answering questions truthfully. However, deception is generally considered detrimental both to the person who is lying and to the person being told the lie.

ACCOUNTABILITY AND RESPONSIBILITY

A nurse is **accountable** when accepting responsibility for his or her own actions. **Responsibility** involves behaving in a reliable and dependable manner. The eth-

---

Critical Thinking and Reflection

How do you feel about confidentiality? How do you maintain patient confidentiality when preparing for clinical or debriefing with friends following a clinical experience? Have there been times you have breached confidentiality? How would you feel if confidential information about your health was discussed in a post-clinical conference?

How do you feel about telling the truth to patients? Do you feel that the truth is always necessary? Are there times that telling the truth may cause undue suffering? How would you feel if the truth about your health was withheld from you?

ical principles outlined thus far rely heavily on the nurse's autonomy and willingness to accept responsibility and behave in a reliable and dependable manner. Accountability and responsibility are guided by values. While superiors may dictate rules of conduct, it is the individual nurse who chooses to think or act in accordance with valued beliefs. Nurses who advocate that they were "just following orders" are abdicating their responsibility to make autonomous decisions. History has dictated that this defense is not adequate and may represent a "moral cop-out" for those who try to justify their behavior by abdicating responsibility. The case of Martin Bormann provides the most notable example of this type of defense during the Nuremberg trials when he argued that he was "just following orders" (Barry, 1982).

Johnstone (1999) provides a guideline nurses can use to avoid abdicating responsibility. The author asserts the nurse must "draw a firm distinction between ethics and following the orders of a superior, and to recognize that moral demands are always the overriding consideration, irrespective of a superior's orders" (p. 61). Decisions to consciously object to orders given by a superior may bring great personal and professional risks. Nurses have been terminated or forced to resign when they have refused to participate in certain medical procedures.

Values

A **value** is a personal belief about the worth or quality of something that makes it desirable or useful. Individuals develop **value systems** or sets of related values. Values represent individual, community, or social convictions concerning the importance of an object, belief, idea, or attitude. Values form the basis for behavior, and value systems are a result of prioritizing values from most important to least important. Values are learned and influenced by an individual's sociocultural environment. **Professional values** are standards of a professional group that provide a framework from which to evaluate action or behavior (e.g., integrity, honesty, or autonomy).

Values guide and motivate individual and professional behavior. "Individuals take risks, overcome barriers, relinquish their own comfort and security, and generate extraordinary effort because of their values" (Tappen, Weiss, & Whitehead, 1998, p. 159). In the terrorist attacks of September 11, 2001, many individuals risked their lives and overcame barriers to save others. Professional firefighters and police as well as untrained individuals sought to rescue victims of the disaster. The rescuers gave up personal comfort and security, generated extraordinary effort, and in many cases lost their own lives because of their commitment to saving others.

Values are learned (Wright, 1987). They can be taught directly or learned indirectly by observing the behavior of others. Developmentally, an individual's values may change and evolve with experience and maturity. Young children value things such as a favorite blanket or toy, while older children value events, including campouts or a trip to the circus. Later, as individuals enter adolescence, peer group values become a priority. With growing maturity, young adults learn to value ideals, such as beauty or heroism. The values of the

All humans make mistakes and superiors make some of these mistakes. Have you ever been faced with feelings of moral conflict when a superior has written an order and you feel a more appropriate mode of therapy is available? Have you even seen a patient's pain be unrelieved because the prescribed narcotic was inadequate? What action did you take? Did you seek a different treatment regime or did you "morally cop out" and wait for time to lapse so that additional medication could be provided? What actions do you plan to take once you are the registered nurse?

mature adult represent a composite of all things valued over a lifetime (Tappen, Weiss, & Whitehead, 1998). Nurses must take into account the developmental importance of values when planning care. The nurse may teach a young child using valued reinforcement items (e.g., stickers, stamps, or other small tokens); conversely, when teaching a young adult learning may be more effectively reinforced by stressing an ideal such as autonomy or individuality. Consider, for example, a young child requiring daily insulin injections. A reinforcement chart could be effective for teaching rotating sites. The child could place a sticker or stamp on rotating sites as a reminder. A young adult learning the same procedure may value the autonomy gained by mastering the skill and, thus, the nurse reinforces the value of independent living that results when the skill is mastered.

While values are important, they are less important than the choices the individual makes in response to values. For example, adolescence is a very difficult time. If a peer group values high-risk behavior and social defiance, a teen may choose to act out these values through the use of drugs, alcohol, or other destructive behaviors. Individuals choose activities, spend money, select careers, pick friends, and decide on a mate based on personal values. Values are significant to nursing care because increasingly nurses are making decisions about value-laden practice dilemmas. In order to respond to ethical dilemmas in an effective way, an understanding of professional values or values clarification is crucial.

Values Clarification and Values Conflict

Values clarification is a process used to increase self-awareness about what is most important to an individual. Values clarification represents a thoughtful procedure whereby a person seeks to better understand his or her own values; it is not a random process of decision-making. Nurses, particularly new graduates or novice nurses, need to be aware of what they value. These values will be challenged as new nurses transition from the sheltered, structured educational environment to the competitive, demanding professional workplace. The nurse's intrinsic, extrinsic, personal, and professional values will be challenged as he or she uses them in decision-making. Nurses who recognize what they value and know when these values are in conflict with the prevailing environment are better prepared to engage in communal dialogue that leads to problem solving and decision-making that promotes relationships without compromising values.

Burkhardt and Nathaniel (2002) suggest keeping a diary or journal of experiences and personal reactions to situations as a way of developing greater awareness of personal values. **Values conflict** occurs when "personal values are at odds with those of patients, colleagues, or the institution" (Burkhardt & Nathaniel, 2002, p. 72). To effectively deal with this type of conflict, the nurse must first recognize what is valued personally and professionally. Journaling is one mechanism for increasing awareness of values. It is a very personal process in which the author of the journal can engage in purposeful, free-flowing written thought regarding an event and one's personal reaction to the situation. Since most adults have little experience with journaling, the format provided in Box 5–1 may provide a useful guide for initiating the process.

As indicated by the questions asked in Box 5–1, journaling should be more than a "rehash" of an event or situation. Journaling is a mechanism for reflective analysis of an event or situation with the focus on identifying values, recognizing patterns of behavior, and addressing change when appropriate.

Case reviews of ethical dilemmas offer another method for increasing self-awareness and reflective thinking on personal and professional values. Most individuals don't routinely think about their values. They are most likely to reflect on them when confronted with conflict over a difficult decision. Case scenarios that pose ethical dilemmas and conflicts in value systems help promote identification of personal and professional values that guide decision-making. This process can also facilitate an understanding of different perceptions and the various actions driven by alternative values.

American Association of Colleges of Nursing Professional Values

The American Association of Colleges of Nursing (AACN) outlines professional values or ethical principles of nursing practice in the *Essentials* document. Baccalaureate education facilitates the development of professional values and professional behavior that serve as a "foundation for practice" and a guide to interactions with patients, colleagues, other professionals, and the public. "Values provide the framework for commitment to patient welfare, fundamental to professional practice" (AACN, 1998, p. 8). The caring, professional nurse uses values to guide "ethical behaviors in the provision of safe, humanistic health care" (AACN, 1998, p. 8).

As stated in the *Essentials* document, professional values "epitomize the caring, professional nurse" (AACN, 1998, p. 8). Baccalaureate education for professional nurses is designed to:

Box 5-1　Journaling for Values Awareness

- Describe a situation in your personal or professional experience in which you felt uncomfortable or felt that your belief or values were being challenged, or in which you felt your values were different from others involved.
- As you record the situation, include how you felt physically and emotionally at the time you experienced the situation.
- Write down your feelings as you remember the situation. Are your reactions now any different from when you were actually in this situation?
- What personal values do you identify in the situation? Try to remember where and from whom you learned these values. Do you totally agree with the values, or is there something about them that you question or do you wonder about their validity?
- What values do you think were being expressed by others involved? Are they similar to or different from your own values?
- What do you think you reacted to in the situation?
- Can you remember having similar reactions in other situations? If yes, how were the situations similar or different?
- How do you feel about your response to the situation? Is there anything you would change if you could repeat the scene? Rewrite the scene with the changes. What might be the consequences of these changes?
- How do you feel with the new scenario?
- What do you need to do to reinforce behaviors, ideals, beliefs, or qualities that you have identified as personal values in this situation? When and how can you do this?

Reprinted with permission from Burkhardt, M. A., & Nathaniel, A. K. (2002). *Ethics and issues in contemporary nursing* (2nd ed.) (p. 71). Albany, NY: Delmar Thomson Learning.

- Build on and/or help the professional nursing student modify values and behavior patterns learned in early life.
- Promote and reward honesty and accountability.
- Increase awareness of social and ethical issues.
- Nurture and increase the nursing student's awareness of his or her own value system as well as the value system of other individuals, groups, and communities (AACN, 1998, p. 9).

The core professional values outlined in the *Essentials* document include altruism, autonomy, human dignity, integrity, and social justice are summarized in Table 5–5.

ALTRUISM

Altruism, as defined by the AACN, is "a concern for the welfare and well-being of others" and is typified by the golden rule—treat others as you would want to be treated. In professional practice, altruism is reflected by nursing's concern for the welfare of patients, nursing peers, and other health care providers (AACN, 1998). The absence of concern for others may reflect a nurse's apathy toward patients as well as indifference toward him- or herself as an individual and a nurse. Every nurse should examine his or her own life and give careful thought to self-nurturing behavior. This self-examination can profoundly impact not only the nurse's self-interest but also the interest of the patient. Simply put,

nurses who care for themselves are most capable of effectively caring for others.

AUTONOMY

Self-determination, independence, and freedom define what it means to be autonomous (Aiken & Catalono, 1994). Husted and Husted (2003) characterize **autonomy** as the uniqueness of all human beings and their right to self-determination. Autonomy within the health care system involves the patient's right to make decisions about his or her own health care. The ethical principle of autonomy is closely tied to informed consent, which requires that all patients be provided clear and sufficient information about their condition and treatment options so as to be able to make rational decisions. Recognizing the inherent right of (competent) individuals to autonomy implies that health care providers are also obligated to educate and encourage patients to participate in their care. While a nurse may not agree with a (competent) patient's decision, the nurse is obligated to respect the patient's decision.

Any failure to respect a patient's autonomy is a danger-signal, warning a nurse about possible contempt for not only the autonomy of a patient, but a lack of respect for their own autonomy as a professional nurse. Autonomy implies respect for others and a willingness to treat all individuals equally (Davis et al., 1997).

Table 5-5 AACN Professional Values

Professional Value	Definition	Sample Behavior
Altruism	Concern for the welfare and well-being of others (e.g., patients, other nurses, and other health care providers).	• Demonstrates understanding of cultures, beliefs, and perspectives of others. • Advocates for patients, particularly the most vulnerable. • Takes risks on behalf of patients and colleagues. • Mentors other professionals.
Autonomy	Accepting the right to self-determination as reflected respect for the patient's right to make decisions about health care.	• Plans care in partnership with patients. • Honors the right of patients and families to make decisions about health care. • Provides information so patients can make informed choices.
Human dignity	Respecting the inherent worth and uniqueness of individuals and populations; value and respect of all patients and colleagues.	• Provides culturally competent and sensitive care. • Protects the patient's privacy. • Preserves the confidentiality of patients and health care providers. • Designs care with sensitivity to individual patient needs.
Integrity	Acting in accordance with an appropriate code of ethics and accepted standard of practice.	• Provides honest information to patients and the public. • Documents care accurately and honestly. • Seeks to remedy errors made by self or others. • Demonstrates accountability for actions.
Social justice	Upholding moral, legal, and humanistic principles to assure equal treatment under the law and equal access to quality health care.	• Supports fairness and nondiscrimination in the delivery of care. • Promotes universal access to health care. • Encourages legislation and policy consistent with the advancement of nursing care and health care.

Adapted with permission from AACN, *The Essentials of Baccalaureate Education for Professional Nursing Practice,* 1998, Washington, DC, pp. 8–9.

HUMAN DIGNITY

Human dignity is exercised and strengthened when a nurse "respects . . . the inherent worth and uniqueness of individuals . . ." (AACN, 1998, p. 9). According to the Code of Ethics for Nurses (ANA, 2001), nurses practice with respect for the inherent dignity of all human beings in all professional relationships. The value of human dignity as applied to all individuals is demonstrated by a sensitivity to needs, values, and choices without exploitation of the patient. Respect for human dignity is also demonstrated when the nurse is respectful of privacy, honors patient requests, advocates for patients when others fail to respect the dignity of the patient, and promotes health and social conditions that promote human dignity.

INTEGRITY

"**Integrity** is acting in accordance with an appropriate code of ethics and accepted standards of practice" (AACN, 1998, p. 9). Integrity involves "the ability to integrate the various dimensions of one's personal and professional life in such a way that the nurse is morally whole, consistent, and trustworthy" (Volbrecht, 2002, p. 104). The behavior implied by this reveals a nurse's fidelity to the patient, the profession, and the self. Integrity is in a nurse's professional and personal self-interest. Two of the nine provisions of the Code of Ethics for Nurses address integrity (ANA, 2001). One focuses on a nurse's duty, to self and others, to preserve integrity and safety through maintaining professional competence. The other addresses maintaining the integrity of the nursing profession by participating to shape social policy as it relates to health care.

SOCIAL JUSTICE

"**Social justice** is upholding moral, legal, and humanistic principles" (AACN, 1998, p. 9). It requires that a nurse "build upon, and as appropriate, modify values and behavior patterns developed early in life" (AACN, 1998, p. 9). **Justice** deals with "fair, equitable, and appropriate treatment in light of what is due or owed to persons, recognizing that giving to some will deny receipt to others who might otherwise have received these things" (Burkhardt & Nathaniel, 2002, p. 57). Within the context of health care ethics, Burkhardt and Nathaniel (2002) further describe justice in terms of distributive application or distributive justice.

Distributive justice refers to the fair and equitable distribution of resources. Health care resources include available providers (e.g., physicians, nurses, and other personnel), equipment, technology, procedures, and supplies. Private, institutional, and government funding are also health resources. Distributive justice implies that all individuals have the right to equal health care resources regardless of race, sex, marital status, medical diagnosis, social standing, or religious belief. When health care resources are limited, governing systems often ensure a fair distribution of resources. Regarding health care resources and distributive justice, questions to consider when resources are limited include (a) What percentage of resources should be allocated to health care? (b) What aspect of health care should receive the greatest allocation of available resources? and (c) What patients should benefit from available resources? (Burkhardt & Nathaniel, 2002). Burkhardt and Nathaniel (2002) point out that resources can be issued either:

- Equally to each individual
- According to need
- According to merit
- According to social contribution
- According to the rights of the individual
- According to the effort of the individual
- As decided by the decision maker
- According to the greatest good for the greatest number

Questions that pose an ethical dilemma cannot be solved by a single person or government entity. Ethical decision-making requires communal dialogue. Ideally, dialogue between health care providers; consumers; government, education, and commercial entities; and

social institutions will lead to recommendations for appropriate distribution of resources.

Ethical Perspectives and Decision Making

Ethical issues and questions of ethical behavior have confronted nurses since ancient times. Providing patient care inherently means that nurses will make decisions that impact the life of the individual. Many health care decisions create "conflicts of values, priorities, and duties related to what is 'good' or 'right' for individuals, families, communities, and society as well as the nursing profession" (Davis et al., 1997, p. 45). Only recently have health care providers become acutely aware of the need to be skilled in ethical decision-making. Technological advances, cost-containment efforts, and other changes in health care delivery have made ethical conflict more visible in society. Even the simplest clinical decisions a nurse makes may have ethical implications. For example, when a nurse administers medication, the process clearly involves providing the right medication to the right patient, at the right time, in the right dose, via the right route. Though a simple process, the steps in medication administration also involve an ethical dimension as the patient maintains the right to decide whether or not to take the medication.

More complex situations do not offer such simple ethical or legal answers. Decisions involving allocation of health care services, end-of-life decisions, and more recent concerns regarding genetic engineering are complex and often engender ethical debate. In these cases, ethical decisions are made based on communal dialogue between health care providers, scientists, society as a whole, individual patients, and political leaders.

Ethical theories build on principles and values and serve as a framework for ethical analysis, decision-making, and action. Steps for ethical decision making are presented in Box 5–2. Initially, ethical decision-making involves identifying the problem. Problem identification is not always easy; however, until the problem is accurately defined, a solution cannot be advanced. It is important to recognize who the stakeholders of a problem are. Stakeholders are those individuals affected by the problem and its solutions. Contextual factors that influence the problem and its resolution must also be identified. These factors may include cultural, political, organizational, and/or legal factors. The impact of these factors needs to be considered as options are explored to resolve the dilemma.

In exploring alternatives, all relevant options should be considered. In the exploratory phase, all

Box 5–2   The Ethical Decision-Making Process

1. Identify the problem
2. Analyze the context
3. Explore options

4. Apply relevant ethical theory
5. Implement the plan
6. Evaluate the results

choices, however implausible, should be considered. The least helpful or least practical solutions will ultimately be disregarded. As options are selected and applied to the ethical decision-making process, more appropriate choices may become apparent.

Nurses find that moral dilemmas are more easily resolved when an ethical model is employed in the decision-making process. In some cases, more than one ethical perspective may be used to reach a solution, while in others a single ethical perspective will suffice. Once a plan is implemented to resolve the dilemma, the results should be evaluated. The traditional rule-based ethics will be presented.

Rule-Based Ethics

Rule-based ethics has dominated the study of moral philosophy since its delineation in the eighteenth and nineteenth centuries. Simply stated, **rule-based ethics** are designed to outline an individual's moral duties and obligations through adherence to a set of rules. A summary of the rules considered relevant to nursing practice is found in Box 5–3. Deontology and utilitarianism represent two rule-based ethical approaches to problem solving. Each approach adheres to a similar set of rules, although different justifications for application of rules are used.

KANTIAN ETHICS OR DEONTOLOGY—A DUTY ETHIC

Immanuel Kant (1724–1804) served as most influential to modern deontologists. A **deontologist** justifies actions as right or wrong based on whether the act is "just, respects autonomy, and provides good" (Potter & Perry, 2001, p. 411). The consequences of action are not relevant to the ethical decision. **Deontology** is "the theory that action in conformance with formal rules of ethical conduct, are obligatory regardless of their result" (Angeles, 1992, p. 60). A deontological theory of ethics is "one which holds that at least some acts are

morally obligatory regardless of their consequences for human health or woe" (Edwards, 1972, p. 343).

Deontology emphasizes what individuals "should" do in terms of duty. Kant emphasized that an action is "good" if it is done for the sake of carrying out one's duty—one's prime directive. The fact that an action would improve a patient's well-being does not inherently make the action ethical—the action must also be consistent with professional duty. Kant maintained that some actions are simply right or wrong regardless of the potential outcome. Donagan (1977) summarized Kant's basic belief that one should act respectfully in relation to him- or herself and every other individual. While Kant believed there were ethical rules that should never be broken, most contemporary deontologists agree that situational influences may be considered. Modern deontologists contend that ethical rules are intended to protect and benefit society; therefore, unusual circumstances may require an ethical rule be broken in order to avert a catastrophe.

UTILITARIANISM—AN ETHIC OF UTILITY

John Stuart Mill (1806–1874), a British philosopher and commentator, first proposed an ethic of utility or a teleological approach to decision-making. The basic premise of this position is the principle of **utilitarianism**, which suggests that "one should act so as to promote the greatest good of the greatest number of people" (Angeles, 1992, p. 307). It is a theory in which value or justification is determined by usefulness; the ends justify the means (Gibson, 1993). Consequences alone are of little importance. From a utilitarian perspective, acting morally should result in a better place to live and increased human happiness for all (Volbrecht, 2002).

The difference between utilitarianism and deontology is the focus on usefulness, consequences, and outcomes. Utilitarianism looks to outcome whereas deontology looks to "rightness" of the action and the adherence to principles. While the concepts that guide utilitarian thought provide guidance, they do not guide

Box 5–3   Moral Rules Relevant to Nursing Practice

Requirement of Nonmaleficence: Do Not Intentionally Inflict Harm

- Do not kill or physically harm others without justified cause (e.g., self-defense or the use of physically harmful treatment as a necessary and consented means to promoting patient welfare).
- Do not impose unreasonable risks of harm. Negligence is conduct that falls below a standard of due care.
- Do not harm others by slander, insult, or ridicule.
- Do not break a freely made promise or contract to do something in itself morally permissible.
- Do not engage in sexual acts that are exploitative or life diminishing. This includes all sex with patients.
- Do not steal the legitimately obtained property of others, including their intellectual property (e.g., published ideas, research data, and computer programs).

Respect for Autonomy: Respect the Ability of Competent Patients to Hold Views, Make Choices, and Take Actions Based on Personal Values and Beliefs

- Respect the choice of competent patients to refuse medical treatment and/or nursing care.
- It is impermissible to lie to patients or to withhold information necessary for an adequate understanding of their conditions.
- It is impermissible to treat competent patients without their adequately informed consent. Such consent requires disclosure of relevant information, probing for and ensuring understanding and voluntariness, and fostering adequate decision-making.
- Establish a clear process for the identification of surrogate decision makers in the case of incompetent patients.
- Respect and protect patient privacy and confidentiality, providing confidential information to others only as required by law or to prevent grave harm to others.

Requirement of Beneficence: Promote the Well-Being of Others and Oneself, Using Morally Permissible Means, Insofar as One Can Do So Without Disproportionate Costs

- Maintain one's competence in nursing; participate in efforts to maintain and improve standards of nursing; participate in efforts to maintain working conditions that support quality nursing care; support the development of nursing's body of knowledge.
- Make reasonable efforts to protect patients and the public from harm due to incompetent or unethical practice by other health care professionals.
- Participate in efforts to promote the health needs of one's community.
- Promote one's own mental, physical, emotional, and spiritual development.

Requirement of Justice: Distribute Benefits, Resources, and Burdens Fairly

- Nursing resources should be allocated fairly among patients served.
- Communities should develop processes for the fair access and allocation of health care to all members of the community.
- Workplaces should ensure that all health care providers receive fair compensation for their work and that appropriate appeal processes are in place to ensure fair distribution of wages, compensation, and workloads.

Volbrecht, R. M. (2002). *Nursing ethics: Communities in dialogue.* Reprinted by permission of Pearson Education, Inc., Upper Saddle River, NJ.

the process that leads to the outcome. Utilitarianism is not concerned with specific needs and desires of individuals. Some would say that since nurses deal with individual patients, a utilitarian standard would not be suited for nursing; however, nurses also serve groups, communities, and humanity at large—looking to the greater good for the aggregate as a whole.

A Professional Code of Ethics for Nurses

Caring is the ethical ideal of nursing—the moral virtue of nursing. Caring cultivates relationships, understanding, commitment, trust, creative individualization, and concern for quality of life. An ethic of care implies that patients matter as unique persons—the meaning of

A value is a personal belief about the worth or quality of something that makes it desirable or useful. Cultural differences are reflected in values assigned to ethical issues such as truth telling, autonomy, and end-of-life decisions. Miscommunication, disagreement, and conflict can arise when the cultural frame of reference of a health care provider is different from that of a patient. Culhane-Pera and Vawter (1998) designed a study to elicit professional health care perspectives and evaluate the influence of culture in a cross-cultural ethical conflict.

MH was a healthy 70-year-old Hmong female with an asymptomatic goiter who presented to the emergency room with acute shortness of breath. Endotracheal intubation was necessary; tracheal compression secondary to a ruptured thyroid cyst was occluding the airway. Permission for the procedure was obtained from the patient and family with the assistance of a trained interpreter. A surgical team prepared to evacuate blood, remove the thyroid, and provide access for a tracheotomy. The patient and family refused the surgery opting to monitor the woman's progress. The patient and family cited concerns for her body and soul. Two days later the patient and family requested the endotracheal tube be removed for physical, social, and spiritual reasons; the physicians refused anticipating a 90% chance the patient would die without airway support.

An ethics case consultation was conducted, the hospital attorney consulted, and a laryngoscopy performed. The ethics consultation supported the position of MH and her family to have the endotracheal tube removed despite the hazard. The decision was based on the ethical principle of autonomy and thus the patient's right to make decisions. The attending surgeons transferred the case and the endotracheal tube was removed. Initially, MH experienced respiratory distress but she could ultimately be discharged 2 days later.

The case of MH was presented at seven conferences and participants were asked to respond to a questionnaire after hearing the case's presentation and ethical dilemma. Respondents were provided cultural information. The study was designed to determine if this information would influence decision-making. Of those responding, 75% indicated they would have supported MH's decision to have the endotracheal tube removed based on a respect for cultural beliefs. The remaining respondents supported the medical decision based on the belief that neither the patient nor her family was capable of making an informed decision. These participants also cited professional integrity and personal moral beliefs as rational to support the medical intervention against the wishes of the patient.

In this study, the cultural information was found to have the greatest effect on health care providers with an orientation of respect for cultural differences. Those health care providers who "believed in the superiority of their biomedical perspective" were not influenced by the cultural information.

---

health or illness experiences holds special significance for the ethics of each patient care situation.

A code of ethics serves as a public expression of this virtuous, ethical ideal and is considered a profession's agreement with the society in which it practices. It serves as a short statement of the obligations and duties a profession has to those it serves. As written, a code provides non-negotiable standards by which the profession functions. A code of ethics expresses the profession's understanding of the commitment it has to the society served. A written code of ethics is often a dynamic document, which is subject to change as the profession and society change.

Within the context of a caring ethics perspective, how are decisions regarding euthanasia and abortion made? To answer this question, the situation should be reviewed, the related connectedness between involved parties analyzed (e.g., fetus and pregnant woman, family and dying patient), and the responsibility and ability to provide care discussed. What conflicts might arise, and how can resolution strengthen connectedness?

Box 5–4   Nightingale Pledge

I solemnly pledge myself before God and in the presence of this assembly:

To pass my life in purity and to practice my profession faithfully.

I will abstain from whatever is deleterious and mischievous, and will not take and knowingly administer any harmful drug.

I will do all in my power to maintain and elevate the standard of my profession, and will hold in confidence all personal matters committed to my keeping and all family affairs coming to my knowledge in the practice of my profession.

With loyalty will I endeavor to aid the physician in his work, and devote myself to the welfare of those committed to my care.

While the values and goals of nursing have remained rather static in recent history, the implementation of nursing practice has been influenced by social change. With the feminist movement of the 1960s, the role of women in society became more collaborative. No longer did professional nurses view their discipline as subordinate to medicine. The changing societal view of women was reflected in ethical dialogue; nurses became more politically active and recognized their ethical responsibility to society (e.g., to improve immigrant health, change child labor laws, and increase awareness of and decrease family violence).

The first attempt to outline the ideal of what a professional nurse should be was written by Mrs. L. E. Gretter, Principal of the Farrand Training School for Nurses (now known as the Harper Hospital School of Nursing). In 1893, she wrote the Nightingale Pledge (Box 5–4), which provided nurses with a document, similar to the Hippocratic oath. The pledge served as a guide to professional practice. Though this pledge was well received across the country and administered at graduation ceremonies nationwide, it was never adopted as an official code of ethics due to the subservient overtones regarding loyalty to physicians.

North American nurses were some of the first to demand a written statement outlining the ethical position of nursing. They turned to the newly formed professional organization, the American Nurses Association, for leadership in establishing a public statement to guide ethical decisions in nursing prac-

tice. The earliest versions of a code for nurses were drafted in 1926, 1940, and 1949; however, the ANA did not approve an official code of ethics until 1950. Canadian nurses also struggled with the task of developing a code of ethics. In 1953 the Canadian Nurses Association (CAN) published the International Council of Nurses (ICN) Code of Ethics. In 1983 this document was revised as the Code of Ethics for Registered Nurses.

Early ethical standards focused on the "appropriate character of nurses and the virtues that were seen as essential to the profession" (Volbrecht, 2002, p. 3). As Volbrecht (2002) notes, initial ethical discussions were unable to separate a nurse's professional behavior from moral character. Social responsibility has consistently been a thread in discussions involving professional behavior (Fowler, 1997). Early versions of the ANA code of ethics focused on virtue and character. Not until 1968 did the language shift to a duty-based ethical focus. The most recent version of the Code of Ethics for Nurses has blended duty-based ethics with a historical focus on character and virtue. Ethical codes represent dynamic documents that reflect societal change. A review of past and present documents clearly depicts this evolution. Copies of the Code of Ethics for Nurses (ANA, 2001) (Appendix A), the International Council of Nurses Code of Ethics for Nurses (ICN, 2000) (Appendix B), and the Code of Ethics for Registered Nurses (CAN, 2002) (Appendix C) are included in the Appendices of this text.

TRANSITION INTO PRACTICE

As a movement, feminism values women and systematically confronts injustice based on gender (Chinn & Wheeler, 1985). Feminists work to bring about social change as they reject the way women have been criti-

cized, ignored, and devalued. The study of ethics has not been immune to gender bias and thus has supported the subordination of women. Though ethical theories presented in this chapter recognize the equality of men and women, they do not take into account the gender bias that has historically influenced the role of women in society. Feminist ethics not only recognizes the equality of men and women, but also serves to eliminate the subordination of women.

The ultimate goal of feminist ethics is social transformation. As Volbrecht (2002) points out, "Feminist ethics begins from the conviction that the subordination of women is morally wrong and works to uncover institutionalized practices that form the web of oppression" (p. 161). Furthermore, there is a commitment to designing alternative ways to restructure relationships, social practices, and institutions.

Many underestimate the impact gender bias continues to exert. The public generally recognizes unequal division of labor within family households, differential expectations of male and female children, or the role women play as care providers for elderly parents. More subtle gender bias has been pointed out by researchers such as Faden, Kass, and McGraw (1996), who note that AIDS research, until very recently, has focused on the role women play as transmitters of the disease either through sexual contact or reproduction rather than on the health implications of AIDS to women.

Many nurses and women in general have difficulty with feminist ideology. Despite these differences, feminists and nurses have a shared history. Feminists have sought to support and expand the role of women not only in nursing but also throughout the workplace. Nurses in turn have promoted women's health and thus have endorsed a feminist perspective. No longer is women's health consistent with reproduction. Women more often than men seek health care and demand a role in that care. Nurses have served as advocates in support of the woman's right to shared decision-making in health care.

Gilligan's ethic of caring has been instrumental in unmasking the tendency of Western ethicists to equate the male experience with the ethical norm. The harm in this type of thinking is not only the failure to explore the female experience, but the use of male experiences as a normative standard by which women fall short. As nursing students enter the historically male dominated health care domain, it is important for them to be empowered by understanding the cycle that has oppressed nurses. Roberts (2000) suggests five steps nurses can take to gain liberation:

- Recognize and discuss domination of nurses in health care.
- Develop pride in the history of nursing.
- Become a cohesive group and support nurse leaders within and outside of administration.
- Work in interdisciplinary groups and evaluate one another as individuals.
- Identify activities to promote social justice and change the hierarchical structure of health care.

KEY POINTS

1. To adequately address changes in health care delivery and the ethical questions raised, nurses; other health care providers; consumers; and government, educational, commercial, and social institutions should be heavily involved in communal dialogue to guide restructuring.
2. The intimate, trusting relationship that exists between a nurse and patient serves as the core for ethical decision-making.
3. Ethics, a process of reflecting consciously on our moral beliefs, consists of an ongoing dialogue about what communities value and what they should do in light of these values.

4. A value is a personal belief about the worth or quality of something that makes it more desirable or useful; values guide and motivate behavior.
5. Values clarification is a method individuals use to become more aware of what they believe to be important.
6. The core values as outlined by the AACN include altruism, autonomy, human dignity, integrity, and social justice.
7. Ethical principles or moral truths guide an individual's actions and deliberations. These include fidelity, beneficence, nonmaleficence, confidentiality, and veracity.

EXPLORE MediaLink

Critical thinking questions, essay questions, key terms, web links, activities, NCLEX review questions, and more interactive resources can be found on the Companion Website at www.prenhall.com/haynes. Click on Chapter 5 to select activities for this chapter.

REFERENCES

Achterberg, J. (1990). *Woman as healer*. Boston: Shambhala.

Aiken, T. D., & Catalono, J. T. (1994). *Legal, ethical, and political issues in nursing*. Philadelphia, PA: F. A. Davis.

American Association of Colleges of Nursing. (1998). *The essentials of baccalaureate education for professional nursing practice*. Washington, DC: Author.

American Nurses Association. (2001). *Code of ethics for nurses with interpretive statements*. Washington, DC: Author.

Angeles, P. A. (1992). *Dictionary of philosophy* (2nd ed.). New York: HarperCollins.

Barry, V. (1982). *Moral aspects of health care*. Belmont, CA: Wadsworth.

Burkhardt, M. A., & Nathaniel, A. K. (2002). *Ethics and issues in contemporary nursing* (2nd ed.). Boston: Delmar Publishers.

Canadian Nurses Association. (2002). *Code of ethics for registered nurses*. Ottawa, ON: Author.

Chinn, P. L., & Wheeler, C. E. (1985). Feminism and nursing: Can nursing afford to remain aloof from the women's movement? *Nursing Outlook, 33*(2), 74–77.

Culhane-Pera, K. A., & Vawter, D. E. (1998). A study of healthcare professionals' perspective about a cross-cultural ethical conflict involving a Hmong patient and her family. *Journal of Clinical Ethics, 9*(2), 179–190.

Davis, A. J., Aroskar, M. A., Liaschenko, J., & Drought, T. S. (1997). *Ethical dilemmas and nursing practice* (4th ed.). Stamford, CT: Appleton & Lange.

Donagan, A. (1977). *The theory of morality*. Chicago, IL: University of Chicago Press.

Donahue, M. P. (1996). *Nursing: The finest art*. St. Louis, MO: Mosby.

Edwards, P. (Ed.). (1972). *Dictionary of philosophy* (Vol. 2). New York: Macmillan.

Faden, R., Kass, N., & McGraw, D. (1996). Gender, feminism, and death: Physician-assisted suicide and euthanasia. In S. M. Worf (Ed.), *Feminism and bioethics: Beyond reproduction* (pp. 252–281). New York: Oxford University Press.

Farley, J. (Ed.). (2001). *Ethics and conflict*. Thorofare, NJ: Slack Incorporated.

Fowler, M. (1997). Nursing's ethics. In A. Davis, M. A. Aroskar, J. Liaschenko, & T. S. Drought (Eds.), *Ethical dilemmas and nursing practice* (4th ed.) (pp. 17–34). Stamford, CT: Appleton & Lange.

Garbarino, J., & Bronferbrenner, U. (1976). The socialization of moral judgment and behavior in cross-sectional perspective. In T. Likona (Ed.), *Moral development and behavior: Theory, research, and social issues* (pp. 70–83). New York: Holt Rinehart & Winston.

Gibbs, J. C., & Schnell, S. U. (1985), Moral development "versus" socialization: A critique. *American Psychologist, 40*(10), 1071–1080.

Gibson, C. H. (1993). Underpinnings of ethical reasoning in nursing. *Journal of Advanced Nursing, 18*(12), 2003–2007.

Gilligan, C. (1982). *In a different voice: Psychological theory and women's development*. Cambridge, MA: Harvard University Press.

Gilligan, C. (1987). Moral orientation and moral development. In E. F. Kittay & D. T. Meyers (Eds.), *Women and moral theory* (pp. 19–33). Savage, MD: Rowman and Littlefield.

Gostin, L. O. (1995). Informed consent, cultural sensitivity, and respect for persons. *Journal of the American Medical Association, 274*(10), 844–855.

Husted, G. L., & Husted, J. H. (2003). *Ethical decision-making in nursing and health care: The symphonological approach* (3rd ed.). New York: Springer.

International Council of Nurses. (2000). *The ICN code of ethics for nurses*. Geneva, Switzerland: Author.

Johnstone, M. (1999). *Bioethics: A nursing perspective* (3rd ed.). Orlando: Harcourt Saunders.

Kohlberg, M. (1963). The development of children's orientation toward moral order: Sequence in the development of moral thought. *Vita Human, 6*(1–2), 11–33.

Kohlberg, M. (1969). Stage and sequence: The cognitive-development approach to socialization. In D. A. Goslin (Ed.), *Handbook of socialization theory and research* (pp. 346–480). Chicago, IL: Rand McNally.

Kohlberg, M. (1976). Moral stages and moralization: The cognitive-developmental approach. In T. Lickona (Ed.), *Moral development and behavior: Theory, research, and social issues* (pp. 31–53). New York: Holt Rinehart & Winston.

Kohlberg, L. (1981). *The philosophy of moral development*. New York: Harper and Row.

Piaget, J. (1963). *The origins of intelligence in children* (M. Cook, Trans.). New York: Norton.

Potter, P. A., & Perry, A. G. (2001). *Fundamentals of nursing* (5th ed.). St. Louis, MO: Mosby.

Roberts, S. J. (2000). Development of a positive professional identify: Liberating oneself from the oppressor within. *Advances in Nursing Science, 22*(4), 71–82.

Simpson, E. (1976). A holistic approach to moral development and behavior. In T. Lickona (Ed.), *Moral development and behavior: Theory, research, and social issues* (pp. 159–170). New York: Holt Rinehart & Winston.

Tappen, R. M., Weiss, S. A., & Whitehead, D. K. (1998). *Essentials of nursing leadership and management*. Philadelphia, PA: F. A. Davis.

Volbrecht, R. M. (2002). *Nursing ethics: Communities in dialogue*. Upper Saddle River, NJ: Prentice Hall.

Wright, R. A. (1987). *Human values in health care*. St. Louis, MO: McGraw-Hill.

SUGGESTED READINGS

Gilligan, C., Ward, J. V., Taylor, J. M., & Bardige, B. (1988). *Mapping the moral domain*. Cambridge, MA: Harvard University Press.

Husted, G. L., & Husted, J. H. (2001, in press). *Ethical decision-making in nursing and health care: The symphonological approach* (3rd ed.). New York: Springer.

Husted, J. H., & Husted, G. L. (1993). Personal and impersonal values in bioethical decision-making. *Journal of Home Health Care Practice, 5*(4), 59–65.

Husted, J. H., & Husted, G. L. (1999). Agreement: The origin of ethical action. *Critical Care Nursing, 22*(3), 12–18.

Kikuchi, J. F. (1996). Multicultural ethics in nursing education: A potential threat to responsible practice. *Journal of Professional Nursing, 12*, 159–165.

McKeon, R. (Ed.). (1941). *The basic works of Aristotle*. New York: Random House.

Rice, V. H., Beck, C., & Stevenson, J. S. (1997). Ethical issues relative to autonomy and personal control in independent and cognitively impaired elders. *Nursing Outlook, 45*, 27–34.

Sayers, G. M., Barratte, D., Gothard, C., & Onnie, C. (2001). The value of taking an "ethics history." *Journal of Medical Ethics, 27*, 114–117.

Scott, P. A. (1998). Professional ethics: Are we on the wrong track? *Nursing Ethics, 5*(6), 477–485.

Tannsjo, T. (1999). Informal coercion in the physical care of patients suffering from senile dementia or mental retardation. *Nursing Ethics, 6*, 327–336.

Tschudin, V. (1998). Myths, magic and reality in nursing ethics: A personal perspective. *Nursing Ethics, 5*(1), 52–58.

6

Making Caring Visible

HOWARD K. BUTCHER

No professional program introduces caring to students for the first time. Individuals care because they are human beings, and they select particular professions because they care. The capacity to care is rooted in their very nature. While the ability to exercise and express this capacity is influenced by many factors from prenatal life onward, educational experiences and opportunity is a strong determinant of the quality of caring manifested in their future professional lives. The capacity to care can be enhanced, called forth, or inhibited by educational experience of the student, and most importantly, by the presence or absence of caring models.

Sister M. Simone Roach, 1992

LEARNING OBJECTIVES

AT THE COMPLETION OF THIS CHAPTER, THE READER WILL BE ABLE TO:

- Examine the invisible nature of caring and the service provided by nurses.
- Explain the increased emphasis on caring in nursing education and practice.
- Understand how caring is a reflection of nursing aesthetics.
- Describe conceptualizations of caring unique to nursing.
- List the attributes, ingredients, and values of caring.
- Explain how caring can be made more visible.

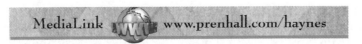

MediaLink   www.prenhall.com/haynes

Additional online resources including NCLEX review questions, critical thinking questions, and real-world activities for this chapter can be found on the Companion Website at www.prenhall.com/haynes.

$\mathcal{C}$aring has long been recognized as central to the history, scholarship, and practice of nursing. Many nurses indicate caring is what attracted them to nursing. While all humans have the ability to care, caring holds a unique meaning for nurses. The capacity of nurses to care guides clinical practice. Despite the application of caring to all facets of patient care, students, nurses, and nurse educators often devalue caring as a focus for study. Caring is generally assumed to be an integral, interwoven aspect of patient care and is rarely explicitly taught as ethical or theoretical content. Caring and the service provided by nurses are generally invisible, hidden, and unrecognized by both the public and other health care professionals. The purpose of this chapter is to "make visible" the nature of caring in nursing by presenting current conceptualizations of caring that aid to define the distinctive nature of caring within the discipline of nursing.

Caring and Service

The Invisibility of Caring

Suzanne Gordon (1997) described nursing as "one of the most invisible arts, sciences, and certainly one of the most invisible parts of our health care system" (p. xi). Nurses are involved in the most private aspects of the lives of their patients. They are the compassionate "strangers" who share the secrets of patients and families during their most vulnerable moments. Nurses remain with patients as they experience pain and suffering, are overwhelmed, and feel out of control (Benner & Wrubel, 1989). The hidden nature of nursing and caring often serves to preserve the patient's integrity and privacy during times of vulnerability.

Intimacy is both invisible and vital to nursing care. Caring is culturally invisible and devalued partially because caring is associated with "woman's work"; historically, women's work has been devalued and often unpaid. Reverby (1987) rightly points out that the crucial dilemma in contemporary nursing is that nurses are obligated to care in a society that does not value caring. While neither nursing nor caring need be specific to gender, caring is viewed by society as the work of women (Benner & Wrubel, 1989). Within the popular mind and deep psyche of the male-orientated worldview, not only does *nurse equal women*, but on an even more profound mythological level, *women equals nurse* (Fiedler, 1987). Women's caring work becomes subsumed under the "important" work of men (medicine) within the patriarchal health care system. Caring, as a core value, is hidden from public view because the work of women is not valued in the dominant worldview (Watson, 1999).

Many moral failures of the current health care system can be attributed to the lack of a caring consciousness among health care policy makers (Phillips, 1994). Depersonalizing procedures, technological problem-solving, and market-driven economics are eclipsing the importance of caring. Caregivers are rewarded for efficiency, technical skill, and measurable outcomes, while concern, attentiveness, and human engagement go unnoticed by profit-driven corporate health care institutions. Many nurses feel frustrated, angry, confused, and even embarrassed by their inability to provide the quality of care patients deserve; simultaneously, patients feel increasingly disenfranchised, depersonalized, and processed.

Evidence of the moral failure of the patriarchal health care system abounds. The current emphasis on power, control, efficiency, technology, cost containment, profitability, oppressive mechanical institutional/bureaucratic practices, and detached standardized treatments that dehumanize patient care all point to moral failures and lack of a caring consciousness in the current health care system (Watson, 1990). The rise in the number of people without health insurance, decreasing access to care, lack of care of the homeless and mentally ill, mistreatment of the elderly, rise in infant mortality among the poor, rise of prison populations while prisons are becoming profit motivated, violence in workplaces and schools, and racist health care practices are but a few of the health care concerns that remain largely ignored by the American health care system. Though the United States is a wealthy country, its medical care statistics are as alarming as those of developing countries. The recent Institute of Medicine

---

Critical Thinking and Reflection

Institutional barriers limit the ability to care. What barriers limit your ability to be caring? In order to overcome these barriers, what strategies will help you be more **caring** in the clinical setting?

(2001) report on the status of health care in America found that there is "abundant evidence that serious and extensive quality problems exist throughout the United States health care system, resulting in harm to many Americans" . . . leading to "years of life lost . . . pain, and suffering" (p. 237).

Through caring, nurses are in an ideal position to rehumanize health care. Nurses comprise the largest single group of health care providers. If nursing is to mobilize its collective power to influence change in health care policy, nurses can begin by overcoming the invisible nature of the service provided. Overcoming invisibility means that nursing's caring values need to be made visible. Restoring and nurturing an ethic of caring, by making caring more explicit within nursing education and the professional socialization of the next generation of nurses, is the best hope for revolutionizing, transforming, and rehumanizing the health *care* system.

Rising Visibility of Caring

Many noted nursing theorists, philosophers, and scholars have written about the role caring plays in nursing. Newman, Sime, and Corcoran-Perry (1991) describe how caring is becoming more prominent in nursing literature. These scholars were among the first to develop a definition of nursing that included caring as a major focus. They proposed that "nursing is the study of caring in the human health experience" (p. 3).

In 1995, the American Nurses Association (ANA) revised *Nursing's Social Policy Statement* to include caring as an important component in the nurse–patient relationship to facilitate health and healing. In addition, the *Essentials of Baccalaureate Education for Professional Nursing Practice* document published by the American Association of Colleges of Nursing (AACN) identified caring as a concept central to the practice of professional nursing. Caring, as defined in the *Essentials* document, "encompasses the nurse's empathy for and connection with the patient, as well as the ability to translate these affective characteristics into compassionate, sensitive, appropriate care" (AACN, 1998, p. 8).

The increasing visibility of caring in nursing can also be attributed to the annual National Caring Conferences that have been held since 1978. The caring conferences have sought to: (a) identify major philosophical, epistemological, and professional dimensions of caring; (b) explicate the nature, scope, functions, and structure of care and its relationship to nursing care; (c) clarify the major components, processes, and patterns of care; and (d) stimulate nurses and others to systematically investigate care and caring and share their findings with other interested colleagues (Leininger, 1981b). In 1989, with the encouragement of nurses from around the world, the conference group became known as the International Association for Human Caring. In 1997, this organization began publishing the peer-reviewed *International Journal for Human Caring*.

In addition to the work of the International Association for Human Caring, organizations such as the American Holistic Nurses Association and the National League for Nursing have advocated for a "Curriculum Revolution" involving the implementation of caring-based curricula in schools of nursing. Graduates from a caring-based curriculum are more likely to be responsive to societal needs, more successful in humanizing a highly technological health care environment, more caring and compassionate, more insightful about ethical issues, more creative, better critical thinkers, and better able to bring about scholarly approaches to the health problems experienced by patients (Bevis & Watson, 1989).

Established in 1986 by Jean Watson, the Center for Human Caring at the University of Colorado Health Science Center School of Nursing has also been instrumental in making caring more visible in nursing. The Center for Human Caring offers a certification program for nurse educators, clinicians, and administrators with a core interdisciplinary curriculum in caring and healing. The Center provides short- and long-term in-residence study programs for scholars from around the world who are interested in the study of human caring. Initiated in 1988, the Denver Nursing Project in Human Caring (DNPHC) is a nurse-managed center devoted to humanistic, holistic, and personalized care of persons with acquired immune deficiency syndrome (AIDS) and human immunodeficiency virus (HIV).

Philosophical Perspectives on Caring

It is our very familiarity with caring, both as an art and as a way of being, that makes it so difficult to either describe or define. Table 6–1 lists some of the common behaviors associated with caring. Gaylin (1976) described caring as an essential ingredient in human development and survival. He goes on to explain that just as stimulation through the senses is essential, so is the need to care and be cared for. Within this context, **to be cared for** involves taking care of; being concerned about and worrying over; and being supervised by, attended to, and loved by others.

Table 6–1   Selected Caring Actions

Comforting	Surveillance	Communion
Compassion	Touch	Reciprocity
Concern	Tenderness	Listening to
Empathy	Being with	Promoting
Enabling	Commitment to	Responsible for
Facilitating	Connectedness	Reflecting
Interest	Doing for	Healing
Involvement	Engrossment in	Sympathy
Helping	Giving to	Understanding
Love	Experiencing with	Watchfulness
Nurturance	Intimacy	Competence
Presence	Kindness	Valuing another
Protecting	Knowing another	Trusting
Sharing	Attention to	Patient teaching
Supporting	Assisting	Advocacy
Bearing witness	Facilitating meaning-making	Cultivating
Empowering	Liberating	Emancipating

Philosopher Martin Heidegger (1996) explained that to *be* is to care. In other words, care is a basic constitutive phenomenon of human existence, which defines one as human. Thus, caring is basic to human existence. Heidegger believed making, doing, seeing, knowing, and understanding are the way we get along in the world. More importantly, the portal to the meaning for existence is opened when we engage in caring practice with others. When we do not care, we lose our sense of *being*; caring is the way back to *being*.

In *On Caring*, Milton Mayeroff explained that caring "is not to be confused with such meanings as wishing well, liking, comforting, and maintaining . . . it is not an isolated feeling or momentary relationship" (Mayeroff, 1971, p. 1). According to Mayeroff, caring is a process for helping others to self-actualize and grow. Helping others grow involves:

- Helping others to care for something or someone apart from themselves
- Encouraging and assisting others to find and create the ability to care
- Allowing others to care for themselves

Mayeroff (1971) described eight major "caring ingredients" (see Table 6–2) useful to explain what caring involves and how one can help another grow.

Virginia Henderson's classic and widely accepted definition of nursing is consistent with the notion of assisting others to grow. Henderson described the unique function of the nurse as follows:

To assist the individual, sick or well, in the performance of those activities contributing to health or its recovery (or peaceful death), that the person would perform unaided given the necessary strength, will, or knowledge. And to do this in such a way as to help the individual gain independence as rapidly as possible (Henderson, 1997, p. 22).

Similarly, Orem (1995) described the goal of a nursing agency as: (a) helping patients accomplish therapeutic self-care demand, (b) helping patients move toward responsible self-care including steadily increasing independence in self-care actions, and (c) helping members of the family or other persons who attend the patient become competent in providing and managing care of the patient.

Noddings's (1984) examination on the nature of caring revealed that the ethical basis for caring is rooted in a deep sense of receptivity, relatedness, and responsiveness. According to Noddings (1984), caring involves: (a) a commitment of self; (b) a risk of becoming overburdened; (c) an appreciation of the reality of another; (d) action, involvement, and engrossment; and (e) a commitment to fully and genuinely being present. In other words, there is a moral obligation or duty to care. The motivation for caring should be the welfare, protection, or enhancement of the patient and not a promise for a grateful response from the patient.

Table 6–2　Mayeroff's (1971) Caring Ingredients

Knowing	Caring requires knowledge of the other. One must be able to understand the other's needs and respond properly to them. Good intentions alone do not guarantee a caring response.
Alternating Rhythms	One learns from one's mistakes and modifies behavior in response to another. An important form of rhythm involves moving back and forth between a narrower and wider frame of reference, so one can move between attending to details and attending to the larger context.
Patience	Having patience is to allow the other to grow in their own time and their own way. Patience is not only allowing time to grow, but also giving the space and room to grow.
Honesty	Honesty involves being open to oneself as well as to the other. The one who is caring needs to be honest enough to accept others as they actually are rather than how the one caring may wish them to be.
Trust	Trust requires faith in the ability of the other to grow and self-actualize in that person's own time and way. Trust is an appreciation of the independent existence of another and involves being able to let go. Trust includes an element of risk and the courage to leap into the unknown.
Humility	Humility involves being willing to learn from the one being cared for. Humility requires overcoming the arrogance that exaggerates the power of the one who is caring, at the expense of the one who is being cared for.
Hope	The hope is that the other will grow through caring. This hope is not based on the hope of an idealized future at the expense of the present, but rather is an expression of a present alive with a sense of possibility.
Courage	Courage is required in order to follow the lead of another into the unknown. This courage is similar to the courage of an artist who rejects conformity in order to create independently and in doing so achieves personal expression.

Research Application

If caring is to be retained as the "essence" of nursing, and if caring research is to advance, then various perspectives of caring need to be clarified, strengths and limitations of the conceptualizations examined, and the applicability of caring as a concept and theory in the practice of nursing identified. It is imperative that caring perspectives be debated, queried, and clarified so that the concept, when developed, is applicable to the art and science of nursing. In an in-depth content analysis of 35 authors whose work either explicitly or implicitly defined or conceptualized caring, the authors (Morse et al., 1990) identified and discussed the strengths and weaknesses of five distinct perspectives on caring in the nursing literature. The first perspective is caring as a trait. As a trait, caring is viewed as a mode of being, part of human nature, and essential to human existence. A second perspective of caring in the nursing literature is caring as a moral imperative or ideal. From this perspective, caring is not viewed as a set of identifiable behaviors, but rather as an adherence to the commitment of maintaining the person's dignity or integrity. In the third perspective, caring as affect, caring is viewed as a feeling of concern, of interest, or protection. Caring was viewed as an aspect of the nurse–patient interpersonal relationship. From this perspective, caring is the foundational essence of the interpersonal relationship. Lastly, caring has also been defined as a therapeutic intervention by some nursing authors. Caring actions as interventions may include active listening, patient teaching, touch, presence, technical competence, or may even include all nursing actions (procedures and interventions). The authors concluded that knowledge development related to caring in nursing is limited by the lack of refinement of caring theory, the lack of definitions of caring attributes, the lack of examining consequences of "uncaring," and the focus of theorists and researchers on the nurse to the exclusion of the patient (Morse et al., 1990).

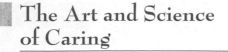

The Art and Science of Caring

Creating Beauty Through Nursing Care

Caring is a way of expressing the beauty of nursing. **Aesthetics** is a branch of philosophy that focuses on the nature and expression of beauty (*American Heritage Dictionary*, 1993). Aesthetics is ordinarily associated with art. Creating art involves skill, raw materials, imagination, and the ability to bring these together as an integral whole. Caring is an art form and all art has a special beauty; thus, all works of caring are works of beauty. Nursing is a special beauty, and caring reflects the beauty and artistry in nursing. Watson (1999) states that "all true works of healing are works of beauty; beauty heals" (p. 193). Mossman (1923) asked nurses to "experience beauty, to see it in commonplace, to learn of books, poems, pictures, and music that interpret beauty and draw from them to fit the needs of those we serve" (p. 319). Caring is an act of beauty "whereby the one-caring connects with and reflects the beauty of the soul to the one-cared-for, one to the other" (Watson, 1999, p. 194). Art is not limited to the fine arts. Chinn and Kramer (1999) explain that art is present in all human activities, which involve putting elements together to create a whole.

Nursing has always been recognized as both an art and a science. Nightingale (1868) long ago wrote that "nursing is an art and if it is to be made an art, it requires as exclusive a devotion, as hard a preparation, as any painter's or sculptor's work" (p. 362). Isabel Stewart (1929) stated that the "real essence of nursing, as any fine art, lies not in the mechanical details of execution, nor in the dexterity of the performer, but in the creative imagination, the sensitive spirit, and the intelligent understanding lying back of those techniques and skills" (p. 1). More recently, Peplau (1988) described nursing as "an art form, not identical to but rather with elements in common with other art forms, such as the performing arts (dance and music) and the plastic or visual arts (painting and sculpture)" (p. 9).

Art does not stand in opposition to science; art is a part of science. Bronowski (1965) explored the commonalities between science and art in his book *Science and Human Values*. Whether our work is science, art, or the daily work of society, Bronowski believed it is only the form by which we explore our experience that is different. Similarly, Rogers (1988) identified nursing as a "learned profession" and a "science and an art" as

she specified the art in nursing is "the imaginative and creative use of knowledge" for the purpose of human service (p. 100).

Caring and art are transformational. Gadamer (1986) explains that one cannot encounter a work of art without being transformed in the process. Likewise, caring is transformative and is at the core of what distinguishes the expert from the gifted professional in all areas of human endeavor. Healing is transformational, and healing occurs through the nurse's acts of caring. Acts of grasping meaning in a situation, establishing a meaningful connection, understanding a patient's situation, intuition, comforting, compassion, empathy, being together in true presence, creating a healing–caring environment, and intentional synchrony of movement are but a few of the ways nurses create beauty through caring acts.

The art of nursing is the capacity of a person to receive another person's expression of feelings and to experience those feelings for oneself. While nursing has long been described as an art, only recently has evidence of a "powerful move toward art in nursing" taken place (Chinn, 1994, p. 20). Carper's (1978) examination of nursing literature identified aesthetics as one of four fundamental and enduring patterns of knowing that nurses value in nursing practice. She described **empathy** as the capacity for participating in or vicariously experiencing the feelings of others. Like caring, the use of empathy, creative resources, and intuition are all examples of nurse artistry.

Expanding on the work of Carper, Chinn and Kramer (1999) elaborated on how aesthetic qualities are reflected in all aspects of nursing practice. **Aesthetics in nursing** is concerned with a deep appreciation of the meaning of a situation. In nursing, aesthetics is a pattern of knowing related to the perception of deep meaning and the use of creative resources that may be expressed through the art form known as nursing practice. For these authors and many nurses, engaging, interpreting, and envisioning are all ways of expressing the aesthetic beauty of nursing.

Chinn (2001) described how Carper's patterns of knowing in nursing gave rise to the ontological elements (nature of being), which describe nursing practice. For example, scientific competence arises from empirical knowing, moral/ethical comportment arises from ethical knowing, the therapeutic use of self arises from personal knowing, and the transformative art/acts of nursing arise from aesthetic knowing. It is aesthetic knowing that brings together the parts of nursing into the integral whole of nursing practice. Art is present in all activities that involve forming elements into a whole (Chinn, 2001). Chinn viewed aesthetics as an integrating pattern, whereby art provides a foundation for transformative art and acts, which in turn integrate moral/ethical comportment, scientific competence, and therapeutic use of self. In other words, nursing art is what brings together all ways of knowing to form the whole of nursing practice.

The work of Johnson and Appleton clarified the meaning of nursing as an art. Their work explored the relationship between caring and nursing aesthetics. In an extensive review of nursing literature, Johnson (1994) identified five conceptualizations or "senses" of nursing as art (see Table 6–3). Caring is embedded within each of Johnson's senses of nursing as art.

Appleton (1994) described artful nursing as the integral connection between caring and aesthetics. The five major themes identified that express the art of nursing include: (a) being there; (b) being with each other in understanding; (c) creating opportunities for fullness of being; (d) transcendent togetherness; and (e) context

of caring. By "being there" nurses are practicing from a humanistic perspective, seeing the patient as a whole, and expressing compassion for the person in need. They are involved in helping the patient through caring. "Artistic nursing care" implies the nurse is sincere, genuine, open, honest, committed, and willing to help. The theme "being-with each other in understanding" captures the intimacy of caring. The nurse strives to make a connection with the patient and seeks to come to know and understand the patient's situation and experience. By being empathetically and intuitively knowing, the nurse is able to individualize caring. As "being-with each other in understanding" deepens, the nurse and patient form a bond based on trust and respect. The theme "creating opportunities for fullness of being" is the welcoming of the patient's feelings, respect for their wishes, and honoring of their self-expression. Nurses prepare patients for transitions by assisting them to make their own decisions and choices; supporting those decisions; making frequent inquiries, contacts, and

Table 6–3 Johnson's (1994) Five Conceptualizations of Nursing as Art

Ability to grasp meaning in patient encounters	1. Attaching significance to patient behavior patterns and cues 2. Tacit knowing or a direct feeling of the experience is how understanding is acquired 3. The ability to grasp meaning is developed through experience 4. Perceptual awareness of the wholeness of a situation
Ability to establish a meaningful connection with the patient	1. Establishing a connection is more than words. It involves gestures and concrete actions in response to a particular patient 2. Connections are expressed as concern, caring, and compassion 3. Is a person-to-person relationship with the patient 4. The connection involves the nurse being authentic
Ability to perform nursing activities skillfully	1. Recognize the nursing needs of a patient and the use of skills to answer the needs 2. Skillfulness can be described as: proficiency, dexterity, finesse, movement, quickness, lightness, strength, endurance, coordination, fluidity, timing, and efficiency 3. Skillfulness refers to the nurse's actions and behaviors 4. Skillfulness can be learned
Ability to determine rationally an appropriate course of nursing action	1. Able to effectively draw valid conclusions from existing knowledge 2. Practical and appropriate actions 3. Involves the rationale use of knowledge 4. Actions are grounded intellectual activity (problem solving) 5. Actions can be evaluated according to a set of standards as being coherent, palatable, and feasible
Ability to conduct one's nursing morally	1. Perform in a way that seeks to cause no harm and is a benefit to the patient 2. Care is guided by moral ideals 3. Care must be competent 4. Involves a commitment to care 5. Care is motivated by altruism

checks; and giving feedback to patients. "Transcendent togetherness" refers to the close bond that forms between caring nurses and their patients. Patients report feeling safe, secure, comfortable, and bonded to nurses who practice artfully (Appleton, 1994).

Patient care encompasses a wide range of skills. Technical skill can be performed with finely tuned style, timing, finesse, and coordination to convey both a sense of artistry and scientific competence. These skills are most effective when balanced with intentional caring. Skills done that only mimic a rote list of steps convey an emptiness that defines nursing care as mechanically technical, without compassion. Intentional caring is a work of beauty. Nurses create beauty in nursing care when the understanding of a patient's experience (e.g., their suffering, illness, stress, and pain) is combined with the use of creative imagination, intuition, and skillfulness.

Illuminations of Caring *in* Nursing

There is a long lineage of nursing scholarship that serves to illuminate and make visible the art of caring in nursing. Caring becomes unique *in* nursing through the expression of philosophies, theories, and beliefs about caring that are used to guide practice. An ever-increasing number of nursing authors have characterized caring as an essential moral value. The moral caring imperative is central to service to society, patients, nurses, and students.

Roach (1992) notes professional programs do not introduce caring to students for the first time. Rather, nurses care because they are human beings; they select nursing as a career because they care. The capacity to care is rooted in the very nature of nurses. While the ability to exercise and express caring is influenced by many factors from prenatal life forward, educational experiences provide a foundation for the quality of caring manifested in future professional lives. The capacity to care is enhanced or inhibited by both educational experiences and the presence or absence of caring models.

Scientific knowledge and technological proficiency are not sufficient to define quality nursing practice. Technology and science used as substitutes for human caring dehumanize. Science and technology are tools of human caring. Caring as a focus of study *must be* made fundamental to nursing education and practice. Several key caring models are presented in this chapter as a way to enhance understanding of the nature of caring *in* nursing.

Nightingale's Caring Arts

Nightingale, the founder of modern nursing and an enduring symbol and exemplar of nursing care, never defined human care or caring in *Notes on Nursing*. Her writings suggest insight into the nature of caring, health, and healing. In Nightingale's view, nature was a curing and restorative force; the role of the nurse was to create a healing environment. Nightingale's (1859) belief in restorative forces and the self-healing capacity of human beings were revolutionary for the time. She emphasized the effect pure air, pure water, effective drainage, food, cleanliness, and light had on restoring health. The nurse's role was to make "habitual" observations and recordings and to monitor the patient's condition and the environment to support the restorative qualities of nature. The emphasis Nightingale placed on monitoring stresses the importance of caring as a therapeutic modality. Nightingale emphasized caring when she noted that nursing is a service to God. Nightingale (1859) described nursing as a "calling" and "God's work."

Watson (1999) clearly illustrated how Nightingale's ideas about the nature of healing are relevant today. Watson explained how Nightingale emphasized each of the five senses in promoting health. For example, Nightingale (1859) stressed the importance of the healing effect of music:

> The effect of music upon the sick has been scarcely at all noticed . . . wind instruments, including the human voice, and stringed instruments, . . . have a beneficent effect . . . with such instruments as have *no* continuity of sound, have just the reverse (Nightingale, 1859, p. 33).

Today, music and sound are used as catalysts to facilitate and enhance self-healing capacities. Tapes that include sounds of nature, wind, waves, chimes, chants, whales, babbling brooks, heartbeats, and symphonic or harmonic music are used to promote relaxation, meditation, and peaceful transitions (e.g., during birth, dying). Nightingale (1859) stressed the importance of beauty and visual arts when she stated "variety and form of brilliancy of color in objects . . . are actual means of recovery" (p. 34) and "the effect in sickness of beautiful objects, of variety of objects and especially of brilliancy of color, is hardly at all appreciated" (p. 33). Nightingale explained the importance of being able to experience pleasant views and the vibrancy of color in flowers, by placing the patient in the most well-lighted spot in a room. She believed that the environment facilitated recovery. Nightingale's special care in the use of color, light, and space continues to be reflected in health care through the design of today's hospitals. Watson (1999) credited Nightingale for the healing color and light, artwork, and images in the redesign of hospitals to create a caring–healing environment. Malkin (1992) lists features used to create a healing environment. A healing environment:

- Creates a mood, lifts spirits, and has cheerful rooms
- Has a variety of wall surfaces, floors, ceilings, furniture, fabrics, and artwork
- Provides views of trees, flowers, mountains, or ocean from patient rooms and lounges
- Offers indoor landscaping
- Has nonglare lighting in patient rooms
- Offers the ability to control intensity of lighting
- Provides adequate places to display personal mementos (family photographs, cards, flowers)
- Has fresh air, a solarium, or a roof garden
- Ensures control of noise

Today's increasing integration of aromatherapy and fragrance in health care is, in part, based on Nightingale's emphasis on pure air. Nurses and others use essential oils, aromas, and familiar scents to promote relaxation, harmony, comfort, balance, and wholeness. Nightingale addressed the importance of food, drink, and taste. Today, attention is given to the gustatory sense and its relationship to diet, nutrition, and basic health lifestyles. The appearance of food, taste, aroma, texture, and atmosphere all need to be considered in the preparation of food for both the sick and the well. Personalized caring makes a difference when seeking to meet the nutritional needs of patients.

Nightingale advocated for restructuring of mental and cognitive thoughts. In 1859, she wrote, "Help the sick to vary their thought . . . Sick children prefer a story to be told to them" (Nightingale, 1859, p. 32) and "You will relieve, more effectually, unreasonable suffering . . . by giving him something new to think of . . . than by all the logic in the world" (Nightingale, 1859, p. 59). Nightingale's consideration of the importance of the imagination and mind in caring and healing supports the use of visualization, imagery, cognitive therapy, dream work, humor, play, story, literature, poetry, affirmations, and journaling designed to promote health and healing.

Models of Caring

Leininger's Care as the Essence of Nursing

Madeleine Leininger was considered among the first to declare caring as the essence of nursing. During the 1976 American Nurses Convention in New Jersey, Leininger and Dr. Jody Gittenberg presented a program on "caring as the essence of nursing." At this convention, Leininger and Gittenberg declared "caring is the central and unifying domain for the body of knowledge and practices in nursing" (Leininger, 1981a, p. 3). This statement continues to be one of the most frequent cited quotes in the nursing literature on caring.

Leininger (1981a) noted the word *care* was used in nursing as a verb, as in *to be cared for, caring for others*, or to *manifest care* with concern, compassion, and interest in another human being. The discipline of nursing has always been concerned about the caring needs of people; however, before Leininger's work became known, caring as a concept remained vaguely defined. Leininger (1991) defined professional nursing care (caring) as:

> formal and cognitively learned professional care knowledge and practice skills obtained through educational institutions that are used to provide assistive, supportive, enabling or facilitative acts to or for another individual or group in order to improve a human health condition (or well-being), disability, lifeway, or work with dying patients (Leininger, 1991, p. 38).

Leininger held that caring behaviors and practices uniquely distinguish nurses from other health care providers. She explained that nursing practices are attempts to nurture or care for and support patients as they heal and grow. She believed caring is the core intellectual, theoretical, heuristic, and central practice of nursing. According to Leininger, no health care profession, other than nursing, is totally concerned with caring behaviors, caring processes, and caring relationships. She defined nursing as:

> A learned humanistic and scientific profession and discipline [that] is focused on human care phenomena and activities in order to assist, support, facilitate, or enable individuals or groups to maintain or regain their well-being (or health) in culturally meaningful and beneficial ways, or to help people face handicaps or death (Leininger, 1991, p. 47).

Her ideas related to caring are based on an anthropological perspective describing caring as a mode of human action and relatedness, which has been present since the beginning of humankind. Caring is uniquely human and is one of the critical features that assist humans through cultural evolution. Table 6–4 lists Leininger's major beliefs concerning care.

Table 6–4   Leininger's Philosophical Claims About Caring and Human Care

1. Care has been essential for human survival, development, and to face critical or recurrent life events such as illness, disability, and death (Leininger, 1985, p. 210).
2. Care (caring) is essential for well-being, health, healing, growth, survival, and to face handicaps or death (Leininger, 1991).
3. There can be no effective cure without care, but there can be care without cure (Leininger, 1985, p. 210).
4. Care expressions, patterns, and lifestyles take on different meanings in different cultural contexts (Leininger, 1985, p. 210).
5. Human care is universal, yet there are diverse expressions, meanings, patterns (or lifestyles), and action modalities (Leininger, 1985, p. 210).
6. Human care patterns, conditions, and actions are largely based upon cultural care values, beliefs, and practices of particular cultures, and of the universal nature of humans as caring beings (Leininger, 1985, p. 210).

Through Leininger's efforts, caring is now a major focus of nursing research and scholarship. She empirically investigated the concept of caring and developed the Theory of Cultural Care Diversity and Universality. Leininger saw a critical need to understand caring from the perspective of different cultures. She envisioned an entire body of essential nursing knowledge related to transcultural nursing care. The Theory of Cultural Care Diversity and Universality was developed to advance and improve nursing practice across cultural barriers. The theory has led to evidence-based knowledge and culturally congruent, safe, and beneficial health care. Leininger encourages nurses to be compassionate and caring in order to help people live peaceful, healthy lives in our complex and diverse world.

Roach and the Five Cs of Caring

Perhaps lesser known, but no less significant works in the caring literature, are the writings of Sister M. Simone Roach. Roach (1992) pointed out that no discipline is seen as so directly and intimately involved in caring needs and behaviors as nursing. Originally, she described caring as a attribute of being human. In her more recent work, she added that caring is a "human mode of being" (Roach, 1992, p. 46). Roach (1992) bases her idea of caring as a human mode of being on the work of Heidegger (1996) as follows:

> Caring, as the human mode of being, entails the capacity or power to care, a capacity linked with and inseparable from our nature as human beings. Caring involves a calling forth of this capacity in ourselves and in others through affirmation of that capacity and through its development. Caring is responsivity, a response to someone/something

who/which matters: a response to a value as the important-in-itself. Caring is the actualization of the capacity or power to care. Caring is expressed in specific moments as particularized in concrete behaviors (p. 47).

Roach is clear about the notion that caring is not unique to any particular profession and therefore caring does not distinguish one profession from another. However, she does assert that caring may be considered unique *in* nursing. Caring is unique *in* nursing through professionalization of human caring. The capacity to care, as a mode of being, is developed and made professional through educational programs. The professionalization of human caring in educational programs involves the development of a student's capacity to care by (a) the teaching of models and theories of caring and (b) providing a learning environment and faculty/mentors/preceptors who model and apply caring concepts and values. Roach (1992) states that the professionalization of human caring occurs through acquisition of knowledge, skills, attitudes, and values. The five Cs of caring are compassion, competence, confidence, conscience, and commitment. Each of the five Cs is considered an attribute of caring.

The idea that compassion is an attribute of caring "hardly needs defending" (Roach, 1992, p. 60). Roach (1992) defined **compassion** as:

> a way of living born out of an awareness of one's relationship to all living creatures; engendering a response of participation in the experience of another; a sensitivity to the pain and brokenness of the other; a quality of presence which allows one to share with and make room for the other (p. 58).

While compassion is indispensable to caring, compassion also depends on competence. Competence without compassion can be brutal and inhumane; however, compassion without competence may be harmful and meaningless. **Competence** is a "state of having the knowledge, judgment, skills, energy, experience and motivation required to respond adequately to the demands of one's professional responsibilities" (Roach, 1992, p. 61). Caring demands competence.

Confidence, the third attribute of caring, is defined as a quality that fosters trusting relationships. Caring is founded on establishing a trusting relationship. Deliberate deception not only shatters the confidence of patients in those they trust to care for them, but also damages the integrity of the profession. Deception destroys confidence; deliberate deception is the antithesis of caring.

Roach views caring as a response to something that matters; a response to a value as important-in-itself. A caring response is intentional, deliberate, meaningful, and rational. **Conscience** is a moral awareness for caring. The conscience directs behavior according to the value fitness of things (Roach, 1992). Conscience involves an attunement to the moral nature of things. Conscience is the "call to care" that leads to the response of caring.

Lastly, **commitment** to caring is a complex affective response. This response is characterized by a convergence of desires with obligations and the deliberate choice to act in accordance with them. Devotion, or commitment, is essential to caring. Commitment is the investment of self in a task, a person, a choice, or a career. Commitment to caring is no longer a burden when it becomes a valued obligation. Commitment is the call to a conscious, willing, and positive course of action (Roach, 1992). Whether a nurse–patient, student–teacher, or researcher–participant relationship, the professional caring relationship involves:

> an interpenetration of experiences, a sharing in the world of the patient (compassion); it always demands the appropriate level of knowledge and skill (competence); it builds on a relationship of trust and loyalty (confidence); it presupposes and nurtures sensitive awareness to the moral and the ethical (conscience); and finally, if it is truly professional, it is marked by a steadfastness of purpose and a devotion to the needs of the other (commitment) (Roach, 1992, p. 124).

Roach suggests that together the five Cs of caring provide a broad framework of human behavior within which professional caring may be expressed. She recommends the five Cs as a focus for professional nursing curriculum so that caring can be taught and assimilated by students.

Gaut's Analysis of Caring

Delores Gaut (1984) views caring as a functional endeavor that can be taught. In her philosophical analysis designed to clarify the meaning of caring, she identified three factors associated with caring: (a) attention and concern; (b) responsibility for or providing for; and (c) regard, fondness, or attachment. She also identified five necessary and sufficient conditions of a caregiver essential to a caring act: (a) awareness of a need for care; (b) knowledge on how to improve the situation; (c) an intention to help; (d) action must be chosen and implemented; and (e) the desired change in the patient is based on what is good for that particular patient rather than some other person or condition. Gaut placed particular emphasis on competent skilled nursing as part of caring actions. She viewed caring as a series of actions that involve setting a goal, choosing a tactic, and implementing the tactic. Gaut offered a description of caring that went beyond the performance of skills to include intention, choices, and judgments.

Watson's Transpersonal Caring–Healing Model

Jean Watson is perhaps the nursing scholar most often associated with the caring movement in nursing. Watson (1985) asserts that human caring is the moral ideal and origin of the professional role of nurse. Like Leininger, Watson (1996) agrees that caring is the essence of nursing and the most central unifying focus for nursing practice. She views caring as the highest form of commitment to oneself, others, society, the environment, and the universe. More significantly, she states that as a discipline, nursing has an ethical, social, and scientific responsibility to develop new theories and knowledge about caring, healing, and health practices.

Watson's (1999) perspective on caring is grounded in humanistic philosophy, existential phenomenology, Eastern philosophy, metaphysics, and more recently postmodernism and quantum field theory. From this perspective, nurses view individuals as greater than and different than the sum of their biopsychosocial spiritual and cultural parts. Nurses place emphasis on the meaning of human health–illness experiences, holism, freedom, choice, responsibility, interconnectedness, processes, values, contextual relationships, and healing.

Nurses who maintain a humanistic perspective are committed to a compassionate approach, attend to the concerns and feelings of others, and are sensitive to culture and lifestyle needs.

Watson's (1997) model helps to distinguish nursing from medicine. Caring is associated with nursing while curing is the focus of medicine. Watson maintains that nurses need to move away from the "nursing-qua-medicine" approach embraced by so many nurses toward a "nursing-qua-nursing" approach grounded in transpersonal caring–healing. She voices concern that the caring values of nurses are eclipsed by the contemporary medical systems dominated by economics rather than a commitment to caring, health, and well-being.

There are several unique and distinct features of Watson's somewhat abstract transpersonal caring–healing model. Emphasis is placed on the existence of the human soul. The soul, according to Watson (1985), "refers to the geist, spirit, inner self, or essence of the person, which is tied to a greater sense of self-awareness, a higher degree of consciousness, an inner strength, and power that can expand human capabilities and allow the person to transcend his or her usual self" (p. 46).

Transpersonal caring is a human-to-human connectedness whereby both the nurse and the patient are touched by the human center, the soul, of the other. "Transpersonal" conveys a concern for the inner life world and subjective meaning of another person. Transpersonal caring–healing moves beyond the ego self to include spiritual concerns, cosmic concerns, and connections that tap into healing possibilities and potentials (Watson, 2001). Watson describes the person as a mind–body–spirit unity.

Watson focuses on the caring-to-caring transpersonal relationship and the healing potential of both the patient and caregiver. Healing, according to Watson, takes place during a "caring occasion/moment" whereby the nurse and others come together by action and choice. Transpersonal caring calls for authenticity, self-reflection, a focus on wholeness, and intentionality to gain harmony within mind, body, and soul.

Watson (1999) describes a "caring consciousness" in nursing, which she traced back to Nightingale. A caring consciousness is reflected in the *presence* of nurses with patients. An authentic caring presence can be cultivated by active listening; an unconditional positive regard and nonjudgmental stance toward the patient; being physically present; seeing, touching, involving, and connecting with patients; and by being mindful. Watson focuses on the relationship between the use of *clinical caritas processes* and the development of a *transpersonal caring relationship* within the context of a *caring occasion* or moment. Clinical caritas processes are listed in Table 6–5. *Caritas* comes from the Greek word

---

Table 6–5   Clinical Caritas Processes

1. Practice of loving kindness and equanimity within the context of caring consciousness.
2. Being authentically present, enabling and sustaining the deep belief system and subjective life-world of self and the one being cared for.
3. Cultivation of one's own spiritual practices and transpersonal self, going beyond ego self, opening to others with sensitivity and compassion.
4. Developing and sustaining a helping–trusting, authentic caring relationship.
5. Being present to, and supportive of, the expression of positive and negative feelings as a connection with deeper spirit of self and the one being cared for.
6. Creative use of self and all ways of knowing as part of the caring process; to engage in artistry of caring–healing practices.
7. Engaging in genuine teaching–learning experiences that attend to unity of being and meaning, attempting to stay with others' frames of reference.
8. Creating healing environment at all levels (physical as well as nonphysical, subtle environment of energy and consciousness, whereby wholeness, beauty, comfort, dignity, and peace are potentiated).
9. Assisting with basic needs, with an intentional caring consciousness, administering "human care essentials," which potentiate alignment of body/mind/spirit, wholeness, and unity of being in all aspects of care, tending to both embodied spirit and evolving spiritual emergence.
10. Opening and attending to spiritual–mysterious, and existential dimensions of one's own life-death; soul care for self and the one being cared for (Watson, 2001).

meaning to cherish, to appreciate, to give special, if not loving, attention to, and it connotes something very fine, indeed even precious (Watson, 2001).

Watson's 10 "clinical caritas processes" give clear direction for integration of caring ideals into nursing practice (see Table 6–5). These practices call for a sense of reverence and sacredness with regard to life and all living things that acknowledges a convergence of art, science, and spirituality.

Boykin and Schoenhofer Nursing as Caring Model

The Nursing as Caring Model was advanced by the work of Anne Boykin and Savina Schoenhofer (2001). Their model serves as the basis for the caring curriculum framework at Florida Atlantic University, in Boca Raton, Florida. The model is designed to serve as an organizing framework for all nursing roles, including practitioner, researcher, administrator, teacher, and developer. The Caring in Nursing theory draws from Mayeroff's caring ingredients (knowing, alternating rhythms, honesty, courage, trust, patience, humility, and hope) and Roach's five Cs of caring (compassion, commitment, confidence, conscience, and competence). Caring is defined as "an altruistic, active expression of love, and intentional and embodied recognition of value and connectedness" (Boykin & Schoenhofer, 2001, p. 393). Similar to Roach, these scholars explain that caring is not the unique province of nursing; however, "as a profession and discipline, nursing uniquely focuses on caring as its central value, primary interest, and the direct intention of its practice" (Boykin & Schoenhofer, 2001, p. 393). A major assumption of this theory is *all humans are caring persons*. Developing the full potential to express caring is an ideal and a lifelong process. According to the theorists, the focus of nursing is the person as living in caring and growing in caring; *the intention of nursing is nurturing persons living and growing in caring*. When entering into a human care situation to offer nursing care, the nurse focuses on coming to know the individual as a caring person, understanding how that person is living and caring uniquely in the moment, and living their dreams and aspirations to grow in caring. The aim of the nurse is to come to know and then to acknowledge, affirm, support, and celebrate the individual as a caring person. Nursing is accomplished by acting on the informed intention to care in personal and meaningful ways (Boykin & Schoenhofer, 2001).

Nursing interventions are a "calling" to care. Calls for nursing are for nurturance through expressions of caring. Intentionality and authentic presence opens the nurse to hearing and responding to calls for nursing. Nursing situations are created when the nurse responds to a call for caring. Nursing situations involve the values, intentions, and actions of two or more persons choosing to engage and live in a nursing relationship. All nursing knowledge and nursing actions occur within the context of the nursing situation. The relationship between the nurse and person being cared for is referred to as "caring between." Caring between is a loving relation in which the patient and nurse enter and co-create the intention to care (Boykin & Schoenhofer, 2001). It is in the context of the nursing situation and caring between that enhances personhood. The theorists are clear that the nurse uses all patterns of knowing in nursing situations. Knowing includes empirical knowing as well as ethical, personal, and aesthetic knowing as nurses practice within a caring context.

It may be difficult for some nurses to accept the commitment to "know" all patients as caring persons. Students will often ask, "how can a person who is a child molester or serial killer be living in caring and how can I come to know the person as caring?" The challenge for nurses is "not to discover what is missing, weakened, or needed in the other, but to come to know the other as a caring person and to nurture that person in situation-specific, creative ways" (Boykin & Schoenhofer, 2001, p. 396). While the individual's actions are not caring, the nurse cares for this individual by virtue of humanness. The authors suggested that Mayeroff's caring ingredients and Roach's five Cs of caring are useful ways to come to know the other as a caring person. These authors suggest that the ethic of caring supersedes all other values and nurses are not called upon to judge or censure another's actions. Undoubtedly, caring for some individuals is difficult and challenging. It is only through the nurse's sustained intention, commitment, study, and reflection that care can be offered in difficult situations. When patients fall short of their commitment to care, condemnation by nurses is inappropriate; rather, there is an opportunity to help the individual care for self, care for others, and grow as an individual.

Swanson's Nursing as Informed Caring Model

In a series of phenomenological studies of caring in perinatal nursing, Swanson (1993) inductively developed a theory of informed caring, which can be applied to all nursing situations. **Informed caring** is a nurturing way of relating to others by knowing the individual's reality. The nurse attempts to understand the patient's reality by being with the patient, doing for the patient, and enabling that patient to achieve an outcome that enhances well-being. Figure 6–1 depicts Swanson's five overlapping processes that are the structure for caring.

Informed caring is based on Swanson's therapeutic interventions "maintaining belief," "knowing," "being with," "doing for," and "enabling." **Maintaining belief** is "sustaining faith in the capacity of others to get through events or transitions and face a future with meaning" (Swanson, 1993, p. 354). Patients are approached with the conviction that there is personal meaning that can be found in the health–illness situation. Maintaining belief fuels nursing and nurses to serve patients and more generally humanity. **Knowing** is "striving to understand events as they have meaning in the life of the other" (Swanson, 1993, p. 355). Knowing includes all knowledge relevant to provide nursing care for the patient. Thus, knowing in nursing situations includes all nursing knowledge from formal and continuing education, as well as knowledge derived from ethical, personal, and aesthetic ways of knowing. Knowing sets the stage for the nurse's actions as therapeutic and effective in promoting well-being.

Being with is "emotional presence . . . a way of sharing the meaning, feelings, and lived experience of the one cared for" (Swanson, 1993, p. 356). Emotional presence is a way of sharing in the meanings and feelings of the patient being cared for and assures the patient's reality is appreciated. Swanson (1993) explained that being with includes "not just the side-by-side physical presence but also the clearly conveyed message of availability and ability to endure with the other" (p. 355). Being with another involves giving authentic presence and time, listening attentively, and providing contingent reflective responses. In many respects, being with is giving of self; the patient feels the commitment, concern, and personal attentiveness of the nurse.

Doing for is "doing for the other what they would do for themselves if it were at all possible" (Swanson, 1993, p. 356). Doing for is consistent with (a) Orem's notion of self-care by doing for patients what they cannot do for themselves and (b) Henderson's notion that nurses assist individuals in the performance of activities they could perform unaided if the patient had the strength, will, and knowledge to do so. Doing for involves actions by the nurse that are performed on behalf of the patient for the purpose of promoting health and well-being. Performing nursing interventions requires nursing knowledge, anticipating needs, competence, timeliness, skillfulness, and above all a caring presence on the part of the nurse.

Enabling is "facilitating the other's passage through life transitions and unfamiliar events" (Swanson, 1993, p. 356). Enabling includes: coaching, informing, explaining, teaching, supporting, helping identify alternatives, guiding, offering feedback, assisting one to focus on important issues, and validating the patient's reality. The goal of enabling is to help the patient achieve well-being. Swanson explained that enabling, like Nightingale's notion of creating an envi-

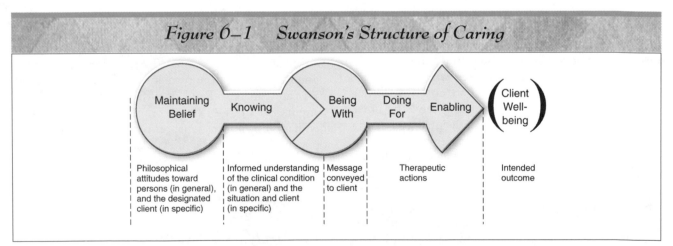

Figure 6–1   Swanson's Structure of Caring

Reprinted with permission from Sigma Theta Tau International from Swanson, K. M. (1993). Nursing as informal caring for the well-being of others. *IMAGE: Journal of Nursing Scholarship, 25*(4), 352–357.

The structure of caring as linked to the nurses' philosophical attitude, informed understandings, message conveyed, therapeutic actions, and intended outcome.

The models of caring that have been presented have practical application. Use Swanson's model of informed caring as you consider a patient you recently cared for. How did you manifest "maintaining belief" in your approach to the patient? What empirical (theoretical), ethical, aesthetic, and per-sonal types of "knowing" guided the care you pro-vided for the patient? In what ways did you use presence when "being with" the patient? What nursing interventions did you use when "doing for" this patient? What "enabling" methods did you use?

ronment so nature's healing effect may act, also involves creating an environment in which self-healing can occur. Within Swanson's (1993) model of informed caring, nursing practice "is the result of blended understandings of the empirical, aesthetic, eth-ical, and intuitive aspects of a given clinical situation and a nexus of maintaining belief in, knowing, being with, doing for and enabling the other" (p. 356) to pass through difficult health-related events and life transitions so well-being may be achieved.

Bringing Caring into the Foreground of Nursing Practice

Caring is a way of *being* in nursing, and in this respect, nursing is caring. Caring is the "art" in nursing practice. Caring is far from ordinary; caring as articulated in this chapter is what makes nursing actions exquisite and extraordinary. The caring perspectives presented in this chapter are not mutually exclusive, rather they are inte-gral to the complex nature of caring. The arc of knowl-edge concerning caring in nursing makes it clear that caring is, all at once, professional nursing's: ethical imperative; moral ideal; essence; central and most unify-ing domain of knowledge and practices; way of being in nursing; way of guiding persons to live and grow in car-ing; and way of informing all aspects of nursing practice.

To the detriment of all, caring and the work of nurses is often invisible. Bringing caring into the fore-ground of nursing will serve to make caring and nurs-ing more visible to all health care professionals and the public. Placing caring at the foreground of nursing practice means bringing caring in from the margins of practice. Bringing caring into the foreground reveals the hiddenness of caring and makes caring clearer, bolder, salient, and more distinguishable to all. When caring is on the forefront of nursing practice, nurses can illuminate the value of caring practices.

Embracing caring as the humanistic philosophical and scientific foundation of nursing means integrating caring into all aspects of nursing education and prac-tice. Basing nursing education and practice on a science of *nursing as caring* does not diminish the need for competence or scientific knowledge. A caring founda-tion places competencies, skills, and scientific knowl-edge within a humanistic context. Caring models are designed to:

- Liberate and enable graduates to be more respon-sive to societal needs
- Assist nurses to be more compassionate and suc-cessful in humanizing the highly technological health care environment
- Enable insightful decisions regarding ethical issues
- Produce creative and capable critical thinking
- Make new graduates more knowledgeable regard-ing cultural diversity while providing culturally sen-sitive care
- Produce more politically active nurses who will advocate on behalf of the health needs of all
- Better prepare nurses for professional roles in this new millennium (Bevis & Watson, 1989)

While all persons are caring, caring is unique in nurs-ing when nursing practice is grounded in and guided by caring. Each caring perspective presented in this chapter offers a unique view of caring *in* nursing and serves as a foundation for teaching, learning, and practicing nursing. This chapter illustrates how the works of Nightingale, Leininger, Watson, Roach, Gaut, Swanson, and Boykin and Schoenhofer demonstrate distinct ways to frame caring in nursing. Each caring perspective offers a way to *create a caring context* for nursing practice by offering specific values, actions, and behaviors associated with caring. Each model describes how to enact practices that exemplify caring in nursing. The caring perspectives presented offer a language and way of articulating how nurses make a difference through caring. Caring serves to *distinguish* nursing from other disciplines. Basing nursing practice on caring models is the first step in

Tell a story about a patient you recently cared for that exemplifies caring in nursing to someone who is unfamiliar with the role of nurses. What caring attributes, values, behaviors, and actions did you use in the caring situation? How did your nursing care make a difference in the situation?

making caring more visible in nursing, more visible in health care, and more visible to society.

The caring–healing arts that can be traced back to Nightingale need to be brought back from the "margins" of health care and into the realm of nursing care. The public commonly uses the healing–caring art of Nightingale and many have been co-opted by nonlicensed practitioners and even by mainstream medicine. In many cases, these healing–caring arts have been used as mere technical (medical) interventions without being grounded in an ethical, philosophical, theoretical, or scientific framework. Caring–healing modalities need to be restored as basic to nursing care and integrated into nursing education and practice. The caring–healing modalities are a rich source for testing in nursing research. The integration of caring–healing modalities into patient care will go far in making nursing visible in the eyes of the public, rehumanizing the current health care system, and in furthering the health and well-being of all.

The integration of caring into nursing education and practice means reclaiming the caring–healing practices/arts. Guided imagery, therapeutic touch, massage, and the use of color, light, movement, and sound are just a few of the caring–healing/arts that have long been advocated by holistic nurses as integral to nursing practice. Nursing students can be taught how to use metaphors, journaling, storytelling, poetry, literature, art, and music to facilitate the patient to find meaning in the health–illness situation and promote health, well-being, and healing. Holistic caring nursing practices distinguish nursing from the traditional medical model that continues to dominate nursing education and practice.

Nurses are obligated to enhance both their own and the public's understanding of the essential contribution nurses make to human health. All nurses need to be continuously engaged in conversations with the public, constantly making clear our unique and invaluable contribution to health care. Nurses need to articulate not just what we do, but explain what it is that nurses know and how we make a difference. Nursing stories are created each day. Nurses practice and have the power to connect the public to the everyday experience of health and illness through these stories. Stories reveal the hidden nature of nursing care, while illuminating how caring is truly the essential process in healing.

To bring caring into the foreground is to make caring *bold*. To rehumanize health care, the next generation of nurses must embrace caring as nursing's moral ideal and use caring knowledge in practice. Suzanne Gordan, a journalist with the Boston Globe, who speaks about increasing the visibility of nursing, asserts that no profession achieves recognition without struggle. Our boldness is mobilized in the expression of our collective moral passion and righteous anger about the policies and politics that impose economic, cultural, and ideological constraints that compromise and limit the nurse's ability to enact caring practices. To be bold and visible is to match the intensity of our politics with the intensity of our caring ethics. Those whom we serve and care for will be the ultimate beneficiaries of our care.

TRANSITION INTO PRACTICE

The nurse's *presence* with patients is a common theme that runs through all the conceptualizations of caring presented in this chapter. Presence is associated with existing in a situation, closeness, being there, being with another, feeling something, existence, influence, and caring. One of the deepest expressions of caring and compassion can be found in Parse's description of "true presence." Parse (1998) reaches beyond traditional definitions of presence and offers nurses a unique way of journeying and sojourning in the personal worlds of patients. According to Parse (1998), true presence is a "special way of 'being with' in which the nurse is attentive to moment-to-moment changes in meaning as she or he *bears witness* to the person's or group's own living of value priorities" (p. 71). Parse (1998) described bearing witness as an interpersonal art, "an intentional reflective love" and a "free flowing attentiveness" (p. 71). Thus, in true presence, the nurse offers presence in the patient's universe unconditionally, is open to the reality the patient lives (Cody, 1995), and is available to bear witness without judging or labeling. Bearing witness is to acknowledge, to be present with, and to testify to the authenticity of another's experience; to demonstrate respect for another's truth is one of the basic processes of human-to-human relating (Cody, 2001). In bearing witness, the nurse attests to a person's authenticity through personal presence while being flexible, graceful, and fully with a patient. To bear witness to a patient's experience may involve attentively listening to the patient tell their story or the story may be conveyed in silence. The nurse does not "dig" for meaning, nor seek to express or explain an attitude or feeling that the patient leaves unspoken, but rather abides in the moment truly with the patient (Cody, 1995). The patient is energized by the courage to be oneself, knows what is right, and chooses how to live from making choices among an infinite number of possibilities co-created with others.

An important distinction in true presence from traditional caring models is the idea that in true presence the nurse reflects the belief that somewhere within themselves the patient knows "the way." In other words, rather than trying to explain, direct, guide, do for, or facilitate the patient's moving in a particular direction, the nurse reveres and honors the patient's own timing, values, choices, and pace co-creating rhythms in tune with what is right for him or her. True presence is not based on some kind of predefined schema because choices and outcomes are unpredictable. Instead, the nurse bears witness to the person's truths and moves with the person's struggle wherever it may lead. This way of being present with the patient is valuing the other's human dignity and freedom to choose.

True presence is a deep expression of caring for persons who want to tell their story of living health, suffering, and/or dying. According to Parse (1998), the nurse's true presence involves face-to-face discussions, silent immersion, and lingering presence. Face-to-face discussions may be through listening to one's story of health or may include dialogue about films, drawings, photographs, music, and metaphors that represent the patient's thoughts for the moment on their health. Silent immersion is a "deep place of no words that symbolizes much, a soundless hush of wordless stillness" (Parse, 1998, p. 73) in which the nurse in rhythm with the patient's experience bears witness to their becoming. Lingering presence is the recalling of a moment with a patient that arises after an immediate engagement. Ideas and glimpses of understanding may surface moments, days, or even years later. True presence transcends traditional caring models toward a deeper way of being with persons during the ups and downs, struggles, moments of joy, and the day-to-day living of their health. Bearing witness in true presence is an indispensable foundation for the genuine and lasting enhancement of the quality of life for the patients we serve.

KEY POINTS

1. The American Association of Colleges of Nursing's *Essentials of Baccalaureate Education for Professional Nursing Practice* document, the revised American Nurses Association Social Policy Statement, and the call for a "curriculum revolution" by the National League for Nursing all indicate there is an increasing emphasis on caring as a central concept and core value in nursing.

2. Nursing is in an ideal position to rehumanize health care. Nurses are the largest single group of health care providers. If nursing is ever to mobilize its collective power to influence change in public health care policy, nurses will need to first overcome the invisible nature of caring and restore caring as a central ethic for nursing.

3. A nurse's capacity to care can be enhanced, called forth, or inhibited by the educational experience of the student and, most importantly, by the presence or absence of theoretical conceptualizations of caring.

4. Caring is not unique to nursing, but is unique *in* nursing. Caring is unique in nursing when caring is informed and guided by philosophical, theoretical, and evidence-based knowledge.

5. Caring is a way of expressing the beauty of nursing and is a reflection of nursing aesthetics.

6. Caring is, all at once, professional nursing's: ethical imperative; moral ideal; essence; central and most unifying domain of knowledge and practices; a way of being in nursing; a way of guiding persons to live and grow in caring; and a way of informing all aspects of nursing practice.

7. Each caring in nursing perspective offers a way to create a caring context for nursing practice by pro-

viding specific values, actions, and behaviors concerning what it means and how to be caring in all nursing situations.

8. The conceptualizations of caring in nursing are designed to liberate and enable graduates to be more responsive to societal needs, more compassionate and successful in humanizing the highly technological health care environment, more insightful about ethical issues, more creative and capable of critical thinking, more knowledgeable about cultural diversity while providing culturally sensitive care, more politically active on behalf of the health needs of all, and better prepared for professional roles in this new millennium.

EXPLORE MediaLink

Critical thinking questions, essay questions, key terms, web links, activities, NCLEX review questions, and more interactive resources can be found on the Companion Website at www.prenhall.com/haynes. Click on Chapter 6 to select activities for this chapter.

REFERENCES

American Association of Colleges of Nursing. (1998). *Essentials of baccalaureate education for professional nursing practice*. Washington, DC: Author.

American Heritage Dictionary (Vol. 3) (1993). Boston: Houghton Mifflin Company.

American Nurses Association. (1995). *Nursing's social policy statement*. Washington, DC: Author.

Appleton, C. (1994). The gift of self: A paradigm for originating nursing as art. In P. C. J. Watson (Ed.), *Art & aesthetics in nursing* (pp. 91–114). New York: National League for Nursing.

Benner, P., & Wrubel, J. (1989). *The primacy of caring: Stress and coping in health and illness*. Reading, MA: Addison-Wesley.

Bevis, E. M., & Watson, J. (1989). *Toward a caring curriculum: A new pedagogy for nursing*. New York: National League for Nursing.

Boykin, A., & Schoenhofer, S. (2001). Anne Boykin and Savina O. Schoenhofer nursing as caring. In M. Parker (Ed.), *Nursing theories and nursing practice* (pp. 391–402). Philadelphia, PA: F. A. Davis.

Bronowski, J. (1965). *Science and human values*. New York: Perennial Library.

Carper, B. (1978). Fundamental patterns of knowing in nursing. *Advances in Nursing Science, 1*(1), 13–23.

Chinn, P. L. (1994). Developing a method for aesthetic knowing in nursing. In P. L. Chinn & J. Watson (Eds.), *Art & aesthetics in nursing* (pp. 19–40). New York: National League for Nursing.

Chinn, P. L. (2001). Toward a theory of nursing art. In N. L. Chaska (Ed.), *The nursing profession: Tomorrow and beyond* (pp. 287–298). Thousand Oaks, CA: Sage.

Chinn, P. L., & Kramer, M. K. (1999). *Theory and nursing: Integrated knowledge development* (5th ed.). St. Louis, MO: Mosby.

Cody, W. K. (1995). True presence with families living with HIV disease. In R. R. Parse (Ed.), *Illuminations: The human becoming theory in practice and research* (pp. 115–133). New York: National League for Nursing.

Fiedler, L. (1987). Images of the nurse in fiction and popular culture. In A. H. Jones (Ed.), *Images of nurses* (pp. 100–112). Philadelphia, PA: University of Pennsylvania Press.

Gadamer, H. G. (1986). *The relevance of the beautiful and other essays* (N. W. R. Bernasconi, Trans.).

Gaut, D. (1984). A philosophic orientation to caring research. In M. Leininger (Ed.), *Care: The essence of nursing and health* (pp. 17–44). Thorofare, NJ: Slack.

Gaylin, W. (1976). *Caring*. New York: Knopf.

Gordon, S. (1997). *Life support: Three nurses on the front lines*. Boston: Little, Brown and Company.

Heidegger, M. (1996). *Being and time: A translation of Sein and Zeit* (J. Stambaugh, Trans.). New York: State University of New York Press.

Henderson, V. (1997). *Basic principles of nursing care* (rev. ed.). Geneva, Switzerland: International Council of Nurses.

Institute of Medicine. (2001). *Crossing the quality chasm: A new health system for the 21st century*. Washington, DC: Institute of Medicine.

Johnson, J. L. (1994). A dialectical examination of nursing art. *Advances in Nursing Science, 17*(7), 1–14.

Leininger, M. (1981a). Foreword. In M. Leininger (Ed.), *Caring: An essential human need*. Thorofare, NJ: Slack.

Leininger, M. (1981b). The phenomenon of caring: Importance, research questions and theoretical considerations. In M. Leininger (Ed.), *Caring: An essential human need*. Thorofare, NJ: Slack.

Leininger, M. (1985). *Qualitative research methods in nursing*. Orlando: Grune & Stratton.

Leininger, M. (1991). *Culture care diversity and universality: A theory of nursing*. New York: National League for Nursing.

Malkin, J. (1992). Developing a healing environment. In J. Malkin (Ed.), *Hospital interior architecure*. New York: Wiley.

Mayeroff, M. (1971). *On caring*. New York: Harper Prennial.

Morse, J. M., Solberg, S. M., Neander, W. L., Bottorff, J. L., & Johnson, J. L. (1990). Concepts of caring and caring as a concept. *Advances in Nursing Science, 13*(1), 1–14.

Mossman, L. C. (1923). The place of beauty in life. *Trained Nurse and Hospital Review 81*.

Newman, M., Sime, A. M., & Corcoran-Perry, S. (1991). The focus of the discipline of nursing. *Advances in Nursing Science, 14*(1), 1–6.

Nightingale, F. (1859). *Notes on nursing*. London: Harrison and Sons.

Nightingale, F. (1868, June). Una and the lion. *Good Works*.

Noddings, N. (1984). *Caring: A feminine approach to ethics & moral education*. Berkeley, CA: University of California Press.

Orem, D. (1995). *Nursing: Concepts of practice* (5th ed.). St. Louis, MO: Mosby.

Parse, R. R. (1998). *The human becoming school of thought*. Thousand Oaks, CA: Sage.

Peplau, H. (1988). Perspectives on nursing science. *Nursing Science Quarterly, 1*, 80–85.

Phillips, S. S. (1994). Introduction. In S. Phillips & P. Benner (Eds.), *The crisis of care: Affirming and restoring caring practices in the helping professions*. Washington, DC: Georgetown University Press.

Reverby, S. M. (1987). *Ordered to care: The dilemma of American nursing*. Cambridge: Cambridge University Press.

Roach, M. S. (1992). *The human act of caring: A blueprint for the health professions* (rev. ed.). Ottawa, Canada: Canadian Hospital Association Press.

Rogers, M. E. (1988). Nursing science and art: A prospective. *Nursing Science Quarterly, 1*, 99–102.

Stewart, I. (1929). The science and art of nursing (Editorial). *Nursing Education Review, 2*, 1.

Swanson, K. M. (1993). Nursing as informed caring for the well-being of others. *Image: The Journal of Nursing Scholarship, 25*, 352–357.

Watson, J. (1985). *Nursing: Human science and human care*. Norwalk, CT: Appleton-Century-Crofts.

Watson, J. (1990). The moral failure of the patriarchy. *Nursing Outlook, 38*(2), 62–66.

Watson, J. (1996). Watson's theory of transpersonal caring. In P. Hinton-Walker & B. Neuman (Eds.), *Blueprint for use of nursing models* (pp. 141–194). New York: National League for Nursing.

Watson, J. (1997). The theory of human caring: Retrospective and prospective. *Nursing Science Quarterly, 10*, 20–26.

Watson, J. (1999). *Postmodern nursing and beyond*. Edinburgh: Churchill Livingstone.

Watson, J. (2001). Jean Watson theory of human caring. In M. Parker (Ed.), *Nursing theories and nursing practice* (pp. 343–354). Philadelphia, PA: F. A. Davis.

SUGGESTED READINGS

Benner, P., & Wrubel, J. (1989). *The primacy of caring: Stress and coping in health and illness*. Reading, MA: Addison-Wesley.

Bevis, E. M., & Watson, J. (1989). *Toward a caring curriculum: A new pedagogy for nursing*. New York: National League for Nursing.

Boykin, A., & Schoenhofer, S. (2001). Anne Boykin and Savina O. Schoenhofer nursing as caring. In M. Parker (Ed.), *Nursing theories and nursing practice* (pp. 391–402). Philadelphia, PA: F. A. Davis.

Leininger, M. (1991). *Culture care diversity and universality: A theory of nursing*. New York: National League for Nursing.

Mayeroff, M. (1971). *On caring*. New York: Harper Prennial.

Roach, S. M. (1992). *The human act of caring: A blueprint for the health professions* (rev. ed.). Ottawa, Canada: Canadian Hospital Association Press.

Swanson, K. M. (1993). Nursing as informed caring for the well-being of others. *Image: The Journal of Nursing Scholarship, 25*, 352–357.

Watson, J. (1999). *Postmodern nursing and beyond*. Edinburgh: Churchill Livingstone.

Watson, J. (2001). Jean Watson theory of human caring. In M. Parker (Ed.), *Nursing theories and nursing practice* (pp. 343–354). Philadelphia, PA: F. A. Davis

7

Reflective Clinical Reasoning

DANIEL J. PESUT

> *Clinicians learn on the job by managing patients. Experience teaches reality, but it can be a slow teacher if what goes on is not examined, closely, accurately, and thoughtfully. And experience can be an inaccurate teacher if the events remain unnoticed, disregarded or consistently misinterpreted. Reflection can integrate the past, present and future—in this case with what happened in the previous case and what to do in future cases. Reflection can look in many directions.*
>
> Ken Cox (1999)

LEARNING OBJECTIVES

AT THE COMPLETION OF THIS CHAPTER, THE READER WILL BE ABLE TO:

- Discuss differences in academic, practical, successful, and nursing intelligence.
- Explain the value of knowing learning style strengths and compensatory needs.
- Describe how critical, creative, and systems thinking support clinical reasoning.

- Explain the Outcome–Present State–Test (OPT) model of reflective clinical reasoning.
- Discuss the importance of clinical reflection as a source of learning and power.
- Explain ways to develop the capacity for reflection in-and-on professional actions.

MediaLink   www.prenhall.com/haynes

Additional online resources including NCLEX review questions, critical thinking questions, and real-world activities for this chapter can be found on the Companion Website at www.prenhall.com/haynes.

*K*nowledge and experience offer nurses an avenue for achieving professional power. This power is derived from reflectively thinking (about relationships between and among problems, interventions, and outcomes), acting (in accordance with identity, intention, knowledge, values, and beliefs), and doing (whatever action is needed in order to derive a meaningful judgment about outcome achievements). While experience helps the new nurse integrate academic knowledge with practical know how, knowledge acquisition and professional development require intentional focus and the ability/willingness to learn. Learning is best achieved when individuals understand how they learn, what their learning strengths and weaknesses are, and existing developmental needs. The more personal insight a nurse has regarding their own learning style, the greater the likelihood for learning. Furthermore, experience supports effective, timely learning and acquisition of clinical reasoning, decision-making, and judgment skills.

Concepts, models, and tools described in this chapter suggest ways to develop and master the power of reflective clinical reasoning. A model of learning and the role learning styles play in the development of self and team learning is discussed. Academic, practical, successful, and nursing intelligence will be defined. Dimensions of critical thinking are highlighted. Questions to stimulate reflection and reasoning are posed.

Academic and Practical Intelligence

Nurses need both academic and practical intelligence to deliver and provide quality care. Psychologist Robert Sternberg (1996) defines **intelligence** as the ability to cope with demands created by novel situations and new problems. Nurses deal with novel situations and new problems every day. Intelligence, then, is the application of experience. Use of reasoning and inference are tools used to guide intelligence. There are many kinds of intelligence; Sternberg (1985, 1988, 1996) makes distinctions among academic, practical, creative, and successful intelligence. **Academic intelligence** is measured by intelligence quotient (IQ) tests. Academic intelligence is knowledge focused on what "should" work. Academic problems are well defined, formulated by others, and usually come with all the information that is necessary for problem-solving. Generally, academic problems have only one correct answer and

method for obtaining the answer. Often, academic problems are unrelated to everyday experience.

In contrast, **practical intelligence** is the ability to apply mental abilities to everyday situations. One of the major challenges novice nurses face as they enter the world of professional practice is the translation of academic intelligence into practical intelligence. Practical intelligence involves learning to manage oneself, others, and tasks. The "street smarts" of practical intelligence are implied or silent and embedded in experience. Sternberg (1988) suggests practical problems differ from academic problems in five ways. First, practical problems are not well defined and are not formulated by others. Second, one often does not have all the information needed to solve the problem. Third, there is rarely a single solution to practical problems. Fourth, everyday experience is used to solve practical problems. Fifth, practical intelligence is knowledge focused on what "does work."

Know What and How

By talking with nurses, Patricia Benner (1984) "uncovered" the kind of practical intelligence needed to be successful in nursing. She asked nurses what they actually did in day-to-day practice situations. Benner (1984) identified the following practical domains of nursing: (a) the helping role, (b) the teaching–coaching function, (c) the diagnostic and patient monitoring function, (d) the effective management of rapidly changing situations, (e) the administration and monitoring of therapeutic interventions and regimens, (f) the monitoring and ensuring the quality of health care practices, and (g) organization and work role competence.

Benner (1984) makes distinctions between "knowing that" and "knowing how." She suggests practical knowledge eludes scientific formulations. She believes knowledge development in an applied discipline consists of extending practical "know how" through theory-based scientific investigations and through sharing the existent "know how" developed with clinical experience. Practical experiences derived from clinical thinking combined with academic experiences build nursing knowledge and enhance individual, collective, and practical nursing intelligence. The challenge for most clinicians is to turn "knowing about" into the working knowledge of "knowing what to do" (Cox, 1999). Knowing what to do requires the development of practical nursing science (knowledge) and successful nursing intelligence.

Were Benner's practical domains of nursing clearly identified in your nursing curriculum? Do you

organize your thinking and/or reasoning around the concepts contained in these domains?

In reality, there are three kinds of nursing science: (a) basic, (b) applied, and (c) practical. Traditional nursing education is concerned with basic and applied nursing science. **Basic science** refers to knowledge that is developed purely for the sake of knowing. This knowledge adds to our sense of understanding about people. It is generally understood the knowledge may be useful one day. **Applied science** is knowledge used in caring directly for patients. Both basic and applied science serves as the foundation for clinical thinking and reasoning (Pesut & Herman, 1999).

Nursing Art and Science

Johnson (1991) argues for a third type of nursing science. She calls this practical science. **Practical science** combines the science and art of nursing. In nursing, more attention is often paid to the topic of science rather than art. However, Johnson (1994) believes "science alone will not solve all the problems of nursing" (p. 1). As novice nurses transition into practice, they face the challenge of developing both the science and art of nursing.

Johnson (1994) argues "art" in nursing involves the ability (a) to grasp meaning in patient encounters, (b) to establish a meaningful connection with patients, (c) to skillfully perform nursing activities, (d) to rationally determine an appropriate course of action, and (e) to morally conduct one's nursing practice. Such "art" is developed with experience and supports the development of practical intelligence. Novice nurses face the challenge of learning how to use the science and art of nursing as they successfully transition from student to professional nurse.

Successful Intelligence

A focus on the practical science of nursing leads to the development of successful intelligence. Psychologist Robert Sternberg (1996) states, "**Successful intelligence** is the kind of intelligence used to achieve important goals. People who succeed, whether by their own standards or by other people's are those who have managed to acquire, develop, and apply a full range of intel-

lectual skills, rather than relying on the inert intelligence that schools value. These individuals may or may not succeed on conventional tests, but they have something in common that is more important than high test scores. They know their strengths; they know their weaknesses. They capitalize on their strengths; they compensate for or correct their weaknesses. That's it" (p. 12).

Sternberg's (1996) research has resulted in the following profile of successfully intelligent people. In general successfully intelligent people:

- Don't wait for problems to hit them over the head. They recognize their existence before they get out of hand and begin the process of solving them.
- Define problems correctly and thereby solve those problems that really confront them, rather than extraneous ones. In this way, the same problems don't keep coming back into their lives. They also make the effort to decide which problems are worth solving in the first place and which are not.
- Carefully formulate strategies for problem-solving. In particular they focus on long-range planning rather than rushing in and later having to rethink their strategies.
- Represent information about a problem as accurately as possible, with a focus on how they can use that information effectively.
- Think carefully about allocating resources for both the short term and long term. They consider risk–reward ratios and then choose the allocations they believe will maximize their return.
- Do not always make the correct decisions, but they monitor and evaluate their decisions and then correct their errors as they discover them.

How do the characteristics of successfully intelligent people apply to individual nurses? Anticipating problems, monitoring responses, framing problems correctly, evaluating and self-correcting decisions, juggling short- and long-term consequences, and balancing risks and rewards are strategies that develop as a result of practical experiences in the world. As one applies the elements of successful intelligence to nursing one develops nursing intelligence.

Nursing Intelligence and Professional Power

Nursing intelligence (NI) is a blend of academic, practical, and successful intelligence acquired through experiences and reflection in and on those experiences (Pesut & Herman, 1999).

- Develops over time and is derived from nursing care experiences that have been subjected to reason and reflection
- Knowing what outcomes are most likely in a given situation or context
- Making clinical decisions and organizing care to achieve those outcomes
- Knowing what to do and how to do it
- Knowing what, how, and why
- Using pattern recognition and intuition

Curiosity supports the development of NI. As NI develops, professional power and expertise grow.

There are many ways to achieve professional goals, maximize practical experiences, and develop professional expert power. Practical experiences contribute to the development of professional power when an individual understands self, values personal learning style strengths, and has insights into compensatory and developmental learning style needs. Practical experiences contribute to the development of professional power when the nurse:

- Understands how critical, creative, and systems thinking support clinical thinking and reasoning
- Realizes that success in contemporary health care requires a focus on outcomes rather than problems
- Gains support for the development of a repertoire of skills and abilities needed to act and react in uncertain situations
- Develops from active **reflection** on practical experiences

Growth and insights gained through reflection enable practitioners to understand, take action, and create new patterns of relating with themselves and others who are powerful. Reflection opens the professional nursing world.

- Reflection is a means to integrate past experiences into present learning and future thinking.
- Reflection allows the nurse to build expertise over time.
- Reflection enables a nurse to become creative and thorough in responding to novel situations rather than unresponsive or reactive.
- Reflection supports self-activation and learning versus self-sabotage and helplessness.
- Reflection is concerned with the growth of the powerful self (Johns, 2000).

Becoming a professional requires self-activation and proactive behavior. It further requires accepting the power that comes with being a professional who has knowledge, skills, and abilities to make a difference in people's lives. Reflection increases the nurse's awareness of issues, choices, actions, and the effects of those actions. The capacity to participate knowingly in the nature of change has been defined as power (Caroselli & Barrett, 1998). **Power** is manifested by awareness of choices, freedom to act intentionally, and involvement in creating change. Awareness, choice, and freedom to act with intentions are manifestations of reflection, reason, and successful nursing intelligence. Reflective clinical reasoning skills are positively related to professional power and influence.

Nursing intelligence grows when nurses share reflections and the clinical thinking involved with experience and action. Every patient cared for contributes to the development of clinical thinking skills and thus is a source of learning, successful NI, and professional power. Development of practical, successful NI requires one to "learn about learning" and to "think about thinking."

Critical Thinking and Reflection

How would you describe the current ratio of academic to practical intelligence that you possess? For example, what percentage of academic or practical intelligence do you currently have—60% academic and 40% practical intelligence or some other ratio? What do you think is the ideal or best ratio of academic to practical intelligence? Examine Sternberg's characteristics of successfully intelligent people. How do you rate yourself on each of the characteristics? Do you think there is such a thing as nursing intelligence? If so, how do you define and describe it?

Sources of Power

Learning About Learning

Kolb (1984, 1985) suggest learning cycles through four stages: concrete experience (CE), reflective observation (RO), abstract conceptualization (AC), and active experimentation (AE). This cycle is a good way to think about the development of professional expertise. Experience is a great teacher. Clinical experiences offer nursing students the opportunity to engage in the concrete situations that make classroom concepts real. Once practical experiences are connected with academic intelligence, nurses and nursing students are better prepared to understand the knowledge gained and skills acquired. Reflection on experience enables one to "connect the dots" between theory and practical reality. Once reflections about experiences are linked with explanations, working knowledge develops to guide practice and future clinical thinking.

Kolb (1985) observed that there are individual preferences associated with learning. Some people prefer to jump right in and get the experience. Others reflect more and experiment less. Still others like to generate many ways to approach problems. People tend to value and rely on their learning style preferences. Reliance on one or more learning modes is simultaneously an advantage and a disadvantage as each style has associated with it strengths and weaknesses. Learning strengths support doing what comes naturally. When nurses rely on strengths, they may not grow or engage other aspects of learning that support the development of practical or successful intelligence. Learning style preferences give clues to developmental learning needs.

To be successful it is valuable for nurses to understand their own individual learning style and to actively seek out time, place, people, and experiences to maximize strengths and compensate for weaknesses through personal or professional development efforts. Individuals who have never completed a learning style inventory may find it advantageous to do so because such self-knowledge leads to insights for action. Kolb (1984, 1985) placed the stages of learning along two axes, an active/reflective and concrete/abstract axis. Within the four quadrants created by the two axes, he defines four learning styles: (a) the **accommodator** prefers learning through concrete experience and active experimentation, (b) the **diverger** prefers learning through concrete experience and reflective observation, (c) the **assimilator** prefers learning through a combination of abstract conceptualization and reflective observation,

and (d) the **converger** prefers to learn through a combination of abstract conceptualization and active experimentation. As seen in Figure 7–1, each learning style has strengths and weaknesses. Developing successful intelligence requires personal insight and a conscious plan to develop and compensate for learning weaknesses.

Thinking About Thinking

It is impossible to think critically without thinking about your thinking. Another term for thinking about your thinking is reflection. Linking reflection with experiences allows nurses to develop practical, successful, and nursing intelligence more quickly. Becoming a reflective practitioner and developing a reflective practice in nursing is crucial to professional success (Burns & Bulman, 2000; Johns, 2000). Reflection or **metacognition** (thinking about thinking) contributes to an understanding of the thinking strategies involved in clinical reasoning and clinical judgment (Pesut & Herman, 1992, 1999).

The metacognitive (reflective) activities of self-monitoring, analyzing, predicting, planning, evaluating, and revising provide the groundwork for developing a nursing diagnosis, planning care, and reflecting and reasoning about clinical decisions and judgments (Herman, Pesut, & Conard, 1994). Developing "thinking about thinking" skills or reflection is one thread in the fabric of expert power and a source of nursing intelligence.

Much like Kolb, Gibbs (1988) defines six dimensions and questions that promote inquiry, reflection, and learning. Answering these questions on some consistent basis supports the development of insights and personal learning power. The dimensions and questions to consider include:

- Description—what happened?
- Feeling—what were you thinking?
- Evaluation—what was good and bad about the experience?
- Analysis—what sense can you make of it?
- Conclusion—what else could you have done?
- Action plan—if it arose again, what would you do?

Consider how one might use knowledge of learning styles and Gibbs's questions to learn more, become more conscious of learning from experience, and develop blue prints in one's mind for future action. This knowledge will allow the nurse to derive the learning acquired through daily clinical experiences. Such power is enhanced as the "thinking about thinking" ability is developed.

Figure 7–1   Kolb Learning Styles

The chart below identifies the strengths and weaknesses of each learning style with notes for improvement.

Concrete Experience

Accommodator

Strengths:	Getting things done
	Leadership
	Risk-taking
Too much:	Trivial improvements
	Meaningless activity
Not enough:	Work not completed on time
	Impractical plans
	Not directed to goals

To develop your Accommodative learning skills, practice:

• Committing yourself to objectives
• Seeking new opportunities
• Influencing and leading others
• Being personally involved
• Dealing with people

Diverger

Strengths:	Imaginative ability
	Understanding people
	Recognizing problems
	Brainstorming
Too much:	Paralyzed by alternatives
	Can't make decisions
Not enough:	No ideas
	Can't recognize problems and opportunities

To develop your Divergent learning skills, practice:

• Being sensitive to people's feelings
• Being sensitive to values
• Listening with an open mind
• Gathering information
• Imagining the implications of uncertain situations

Active   Reflective
Experimentation   Observation

Converger

Strengths:	Problem solving
	Decision making
	Deductive reasoning
	Defining problems
Too much:	Solving the wrong problem
	Hasty decision making
Not enough:	Lack of focus
	No shifting of ideas
	Scattered thoughts

To develop your Convergent learning skills, practice:

• Creating new ways of thinking and doing
• Experimenting with new ideas
• Choosing the best solution
• Setting goals
• Making decisions

Assimilator

Strengths:	Planning
	Creating models
	Defining problems
	Developing theories
Too much:	Castles in the air
	No practical application
Not enough:	Unable to learn from mistakes
	No sound basis for work
	No systematic approach

To develop your Assimilative learning skills, practice:

• Organizing information
• Building conceptual models
• Testing theories and ideas
• Designing experiments
• Analyzing quantitative data

Abstract Conceptualization

Robert Reich (1992) suggests twenty-first century "knowledge workers" need to develop four types of thinking skills:

- Abstraction or the ability to discover patterns and meanings in data, information and knowledge, events, and circumstances.
- Systems thinking or an understanding of the complexity of cause-and-effect relationships between problems and solutions in a system.
- Experimentation and testing, which requires curiosity, skepticism, and active analysis and evaluation of data, facts, conclusions, and interpretations and knowing how to make judgments and interpretations from a set of facts.
- Collaboration and communication skills, which are essential for negotiating and working in teams to find answers and achieve outcomes.

Richard Paul (1993) defines **critical thinking** as a unique kind of purposeful thinking, in which the thinker systematically and habitually imposes criteria and intellectual standards to conscious thought. It involves taking charge of one's thinking. When thinking critically, nurses can assess the effectiveness of their thinking by asking themselves the following questions (Paul & Elder, 2001):

- What is the purpose of my thinking?
- What precise question am I trying to answer?
- Within what point of view am I thinking?
- What information am I using?
- How am I interpreting that information?
- What concepts or ideas are central to my thinking?
- What conclusions am I coming to?
- What am I taking for granted, what assumptions am I making?
- If I accept the conclusions, what are the implications?
- What would the consequences be if I put my thought into action?

In order to pose these questions to oneself, the following must be valued: (a) independence of thinking, (b) fair-mindedness, (c) insight into self and others, (d) humility and a nonjudgmental attitude, (e) courage, (f) good faith and integrity, (g) perseverance, (h) confidence in reason, (i) openness and exploration of the thoughts underlying feelings and feelings underlying thoughts, and (j) curiosity (Paul & Elder, 2001).

The 10 characteristics noted above support the development of the type of thinking and feeling required for purposeful self-observation, analysis, reflection, and insight. These characteristics are important critical thinking skills that support the development of self-regulatory judgment.

Critical thinking is purposeful self-regulatory judgment; it involves one's ability to interpret, analyze, infer, explain, evaluate, and self-regulate (Facione & Facione, 1996). Interpretation involves skills related to categorizing, decoding sentences, and clarifying meaning. Analysis requires the ability to examine ideas and identify and analyze arguments. Inference relates to ones ability to query evidence, conjecture alternatives, and draw conclusions. Explanation involves determining results, justifying procedures, and presenting arguments. Evaluation requires one to assess claims, assess arguments, and attribute meaning to evidence. Self-regulation involves self-monitoring, self-evaluation, and self-correction in service of an identified outcome.

Clinical reasoning in nursing involves four threads of logic that need to be woven together at the same time. First, the nurse has to consider relevant patient care needs or nursing diagnoses. Second, the nurse has to know how the patient's needs fit into the care processes. Third, the nurse has to monitor the logic of one's own thinking about the diagnoses and related care planning processes. Fourth, the nurse has to take into consideration the system in which he or she operates. The logic embedded in these threads requires the nurse to think about and structure many things simultaneously.

Traditional nursing process models support a piece-by-piece, stepwise way of thinking. As nursing students transition into professional practice, they will be required to weave multiple threads together into a fabric of care. Clinical reasoning is a process in which clinicians interact with others in a given context to

Critical Thinking and Reflection

How do you rate yourself in regard to Reich's essential skills? What are your greatest strengths? Which of these skills would benefit from developmental work on your part? Thinking about your thinking adds to your practical, successful, nursing intelligence and professional power.

structure and give meaning to goals and health management strategies based on data, professional judgment, and knowledge (Higgs & Jones, 2000).

Clinical Experience

In the book, *Sources of Power: How People Make Decisions*, author Gary Klein (1999) describes several sources of power derived from the study of naturalistic decision-making. Klein's research focuses on the decision-making processes of people who make decisions under time constraints, where there is often inadequate information and there are poorly defined, constantly changing conditions. Based on studies with firemen, policemen, military personnel, and nurses, Klein concludes there are several sources of power in the decision-making process. Some of these sources of power include: situation awareness, understanding the big picture, pattern recognition, and intuition. Another source of power is mental simulation or seeing the past and future. For example, many nurses know what to do in a Code Blue situation because once they have had the experience they can replay it in their mind like a movie. Thus, the experience enables them to call up and use this "mental movie making" ability to know what the sequence of events is and how the drama of the Code plays out. Klein's Concept Map (Figure 7–2) provides a picture representation of the elements of expert thinking derived from clinical experience.

Every clinical encounter contains a patient's story. Over time, stories contribute to the development of patterns. Pattern recognition leads to action. As nurses share stories, they develop scenarios or mental movies about how the events of the story unfold. Nurses who have extensive experience have access to multiple scripts and story lines and are more prepared to know how the story unfolds. There may be deviations from an expected course of action and so nurses develop intuitive knowing that informs them of what to expect in specific individual cases. These experiences support memory, anticipation, and detection of problems before they even occur. With practical experiences, nurses learn to recognize typical cases, detect anomalies, and make fine discriminations. Such learning enables nurses to improvise and develop tricks of the trade as they spot leverage points, which contribute to the solvability of a problem.

Active Reflecting

Embedded in the stories nurses share with one another is learning that contributes to professional power.

Actively reflecting and organizing experience over time helps develop expertise and successful NI. Never underestimate the value of reflecting on a clinical story. Klein (1999) suggests storytelling organizes events into meaningful frameworks. Storytelling helps make sense of things. Good stories blend the following ingredients:

- Agents—the people who figure in the story
- Predicaments—the problems the agents are trying to solve
- Intentions—what the agents are trying to do
- Actions—what agents do to achieve their intentions
- Objects or tools that agents use
- Causality—the effects of carrying out actions
- Context—the details surrounding the agents and actions
- Surprises or unexpected turns of events

When nurses stop to think, they realize each nursing care situation contains all the elements of a good story. As nurses share and tell stories, NI and professional power develop. Stories are natural experiments that link a network of causes to their effects. Stories can become mental simulations or movies that help people reflect, reason, explain, and evaluate a course of action. Stories can be used to extract and communicate subtle aspects of expertise.

Active reflection enables a novice nurse to learn more than can be expressed. Story sharing connects nurses with experiences. Nurses learn from experience. Experience contributes to NI, professional expertise, and knowing. Nurses use experiences through time to make judgments while comparing and contrasting what they know with what they do not know. Reflective clinical reasoning is one way to recognize connections between stories and build expertise in clinical reasoning, clinical decision-making, and clinical judgment. It is useful to have a way to think about these stories and structure clinical reasoning activities.

Experts have extensive mental models, simulations, or movies in their heads. Experiences add to their mental film library. When confronted with new or difficult situations, they rely on their abilities to retrieve scenarios or simulations of past events so they can apply what they know about action needed in new situations. These "mental models" or "archived movies in their heads" build memories and unique, expert ways of thinking and knowing.

These simulations support perceptual discrimination and help nurses know what to expect in uncertain situations. Such experiences enable nurses to see what others do not see or to sense what is not presently evi-

Figure 7–2   Sources of Power Concept Map

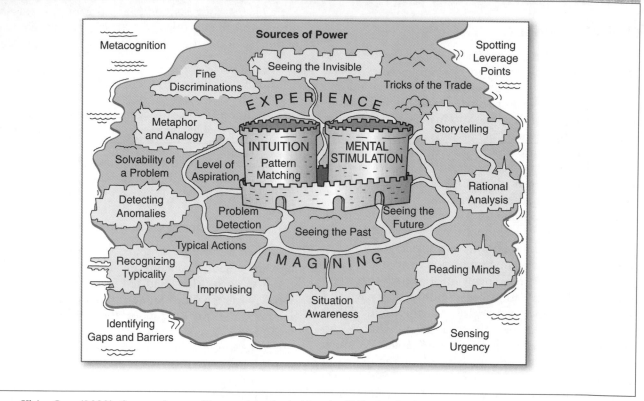

Source: Klein, Gary (1998). *Sources of power: How people make decisions* (p. 289). Cambridge, MA: MIT Press.

dent. Sometimes the use of different forms of thinking and reasoning (e.g., using metaphors) help develop understanding and explanation.

For example, a group of nurses who have gone through several difficult situations may come to refer to a set of circumstances with a code name (e.g., the "Jones disaster" or the "Kelly miracle"). Such references are often concrete memories of specific stories about specific patients or crises. A patient's story provides important information. The story provides the context and major issues for clinical reasoning. Listening to patients, connecting with them in meaningful ways, attributing meaning to their story, and getting the facts of their situation is the art of nursing (Johnson, 1994).

Stories are a key element of clinical reasoning. The more stories you have that support your clinical thinking and reasoning, the greater your professional understanding, insights, and expertise. This expertise evolves over time and is derived from simultaneously thinking

consciously and unconsciously about the sources of power outlined in Klein's Concept Map (Figure 7–2).

REFLECTION-IN-ACTION AND REFLECTION-ON-ACTION

Reflection-in-action is a term used by Donald Schon (1983) to describe the process by which professionals think and act. Reflection-in-action is self-talk. Reflection-in-action is the process whereby a clinician recognizes and thinks about a new situation as he or she is engaged in that situation. **Reflection-on-action** is retrospective and also provides an opportunity to access and uncover the knowledge used in the situations and how the situation might have been handled differently and what other knowledge might have been useful (Burns & Bulman, 2000).

Reflection helps nurses figure out what works and also what does not work. What doesn't work should become a point of curiosity and further inquiry. When someone reflects on action, he becomes a student of his own learning and thus enhances his academic, practical, successful, and nursing intelligence.

ELEMENTS OF REFLECTION

Johns (2000) notes the elements of reflection are contained within the following 10 Cs: commitment, contradiction, conflict, challenge and support, catharsis, creation, connection, caring, congruence, and constructing personal knowing in practice.

- Commitment involves a belief in oneself and in the value of practice. Commitment requires openness, curiosity, and a willingness to challenge norms and the status quo.
- Contradiction requires negotiation of the tensions that exist between the ideals and the realties of practice.
- Conflict involves managing the tensions that exist between competing commitments, and using that tension and energy to create new options. Such conflict can be helpful if challenges are linked with support.
- Catharsis involves working through negative feelings.
- Creation involves holding the tension of contradictions and opposites long enough for something new to emerge from the tension.
- Connection involves linking new insights with past learning and bringing past learning to new situations and connecting the dots associated with pattern recognition and intuition.
- Caring is the energy that fuels desirable practice as an everyday reality.
- Congruence requires alignment of thoughts, feelings, and actions, and is facilitated through reflective practice.
- Constructing personal knowing in practice involves spinning and weaving the threads of personal knowledge with theory in constructing knowledge that builds on academic, practical, successful, and nursing intelligence.

The experiences of nurses provide opportunities for reflection-in-action and reflection-on-action. Such reflection supports learning and is a source of power. If nurses begin to recognize the importance of learning about learning and thinking about thinking and develop the capacity for reflection in and on the stories they experience on a daily basis, they will develop practical intelligence. This practical intelligence becomes a source of professional power.

This chapter has described and discussed a number of tools and techniques nurses can use to enhance reflection in and on their thinking and practice. Learning about learning, and thinking about thinking support the development of reflection. The Kolb Learning Styles Inventory helps a nurse to pinpoint learning style strengths and developmental needs. Appreciating learning style differences supports and underscores the importance of individual and team learning. The Six Questions developed by Gibbs (1988) helps one actively reflect on clinical experiences and supports thinking about how patient cases are the same and how they are different. Such reflection supports learning from one case and taking the learning from that case into the future. The OPT model structure (Pesut & Herman, 1999) and the Concept Map developed by Klein (1999) provide ways to think about clinical reasoning, clinical decision-making, and clinical judgment. Based on the facts of the situation, choices are made in order to achieve outcomes defined. The first challenge of clinical reasoning is to represent all the issues and needs that patients reveal. The second challenge is to consider how all these issues are related to one another. The third challenge is to find the keystone issue that organizes the focus of care based on the patient's story. Once the keystone issue is identified, other diagnostic concerns may be resolved through activities surrounding the keystone issue. Through stories and the development of mental simulations, nurses come to recognize patterns, develop intuition, and have a sense of how uncertain situations unfold toward some resolution. Reflection in and on experiences is a source of professional power.

Critical Thinking and Reflection

Think back to a crisis situation you have experienced. Replay the movie in your head. First play it forward from beginning to end. Now rewind the movie and play it backwards from the end to the beginning. Such mental simulations help create a library of clinical simulations in your own head.

Actively running these scenarios over and over helps one develop the capacity to learn and respond. Acquisition of these experiences and actively filing them away over time becomes a source of practical, successful, and nursing intelligence as well as a source of professional expert power.

Cox (1999) states reflection requires looking in many directions. One can reflect during a clinical encounter and try to capture the clinical thinking that takes place at the bedside. One can reflect backwards at the clinical evidence found in a case to test interpretations, inferences, and hunches and compare these with past personal experiences with patients and to review how past situations were handled. Reflection can focus on an inward direction and ascertain what the health–illness experience means for the patient and/or clinician. Reflection can focus beneath an issue and go below the surface to find explanations and new knowledge or evidence about current theories and research findings. Reflection can go forward to build blueprints for future action or decision rules on what to do next time and to learn from past mistakes or successes. Each of these directions for reflection has its own logic and dynamic. Each contributes to the development of practical intelligence as a source of power.

The OPT Model of Reflective Clinical Reasoning

The traditional nursing process has changed over time and has moved from a focus on problems to outcomes. Today the health industry is most interested in specification and measurement of outcomes rather than the assessment and identification of problems. Nursing care that is problem focused is not necessarily outcome specific. Outcomes focus on an end result or desired states. Outcome specification is central to care and case management (Oerman & Huber, 1999). The most recent version of the American Nurses Association (ANA) (1995) Social Policy Statement advocates attention to outcomes and deemphasizes a problem-focused approach to nursing care.

Nursing process models of the past did not explicitly deal with outcome specification (Pesut, 1989).

Consider how the nursing process has changed over time. The first generation (1950–1970) focused on problems and process. The second generation (1970–1990) highlighted diagnosis and reasoning. The third generation nursing process models will manage the juxtapositions of both problems and outcomes at the same time; nursing will recognize this crucial skill (Pesut & Herman, 1998). Clinical reasoning that focuses on outcomes is more valuable and cost-effective than clinical reasoning that focuses on problems.

The Outcome–Present State–Test (OPT) model of reflective clinical reasoning (Figure 7–3) is a third generation nursing process model that emphasizes reflection, outcome specification, and tests of judgment within the context of individual patient stories. The OPT model (Pesut & Herman, 1999) builds on the heritage of the nursing process and fits contemporary nursing practice needs. The OPT model provides a structure for clinical thinking. The model suggests nurses simultaneously consider relationships among diagnoses, interventions, and outcomes with attention to the evidence used to make judgments. The model is not a step-by-step problem-solving model that focuses on one problem at a time. The OPT requires one to consider many problems at the same time, and discern which problem or issue is most important. Once this "keystone issue" is determined, efforts are put into specifying the outcomes that are derived from problems or presenting state conditions. Next, the nurse identifies the evidence for outcome achievement. Interventions are chosen, then applied, and reflection and judgment about the results of those interventions or clinical decisions are made.

The model uses the facts associated with a patient's story to frame the context and content for clinical reasoning. **Clinical decision-making** in this model is defined as choosing nursing actions. **Clinical judgment** is the conclusion or meaning one gives data drawn from a comparison of patient present state data to specified outcome criteria. Reflection on judgments suggests the need for reframing situations or creating new tests, making different intervention decisions or choices. Clinical reasoning involves concurrent, creative, critical, and sys-

Critical Thinking and Reflection

How is the model similar or different from the way you currently structure your clinical thinking? Does this model make more explicit how you think about your own thinking? What parts of the model are clear and familiar? What aspects of the model are confusing to you? How might you use this model to structure your clinical thinking about multiple problems and outcomes associated with a particular patient story and context?

Figure 7–3   OPT Model of Reflective Clinical Reasoning

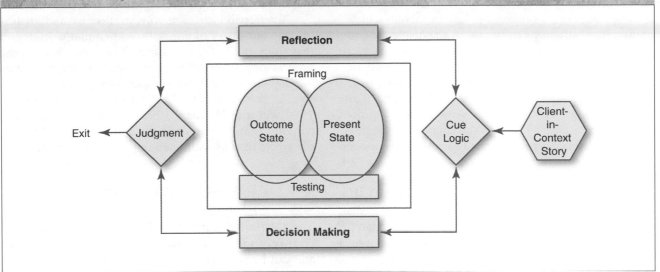

From *Clinical Reasoning: The art and science of critical and creative thinking*, by D. Pesut and J. Herman. © 1999. Reprinted with permission of Delmar, a division of Thomson Learning. Fax 800-730-2215.

tems thinking. Clinical reasoning is supported by higher-order critical thinking skills and lower order thinking strategies. The thinking strategies that enable one to perform clinical reasoning are gained through practice and conscious reflections on that practice.

In the OPT model, reflection is a component of executive thinking processes (thinking about thinking) and consists of the simultaneous application of critical, creative, and systems thinking. Reflection is the process of observing one's own thinking while simultaneously thinking about patient situations. A large part of clinical reasoning involves observing and talking to one's self as one thinks through all the elements of a complex, uncertain situation. The goal of reflection is to achieve the best possible clinical thinking. The greater the self-observation and monitoring, the more likely one is able to attend to the quality of care delivered because self-consciousness helps to focus the issues and situational dynamics.

Clinical reasoning requires the simultaneous application of three types of thinking: critical, creative, and systems. Critical thinking is an aspect of reflection that supports nursing as science. **Creative thinking** is an aspect of reflection that supports nursing as art. **Systems thinking** suggests when many elements stand in relationship to each other there is a balancing and reinforcing loop that supports the dynamics of the situation. Systems thinking requires attention to induction, deduction, and dialectic thinking.

Induction is forward reasoning and involves reasoning from specific cues toward a general judgment. **Deduction** involves reasoning from a general premise toward a conclusion. Deduction can also be considered backward reasoning as one can reason backward from a conclusion to a premise. **Dialectic thinking** considers both the deductive and inductive aspects of a situation in terms of an open system subject to feedback and change. Dialectic thinking requires both forward and backward reasoning.

Another component of the model is cue logic. **Cue logic** is the deliberate structuring of patient data to discern the meaning for nursing care. Cue logic contributes information that helps set up, structure, or frame a situation. Framing involves thinking about the meaning of cue connections through some lens or frames of meaning. This "frame" could be a specific nursing theory, a particular model, a developmental perspective, or a set of policies and procedures.

Success in practice requires one to reason forward from a problem to an outcome and also backwards from the outcome or effect to the current state. **Present states** (P) represent where the patient is in present time given the context. **Outcomes** (O) are desired or end states that you want the patient to achieve in future time.

Through the use of creative, critical, systems, and reflective thinking (that occur simultaneously) nurses create future time outcomes, using current present state data, and establish side-by-side comparisons. This side-by-side comparison of present to desired future states creates a "test" or an evidence gap that needs to be filled in order to make a judgment about achievement of the outcome. This "test" is the deliberate comparison of the present state to the outcome state. To know whether the outcome has been achieved one needs a measure to note changes in the evidence or criteria used to determine success. For example, if the nurse is taking care of a diabetic patient and has gotten blood glucose level back from the lab of 290, the nurse mentally creates a "test" in her head when comparing this result to the known normal value of 80 to 120. Thus the juxtaposition of the present state of 290 is compared with the desired outcome of 80 to 120. The difference in blood glucose is 170 points greater than the desired outcome. The "test" is like a gap analysis. Thus, the test or gap in this example is the difference between the actual and desired blood glucose. A judgment is the nurse's conclusion about what a blood glucose of 290 means for this particular patient, given the context of the story.

The goal of nursing care is to bridge gaps between patient present states and desired outcome states. For example, how does one help the patient achieve a desired state of a normal blood glucose level? Clinical decision-making is the selection of interventions and actions that move patients from a presenting state to a specified or desired outcome state. Decision-making is the process of selecting interventions from a repertoire of actions that facilitate the achievement of a desired outcome state. In other words, the nurse considers what interventions and actions are necessary to bring about the desired outcome? There are many nursing intervention choices the nurse can make when working with the diabetic patient. These represent clinical decisions based on the context of the story.

As noted, clinical judgment is the process of drawing conclusions based on the test of the comparison of present state (blood glucose of 290) to a specified outcome state (normal blood glucose 80 to 120). Judgment involves evidence and meaning. Judgments result in reflective action and reasoning about clinical decisions. Reflection and clinical decision-making continue until there is a satisfactory judgment that supports a match between the evidence of achieving a patient's desired outcome state and present state. If a match exists, the nurse concludes she or he has achieved the outcome and exits the reasoning task. The OPT model is unique in terms of its explicit focus on outcomes. Side-by-side comparisons of outcomes with present state information of patients creates a contrast state or test condition from which evidence can be derived and meanings attributed to the evidence. Such judgment can then be subjected to a reflection check.

A **reflection check** involves reflecting and analyzing the critical thinking skills and thinking strategies that support clinical reasoning. Reflection check is the process of self-monitoring, self-correcting, self-reinforcing, and self-evaluating ones own thinking about a specific task or situation (Herman, Pesut, & Conard, 1994; Pesut & Herman, 1992). A reflection check can pinpoint things done correctly and also can help identify errors thus providing an opportunity to fix them.

THE OPT MODEL AND NURSING NOMENCLATURE

The OPT model supports the application of critical, creative, and systems thinking skills in clinical practice and can be used as a structure and framework to integrate and link the content contained in the North American Nursing Diagnosis Association (NANDA) (2001), *Nursing Interventions Classification (NIC)* (McCloskey & Bulechek, 2000), and *Nursing Outcomes Classification (NOC)* (Johnson, Maas, & Morehead, 2000) nursing classification systems. For example, consider how the OPT model provides a structure for linking nursing diagnoses, interventions, and outcomes. When using the OPT model structure, nursing diagnoses lend themselves to present states, nursing outcomes lend themselves to desired outcome states, and nursing interventions are clinical decisions or choices among alternatives that help transition patients from present states to desired outcome states. The clinical indicators associated with outcome measures provide measures for the testing and judgment phases of the OPT model clinical reasoning processes.

For example, consider the nursing diagnosis of Anxiety (NANDA, 2001, p. 19). Based on analysis and reflection of a particular patient's story, anxiety might be deemed the present state or nursing diagnosis of concern. Anxiety Control is the outcome. There are several clinical indicators of Anxiety Control listed in the NOC (Johnson et al., 2000, p. 116) classification system. Each of these indicators is scaled on a 1 to 5 scale that ranges from 1 (never demonstrated) to 5 (consistently demonstrated). For example, two such indicators are: reports adequate sleep or maintains concentration. The clinical indicators are exemplars of outcome criteria and provide evidence of outcome achievement. Scaling these indicators helps measure achievement of anxiety control.

Nursing interventions are clinical decisions or

The purpose of this educational intervention was to enhance the clinical reasoning and critical thinking abilities of the nurse to enhance expert practice and quality patient care outcomes at Mount Sinai Hospital in New York City. Ongoing quality improvement efforts at the hospital led to the creation of an Educational Intervention Task Force. The Task Force was charged to create, investigate, develop, and evaluate strategies to expand knowledge, enhance clinical reasoning, and develop clinical thinking skills of staff nurses. A variety of educational programs were developed. Programs included nursing grand rounds, small group workshops for directors of nursing, clinical nurse managers, nurse educators, and clinical nurses.

An educational research demonstration project was developed to test the effects of a focused education intervention with nurses who worked on four pilot units. It was hypothesized that the intervention would enhance the clinical reasoning skills of the nursing staff. The assumption was that improved clinical reasoning would lead to more outcome-based thinking in service of patient care. A convenience sample of practicing nurses on three medical–surgical units and one intensive care unit within an academic health science center setting participated in the study. Pre-workshop and post-intervention questionnaires were administered to the clinical nurses on the selected units using the *Reflective Clinical Reasoning* and the *Barrett Power as Knowing: Participation in Change* tools.

The OPT model of reflective clinical reasoning, created by Pesut and Herman (1999), was used as the conceptual framework for the educational intervention. The OPT model provides a unique structure and strategies that focus on the complexity of clinical reasoning, decision-making, and judgment. The OPT model employs critical, creative, and systems thinking in the analysis of patient stories and the specification of outcomes and clinical judgments. The importance of reflection and an outcome rather than problem-oriented approach to care is highlighted in the OPT model.

The Clinical Reasoning Initiative at The Mount Sinai Hospital in New York presented opportunities for nurses to talk about their practice and share what they "know" in an arena of didactic and unit work. This initiative became centered in Reflection and Reasoning Rounds. These rounds assisted nurses to understand better what they "do" and improved dialogue between newer nurses and experts. Using a model of clinical reasoning and decision-making rather than a task-based approach, nurses were better able to use self-reflective strategies and outcome-based methods in their daily practice.

Pre- and post-intervention data was collected using the *Reflective Clinical Reasoning* and the *Barrett Power as Knowing: Participation in Change* tools. The hypothesis that the clinical reasoning initiative would increase nurses' perceived power as measured by the *Barrett Power as Knowing: Participation in Change* tool was supported. Significant differences in pre and post data were evident on the Barrett measure. Specifically, statistically significant differences were noted pre to post test on total scores of the tool ($F = 12.8$, 1df, $p = 0.0040$) and three of four of the tool factors: intentionality ($H = 9.91$, 1 df, $p = 0.0016$), awareness ($F = 5.43$, df = 1, $p = 0.0207$), and change ($F = 12.8$, 1df, $p = 0.0004$). The intervention did seem to have an effect on nurses' attention to clinical reasoning related to these factors and variables. The factor of choices was not significantly different ($H = 1.51$, df = 1, $p = 0.286$). Iterative factor analysis of the *Reflective Clinical Reasoning* tool is ongoing.

Source: Smith, T., McEvoy, M. D., & Vezina, M. (2002). *Preliminary results of the clinical reasoning initiative.* Unpublished manuscript. The Mount Sinai Hospital Department of Nursing. New York, NY.

choices of interventions that may be used to facilitate the transition from present to desired state. The NIC (McCloskey & Bulechek, 2000) interventions of Calming Techniques (p. 194), Coping Enhancement (p. 234), Anxiety Reduction (p. 146), and Decision-Making Support (p. 243), or Progressive Muscle Relaxation (p. 539) are all interventions that may or may not be appropriate given the context and content of the patient story. One has to make clinical decisions about the appropriate choice of an intervention.

Using the NOC (Johnson et al., 2000) clinical indicator scales provides evidence and a measure of outcome achievement. However, the meaning of the scale scores requires some reflection and clinical judgment that in turn leads to additional clinical decisions, reframing, or the identification of a different nursing diagnosis—outcome intervention priority.

APPLICATION OF THE OPT MODEL

Following are some guidelines and questions that help in application of the OPT model structure:

- What is the patient's story?
- How are you thinking about the patient's situation?
- What diagnoses have you generated as a result of your thinking?
- What evidence supports those diagnoses?
- How are the diagnoses related to one another?
- As you consider the whole story, are there themes that emerge?
- How are you framing this situation? What assumptions have you made?

- How have you defined the present state?
- What is the desired outcome?
- What is the gap between the outcome and the present state?
- What evidence will fill the gap?
- How will you know the outcome is achieved?
- What clinical decisions or interventions are you going to make to help move the patient from the present to the desired state?
- How and why are you considering these choices? What are the risks and benefits and short-term and long-term gains for each?
- Are these decisions and choices within your span of control? If they involve others, how will you negotiate participation and action?
- Have you had experiences similar to this before? If so, what was successful then? Do you think it can be applied in this situation?
- What clinical judgments are called for?
- How will this experience help you with similar cases in the future?

TRANSITION INTO PRACTICE

If you want to maximize learning through reflection consider using the questions in the Gibbs (1988) reflective learning cycle to analyze your experiences on a day-to-day basis. Put the questions on a bulletin board in your home or use them as a structure or outline for keeping a professional journal about your critical learning experiences.

Description: What happened?
Feelings: What were you thinking and feeling?
Evaluation: What was good and bad about the experience?
Analysis: What sense do you make of the situation?
Conclusion: What else could have been done?
Action Plan: If it arose again what would you do?

Take a moment and think about one or two stories from your own clinical experiences that were important learning for you. Using Klein's set of ingredients, identify the agents—the people who figure in the story. Describe the predicaments or the problems that you were trying to solve. What were your intentions? What were you trying to do? What actions did you undertake to achieve your intentions? What objects or tools are contained in the story? What were the intended and unintended effects of carrying out the actions in the story? How did the context or the details associated with the agents or actions influence the story? Finally, what surprises or unexpected things happened?

KEY POINTS

1. Academic, practical, successful, and nursing intelligence are needed to perform effectively in real world settings.
2. Nursing intelligence (NI) is a blend of academic, practical, and successful intelligence acquired

through experiences and reflection-in-actions and reflection-on-actions of those experiences. NI is derived from nursing care experiences that have been subjected to reason and reflection.
3. NI involves knowing what outcomes are most likely

in a given situation or context. NI is about how to make clinical decisions and organize care to achieve those outcomes.

4. Developing successful intelligence requires personal insight of learning style strengths and a conscious development of a plan to develop and compensate for learning style weaknesses.

5. Critical thinking is purposeful self-regulatory judgment and consists of one's ability to interpret, analyze, infer, explain, evaluate, and self-regulate. Self-regulation involves self-monitoring, self-evaluation, and self-correction in service of an identified outcome.

6. Reflection is a means to integrate past experiences into present learning and future thinking.

Reflection supports self-activation and learning versus self-sabotage and helplessness. Reflection supports the growth of the powerful professional self.

7. The OPT model provides a structure for clinical reasoning that includes both problems and outcomes and the application of the critical, creative, and systems thinking skills that are embedded in nursing practice contexts.

8. Stories connect us with our experiences. Over time, professionals build mental models of thinking, acting, and behaving that are derived from experiences. Such experiences contribute to the growth and development of practical, successful, and nursing intelligence; expertise; and professional power.

EXPLORE MediaLink

Critical thinking questions, essay questions, key terms, web links, activities, NCLEX review questions, and more interactive resources can be found on the Companion Website at www.prenhall.com/haynes. Click on Chapter 7 to select activities for this chapter.

REFERENCES

American Nurses Association. (1995). *Nursing's social policy statement.* Washington, DC: American Nurses Association.

Benner, P. (1984). *From novice to expert: Power and excellence in nursing practice.* Menlo Park, CA: Addison-Wesley.

Burns, S., & Bulman, C. (2000). *Reflective practice in nursing: The growth of the professional practitioner* (2nd ed.). London, England: Blackwell Science.

Caroselli, C., & Barrett, E. (1998). A review of the power as knowing participation in change literature. *Nursing Science Quarterly, 11,* 9–16.

Cox, K. (1999). *Exploring clinical thinking.* Sydney, Australia: University of New South Wales Press Ltd.

Facione, N., & Facione, P. (1996). Externalizing the critical thinking in knowledge development and clinical judgment. *Nursing Outlook, 44(3),* 129–136.

Gibbs, G. (1988). *Learning by doing: A guide to teaching and learning methods.* Oxford, United Kingdom: Oxford Brookes University.

Herman, J. A., Pesut, D. J., & Conard, L. (1994). Using metacognitive skills: The quality audit. *Nursing Diagnosis, 5(2),* 56–64.

Higgs, J., & Jones, M. (2000). *Clinical reasoning in the health professions.* Boston, MA: Butterworth-Heinemann.

Johns, C. (2000). *Becoming a reflective practitioner.* London, England: Blackwell Science.

Johnson, J. (1991). Nursing science: Basic, applied, or practical? Implications for the art of nursing. *Advances in Nursing Science, 14(1),* 7–16.

Johnson, J. (1994). A dialectical examination of nursing art. *Advances in Nursing Science, 17(1),* 1–14.

Johnson, M., Maas, M., & Moorehead, S. (2001). *Nursing outcomes classification (NOC)* (2nd ed.). St. Louis, MO: Mosby.

Klein, G. (1999). *Sources of power: How people make decisions.* Cambridge, MA: MIT Press.

Kolb, D. A. (1984). *Experiential learning: Experience as the source of learning and development.* Englewood Cliffs, NJ: Prentice Hall.

Kolb, D. A. (1985). *Learning style inventory.* Boston, MA: McBer & Co.

McCloskey, J., & Bulechek, G. (2000). *Nursing interventions classification (NIC)* (3rd ed.). St. Louis, MO: Mosby.

North American Nursing Diagnosis Association (NANDA). (2001). *Nursing diagnoses: Definitions and classifications 2001–2002.* Philadelphia, PA: Author.

Oerman, M., & Huber, D. (1999). Patient outcomes: A measure of nursing's value. *American Journal of Nursing, 99(9),* 40–48.

Paul, R. (1993). *Critical thinking: How to prepare students for a rapidly changing world.* Santa Rosa, CA: Foundation for Critical Thinking.

Paul, R., & Elder, L. (2001). *Critical thinking: Tools for taking charge of your learning and your life*. Upper Saddle River, NJ: Prentice Hall.

Pesut, D. J. (1989). Aim versus blame: Using an outcome specification model. *Journal of Psychosocial Nursing and Mental Health Services, 27*(5), 26–30.

Pesut, D. J., & Herman, J. A. (1992). Metacognitive skills in diagnostic reasoning. *Nursing Diagnosis, 3*(4), 148–154.

Pesut, D. J., & Herman, J. A. (1998). OPT: Transformation of nursing process for contemporary practice. *Nursing Outlook, 46*(1), 29–36.

Pesut, D. J., & Herman, J. A. (1999). *Clinical reasoning: The art and science of critical and creative thinking*. New York: Delmar.

Reich, R. (1992). *The work of nations*. New York: Vintage Books.

Schon, D. (1983). *The reflective practitioner: How professionals think in action*. New York: Basic Books.

Smith, T., McEvoy, M. D., & Vezina, M. (2002). *Preliminary results of the clinical reasoning initiative*. Unpublished manuscript. New York: The Mount Sinai Hospital Department of Nursing.

Sternberg, R. (1985). Implicit theories of intelligence, creativity, and wisdom. *Journal of Personality and Social Psychology, 49*, 607–627.

Sternberg, R. (1988). *The triarchic mind: A new theory of human intelligence*. New York: Viking.

Sternberg, R. (1996). *Successful intelligence*. New York: Simon & Schuster.

SUGGESTED READINGS

Benner, P. A., Tanner, C. A., & Chesla, C. A. (1996). *Expertise in nursing practice: Caring, clinical judgment, and ethics*. New York: Springer.

Bolman, L., & Deal, T. (2000). *Escape from cluelessness: A guide for the organizationally challenged*. New York: American Management Association (AMACOM).

Buzan, T., & Buzan, B. (1994). *The mind map book: How to use radiant thinking to maximize your brain's untapped potential*. New York: Plume Books.

Bower, F. (2000). *Nurses taking the lead: Personal qualities of effective leadership*. Philadelphia, PA: W. B. Saunders.

Fowler, L. (1997). Clinical reasoning strategies used during care planning. *Clinical Nursing Research, 6*(4), 349–361.

Gordon, S. (1998). *Life support: Three nurses on the front line*. Boston, MA: Little, Brown & Company.

Johns, C. (1995). Framing learning through reflection within Carper's fundamental ways of knowing. *Journal of Advanced Nursing, 22*(2), 226–234.

Johnson, M., Bulechek, G., Dochterman, J. M., Maas, M., & Moorehead, S. (2001). *Nursing diagnoses, outcomes, and interventions: NANDA, NOC, and NIC linkages*. St. Louis, MO: Mosby.

O'Connor, J., & McDermott, I. (1997). *The art of systems thinking: Essential skills for creativity and problem-solving*. San Francisco, CA: Thorsons.

8

Information Technology

Toni Hebda
Patricia Czar
Cynthia Mascara

A growing body of evidence supports the conclusion that various types of IT applications lead to improvements in safety, effectiveness, patient-centeredness, timeliness, efficiency, and equity . . . Nonetheless IT has barely touched patient care.

Institute of Medicine, 2001

LEARNING OBJECTIVES

AT THE COMPLETION OF THIS CHAPTER, THE READER WILL BE ABLE TO:

➤ Discuss the concepts of computer and information literacy.

➤ Recognize factors driving the implementation of information technology (IT) in health care delivery, education, research, and practice.

➤ Identify why the implementation of the computerized patient record (CPR) is needed to achieve improved quality and efficiency in health care delivery.

➤ Describe how computerized physician order entry (CPOE) can improve patient care and decrease errors.

➤ Recognize the utility of benchmarking to improve quality of care and promote cost reduction.

➤ Identify examples of telenursing and related issues.

➤ Evaluate health-focused Web sites.

➤ Discuss issues related to the use of IT in health care delivery, research, administration, and education.

MediaLink   www.prenhall.com/haynes

Additional online resources including NCLEX review questions, critical thinking questions, and real-world activities for this chapter can be found on the Companion Website at www.prenhall.com/haynes.

*T*oday's nurse must interface with both patients and technology. They need to have basic competencies in both patient care and information management in order to meet patient needs (Berke, 2002; Hobbs, 2002). This chapter reviews ways that technology can support nursing and health care delivery.

Employers and consumers expect nurses to be increasingly computer literate (American Association of Colleges of Nursing [AACN], 1998; Graveley, Lust, & Fullerton, 1999; Petro-Nustas, Mikhail, & Baker, 2002; Yee, 2002). **Computer literacy** is a popular term used to refer to a familiarity with the use of personal computers, including the use of software tools such as word processing, spreadsheets, databases, presentation graphics, and e-mail. In recognition of these expectations, the AACN identifies **information management** as a skill needed by baccalaureate nursing graduates. More specifically, baccalaureate graduates must (a) remain abreast of the evolving changes in information technology and (b) be able to use technology to discover, retrieve, and use information in practice. To do this requires advanced, broad-based computer literacy. Nursing programs now offer courses and/or require knowledge in basic computer literacy as a gateway to information management. This knowledge provides a foundation for managing patient information via hospital and nursing information systems.

Information literacy is an important aspect of information management. **Information literacy** or **fluency** is the ability to recognize when information is needed as well as the skills to find, evaluate, and use information effectively (ACRL, 2002). Information literacy is particularly important in today's dynamic environment where technology changes rapidly and more information is constantly made available. With information coming from many sources and in a variety of formats (e.g., text, graphics, and audio) basic computer literacy is a prerequisite for all health care providers.

Information technology (IT) is a term used to refer to the management and processing of information with the assistance of computers. The **nurse informatics specialist** has specialized knowledge related to the management and processing of information. The American Nurses Association (ANA) (2001) provides the following comprehensive definition of **nursing informatics:**

> Nursing informatics is a specialty that integrates nursing science, computer science, and information science to manage and communicate data, information, and knowledge in nursing practice. Nursing informatics facilitates the integration of

data, information and knowledge to support patients, nurses, and other providers in their decision-making in all roles and settings. This support is accomplished through the use of information structures, information processes, and information technology (ANA, 2001, p. 17).

Staggers, Gassert, and Curran (2001) identify four levels of information technology competency (Bickford, 2002). The **beginning nurse** has fundamental information management skills and can use information systems. The **experienced nurse** (a) is proficient in his or her area of specialization and highly skilled in the use of information technology and computers to support that area of practice, (b) sees the relationship between data elements and makes judgments based on observed trends and patterns, and (c) uses information systems and works with the informatics specialist to enact improvements in information systems. The **informatics nurse specialist** has advanced preparation in information management, focuses on informatics applications that support all areas of nursing practice, and uses skills in critical thinking, data management and processing, decision-making, and system development and computer skills. The **innovator nurse** is educationally prepared to conduct informatics research and generate informatics theory, holds the vision of what is possible, has the ability to make things happen, is creative in developing solutions, and possesses a sophisticated level of understanding and skills in information management and computer technology.

Driving Forces for Health Care Technology

A number of forces have lead to the development and use of technology to support patient care. These driving forces include the nursing shortage, the rapid growth of knowledge, concern for patient safety, and consumer demands for quality and cost-effective care based on research findings.

These driving forces became public knowledge when the Institute of Medicine (IOM), a division of the National Academy of Sciences, published the landmark reports, *To Err Is Human: Building a Safety Health System* (IOM, 1999) and *Crossing the Quality Chasm: A New Health System for the 21st Century* (IOM, 2001). The National Academy of Sciences was created to advise the government in scientific and technical matters. Recent initiatives on health care quality (e.g., the IOM Committee on the Quality of Health

Care in America, formed in 1998) have led to the development of strategies that would result in substantial improvement in the quality of health care over a 10-year period.

The National Advisory Council on Nurse Education and Practice (NACNEP) and the Council on Graduate Medical Education (COGME) met jointly following the release of the *To Error Is Human* report and subsequently released their findings in a report entitled *Collaborative Education to Ensure Patient Safety* (2000). This report called for sweeping changes in the education of providers and delivery of health care that includes technology as a means to simulate clinical situations for training purposes as well as for the prevention and detection of errors. Furthermore, the Joint Commission for Accreditation of Health Care Organizations (JCAHO) has revised standards for accreditation to better support patient safety and thus reduce errors by encouraging internal reporting and analysis of errors. To that end, concerns for patient safety have led to the design and development of information systems that support ordering, dispensing, and documentation of medications.

The IOM Committee on the Quality of Health Care in America espouses the belief that improvements in health care will depend on new system designs that are intended to provide care that is "safe, effective, patient-centered, timely, efficient and equitable" (IOM, 2001, p. 7). The IOM calls for the creation of a health information infrastructure that will support health care delivery, consumer health, quality measurement and improvement, accountability, clinical and health services research, and clinical education (IOM, 2001). The existence of such an infrastructure requires the use of IT as a means to automate and share information. The IOM sees the need to use standardized approaches to achieve this vision. Examples of standardized approaches include the ability to exchange information for research, error reporting, outcome measurement, and benchmarking.

Ten domains or areas of concern (e.g., leadership and planning, economic value, delivery systems, work environment, legislation/regulation/policy, public relations/communication, professional/nursing culture, education, recruitment/retention, and diversity) have been identified that demand attention in order to bring about positive changes for nurses and health care systems (IOM, 2001). Technologic advances in each of these domains can support and enhance the work in light of the current nursing shortage. The development of technology and information systems is expected to reduce a nurse's workload and improve efficiency.

Technology cannot solve problems that result from staffing shortages, but it can help prevent errors by giving busy nurses a system of double checks.

Patient Safety

The issue of patient safety is primarily related to the prevention of medication errors and adverse events. According to the IOM (1999), at least 44,000 to 98,000 deaths per year in U.S. hospitals are due to medication errors. This rate of errors has driven health care providers to design and develop information systems that support ordering, dispensing, administering, and documenting of medication administration. Additionally, technology can help prevent patient-related **sentinel events** (e.g., adverse drug interactions, inappropriate doses, and adverse effects) when health care providers have readily available current information (Simpson, 2002).

Rapid Growth of Knowledge

Health care professionals need to know more today to perform their daily jobs than at any previous point in history. Among these professionals, nurses are the largest group of "knowledge workers" in the health care delivery system (Pittman, 2000; Robert Wood Johnson Foundation, 1996; Snyder-Halpern, Corcoran-Perry, & Narayan, 2001). Advancements in knowledge, skills, interventions, and medications are growing at an exponential rate. These advances make it impossible for any one individual to keep up with all information needed to practice nursing without supportive technology and continuing education. Unfortunately, the present health care delivery system fails to consistently translate new knowledge into practice and apply new technologies safely and appropriately (IOM, 2001). A lapse of several years is typical before new advancements make it into the clinical setting. Technology offers a mechanism for conveying information and new knowledge to the bedside in a more timely fashion than ever available in history.

Consumer Demands for Quality and Cost-Effective Care

Consumers want options, demand quality, and expect cost-effective care. The current system does not typically provide these and does not consistently make the best use of its resources. It is a highly fragmented and often wasteful system that creates unnecessary duplication of services (IOM, 2001). In today's health care systems, consumers are asked to provide the same information over and over because that information is not conveyed to all providers. As a consequence, providers are often forced to act without complete information; thus, increasing the incidence of treatment errors. The IOM states that safety and quality problems occur largely because of an ongoing reliance on outmoded work systems that set providers up to fail despite their best efforts. Correction of this situation requires redesign of work processes through the development of new technology.

Quality and cost-effective care should be based on research- or evidence-based practice. **Evidence-based practice** is the process by which nurses and other health care practitioners use the best available research evidence, clinical expertise, and patient preferences to make clinical decisions (DiCenso, Cullum, & Ciliska, 1998). Evidence-based practice represents the ideal. Unfortunately, the domain of reliable data that nursing can depend on for informed decision-making is limited.

A significant number of individuals have chronic diseases. These individuals use a disproportionate amount of the overall available health care dollars. **Disease management** as defined by the Disease Management Association of America (1999), is a multidisciplinary, continuum-based approach to care that proactively identifies populations with, or at risk for, established medical conditions. This continuum-based approach:

- Supports the physician–patient relationship and plan of care
- Emphasizes prevention of exacerbations and complications using cost-effective evidence-based practice guidelines and patient empowerment strategies such as self-management education
- Evaluates clinical, humanistic, and economic outcomes with the goal of improving overall health (p. 4).

Careful management of individuals with these chronic conditions can minimize complications and reduce health care costs. Technology will provide tools that can help nurses deliver individualized care based on patient health status and evidence-based guidelines.

Health Care Technology Solutions

Prior to a discussion of IT solutions it is important to define and discuss some basic terms. First it is important to understand the difference between data, information, and knowledge. **Data** involves the collection of numbers, characters, or facts gathered according to

some perceived need (Anderson, 1992). One piece of data has little or no meaning when it stands alone. A blood pressure reading is an example of a single piece of data. Collecting data can be studied for patterns and structure, which can then be interpreted (Saba & McCormick, 1996; Warman, 1993). Interpretation occurs when nurses use other assessment findings and prior learning to give meaning or context to the data. Once interpretation occurs, data become **information** that can be acted on. When several blood pressure readings for one person are reviewed and compared with normal values, it may be determined that the individual has hypertension, which is an adverse reaction or an underlying physical condition that raises the blood pressure.

Knowledge is a more complex concept that requires the nurse to integrate information obtained from several sources and formulate one or more ideas about the situation. Sources for this information may come from formal and informal learning opportunities, assessment findings, patient histories, and diagnostic test results to name a few. Knowledge uses analysis to provide order to thoughts and reduce uncertainty (Ayer, 1966; Engelhardt, 1980). As a nurse, or student of nursing, one begins to search for the significance of individual patient findings in relationship to nursing knowledge. Additional information may be needed. Patient history, physical findings, a review of current medications, emotional status, test results, and recent events provide additional clues to formulate an appropriate plan of care. Computer technology can aid the collection and analysis of data. Information that has been validated provides knowledge that can be used again.

Information overload is stress generated by an overwhelming amount of input that must be processed and/or acted on. Most often used in the context of workplace stress, information overload results from increasing technological advances and input from multiple sources including e-mail, voice mail, cellular telephones, pagers, the Internet, and faxes.

Data Capture

During the course of a single day, nurses routinely collect, process, document, retrieve, and share large amounts of data and information. Data is gathered when nurses interview patients, perform physical assessments, measure vital signs, schedule diagnostic tests, review test results and records, perform treatments, conduct patient education, and talk with family members and other health care professionals. Much of the information collected is directly related to the care of individual patients and supports decisions made at the point of care.

Other sets of information facilitate day-to-day operation of the health care facility. This may include composite information collected from groups of patients to (a) assure the deliverance of quality care, (b) assist in formal research, and (c) identify trends to help guide the decision-making of administrators, public health professionals, and policy makers (Ammenwerth & Haux, 2000).

Nurses should not have to worry about technical aspects of data collection, retrieval, and comparison as they perform their daily work. These abilities are contingent upon the adoption and use of terms and language that have been standardized so that all users share the same understanding. The American Nurse's Association Steering Committee on Databases to Support Clinical Nursing Practice has developed criteria for the development and recognition of standardized nursing language systems for inclusion in the National Library of Medicine's Unified Medical Language System (UMLS) (Coenen, McNeil, Bakken, Bickford, & Warren, 2001). While work continues on the evolution of these languages, the ANA recognizes several systems at this time. Box 8–1 lists standardized languages that are recognized at this time.

Box 8–2 identifies some terms and concepts that must be considered to capture data. In particular, all units of data or data elements must be defined to pave the way for implementation of the computer-based patient record (CPR). Nursing has been plagued with inconsistent use of language for the description of clinical problems and treatments. Data exchange standards can ensure that information can pass between different hospital information systems such as registration, order entry, radiology, laboratory, nursing information, and billing systems. Health Level 7 (HL7) is a standard for the exchange of clinical information between systems. Although it is widely accepted as a standard, vendors have introduced their own variations.

Health care delivery systems are knowledge-intensive settings with nurses as the largest group of knowledge workers (Snyder-Halpern et al., 2001). Daily work is accomplished as nurses assume several roles. Each role requires a different level of decision-making and a different type of decision support. These nurse serves as a:

- **Data gatherer**, one who collects clinical data such as vital signs
- **Information user**, one who interprets and structures clinical data such as a patient's report of experienced pain into information that can then be used to aid clinical decision-making and patient monitoring over time
- **Knowledge user**, one who applies information or individual patient data to provide a service
- **Knowledge builder**, one who combines clinical data and demonstrates patterns across patients that are then be interpreted within the context of existing nursing knowledge.

The Computerized Patient Record

Costs associated with health care delivery and record management, malpractice and the implementation of regulatory requirements, and the drive to improve the quality of care represent driving forces for the implementation of automated records. In addition, the majority of potential benefits that technology offers to

---

Box 8–1   American Nurses Association Recognized Standardized Languages

Nursing Management Minimum Data Set	Nursing Interventions Classification
Nursing Minimum Data Set	Nursing Outcomes Classification
Complete Complementary Alternative Medicine	Omaha System
Billing and Coding Reference	Patient Care Data Set
Home Health Care Classification	Perioperative Nursing Data Set
North American Nursing Diagnosis Association	International Classification for Nursing Practice
Taxonomy (NANDA)	SNOMED

Adapted from Coenen, A., McNeil, B., Bakken, S., Bickford, C., & Warren, J. J. (2001). Toward comparable nursing data: American Nurses Association criteria for data sets, classification systems, and nomenclatures. *Computers in Nursing, 19*(6), 240–246. Reprinted with permission from Lippincott Williams & Wilkins.

Box 8–2   Key Terms for Data Exchange

Data. A collection of numbers, characters, or facts that are gathered according to a perceived need for analysis and the possibility for action at a later point in time.

Database. A computer file structure that supports the storage of data in an organized fashion so that it can be retrieved as meaningful information.

Data dictionary. A reference tool that defines terms used in an automated system to guarantee consistent understanding and application among all users within an organization. This process may be performed through the use of an interface engine.

Data element. A small piece of data that cannot be further divided. It should be defined in the data dictionary. An example might be a particular lab value or patient's sex.

Data integrity. The ability to collect, store, and retrieve correct, comprehensive, current data so that it is available to authorized users when it is needed.

Data management. Process of controlling the storage, retrieval, and use of data to optimize accuracy and utility while safeguarding integrity.

Data mining. Process used to search for previously unknown information patterns in large data sets that have already been collected and stored in data warehouses.

Data repository. Centralized database that contains diagrams of data flows, definitions, and data structure to facilitate the storage and use of information within a system.

Data warehouse. Collection of data that can be used to support management decision-making processes.

Data exchange standards. A set of agreed-upon rules that permit the uniform capture and interchange of data between information systems from different vendors and between different health care providers.

Electronic data interchange (EDI). The communication of data in binary code from one computer to another.

Health Level 7 (HL7). An EDI standard for clinical data that relies on an extensive set of rules.

Interface engine. A software application that allows users of different computer systems to access and exchange information without the need for any special effort on the part of the user, customization of equipment, or special programming.

Standardized Nursing Language. A structured vocabulary that provides nurses with a common means of communication.

health care relies on the computerization of patient records. Changing requirements for the management and use of patient information make the paper record inadequate. The Institute of Medicine (IOM) (1991) Committee on Improving the Patient Record recommended adoption of a computer-based record.

Historically, the prime function of the patient record has been to support care. Traditional users of the patient record include all health care practitioners who are involved in the treatment of the patient. Researchers comprise another group of users who may not provide direct care but use chart information. The paper record is a rich source of information, but locating or extracting that information is time consuming and difficult, particularly when materials are not on the chart, in the wrong section, or even on the wrong chart. Other drawbacks associated with paper records include access issues, the episodic nature of the record, and legibility (Hebda, Czar, & Mascara, 2001). Simply locating the paper record can be difficult. It may or

may not be with the patient. Often, several users need the patient record at one time causing delays in treatment and time lost to waiting.

One record generally chronicles a single visit to a health care facility or provider with no mechanism to ensure that important information such as patient allergies is carried over from one health care visit to the next. There is also the possibility that the patient has been treated at other facilities and locations and these records may not be available. As a result, the current health care record is a series of disconnected reports from various practitioners, clinics, inpatient and outpatient visits, and emergency room admissions. Even if all of these separate records can be assembled for review, it is highly likely that conflicting information will be found and that a situation will arise that can cause treatment errors.

There are also unanswered questions about responsibility for ensuring that the information is correct in all of these disjointed accounts. By contrast, computerized records can reduce problems associated with paper records and offer benefits to help reduce errors, measure patient outcomes, and improve the working environment for health care professionals.

The terms electronic medical record and computer-based patient record are often used interchangeably but are not the same. The **electronic medical record (EMR)** is an electronic version of the paper patient record. It includes unstructured data, which is data that does not follow particular formatting, for example, text report or history and physical. The EMR also includes structured data, with predefined data elements such as lab results. Moreover, the EMR represents a single treatment episode (Hebda, Czar, & Mascara, 2001).

The **computer-based patient record (CPR)** is more than an automated record. It is also an information system developed to support patient care. The Institute of Medicine requires that a true CPR system provide an integrated view of patient data across individual treatment episodes; afford access to knowledge resources, physician order entry, and clinician data entry; and provide communications and clinical decision support. The IOM also delineated defining attributes for the CPR (Andrew, 2002). These include the following:

- A problem list of the patient's clinical problems for each encounter as well as the current status of each problem
- An evaluation and record of health status and functional levels using accepted measures
- Documentation of the clinical reasoning/rationale for diagnoses and conclusions to allow sharing of clinical reasoning with other caregivers, thus automating and tracking decision-making
- A longitudinal or lifetime record that links data from previous encounters
- Support for confidentiality, privacy, and audit
- Access to authorized users at any time
- Simultaneous and customized views of the patient data for individuals, departments, or enterprises
- Links to local or remote information resources, such as various databases using electronic mail, CD-ROM, or hard disk
- Decision analysis tools to support clinical problem solving
- Support for direct entry of patient data by physicians
- Mechanisms for measuring the cost and quality of care
- Support for evolving clinical needs by being flexible and expandable

ADVANTAGES ASSOCIATED WITH THE CPR

It will take time before these advantages can be fully realized in all settings. Implementation of the CPR is an essential step to achieving the majority of benefits that IT can offer. These benefits include:

- Improved data integrity, since information is more readable, better organized, and more accurate and complete.
- Increased productivity. Caregivers are able to access patient information whenever it is needed, and at multiple convenient locations. This can result in improved patient care due to the ability to make timely decisions based on appropriate data.
- Improved quality of care. The CPR supports clinical decision-making processes for physicians and nurses.
- Increased satisfaction for caregivers. Caregivers are able to take advantage of easy access to patient data as well as other services including drug information sources, rules-based decision support, and literature searches (Amatayakul, 1997).
- Current data and data from previous events are easily compared.
- An ongoing record of the patient's education and learning responses across encounters.
- Baseline demographic and assessment data does not have to be repeated for each encounter.
- Data that has been entered is universally available to all that have access to the CPR.
- Data for research is more readily available and of better quality.
- Prompts ensure administration and documentation of medications and treatments.
- Facilitates automation of critical and clinical pathways.
- Multiple users can access the patient record simultaneously.
- Chart access is faster. No need to wait for old records to be delivered from the medical records department.
- Trends and clinical graphics are available on demand.
- Patient record security is improved (McFall, 1993).
- Less space is needed for record storage (For your files, 2001).
- Improved access and quality of documentation helps to lower the incidence of expensive duplicative tests (Kondro, 1999).
- Supports comparative assessments on efficacy of alternative forms of treatment tests (Kondro, 1999).

- The medical record department saves costs because of decreased need for pulling, filing, and copying of charts (Sickenberger, 2001).
- Patient eligibility for coverage in managed care settings is easily verified (Amatayakul, 1997).
- Cost evaluation is improved based on clinical outcomes and resource utilization data.

OBSTACLES AND CONCERNS TO THE IMPLEMENTATION OF THE CPR

An area of major concern today is protecting the privacy of individual patients. While the terms privacy, confidentiality, and information privacy are often used interchangeably, they are not the same. **Privacy** is a state of mind, a specific place, freedom from intrusion, or control over the exposure of self or of personal information (Kmentt, 1987; Windslade, 1982). **Confidentiality** occurs after a relationship has been established and private information is shared (Romano, 1987). Confidentiality is necessary for the accurate assessment, diagnosis, and treatment of health problems. Once confidential information is shared, control over its redisclosure lies with the persons who access it. Inappropriate redisclosure may be extremely damaging. **Information privacy** is the right to choose the conditions and extent to which information and beliefs are shared (Murdock, 1980). One example of this concept

Research Application

There are numerous claims that the use of IT in health care delivery can help nurses to perform their work more effectively, improve the quality of documentation, and improve patient satisfaction. There are a number of variables to consider when examining these claims. These variables include participation of nurses in the design of information systems, the types of systems used, access to and placement of computers, the type of measurement tool used, how the comparison was made, and whether or not work processes were reengineered for a better flow and improved productivity. Empirical evidence to support these claims demonstrates mixed results. The majority of research reports a positive correlation between automation and quality of documentation. The relationship between automated documentation and patient satisfaction is less clear.

Nahm and Poston (2000) sought to demonstrate that the implementation of the integrated ULTICARE hospital information system at one facility would improve the quality of nursing documentation and increase patient satisfaction. Four different nursing units were included in the study. Implementation was staggered over a 2-month period with measures taken at 6-, 12-, and 18-month intervals on each unit. Two researchers measured the quality of nursing documentation against 35 items from the Joint Commission on Accreditation of Healthcare Organizations (JCAHO) Closed Medical Review Tool. A sample of 288 charts was used. The first chart audit (n = 61) was done 3 months prior to implementation with 67 at 6 months, 82 at 12 months, and 78 at 18 months after implementation. The quality of documentation improved. There was a 13% increase in compliance to JCAHO standards after automation.

A revision of the Risser Patient Satisfaction Scale was distributed to subjects to measure satisfaction. There were 108 participants. There were 49 participants who completed the tool prior to implementation. There were 30 participants in the 6-month group and 29 in the 18-month group. A one-way analysis of variance was done to compare pre- and postimplementation data. There was no statistical evidence to support an increase in patient satisfaction.

In a discussion of their findings, Nahm and Poston (2000) noted that this documentation system contained several attributes to encourage quality charting. These attributes included prompts, the ability to collect and record data at the bedside, mandatory completion of certain fields for progression, notification of missed tasks, and historical data was carried forward. Nahm and Poston also noted that staff needed time to become accustomed to a new system. They concluded that the failure to demonstrate an increase in patient satisfaction might be attributed to the use of a convenience sample. Nahm and Poston also call for further research to help refine the practice of nursing by using data accumulated from information systems.

is the requirement in practice to obtain informed consent for the release of specific information. Information privacy also includes the right to ensure accuracy of information collected by an organization (Murdock, 1980).

Information security, on the other hand, is the protection of information against threats to its integrity or inadvertent disclosure. Information systems can improve protection for patient information in some ways and endanger it in others. Unlike the paper record that can be read by anyone, the automated record cannot easily be viewed without an access code. Poorly secured information systems threaten record confidentiality because they may be accessed from multiple sites with immediate dissemination of information. This makes patients highly vulnerable to the redisclosure of sensitive information.

Information system vendors as well as health care providers are aware of the pressing need to develop and establish security of CPR. The necessity for creating an electronic infrastructure and the cost of development are the major impediments to achieving a fully functional CPR. Other impediments include the lack of a common vocabulary and resistance among caregivers to accept the CPR.

Electronic Infrastructure Health care facilities, payers (e.g., insurance providers), and physicians all need the ability to access and update the record. Access requires electronic links, or a network infrastructure, for the information systems that support these stakeholders (Anderson & Bunschoten, 1996). All participants must first reach agreements regarding the nature and format of patient data to be stored and the mechanisms for data exchange, storage, and retrieval. This requires the use of common data communication standards. Adoption of a universal patient identifier, such as a Social Security number, is essential to associate all patient data with the correct patient. Concerns related to the privacy and confidentiality of

health care records have made the adoption of a universal patient identifier a hotly contested issue.

Costs Another impediment is cost (Dick & Steen, 1991). The development of the electronic links forming the infrastructure is costly and fiscal responsibilities are unclear. Traditionally, each health care enterprise or system has paid for its own electronic medical record development. Links to other facilities and agencies have been primarily limited to provider–payer arrangements.

Vocabulary Standardization Little standardization exists in health care settings regarding the medical vocabulary or language used in patient records. This lack of standards impedes the integration of discrete and disparate data from several sources into one complete record (Anderson & Bunschoten, 1996). Progress in the development of a universal language will support the development of the CPR.

Caregiver Resistance Resistance on the part of caregivers represents another impediment (Stetson & Andrew, 1996). The fully developed CPR mandates the use of computers by all caregivers as a part of their daily routine. This may be difficult for some individuals because computers are not readily available, software is complex, and users resist changes in work patterns. Some nurses and physicians may feel that data entry requires more time than handwritten notes thus detracting from patient care.

Decision Support

No other industry requires as many front-line workers to make as many high-risk decisions that require judgment and choices involving so many variables as does the health care industry (Valusek, 2002). For this reason, decision support is identified in three IOM reports as a major tool to achieve more effective and safer clin-

---

Critical Thinking and Reflection

A review of the literature on privacy and confidentiality of health care information generally concludes that clinicians are ultimately responsible for the safety of patient data committed to electronic transfer or storage. Identify measures that should be used to safeguard patient data that is maintained on automated systems. Talk about behaviors you have observed among students and professionals using information systems that you feel violate information privacy and patient confidentiality and state why these behaviors constitute violations.

Advocates for the CPR purport that it supports the delivery of safer patient care. Discuss various means in which a birth-to-death record that is integrated with other hospital systems supports safety.

ical decisions. Consumer groups, such as the Leapfrog Group, also demand decision support as a means to help prevent accidents.

A decision is the result of a process that involves problem detection, generation of alternatives, analysis including cost/benefit judgments, selection among alternatives, and implementation (Valusek, 2002). In order to be helpful, decision support needs to be readily accessible, available immediately in high-risk environments, and easy to use. Decision support requires good design and use of a database, models or algorithms, and dialogue. Users need to be extensively involved in the modeling of the decision process and system design. Good data are critical for good decision support. Questionable data raise doubt about the utility of available decision support.

Decision support applications are touted as a means to improve the quality of patient care. This is particularly important since it is impossible for any individual health care practitioner to know and recall all information relative to the care of a particular health care problem at any one time. Decision support systems are computer software applications that organize information to aid decision-making relative to patient care or administrative issues. Decision support along with the automation of guidelines for care decrease strain on the health care worker. The health care industry has not yet adequately addressed the fundamental issue of how to use data to support knowledge. The question as to what data is needed, at what point, and how it will be used must be addressed in the design of information systems for decision support (Amatayakul, 2000). At the same time that the importance of decision support is noted (Snyder-Halpern et al., 2001), one must note that the fluid, immature nature of nursing knowledge makes it very difficult to transfer knowledge to automated decision support and that some nursing knowledge cannot be readily committed to an automated database. It is also important not to impose excessive standardization in decision support systems so that nurses can exercise options that may need to be tailored to a particular patient. Therefore, as further technical impediments are removed, additional efforts are needed to provide more support for the more complex information roles (Snyder-Halpern et al., 2001).

Decision support is a key component of computerized physician order entry (CPOE) as a means to warn physicians that ordered drugs or doses are not appropriate for a particular patient because of dosage errors, allergies or drug interactions, or that a better drug is available at a lower cost (Ferren, 2002; Simpson, 2002). This is sometimes known as knowledge-based system (KBS). KBSs are designed to interact with users as they provide care by providing warnings when lab values fall out of normal range or when particular actions may be inappropriate. Knowledge-based order entry (KBOE) on the front end of the medication ordering and administration process along with bar coding used by the nurse at the patient's bedside have the potential to greatly improve the quality and safety of medication administration (Valusek, 2002). Unfortunately, cost often limits institutional use to one system rather than a combination of systems, which would further decrease the likelihood of errors.

Disease Management

Disease management programs can also benefit from appropriate use of IT software, data registries, automated decision support tools, and callback systems. IT can allow fewer health care professionals to manage a larger patient load. Programs should provide:

- Routine reporting/feedback loop (may include communication with patient, physician, health plan and ancillary providers, and practice profiling)
- A process to identify the population
- Evidence-based practice guidelines
- A collaborative practice model that includes physician and other health care providers
- The identification of risks and matching of interventions with need
- Self-management education for patients (e.g., primary prevention, behavior modification, and compliance or surveillance programs)
- Process and outcomes measurement, evaluation, and management

Despite the advantages that IT offers for disease management, its adoption among organizations conducting these programs has been slow. Barriers to its use include cost and resistance to the use of technology by elderly and/or chronically ill persons. The cost barrier comes from the need to create and maintain the electronic infrastructure for use in disease management and to train staff to use the technology (Kelly, 2002). There are also unanswered questions about who should bear the cost of the required IT investments. In some cases, institutions opt to outsource disease management services to avoid the costs associated with setup and maintenance.

The Internet provides an excellent tool for disease management programs (Joch, 2000). It allows programs to be launched and customized quickly. Disease-specific information can be offered, eliminating the need for patients to search the entire Web for information, which may be of questionable quality. Unfortunately, Internet access is not available to all participants. Some organizations still use the telephone for patients to report data because it is more readily available and better accepted. Meanwhile, IT is used to record data or generate alerts for values that fall out of normal range.

Other Decision Support Tools

In addition to decision support software, there are a number of tools that help health care personnel, particularly administrators, collect and interpret information and subsequently make decisions. These include reports, query tools, information visualization, and data mining. Hospital information systems, nursing information systems, and ancillary systems generally provide report capability. Static reports provide snapshots of designated performance areas at prescribed frequencies for a designated period. In common practice, managers often view reports for a specified time period. Reports may be designed and provided by the information services department or available for review online. As a consequence, needed information may not be available or may not be available when it is needed.

Query tools allow the query user to access relatively small sections of the database, particularly if the database contains preaggregated, summarized data. The query user has a specific set of questions in mind.

Information visualization is a process that uses visual mechanisms to clearly and quickly communicate the structure of data, information, and knowledge to the user (Gershon & Page, 2001; Hawkins, 1999; Pack, 1998). It uses research on human–computer interaction and storage and retrieval of information in large databases (Hawkins, 1999). Information visualization technology is useful when traditional data analysis methods are no longer enough (Mahoney, 2000). Information visualization is suited for massive streams of information and data that arrive in real time from existing sources. The user needs to integrate those streams, understand them, and make decisions in a timely fashion. The advantage to visualization is that it provides an overview more quickly than can be gleaned from a text explanation.

Data mining is the search for previously unknown information patterns in large data sets that have already been collected. The data miner does not start with specific questions. Visualization is an important tool to use in conjunction with data mining as it creates visual displays of normal and abnormal patterns and relationships. Individuals interested in retrieval of information for scientific purposes need to be aware of data mining and information visualization (Blake, 2000). Ultimately, the value of information tools is based on the assumption that one started with quality data.

Computerized Physician Order Entry

Computerized physician order entry is the process by which the physician enters orders for patient care into a hospital information system that provides clinical decision support to help the physician avoid adverse drug reactions (Ball & Douglas, 2002; Eisenberg & Barbell, 2002). This support integrates patient information from separate systems (e.g., pharmacy and laboratory) with drug databases to warn physicians of potential problems with dosages, potential drug interactions, allergies, and contraindications to use, such as pregnancy or other health conditions. This order entry system is designed to improve patient safety and reduce medication errors. The Leapfrog Group and Institute for Safe Medication Practices have placed demands on the health care delivery system to enact changes to provide safer, more effective care. The Leapfrog Group is a coalition of large corporations that have mobilized their purchasing power to promote changes in the health care delivery system by channeling patients to facilities that meet specified safety standards that include CPOE (Ferren, 2002).

Computerized physician order entry sends orders entered by the physician directly to the appropriate ancillary system. Orders cannot be completed until the physician completes mandatory fields or addresses prompts and alerts. It is hoped that CPOE will significantly cut medication errors; however, it may also introduce new sources of errors since physicians are not accustomed to selecting the correct patient in a hospital information system for order entry. For this reason, it is recommended that additional safeguards be used to verify patient identity. The primary barrier to the acceptance and use of CPOE is resistance on the part of physicians who see CPOE as overly demanding of their time. Advocates for CPOE claim that it streamlines the ordering process, expedites patient care, eliminates transcription errors, reduces duplication, lowers the incidence of adverse drug reaction, and lowers costs for drugs.

Error Reporting/Patient Safety

The ANA (1995) supports the position that nurses should feel safe to report errors and near misses without fear of punitive action. This requires institutions to adopt policies that encourage open error reporting (Simpson, 2002). There are several mechanisms to report errors, including national reporting programs for adverse drug events (ADEs). Data provided by these national reporting programs can be used to help prevent additional medication errors and adverse drug reactions. The following is a list of the national reporting programs now available:

- The Medication Errors Reporting Program (MERP) is operated by the United States Pharmacopeia (USP). Medication errors are voluntarily submitted by practitioners and independently reviewed by The Institute for Safe Medication Practices (ISMP), a nonprofit organization that works with health care practitioners and institutions, regulatory agencies, professional organizations, and the pharmaceutical industry to provide education about adverse drug events and their prevention. ISMP also works with the Food and Drug Administration (FDA) to reduce medication errors. Identifying information remains confidential from outside parties.
- MedWatch is an FDA Safety Information and Adverse Event Reporting Program that provides a means for health care professionals and consumers

to report suspected problems with drugs and medical devices that they prescribe, dispense, or use. Reporting can be done online or by phone, mail, or fax.
- MedMARx was developed by the USP. This program allows hospitals to anonymously report and track medication errors in a standard format via the Internet. MedMARx offers organizations the ability to track errors and error prevention strategies within their organization and learn from the experiences of others by searching an aggregate database. MedMARx is intended to supplement rather than replace MERP and MedWatch.

Benchmarking

Benchmarking is the process of continually measuring services and practices against the toughest competitors in the industry. The intent of benchmarking is to compare data for the purpose of self-assessment and improvement (Betzold, 1999). Benchmarking is gaining popularity as more institutions seek to establish data-driven performance measurement strategies. It provides a means to identify areas needing attention and improvement as well as highlight areas that excel. Comparison with similar facilities also provides data that can be used for marketing purposes.

Bar Coding

Bar coding provides a means to capture data automatically. While it has been used previously for inventory control and for recording and filing costs, current interest centers on the use of bar coding medication administration. Patients receive a unique bar code that is affixed to their wristband and record. Once a treatment or medication has been ordered, the bar code is scanned with an optical scanner and patient details are automatically entered into the hospital information system. This eliminates the need for redundant data entry as well as the opportunity for transcription errors. It also allows staff at the bedside to verify a match between patient identity and ordered medications prior

Critical Thinking and Reflection

Computerized physician order entry (CPOE) has been identified as a measure to decrease medication errors. Compare and contrast the CPOE against transcription of handwritten orders to identify how medication errors may be reduced.

The use of bar coding in medication administration has been hailed as a means to help harried nurses perform their duties more safely and efficiently. Identify how bar coding may realize that potential.

to administration, reducing stress over potential errors and streamlining workflow. The use of bar code medication administration (BCMA) can also eliminate communication delays that occur when medication orders are changed. As a result of its benefits large corporations are pressuring hospitals to implement bar code technology (Rosser, 1997; Shapiro, 2000; Simpson, 2002; 2-D Barcodes, 1998).

Telehealth

Telemedicine allows health care professionals to consult with colleagues, conduct interviews, assess and monitor patients, facilitate computer-based support groups, view diagnostic images, and review slides and lab reports (Cudney & Weinert, 2000; Davis, 1996; McGee & Tangalos, 1994; Perednia & Allen, 1995; Zurier, 1995). **Telenursing** is the delivery of nursing care via telecommunications and computer applications. The terms *telehealth* and *telemedicine* are often used interchangeably. The term **telemedicine** has been in use longer. It is the use of telecommunication technologies and computers to provide medical information and services to patients at another location. These technologies may range from low-technology applications via the telephone to the incorporation of videoconferences and monitoring devices via the use of computers. Distant practitioners and patients benefit from the skills and knowledge of the consultants without the need to travel to regional referral centers. Health care consumers benefit through improved access to personalized care when they need it without traditional delays (Binns & Homan, 2001).

Some of the biggest issues relative to the practice of telemedicine and telenursing center on reimbursement, licensure, and liability issues. There have been problems getting health insurance companies to pay for telehealth applications, even though such technology expands consumer options and can help to reduce overall costs for patient care. This situation is changing as telehealth becomes more prevalent. Licensure can be an issue when nurses and other health care professionals practice across state lines unless they are also licensed to practice in the same state in which the consumer resides. Telehealth advocates want to enact changes that would lead to nationwide licensure or changes in state practice acts that would allow practitioners from any state to consult with practitioners from another state without the need to be licensed in the second state (Hebda, Czar, & Mascara, 2001).

Research with IT

Computers and IT have the potential to facilitate research. This can range from the identification of areas in need of further research to the rapid dissemination of study findings. Topics for further research can be discovered through discussion groups, chats, and e-mail as well as reading recent research findings on the Web (Hebda, Czar, & Mascara, 2001). There are also online databases. The Cumulative Index for Nursing and Allied Health Literature (CINAHL) and Medline are the primary databases for searching nursing literature. There are also other databases that provide full-text retrieval. Instruments for traditional or online data collection can be located via Internet and online literature searches.

However, many Internet users are not very proficient at searching the Web (Kent, 2001). Effective Web searches require an understanding of how Web search tools work and the different types of search instruments available. **Search engines** are tools that maintain an index of information on the Web. Each search engine maintains its own organization. Search results vary from tool to tool each time a search is done because of differences in index systems, the fact that information is stored on several computers, and some tools may be down for maintenance activities at the time a search is done. Meta search engines pull data from several search sites at once saving search time and often have the capacity to eliminate redundant results.

Search tools can also be found for particular topics. The choice of keywords and the manner in which keywords are entered determine search results. Additional keywords help to improve the relevance of findings. By default, search tools return all results containing any of the keywords entered. Boolean operators with keywords (e.g., "AND" and "OR") can further improve search results. Connecting keywords with the "AND" ensures that results contain both keywords, while "OR" will display results containing either of the keywords. Moreover, in the event that no suitable data collection tool is found, the Internet can be used to collaboratively design a new tool and solicit expert feedback on its design and content.

Online data collection offers several advantages (Duffy, 2000; Jamieson, 2002; Miller, 2001; Thomas, Stamler, Lafreniere, & Dumala, 2000). It is quick, easy, cost effective, relatively anonymous, supports quantitative and qualitative research, and allows researchers to reach large numbers of participants from anywhere in the world. Large sample sizes help to decrease sampling errors. The Web even provides a means to recruit study participants quickly and inexpensively. Online data collection also facilitates data analysis and provides a convenient forum for dissemination of results. For example, in the case of qualitative research wherein respondents are asked to maintain diaries, information can be entered into a program on a password-protected Web site instead. The advantages of online data collection make it likely that its popularity as a research tool will increase. Research firms are going online with their qualitative research as a way to save time and money.

Technology and online data collection also brings with it disadvantages or new issues to be resolved. Disadvantages include (a) the potential for one individual to reply more than once, (b) a population that is skewed toward the more affluent and educated who have computers and Internet access, and (c) observations that once relied on gestures and facial expressions must rely solely on words instead (Yoffle, 2000). The success of online data collection may also be adversely affected by poor Web site design (Miller, 2001). The appearance of online surveys can differ by monitor size and type, resolution, and browser. Additional factors that may impact user response include distortion of the rating scale, transmission time, and the need to scroll or use extra keystrokes to view the entire data collection tool. Critics state that additional research is needed with other methods to prove that online research provides comparable results to traditional data collection/research methods.

The Web also provides a means to collaborate with other researchers and to publish study findings quickly via established online publications or as an independent effort. Online publications and journals are increasingly popular for several reasons. These include:

- A shorter turnaround time from study to publication. This is particularly important where information becomes outdated quickly.
- Lower costs associated with printing, layout, and distribution.
- Revisions can be made and distributed quickly.
- Ease of collaboration between researchers or authors from different sites.
- Twenty-four-hour access.

Access to online publications varies. Some are free, while others require subscription. In some cases it is also possible to request specific articles on a fee basis.

The computerized patient record provides the ideal tool for contributing to domain knowledge, and subsequently results in an improved quality of care. There are research issues related to new requirements for research protocols imposed by HIPAA. In particular, there are problems with confidentiality requirements that may significantly harm health research (Nozer, 2000). These include:

- The definition of "de-identified" information. Information that has had personally identifiable information removed may impede the ability to follow individual subjects over time. At this time, demographic and medical information is forwarded to a number of databases known as registries for follow-up study and care. For example, there is a tumor registry, a registry for patients who have had cardiothoracic surgery, and a number of other registries for special populations.
- Transition rules for existing medical records.
- New requirements for research protocols that require individual patient permission rather than a general admission and permission to treat form.

IT Applications in Education

Education is affected by some of the same influences as health care delivery. These include the exponential

---

Critical Thinking and Reflection

The Internet is commonly hailed as a wonderful tool for research. Compare and contrast ways that the Internet can be used to facilitate all aspects of research over traditional methods.

growth of knowledge and demands for quality, cost efficiency, and flexibility to better meet the needs of the individual learner. Computers and electronic communication can help address these demands. **Electronic communication** is the ability to exchange information through the use of computer equipment and software. This is achieved through network connections or the use of a modem. A **modem** is a communication device that transmits data over telephone lines from one computer to another. **Online** is a term that indicates a connection to computer resources such as the Internet (Net). The Internet provides access to information through a variety of services.

- **E-mail** is one of the most frequently used Internet applications. E-mail encourages networking among peers. It is also a convenient way to contact recruiters and send resumes.
- **Listservs** represents an e-mail subscription list. E-mail messages are distributed to subscribers through a central computer that acts as the server. Some groups have a moderator who screens messages for relevance. Listservs are sometimes referred to as discussion groups.
- **News Groups** are similar to listservs in content and diversity. Users can post messages for discussion and reply or passively follow the discussion. Unlike listservs, users neither subscribe nor receive individual messages. Instead, they participate whenever they choose to do so.
- **File Transfer** allows users to download files or send files to others through the File Transfer Protocol (FTP). FTP is a set of instructions that controls both the physical transfer of data across the network and its appearance on the receiving end.
- **Remote Log-on** allows users to access computers at other locations for the purpose of using resources available at those locations.
- **Instant Messaging or Internet Relay Chats (IRCs)** provide the ability to conduct interactive discussions.
- **World Wide Web (Web)** is an information service that allows access to Internet resources by content rather than file names. Users locate content through word searches or by moving from link to link with a mouse click. Links are displayed by highlighted keywords, text, or images.

Along with the ability to access Internet resources comes the responsibility to learn and use netiquette. Netiquette refers to proper etiquette when using Internet resources. General netiquette rules are displayed in Box 8–3.

The Internet offers a number of formal and informal opportunities for education and learning for health care professionals and consumers. In recent years, Web-based education has become extremely popular for stand-alone courses and as a component of traditional classes. Some of these sites are public. In other cases, registration is required to access materials. Box 8–4 displays some terms used that refer to instructional uses of technology. Internet-based learning has become popular as:

- Activities are available 24-hours a day, 7 days a week.
- The learner can proceed at his or her own pace.
- The Internet makes education available without the need to travel to distant sites.
- Incorporated links allow the learner to pursue additional areas of interest.

While the Internet provides unprecedented access to health care information for health care professionals and consumers, it also offers the novice user a variety of challenges regarding validity of information. Though information is often available more quickly than via traditional media and may be viewed by professionals and consumers at the same time, accuracy, readability, depth, diversity, and design of information vary greatly from site to site (Internet Healthcare Coalition, 2002; RAND Health/California HealthCare Foundation, 2001). Relevance of search results also varies because of the differences in the way that individual search tools are set up and subtle differences in search techniques. Nurses need to know how to locate online information and to critically examine it for quality. They have an obligation to help health care consumers to do the same. Online information should be held to the same standards that are applied to other forms of media. Unfortunately, no single agency polices Web sites. Fortunately, help is available to identify quality sites.

Several groups have been working to ensure the quality of information found on health-related Web sites. These groups include but are not limited to the following: the Health Internet Ethics Alliance, Health on the Net Foundation, Health Web and Healthfinder, the Internet Healthcare Coalition, and the American Accreditation Health Care Commission. None of these groups exercise mandatory controls, but instead provide guidelines for Web site content. Several of these organizations list sites online that meet with their approval or provide the means to search for content by topic. Health Internet Ethics, also known as Hi-Ethics, Incorporated, published a set of 14 Principles in 2000 which forms the basis for the American Accreditation Healthcare Commission's (URAC) Health Web Site

Box 8–3   Netiquette Rules

E-mail
- Avoid sarcasm and attempts at humor that may be misunderstood or seen as offensive.
- Avoid flaming or harsh words to attack a discussion participant or sender.
- Do not use e-mail as a substitute for face-to-face communication.
- Avoid overuse of punctuation for emphasis. It may be perceived as irritating.
- Do not include quotes from others without their express permission.
- Limit e-mail recipients to the people who need the information. This keeps the number of messages manageable.
- Choose an accurate description for the subject line. This helps recipients to determine which messages to read first.
- Give e-mail messages and postings for listservs and discussion groups the same consideration given to business correspondence relative to acceptable language, spelling, and content. Persons other than intended recipients may see messages.
- Avoid language that might be perceived as confrontational. E-mail has no corresponding body language to provide help with interpretation of the message.
- Start e-mail with the recipient's name and end it with your signature. Use a formal salutation to address someone that you have not previously met. Include your name, title, and company name, address, and telephone and fax numbers. Many mail programs have the ability to add a signature to messages automatically.
- Keep messages brief and clear. This helps to maintain interest.
- Avoid one-word replies. Recipients may not know what your answer refers to unless the original message is included or the message contains clarifying information.
- Avoid the use of all capital letters. This is perceived as yelling and can be more difficult to read.
- Limit abbreviations to those that are common and easily understood. Avoid acronyms that may not be understood by others.
- Always be polite. Avoid judgment comments and gossip particularly when posting to listservs and discussion groups where large numbers of individuals may be offended.
- Be timely with replies. Long delays may be construed as rude.
- Ensure that recipients have software (and version) required to access attachments. Confirm that they know how to open attachments as well.
- Avoid sending attachments that take a long time to download *unless* they are sent at the specific request of the intended recipient. Consider the use of FTP for transfer of large files.
- Use antivirus software to detect viruses and worms and to avoid sending them out to others.
- Refrain from forwarding jokes and chain e-mail messages *unless* the recipient has indicated that they are wanted. Delete the long list of prior recipients before forwarding chain messages.

Listservs and Discussion Groups
- Apply e-mail netiquette rules plus additional guidelines for these groups.
- Respect listserv and discussion group members. Check for the focus of discussion before asking questions that have already been discussed.
- Avoid posting messages to the group that are intended for an individual within the group. This may occur inadvertently with the use of the "reply" function.
- Don't spam. Spamming is sending out advertisement to newsgroups or large mailing lists.

Accreditation standards. This accreditation requires compliance with more than 50 standards that consider disclosure, site policies and structure, content currency and accuracy, linking, privacy, security, and accountability. URAC-accredited sites carry the URAC seal. Accredited sites must periodically review functionality and appropriateness of links to other sites and provide a means for users to report links that do not work. Consumers also have an opportunity to provide feedback to URAC on whether a Web site's information and disclosures are understandable (American Accreditation Healthcare Commission, 2002). This is the first accreditation program in the nation to review health information sites using quality standards of reference.

Box 8–4   Technology Applications for Education

Web-based instruction (WBI) uses the attributes and resources of the World Wide Web such as links and multimedia for educational purposes. WBI may make use of synchronous discussions that take place in "real time" but there is a trend for discourse in asynchronous mode as participants may span several time zones or work schedules.

Computer-assisted instruction (CAI) uses computers to organize and present instruction materials for use by an individual learner. CAI facilitates learning by actively involving the learner.

E-learning is the delivery of content through electronic media. This term is frequently used to refer to corporate training activities. These may be delivered via the Internet, CD-ROM, or audio/videotapes or broadcasts.

E-mail provides opportunities for formal and informal learning through scholarly dialogue with experts. E-mail can also help facilitate the development of critical thinking (Ribbons & Vance, 2001).

Presentation software is a special type of computer program that allows the presentation of information by computer that may include text, images, and sound. Content may be projected onto a screen, incorporated into WBI or e-learning, or sent as a file attachment with e-mail.

Web Course Development Tools are types of software that provide a shell for course layout and administration. Features include interactive chat capability, e-mail, student tracking capability, and the ability to share files and post and automatically grade examinations. Administrative features also include the ability to limit access to some or all features to a select group of users.

In the event that it is necessary to determine the quality of a site the following areas should be considered (Internet Healthcare Coalition, 2002; Mascara, Czar, & Hebda, 2001):

- The credentials of the author
- The ability to validate information
- Privacy policies when personal information is collected
- Content accuracy
- Date of issue or revision
- Bias or sponsorship
- Comprehensiveness of information
- Agreement with comparable sources
- Intended purpose and audience

Another effort to ensure the relevance and quality of health information on the Web focuses on labeling information appropriately via the use of the HIDDEL vocabulary (Health Information Disclosure, Description and Evaluation Language). This special language was developed by the MedCERTAIN (MedPICS Certification and Rating of Trustworthy and Assessed Health Information on the Net) Consortium, a project funded by the European Union, with the purpose of establishing an international trustmark for health information. The HIDDEL vocabulary is for use by Web page designers to create labels that Web browsers can use to compare against user preferences. MedCERTAIN expresses the intent to establish a fully functional self- and third-party rating system enabling patients and consumers to filter harmful health information and to positively identify and select high-quality information.

More consumers use the Internet each day to obtain health care information (Leaffner & Gonda, 2000). One of the fastest growing consumer groups shopping for information online are senior citizens. Rising costs along with an increasing patient base keep health care professionals busy with less time for patient education. Nurses need to tap Internet resources to redesign patient education and help reinforce counsel-

Critical Thinking and Reflection

Nurses need to be able to use computer and IT. Describe skills that nurses need as well as methods that nurse educators should use to foster the development of those skills.

ing for all patient populations. Incorporation of Internet resources can strengthen the nurse–patient bond and improve health outcomes. Practicing nurses and nursing students need to learn to use the Internet as a tool for patient education as well as their own continuing education.

TRANSITION INTO PRACTICE

In their 1988 article. "Design of Nursing Information Systems: Conceptual and Practice Elements," Graves and Corcoran note the potential for nursing information systems (NIS) to determine the course of clinical practice and influence the development of a body of knowledge unique to nursing. They also note that it is essential for nurses to participate in the design of these systems. An NIS must provide information needed to provide nursing care. The majority of systems evolved from administrative support system. This leads to a situation where systems fail to meet the needs of the nurse providing patient care. There is a shift to design newer systems on a patient care model. Graves and Corcoran caution that NIS must provide access to professional literature and other resources because it is unrealistic to expect that nurses can remember all information needed for patient care. They also note that systems will become more important as nursing practice becomes more knowledge based. They also suggest two models.

In their discussion of these two models, Graves and Corcoran (1988) first envision an integrated system that:

- Stores demographic and clinical data
- Permits documentation of interventions and outcomes

- Allows retrieval of information in accord with user needs
- Supports aggregation of data from individual records
- Provides access to relevant knowledge
- Provides the means to continue to build nursing knowledge

In their second model, Graves and Corcoran (1988) call for the system to consider the discipline itself, professional practice, and the practitioner. This model would incorporate multiple conceptual models and is problematic because of the different taxonomic labels for various areas of concern and differences in interpretation.

Graves and Corcoran (1988) note that for many years nursing data was discarded or archived in a format that was very difficult to retrieve. The appearance of NIS mark the beginning of an era in which data needed to build knowledge is retained in a form that can be accessed. The databases that result open new avenues for research. They reiterate that nurses must be involved in the selection and design of systems. They recognize that differences in practice settings will influence system design.

KEY POINTS

1. Nurses need to interact with both patients and technology. For this reason, they need to have basic competencies in both patient care and information management. These competencies start with computer and information literacy.
2. Nursing informatics integrates nursing science, computer science, and information science to manage and communicate data, information, and knowledge in nursing practice. All nurses need to demonstrate a basic level of informatics skills.
3. There are several factors that drive the development and use of IT in health care. These include the rapid growth of knowledge, the nursing shortage, patient

safety, computerized physician order entry, and demands for quality and cost-effective care based on research findings.
4. IT cannot solve all of the problems that nurses face in their practice, but it can provide a valuable tool that helps to reduce errors, enhance productivity, and make the work environment less stressful.
5. Disease management and telehealth provide mechanisms to expand health care choices and quality through the use of IT.
6. IT has the potential to facilitate all areas of nursing research from the identification of topics to the dissemination of study findings.

7. IT broadens opportunities for informal and formal learning opportunities for health care consumers and professionals.
8. The quality of online information varies widely. Nurses need to be able to evaluate the quality of online information and to help consumers to do the same. Evaluation criteria include the ability to verify the accuracy and completeness of information, whether the site shows bias, contains a date to show currency, or displays credentials of the source.
9. There are several issues pertaining to the use of IT in health care. The single biggest issue is the protection of online patient information.

EXPLORE 〰 MediaLink

Critical thinking questions, essay questions, key terms, web links, activities, NCLEX review questions, and more interactive resources can be found on the Companion Website at www.prenhall.com/haynes. Click on Chapter 8 to select activities for this chapter.

REFERENCES

2-D barcodes speed Spanish prescriptions. Automatic I.D. (1998). *News Europe, 7*(1), 11.

Amatayakul, M. (1997). Making the case for electronic records. *Health Data Management, 5*(5), 56–63.

Amatayakul, M. (2000). The race to standardize medical record information. *MD Computing, 17*(6), 22–24.

American Accreditation Healthcare Commission. (2002). *Health web site standards.* Washington DC: Author.

American Association of Colleges of Nursing (AACN). (1998). *Essentials of baccalaureate education for professional nursing practice.* Washington, DC: Author.

American Nurses Association. (1995). *Position paper on computer-based patient record standards.* Washington, DC: Author.

American Nurses Association. (2001). *Scope and standards of nursing informatics and practice.* Washington, DC: Author.

Ammenwerth, E., & Haux, R. (2000). A compendium of information processing functions in nursing. *Computers in Nursing, 18*(4), 189–196.

Anderson, H. J., & Bunschoten, B. (1996). Creating electronic records: A progress report. *Health Data Management, 4*(9), 36–44.

Anderson, S. (1992). *Computer literacy for health care professionals.* New York: Delmar.

Andrew, W. F. (2002). A new dawn for the CPR. *ADVANCE for Health Information Executives, 6*(4), 22–26.

Association of College and Research Libraries (ACRL). (2002). *Information literacy competency standards for higher education.* Chicago, IL: Author.

Ayer, A. J. (1966). *The problem of knowledge.* Baltimore, MD: Penguin.

Ball, M. J., & Douglas, J. V. (2002). IT, patient safety and quality care. *Journal of Healthcare Information Management, 16*(1), 28–33.

Berke, W. J. (2002). Progressive care units continue to grow in number as the patient acuity gap between critical care and medical/surgical care narrows. *Nursing Management, 33*(2), 27–29.

Betzold, J. (1999). Oryx: Good intentions gone astray. *Behavioral Health Management, 19*(4), 14.

Bickford, C. J. (2002). Informatics compencies for nurse managers and their staffs. *Seminars for Nurse Managers, 10*(3), 215.

Binns, K., & Homan, Q. (2001, January). Consumers demand personalized services to manage their health. *Advances for Health Information Executives,* 87–88, 90.

Blake, P. (2000). Seeing the wood for the decision trees. *Information World Review, 157*(14), 2–3.

Coenen, A., McNeil, B., Bakken, S., Bickford, C., & Warren, J. J. (2001). Toward comparable nursing data: American Nurses Association criteria for data sets, classification systems, and nomenclatures. *Computers in Nursing, 19*(6), 240–246.

Cudney, S. A., & Weinert, C. (2000). Computer-based support groups: Nursing in cyberspace. *Computers in Nursing, 18*(1), 35–43.

Davis, A. W. (1996). Remote control medicine: VARs help doctors make house calls. *Reseller Management, 19*(7), 170–174.

DiCenso, A., Cullum, N., & Ciliska, D. (1998). Implementing evidence based nursing: Some misconceptions [Editorial]. *Evidence Based Nursing, 1,* 38–40.

Dick, R. S., & Steen, E. B. (1991). *The computer.* Washington, DC: National Academy Press.

Disease Management Association of America. (1999). *The Disease Management Association of America releases the first comprehensive definition of disease management.* New York: PR Newswire.

Duffy, M. (2000). Reflections on research: Web-based research: An innovative method for nursing research. *Canadian Oncology Nursing Journal, 10*(2), 45–49.

Eisenberg, F., & Barbell, A. S. (2002). Computerized physician order entry: Eight steps to optimize physician workflow. *Journal of Healthcare Information Management, 16*(1), 16–18.

Engelhardt, H. T., Jr. (1980). Knowing and valuing: Looking for common roots. In H. T. Engelhardt & D. Callahan (Eds.), *Knowing and valuing: The search for common roots* (Vol. 4) (pp. 1–17). New York: Hastings Center.

Ferren, A. L. (2002). Gaining MD buy-in: Physician order entry. *Journal of Healthcare Information Management, 16*(2), 66–70.

For your files. (2001). *Health Management Technology, 22*(20), 58.

Gershon, N., & Page, W. (2001). What storytelling can do for information visualization. *Communications of the ACM, 44*(8), 31.

Graveley, E. A., Lust, B. L., & Fullerton, J. T. (1999). Undergraduate computer literacy: Evaluation and intervention. *Computers in Nursing, 17*(4), 166–170.

Graves, J., & Corcoran, S. (1988). Design of nursing information systems: Conceptual and practice elements. *Journal of Professional Nursing, 4*(3), 168–177.

Hawkins, D. T. (1999). Information visualization: Don't tell me, show me. *Online, 23*(1), 88–90.

Hebda, T., Czar, P., & Mascara, C. (2001). *Handbook of informatics for nurses and health care professionals* (2nd ed.). Upper Saddle River, NJ: Prentice Hall.

Hobbs, S. D. (2002). Measuring nurses' computer competency: An analysis of published instruments. *Computers in Nursing, 20*(2), 63–73.

Institute of Medicine. (1991). *The computer-based patient record: An essential technology for health care.* Washington, DC: National Academy Press.

Institute of Medicine. (1999). *To err is human: Building a safer health system.* Washington, DC: National Academy Press.

Institute of Medicine. (2001). *Crossing the quality chasm: A new health system for the 21st century.* Washington, DC: National Academy Press.

Internet Healthcare Coalition. (2002). *Tips for health consumers: Finding quality health information on the Internet.* Newtown, PA: Author.

Jamieson, D. (2002). Online research gets fewer Euro cheers. *Marketing News, 36*(2), 15.

Joch, A. (2000, March). Can the Web save disease management? *Healthcare Informatics*, 58–60, 62, 64.

Kelly, B. (2002). Obstacles block path to increased use of I.T. in disease management. *Health Data Management, 10*(4), 36–38, 40, 42, 43.

Kent, M. L., (2001). Essential tips for searching the Web. *Public Relations Quarterly, 46*(1), 26.

Kmentt, K. A. (1987). Private medical records: Are they public property? *Medical Trial Technique Quarterly, 33*(Winter), 274–307.

Kondro, W. (1999). Canada must update patient records. *Lancet, 353*(9152), 568.

Leaffner, T., & Gonda, B. (2000). The Internet: An underutilized tool in patient education. *Computers in Nursing, 18*(1), 47–52.

Mahoney, D. P. (2000). Computer, visualize thyself. *Computer Graphics World, 123*(6), 17.

Mascara, C., Czar, P., & Hebda, T. (2001). *Internet resource guide for nurses and health care professionals.* Upper Saddle River, NJ: Prentice Hall.

McFall, E. (1993). An electronic medical record delivering benefits today. *Healthcare Informatics, 10*(10), 76–78.

McGee, R., & Tangalos, E. G. (1994). Delivery of health care to the under served. *Mayo Clinic Proceedings, 69*(12), 1131–1136.

Miller, T. W. (2001). Make the call: Online results are mixed bag. *Marketing News, 35*(20), 30.

Murdock, L. E. (1980). The use and abuse of computerized information: Striking a balance between personal privacy interests and organizational information needs. *Albany Law Review, 44*(3), 589–619.

Nahm, R., & Poston, I. (2000). Measurement of the effects of an integrated, point-of-care computer system on quality of nursing documentation and patient satisfaction. *Computers in Nursing, 18*(5), 220–229.

National Advisory Council on Nurse Education and Practice and the Council on Graduate Medical Education. (2000, December). *Collaborative education to ensure patient safety.* Washington, DC: NAC NEP.

Nozer, R. (2000). Closer scrutiny might lead to changes in HIPAA's final implementation. *Managed Healthcare Executive, 12*(4), 52–54.

Pack, T. (1998). Visualizing information. *Database Magazine, 21*(1), 47.

Perednia, D. A., & Allen, A. (1995). Telemedicine technology and clinical applications. *Journal of the American Medical Association, 273*(6), 483–488.

Petro-Nustas, W., Mikhail, B. I., & Baker, O. G. (2002). Perceptions and expectations of baccalaureate-prepared nurses in Jordan: Community survey. *International Journal of Nursing Practice, 7*(5), 349–358.

Pittman, L. (2000). Dealing with the knowledge explosion. *Australian Nursing Journal, 8*(5), 30.

RAND Health/California HealthCare Foundation. (2001). *Evaluation of English and Spanish health information on the Internet.* Santa Monica, CA: Author.

Ribbons, B., & Vance, S. (2001). Using e-mail to facilitate nursing scholarship. *Computers in Nursing, 19*(3), 105–110.

Robert Wood Johnson Foundation. (1996). *Chronic care in America: A 21st century challenge.* Princeton, NJ: The Robert Wood Johnson Foundation.

Romano, C. (1987). Confidentiality and security of computerized systems: The nursing responsibility. *Computers in Nursing, 5*(3), 99–104.

Rosser, M. (1997). Collaboration offers big savings in healthcare. Automatic I.D. *News Europe, 6*(3), 20.

Saba, V., & McCormick, K. (1996). *Essentials of computers for nurses.* New York: McGraw-Hill.

Shapiro, J. P. (2000). Industry preaches safety in Pittsburgh. *U.S. News & World Report, 129*(3), 56.

Sickenberger, J. (2001). Realizing ROI on an automated records system. *Behavioral Health Management, 21*(3), 18.

Simpson, R. L. (2002). Winning the "blame game." *Nursing Management, 33*(1), 14–16.

Snyder-Halpern, R., Corcoran-Perry, S., & Narayan, S. (2001). Developing clinical practice environments supporting the knowledge work of nurses. *Computers in Nursing, 19*(1), 17–23.

Staggers, N., Gassert, C. A., & Curran, C. (2001). Informatics competencies for nurses at four levels of practice. *The Journal of Nursing Education, 40*(7), 303–316.

Stetson, D. S., & Andrew, P. E. (1996). The CPR: Getting physicians on board. *Healthcare Informatics, 13*(6), 20–24.

Thomas, B., Stamler, L. L., Lafreniere, K., & Dumala, R. (2000). The Internet: An effective tool for nursing research with women. *Computers in Nursing, 18*(1), 13–18.

Valusek, J. R. (2002). Decision support: A paradigm addition for patient safety. *Journal of Healthcare Information Management, 16*(1), 34–39.

Warman, A. R. (1993), *Computer security within organizations*. London: Macmillan.

Windslade, W. J. (1982). Confidentiality of medical records: An overview of concepts and legal policies. *Journal of Legal Medicine, 3*(4), 497–533.

Yee, C. C. (2002). Identifying information technology competencies needed in Singapore nursing education. *Computers in Nursing, 20*(5), 209–214.

Yoffle, A. J. (2000). Web advantages. *Adweek Eastern Edition, 41*(40), 22.

Zurier, S. (1995). Telemedicine is bringing electronic doctors closer. *Government Computer News, 14*(21), 56.

SUGGESTED READINGS

Baldwin, F. D. (2002, March). Making do with less. *Healthcare Informatics*, 37–38, 40.

Beyea, S. (2000). Standardized nursing vocabularies and the perioperative nursing data set. *CIN Plus, 3*(2), 1, 5–6.

Carlon, G. C. (2000). The electronic medical record and the oath of Hippocrates. *Health Management Technology, 21*(5), 16.

Charp, S. (2002, February). Educating the Web community. *T.H.E. Journal*, 8, 10.

Curtin, L., & Simpson, R. L. (2000). Staffing and the quality of care. *Health Management Technology, 21*(5), 42, 45.

Curtin, L., & Simpson, R. L. (2002). Conveying an effective message in voice mail or e-mail. *Health Management Technology, 23*(2), 52.

Flaum, M. (2001). Comorbidity and DM. *Health Management Technology, 22*(10), 28–29.

Goorman, E., & Berg, M. (2000). Modeling nursing activities: Electronic patient records and their discontents. *Nursing Inquiry, 7*(1), 3.

Hallam, K. (2000). Battling medical errors Star Wars style. *Modern Healthcare, 30*(22), 18.

HIT to the rescue: Technology improves patient safety. *HIMSS News, 13*(2), 10.

Saba, V., & McCormick, K. (1996). *Essentials of computers for nurses*. New York: McGraw-Hill.

9

Skill Acquisition and Competency

Janis C. Childs
Frances Strodtbeck
Teresa A. Boese

"Learning is about making connections.

Patricia Cross, 1999"

LEARNING OBJECTIVES

AT THE COMPLETION OF THIS CHAPTER, THE READER WILL BE ABLE TO:

➤ Define competence and competency.

➤ Discuss critical thinking and decision-making as essential nursing skills.

➤ Recognize the necessity for technical skill competence and mastery of core scientific principles.

➤ Recognize divergent expectations of skills competency: faculty versus nursing student and employer versus employee.

➤ Discuss competency and errors in health care.

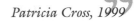

MediaLink   www.prenhall.com/haynes

Additional online resources including NCLEX review questions, critical thinking questions, and real-world activities for this chapter can be found on the Companion Website at www.prenhall.com/haynes.

Nurses today see themselves as partners to physicians and other health care providers in today's rapidly changing health care environment. All have witnessed a worldwide knowledge and technology explosion that began in the late 1990s and continues today. Changes in the American health care system are a representative microcosm of changes that are occurring on a global level (Donner & Wheeler, 2001). With the Internet and other readily accessible resources for information and knowledge, nurses today must be able to keep pace with changes on a grander scale than previously appreciated.

Since it is likely a great deal of knowledge gained in nursing school will be obsolete within five years of graduation, nurses must possess not only fundamental skills, but also expert up-to-date knowledge, clinical competence, creativity, and flexibility in order to control their careers (Donner & Wheeler, 2001). The nurse who is best able to accomplish this is the nurse who possesses a strong scientific foundation for clinical decision-making, a broad set of psychomotor and technical skills, and a willingness to accommodate to the ever-changing health care setting. This nurse must also understand the importance of locating information needed for practice and be skilled in information retrieval from a variety of resources, including the World Wide Web. Professional nurses understand that competency is the sum of all skills (e.g., critical thinking, judgment, delegation, supervision, etc.), not just the technical skills, that define nursing practice. Successful nurses must have a commitment to lifelong learning in order to assure competent and safe professional practice.

Nursing school prepares students to assume entry-level positions as nurse generalists. The complexity of the current health care environment pushes the newly graduated nurse to take on specialty knowledge early in their careers (Wigens & Westwood, 2000). The reali-ties of the clinical practice arena require the novice nurse to assess personal competency for general nursing practice as well as the specialized nature of a chosen job. While graduate nurses may possess many nursing skills, they are usually required to (a) learn additional skills or competencies, (b) adapt existing skills to the uniqueness of the specialty population, and (c) gain proficiency in the ability to perform skills once employed.

Embarking on a job in nursing is the first step on the road to a rewarding career. Throughout the journey, the new nurse will encounter intersections where the road selected determines the next beginning for the nurse's professional life. This chapter will focus on planning for a successful career in nursing. The concepts of competency and career development are discussed to help the novice nurse manage his or her nursing career.

Maintaining Competence While Planning a Career

As the American health care system continues to evolve, the educational standards for nurses are steadily increasing. To maintain competency, individual nurses face the need for continued education, either informal or formal. Educational decisions should be based on a systematic process, which is carefully thought out and planned.

Career planning is "a continuous process of self-assessment and goal setting" (Kleinknecht & Hefferin, 1982, p. 31). According to Donner and Wheeler (2001), career planning is "an integral part of developing as a professional, wherever nurses live and work" and "can play a crucial role at every stage of one's career" (p. 80). The stages a nurse goes through in career development are described in Table 9–1.

Table 9–1 Stages of Career Development in Nursing

Stage	Description
I. Learning	Basic education, which occurs in nursing school
II. Entry	Employment in the first nursing position
III. Commitment	Fine-tuning the nursing job by determining preference for patient population, work setting, city, shift, etc. Occurs 2–5 years after graduation
IV. Consolidation	A period of comfort with the chosen practice area and/or job
V. Withdrawal	Preparing for retirement

While career goals should be identified early in a nurse's career, many nurses fail to do so. As nursing students are exposed to different practice settings and patient populations during their education, they begin to identify practice preferences and, thus, should begin to formulate goals that will help in the selection of their first job. Unfortunately, most nurses make career decisions based on situational factors rather than careful planning.

Nursing students can alter the path trod by past generations of nurses by attending to content on career planning in their nursing school curriculum. They can seek faculty guidance to facilitate the career planning process. Generally, nursing faculty can assist students by helping to link the students' stated interests and goals with clinical sites that enable the students to explore their interests further. Faculty can also assist students by identifying networking opportunities so students can position themselves for future jobs and career opportunities (Donner & Wheeler, 2001).

Engaging in a formal career assessment periodically helps nurses identify and plan future career choices. Although most individuals think of career assessment as an intellectual activity, it is recommended that a formal career assessment be undertaken (DiMauro, 2000; Donner & Wheeler, 2001; O'Halloran, 1996). A career assessment requires each nurse to ask a series of critical questions regarding (a) professional likes and dislikes, (b) the realistic possibility of pursuing further education, and (c) personal and professional goals for the future. Table 9–2 provides a tool for career assessment.

Table 9–2 Career Assessment Tool

Step	Purpose	Activities
1. Reality check and internal inventory	Identify personal career preferences	• Answer the following questions about your current practice: -Do I like my current job? -What experiences do I like the most? -What experiences do I like the least? -What are my strengths as a nurse? -Are these strengths being used in my current position? What can I do to put these strengths to better use? • Make a list of the nursing positions that are a good match according to your reality check.
2. Creating the career vision	Identify the desired position and/or role	• Answer the following questions: -What do I see myself doing in 2 years? 5 years? -What do I need to do to achieve my goals? -What am I willing to do, given my other obligations to family, church, etc.? -How will the change affect my life? My family? • Peruse job opportunities in professional journals, newsletters, and newspapers to identify job possibilities and requirements.
3. Developing a global perspective of the professional marketplace	Become informed about the work environment and health care system in order to anticipate changes that impact your career vision	• Read a variety of journals, magazines, newspapers, etc. about business, legislative, technology, and lifestyle trends that are impacting health care., i.e., *The American Nurse, Wall Street Journal, Time, Newsweek*, etc. • Become a member of an agency/hospital-wide or multidisciplinary committee to broaden your institutional perspective. • Access pertinent information on the Internet on a regular basis.

Table 9–2 (continued)

Step	Purpose	Activities
		• Set up a personal information update service through Web sites such as My Nursing Center (http://www.nursingcenter.com).
4. Developing the Career Strategic Plan	Determine the knowledge, skills, and competencies needed to achieve the desired career goal	• Interview individuals in your desired career. • Check on requirements for the desired career with the appropriate specialty nursing organization. • Build your skills through continuing education, specialty certification, volunteer work, etc.
5. Networking	Linking with potential mentors and others who can facilitate the career plan	• Join listserv discussion groups on topics related to your career plan. • Identify colleagues or role models who may be able to help you with your career plans and talk with them. • Join and participate in professional organizations that can foster your career plans.
6. Marketing the Plan	Promoting yourself within the profession, positioning yourself for advancement	• Establish a professional network. • Acquire a mentor. • Volunteer for positions that can promote yourself and increase your visibility within the institution.

Adapted from Donner & Wheeler, 2001; DiMauro, 2000; O'Halloran, 1996.

Competence and Competency

What is competency? How does one measure practice competence? These are questions being asked by individual nurses, nursing educators, employers, supervisors, and regulators. Schmalenberg and Kramer (1979) define competency as the "possession of the skills, knowledge, and understandings needed to do the job of a nurse" (p. 99). Alspach (1984) defines competence as the "possession of knowledge, skills and abilities necessary to perform the job" (p. 655) and competency as "the employee's ability to actually perform in the [work] environment in accordance with the role and standards of the institution" (p. 656). The National Institutes of Health Clinical Center Nursing Department (1995) defines competency as a general statement that describes the knowledge, skills, and abilities necessary for safe nursing practiced in a specific area. Competency, according to Benner (1984), is "the ability to perform the task with desirable outcomes under the varied circumstances of the real world" (p. 41).

Jeffrey (2000) states that competency is "a written statement established by expert opinion that identifies specific standards and direction for the professional's decision-making in health care" (p. 195).

Recently, the American Nurses Association (ANA) Expert Panel (2000) published the following definitions:

- **Continuing competence**—"ongoing professional nursing competence according to the level of expertise, responsibility, and domains of practice" (p. 5).
- **Professional nursing competence**—"behavior based on beliefs, attitudes, and knowledge matched to and in the context of a set of expected outcomes as defined by nursing scope of practice, policy, *Code for Nurses*, standards, guidelines, and benchmarks that assure safe performance of professional activities" (p. 5).
- **Continuing professional nursing competence**—"ongoing professional nursing competence according to level of expertise, responsibility, and domains of practice as evidenced by behavior based on beliefs, attitudes, and knowledge matched to and in

the context of a set of expected outcomes as defined by nursing scope of practice, policy, *Code of Ethics*, standards, guidelines, and benchmarks that assure safe performance of professional activities" (p. 6).

Competence and competency are two sides of the same coin; **competence** refers to skills and abilities of the individual, while **competency** is the ability of the individual to demonstrate personal skills and abilities in a work setting. Competency is seen as an ongoing process. Employers evaluate competency at the time of initial employment and at periodic intervals for the duration of employment.

Developing Competency

Competency is an essential aspect of nursing and, therefore, nursing education. Educators, clinicians, and nursing students don't always agree as to the appropriate distribution of time between the classroom, the simulated practice lab setting, and the clinical patient care setting. Educators believe the time spent teaching basic skills should be balanced with other areas of the nursing curriculum (e.g., critical thinking strategies, delegation, collaboration). On the other hand, students are anxious to learn psychomotor skills and tend to be dissatisfied when they feel ill prepared to perform skills. This is no surprise as the "doing" part of nursing makes nursing seem much more real than the theoretical underpinnings of education. The "doing" holds the allure and excitement of nursing and, for many students, is the reason they chose to become nurses.

Educators as well as employers recognize the importance of developing the nursing student's and, subsequently, the nurse's ability to incorporate the basic tenets for performing skills with decision-making and critical thinking. New nurses require knowledge and experience but will also ultimately require the ability to supervise and delegate. Learning to supervise and delegate requires more than is implied in the old adage "see one, do one, teach one." Only after developing proficiency as a generalist can the new nurse competently proceed to teaching, delegating, and supervising other care providers.

Making Connections: The Process of Skills Acquisition

Cross (1999) describes learning as a process of making neurological, cognitive, social, and experiential connec-

tions. Acquisition of patient care skills is oversimplified when one assumes simulated demonstration and practice results in mastery. Simulated learning is only one step in the mastery process. Anxiety, unexpected patient behavior/presentation, or even unfamiliar equipment can adversely influence information learned under simulated conditions. To better understand the process of skill acquisition, the importance of developing neurological, cognitive, social, and experiential connections will be discussed.

Neurological Connections

Research indicates the neurocircuitry of the brain is developed very early. At birth, an infant is believed to have 100 billion neurons and associated fibers. Through a process of sensory stimulation these neurons are either retained or, when rarely used, disposed of by the brain. Research has demonstrated that children deprived of sensory stimulation have 20% to 30% smaller brains than age mates (Nash, 1997).

While a great deal is known about learning in young children, data to explain adult learning is less complete. Using data abstracted from individuals who have developed Alzheimer's disease, Diamond advises "the brain grows with deliberate stimulation . . . enrich your own experiences and enlarge your cerebral cortex; deprive yourself of stimulation and the brain will shrink from disuse" (Diamond & Hopson, 1998, p. x).

Cognitive Connections

Unlike neurological connections, cognitive connections cannot be seen and can only be explained hypothetically. Modern cognition scientists postulate cognitive connections are built as a result of mental activity and experience. Activities and experiences lead to the development of schema. A **schema** or **schemata** (pleural form) is a "cognitive structure that consist of facts, ideas, and associations into a meaningful system of relationships" (Cross, 1999, p. 8). A schema does not possess a physical location within the neurological make up of an individual. Rather, a schema is a cognitive representation (e.g., an experience, a skill, a procedure, or a person).

Traditional educators have assumed knowledge could be transferred from the teacher to the learner. Learning has been compared to filling an empty vessel (e.g., the teacher could literally pour information into the learner's head). Cognitive scientists reject this traditional premise for learning, noting the mind is not an empty vessel in which teachers can place knowledge for storage and retrieval. While the empty vessel image for learning may explain how facts are learned, this model does not explain how abstract concepts are formed. Learning complex data occurs through schema formation. For example, knowledge of sterile technique, urinary catheter size, rationale for urinary catheter insertion, anatomical landmarks, and other pieces of information that combine to form the mental structure for catheter insertion each represent schema. These facts or inert ideas, schemata, are used to build connections and understanding and, thus, the complex task of inserting a urinary catheter can be learned (Ramsden, 1992).

As Cross (1999) points out, most contemporary educational systems support surface learning by utilizing "an anxiety-providing assessment system that rewards or tolerates regurgitation of factual information" (p. 10) rather than critical analysis of available data. This condition is clearly exemplified in many traditional nursing simulated learning environments where procedural steps are generally taught and regurgitated without contextual clues that promote critical decision-making. Students and nurses should heed the knowledge gained by cognitive scientists, which suggest skills are best learned when the schema for the skill is allowed to develop and not simply remain a surface fact (e.g., rote memorization of the steps of the skill does not include critical thinking and problem solving). Deeper learning occurs when the student, through mental activity which may include a simulated experience, is able to form connections. Only when these connections are made can the learner really own the knowledge and apply it to patient care.

While a teacher cannot build schemata for a student, students can become "strategic learners" (Cross, 1999, p. 11). Nursing students who learn to be strategic learners will have skills to optimize life long learning experiences. Three basic cognitive strategies for life-long learning include rehearsal, elaboration, and organization (Weinstein & Mayer, 1985). **Rehearsal** brings information into short-term memory. **Elaboration** helps learners connect new information with existing information by paraphrasing, summarizing, creating analogies, and self-quizzing. All of these activities serve to move surface learning into schemata. **Organization** (e.g., outlining, categorizing) helps learners retain and apply meaning to knowledge.

Along with these cognitive strategies, good learners also plan, monitor, and self-regulate. These strategies are highly useful when applied to skill acquisition. Learning a skill requires goal setting, study, and practice. In conjunction with planning, good learners monitor their progress as they gather information. This type of self-regulation helps the learner check and correct behaviors as knowledge is acquired.

Social Connections

Learning involves more than reproducing or regurgitating rote facts. Learning also involves the process of "constructing knowledge through negotiation and agreement among knowledgeable peers" (Cross, 1999, p. 17). As such, learning is also dependent on language and cultural influences. There is a growing educational trend toward collaborative learning with emphasis on socially interactive learning environments in which problem solving and critical thinking are emphasized.

Today's learning theorists agree that the situation in which learning occurs is important. For example, simulated learning results in passive acceptance of ready-made steps for skill acquisition; whereas, learning associated with contextual experiences (e.g., actual patient care) facilitates understanding. Contextual cues (e.g., patient data) promote active learning and build knowledge. Learning goes beyond basic facts to include an understanding of social relationships, consequences of care provided, and many other facets of social relationships. Learning in a socially interactive setting improves acquisition of knowledge, supports retention, and promotes learner satisfaction with the educational experience (Cross, 1999).

It is important for the nurse to remember the value of social connections when teaching patients. Lack of knowledge and understanding of different cultural viewpoints and health beliefs may result in inadequate care. When the nurse understands the patient's context of health, illness, and care, that nurse can provide the patient with meaningful and relevant information. Patients who understand are more likely to be compliant and relate to and share the vision of care. Desired outcomes are also more possible.

Experiential Connections

Clearly, experience enhances learning and improves performance. John Dewey (1967) is credited with emphasizing the importance of "learning by doing" (Ehrlich, 1996). According to Dewey (1967), providing students with the opportunity to use problem solving in a contextual environment increases the effectiveness of the learning.

Nursing students are provided formal instruction, which is followed by simulated learning experiences.

Actual patient care experiences enhance learning. What are the responsibilities of the nursing student, new nurse, and nurse educator for ensuring patient safety as the nurse learner is acquiring skills and faced with applying these skills in patient care situations? What are the benefits of simulated learning experiences? How can simulated learning experiences be created that resemble actual nurse–patient encounters?

Students are then provided with clinical instruction in a health care setting where care of patients is possible. Experiential connections acquired during clinical practice are vital to learning skills. This same plan for instruction can be applied to patients. The patient is provided with formal instruction on an aspect of care (e.g., wound care). The patient may then be allowed to participate in the care.

While logically and traditionally accepted, this stepwise linear approach to nursing education (formal learning to application) does not meet all the educational needs of today's professional nurse. Health care employers expect nurses to also think and analyze problems. Because of the rapid increase in available knowledge in health care today, much of what the new nurse learned in school is quickly outdated. Experiential connections must teach the nurse and the patient to think, analyze, and critique. Through experiential connections the nurse must learn to "learn from experiences, to constantly reflect on what has been learned, to experiment with alternatives, and to evaluate the outcomes" (Cross, 1999, p. 21).

Maintaining Competence

Professional nurses maintain competence in their area of practice. Increased scrutiny by the general public, the government, and other professional groups seek to ensure that health care providers maintain skill competence and evidence-based knowledge as their careers advance. Maintaining competence involves some degree of planning. A variety of factors influence competence of the nurse (e.g., the practice setting, the type of patients cared for, ongoing continuing education, and work experience).

Like many other practice disciplines, nursing is both an art and a science. While the science of nursing is imparted in formal educational programs and continuing education, the art of nursing is more elusive and learned over time. Mastering both dimensions of nursing is a critical aspect of competency. Benner (1984) described process for developing mastery. Her model is summarized in Table 9–3.

A key concept underlying the Benner model is the importance of clinical experience in the development of

Table 9–3   Benner's Stages of Nursing Proficiency

Stage	Nursing Behavior
I. Novice (entry into nursing school)	Learner has little experience of the situation in which performance is expected; rule-governed behavior is typical; expects direction from others.
II. Advanced Beginner	Learner demonstrates marginally acceptable performance; skill acquisition focuses on discriminating and differentiating information.
III. Competent Practitioner (2–3 years' work experience)	Learner begins to feel competent and organized; able to establish priorities and set goals; thinking becomes more analytical and abstract while the learner is able to coordinate several tasks at once.
IV. Proficient Practitioner (3–5 years' work experience)	Learner views patients holistically; recognizes subtle variations in data so as to set priorities and establish long-term goals.
V. Expert Practitioner (after extensive practice experience)	Learner intuitively assesses patient and situation needs; gracefully and efficiently provides care with little excess or wasted effort; integrated nature of responses comes naturally.

expertise. Is it reasonable to expect a nurse who is considered competent by colleagues or an employer in one clinical area to be competent at the onset of employment in another clinical area? Let's assume Nurse A has five years of experience in emergency nursing, while Nurse B has one year of experience in labor and delivery. Both nurses transfer to the same pediatric intensive care unit (PICU). Are they competent nurses? Yes. Are they competent at providing nursing care to children in the PICU? No. Both individuals will require some type of education and skill training before they can become contributing members of the PICU nursing staff. Because of the differences in their work experience to date, each nurse is likely to adapt to the new nursing clinical practice differently. Ideally, individualized orientation programs take into account previous experience.

Fey and Miltner (2000) describe three levels of nursing competencies: core, specialty, and patient care management. **Core competencies** are those required for the minimum safe level of nursing performance. **Specialty competencies** are the skills and knowledge required for the minimum safe level of nursing care to a specific patient population. Specialty competencies are often unit specific. **Patient care management competencies** demonstrate the integration of core and specialty competencies in the provision of safe patient care (Fey & Miltner, 2000). The relationship of these levels is shown in Figure 9–1.

Competencies are often written in two parts—a statement that describes the performance standard and a list of performance criteria (Luttrell, Lenburg, Scherubel, Jacob, & Koch, 1999). Table 9–4 illustrates the difference between the levels of competencies. The competence of a nurses ranges from broad (core competence) to specific (patient care competencies) for a unique patient population.

Essential Competency

A number of professional organizations have sought to define skills essential to patient care. The American Association of Colleges of Nursing (AACN) published the *Essentials* document as a guide to the essential knowledge, values, and professional behaviors required of the baccalaureate nurse graduate (AACN, 1998). The PEW Health Professions Commission (1998) defined the Twenty-one Competencies for the Twenty-first century in their report as a guide for safe practice. The American Nurses Association (ANA) has developed Standards of Care to guide nurses in recognizing expected competencies. Specialty groups such as the American Association of Critical Care Nurses or Association of Operating Room Nurses have further delineated standards for their specialty groups.

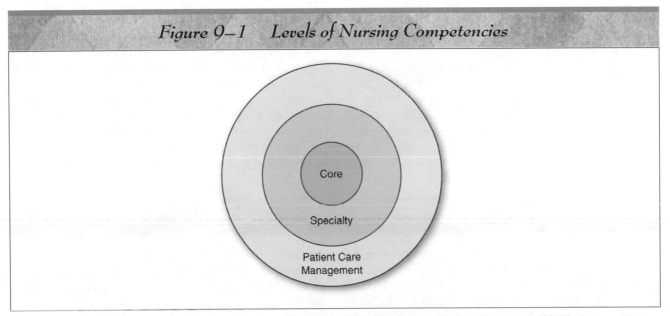

Figure 9–1   Levels of Nursing Competencies

Reprinted with permission from Lippincott, Williams & Wilkins. Modified from Fey, M. K., & Miltner, R. S. (2000). A competency-based orientation program for new graduate nurses. *Journal of Nursing Administration, 30*(3), 126–132.

Table 9–4 Competency Levels Applied to Nursing

	Core Competency	Specialty Competency	Patient Care Management Competency
Performance Standard	The nurse will assess the patient's level of pain.	The nurse will recognize the signs and symptoms of pain in the postoperative patient.	The nurse will provide care for patients in the immediate post-operative period.
Performance Criteria	• The nurse routinely assesses each patient's pain level. • The nurse implements a plan of care to provide pain relief.	• The nurse assesses the post-operative patient for signs and symptoms of pain every hour. • The nurse will initiate non-pharmacological pain interventions per unit protocol.	• The nurse will care for a patient immediately following coronary artery bypass surgery. • The nurse will care for the patient immediately following heart transplant surgery.

Adapted from Fey & Miltner (2000).

American Association of Colleges of Nursing

In 1986, the American Association of Colleges of Nursing (AACN) compiled the first national document that defined the essential knowledge, values, and professional behaviors required of the baccalaureate nursing graduate. That document was revised in 1998. The term **professional nurse** as defined in the *Essentials* document "refers to that individual prepared with a minimum of a baccalaureate in nursing, but is also inclusive of one who enters professional practice with a master's degree in nursing or a nursing doctorate" (AACN, 1998, p. 2). Changes in the health care delivery system, shifting population demographics, and scientific advances have forced nurses to reexamine their role and preparation for practice.

The members of the task force responsible for the *Essentials* document identified five essential components to professional nursing education: (a) liberal education, (b) professional values, (c) core competencies, (d) core knowledge, and (e) role development. Core competencies identified in the document include critical thinking, communication, assessment, and technical skills (Table 9–5). Box 9–1 list technical skills that the AACN has deemed the new graduate nurse must have to deliver safe and efficient patient care.

Pew Health Professions Commission

The Pew Charitable Trusts encourage and sustain individuals and professionals who address critical issues in hope of effecting social change. The trusts consist of seven individual charitable funds whose grant making activities are managed collectively. Within the Pew Charitable Trusts, the Health and Human Services program is designed to promote the health and well being of the American people. The Trusts provided a decade of support to the Pew Health Professions Commission through the Health and Human Services program. The goal was to improve health care and thus the well-being

Critical Thinking and Reflection

When evaluating your own competence, what do you perceive to be your strengths and weaknesses? What are the responsibilities of faculty, staff, and the employer for ensuring your competence and the safety of patients? What are your responsibilities for attaining, maintaining, and sustaining competence in light of ever-changing technology and patient demands? Does the responsibility for competence lie with the profession, the institution, or the individual?

Table 9–5 Essential Skills for Baccalaureate Nursing Graduates

Skill Category	Specific Competencies
Core Competencies	• Critical thinking • Communication • Assessment • Technical skills
Core Knowledge	• Health promotion, risk reduction, and disease prevention • Illness and disease management • Information and health care technologies • Ethics • Human diversity • Global health care • Health care systems and policy
Role Development	• Provider of care • Designer/manager/coordinator of care • Member of a profession

Box 9–1 Technical Skills Deemed Essential for the Graduate of a Baccalaureate Program

- Assess and monitor vital signs, including pulse and respiratory rates, temperature, pulse oximetry, blood pressure, and three-lead electrocardiogram.
- Provide appropriate individual hygiene maintenance.
- Apply infection control measures.
- Assess and manage wounds, including irrigation, application of dressings, and suture/staple removal.
- Provide and teach tracheotomy care.
- Apply heating and cooling devices.
- Apply and teach proper positioning and mobility techniques, including range of motion exercises, transferring, ambulating, and use of assistive devices.
- Provide nursing care using proper safety techniques, including the use of call systems, identification procedures, appropriate use of restraints, and basic fire, radiation, and hazardous materials protection.
- Administer CPR.
- Perform specimen collection techniques.
- Perform accurate intake and output calculations and recording.
- Administer medications by all routes.
- Initiate, assess, and regulate intravenous therapies.
- Demonstrate the proper use and care of various therapeutic tubes and drains.
- Provide comfort and pain reduction measures including positioning and therapeutic touch.
- Provide care of the respiratory system, including chest physiotherapy, oxygen therapy, resuscitation, spirometry, and suctioning.
- Provide teaching, and emotional and physical support in preparation for therapeutic procedures.
- Provide preoperative and postoperative teaching and care.

Reprinted/Adapted with permission from AACN (1998). *Essentials of baccalaureate education for professional nursing practice*, pp. 11–12.

of individuals, families, and communities. Recommendations were directed at health care professionals, professional schools, delivery systems, and policy makers. The Pew Health Professions Commission sought to make health professions and workforce issues "an essential part of the debate about health care change; create a set of competencies for successful health professional education and practice in the emerging health care system; and provide resources and services in the form of research policy analysis, technical assistance, advocacy, grants, and programs to policy makers, institutional leaders, and health professionals as they work to integrate this vision and these competencies into daily practice" (Shugars, O'Neil, & Bader, 1991, p. iii). The commission has issued four major reports. In the first report the commission indicated "the education and training of health professionals is out of step with the evolving needs of the American people" (Shugars, O'Neil, & Bader, 1991, p. iii). Subsequent reports were designed to clarify this statement and provide recommendations for improvement. In the final report the Pew Health Professions Commission (1998–1999) defined the Twenty-one Competencies for the Twenty-First Century designed to balance individual patient needs with system and population constraints

(Box 9–2). These competencies are intended to address future health care needs resulting from nine identified trends, which the Pew Commission anticipated would influence health care and professional practice. These trends include:

- Pressure to control cost
- An oversupply of resources including health care professionals and hospitals
- An aging population
- Increasing availability of information technology
- Advances in the treatment of disease
- A need to improve the quality of current health care services
- The changing role of the health care consumer to include "smart consumer" tactics to demand quality and control costs
- A recognition that disparities exist within the population related to health care
- A broadening definition of health care, which focuses on disease prevention and well as treatment

According to the Pew Commission report, future health care demands will require nursing to produce RNs prepared beyond the ADN and diploma levels.

Box 9–2 *Pew Health Professions Commission: Twenty-One Competencies for the Twenty-First Century*

1. Embrace a personal ethic of social responsibility and service.
2. Exhibit ethical behavior in all professional activities.
3. Provide evidence-based, clinically competent care.
4. Incorporate the multiple determinants of health in clinical care.
5. Apply knowledge of the new sciences.
6. Demonstrate critical thinking, reflection, and problem solving.
7. Understand the role of primary care.
8. Rigorously practice preventive health care.
9. Integrate population-based care and services into practice.
10. Improve access to health care for those with unmet health needs.
11. Practice relationship-centered care with individuals and families.
12. Provide culturally sensitive care to a diverse society.
13. Partner with communities in health care decisions.
14. Use communication and information technology effectively and appropriately.
15. Work in interdisciplinary teams.
16. Ensure care that balances individual, professional, system, and societal needs.
17. Practice leadership.
18. Take responsibility for quality of care and health outcomes at all levels.
19. Contribute to continuous improvement of the health care system.
20. Advocate for public policy that promotes and protects the health of the public.
21. Continue to learn and help others learn.

New graduates will require "critical thinking skills, independent judgment, management and organizational skills, leadership abilities, and technological understanding to operate in diverse settings" (Pew Health Professions Commission, 1998, p. 64). In recognition of the needs, the commission recommended that nursing (a) adjust educational programs to produce the number and types of nurse appropriate to local and regional demands; (b) delineate knowledge and outcome competencies for each level of nursing program; (c) revamp curricula to produce graduates prepared for differentiated practice; and (d) integrate research, teaching, and practice to further the professional and practical goals of the professions.

In summary, the commission's recommendations focused on the values that shape health care delivery and education. These values include the need for universal access to basic health care services, efficient use of resources, creativity and innovation, and choice. The commission offered nursing recommendations, which will require the profession and individual nurses to make hard choices. The challenge for all nurses, new and experienced, will be to adapt new skills and accommodate to the changing health care system. In order to assure this accommodation, nurses must be flexible; the responsibility rests with each nurse to maintain a commitment to lifelong learning and a willingness to adapt.

ANA Standards of Care

Although non-nursing organizations such as accreditation agencies (e.g., Joint Commission on Accreditation of Healthcare Organizations) have mandated competencies for nurses, the majority of nursing competencies are derived from standards of practice developed by professional nursing organizations. The American Nurses Association (ANA) has published a variety of documents that define and describe generalist and specialist nursing competencies. The ANA's *Standards of Clinical Nursing Practice* (ANA, 1998) lists nursing competencies according to (a) Standards of Care and (b) Standards of Professional Performance. The care standards are based on the nursing process (assessment, diagnosis, planning, implementation, and evaluation). Professional performance standards describe skills concerned with quality of care, performance appraisal, education, collegiality, ethics, collaboration, research, and resource utilization. Specialty nursing organizations have further delineated nursing competencies. Specialty organizations are responsible for developing specific standards and clinical guidelines for their respective specialty practice areas (Whittaker, Carson, & Smolenski, 2000).

The ANA and specialty nursing organizations work to update competencies with new knowledge in order to meet the changing needs of the health care system. These organizations play a fundamental role to implement health policy, support research to link nursing interventions to patient outcomes, influence changes in state nurse practice acts and federal legislation, and provide for credentialing of specialty nurse groups (Whittaker, Carson, & Smolenski, 2000; Weinstein, 2000).

Validating Competence

Hospitals are required to document initial competency and the ongoing competence of their nursing staff. Responsibility for validation often falls on the shoulders of nursing staff development personnel and/or unit managers. Validation is essential to assure that the nurse continues to maintain a minimal level of expertise necessary to provide safe care and to assure that the nurse has the knowledge needed to provide care for the particular problems of patients (Gunn, 1999).

The frequency of validation may vary depending on the specific skill. The time interval for skills, such as neonatal resuscitation, is determined by the national standard as set by the Neonatal Resuscitation Program (Bloom, Cropley, AHA/AAP Neonatal Resuscitation Steering Committee, 2000). Other skills are usually validated annually or as required by accreditation criteria set forth by the Joint Commission on Accreditation of Healthcare Organizations (JCAHO).

Competency validation can be achieved through a variety of mechanisms including self-assessment, direct observations of performance, objective examinations, and documentation of the number of technical skills/procedures performed in a given time (Miller, Flynn, & Umadac, 1998). For many skills, a combination of strategies are employed (e.g., neonatal resuscitation), and may include objective and performance evaluations.

Orientation to a New Job or Unit

Traditionally, individual competence of a nurse has been assessed during the interview and hiring process. This assessment consists of checking letters of recommendation, verification of education and state recognition for practice as a registered nurse, and self-report evidenced in the applicant's resume and/or job application, and personal interview(s). Further evidence of competence is gathered during the orientation period (e.g., math and skills competence testing).

Assuring the competency of a nursing staff requires an organized approach to orientation to the unit and a system of verification/validation of the skills and knowledge applied. Since nurses have a variety of educational and experiential backgrounds, the traditional approach of lectures and reading procedure manuals is no longer an efficient and effective orientation strategy (Dunn et al., 2000). Competency-based orientation is the preferred model in many institutions because it allows for individual differences between nurses. It is ideally suited to adult learners (Knowles, 1980).

Competency-based orientation (CBO) involves the integration of knowledge, skills, and attitudes needed to perform in a designated role or setting (Alspach, 1984). Understanding competency-based education (CBE) requires an understanding of what is a competency. A competency consists of three components: knowledge that forms the basis of nursing practice, the performance (psychomotor and problem-solving) skills to apply the knowledge to a clinical situation, and an affective response (Dunn et al., 2000).

A competency-based orientation has many advantages and few disadvantages. A major advantage is a decrease in the length of orientation for experienced nurses (Marrone, 1999; O'Grady & O'Brien, 1992; Stewart & Vitello-Cicciu, 1989). In today's economic environment this can result in significant savings to the unit and institution. Other advantages attributed to CBO are increased quality control since there is consistency in performance standards, measurable performance standards, no repetitive classroom lectures and/or presentations, length of orientation can be flexed to meet the needs of the new graduate and the experienced nurse, the orientee becomes accountable for his/her own learning (or lack of), and orientees are treated as adult learners (Alspach, 1984; Chaisson, 1995; Marrone, 1999; Mikos-Schild, 1999; O'Grady & O'Brien, 1992; Staab, Granneman, & Page-Reahr, 1996). The educator becomes the facilitator of the process rather than the master teacher and gatekeeper of learning (Mikos-Schild, 1999). As unit resources, preceptors serve as expert role models to facilitate the learning of the orientee (Staab, Granneman, & Page-Reahr, 1996).

Competency-based programs are criticized for emphasizing the science of nursing while paying little to no attention to the art of nursing. Communication skills, ethics, creative problem solving, and role development skills inherent in the art of nursing are difficult to quantify and translate into objective, measurable competency statements. The emphasis on skills and the technical aspects of nursing performance may not promote critical thinking and problem-solving skills (Mikos-Schild, 1999). Neary (2001) notes the difficulty in measuring competency due to the subjective nature of evaluation and problems in measurability. Competencies often include a laundry list of skills and knowledge that must be attained. This may prolong orientation for the individual who is not able to set priorities or is not motivated to complete the process (Mikos-Schild, 1999). Despite these disadvantages, competency-based programs are widely used for orientation programs and some academic nursing programs.

Most graduate nurses complete their basic nursing education with little clinical experience in specialty areas of practice such as intensive care, operating room, hospice care, and so on. This places the burden of developing practice competence on the unit, hospital, and/or employer. Because of the current nursing shortage, many specialty areas are employing new graduate nurses in a time when the supply of seasoned nurses may be decreased. The traditional orientation model of classroom learning followed by a period of joint clinical practice with an assigned preceptor may not be possible. As the competition for hiring new graduate nurses intensifies between institutions, many are developing internship or externship programs to lure prospective employees. Internships/externships for the new graduate nurse are a viable option for providing nursing staff for specialty units. Most new graduate nurses recognize the paucity of their knowledge and skills for these units and want some type of formalized educational program to become competent nurses. Depending on the availability of staff development instructors and seasoned nurses who are willing to assume preceptor responsibilities, internship/externship programs may offer a mixture of traditional classroom teaching and competency-based education. In an effort to maximize resources, nurse interns/externs are often combined together for the classroom content. For example, a large tertiary hospital may offer a maternal–child nursing option, while a children's hospital may offer a critical care option. In the former, the interns and externs may sit together for classes on maternity and pediatric nursing. In the latter, the interns may be in class together for critical care core content and then assigned to a preceptor in their work experience in the PICU or the neonatal intensive care unit (NICU).

Competency-based programs are also well suited to orientation for new graduate nurses and experienced nurses who are changing their focus area. The seasoned staff nurse who switches from adult intensive care to pediatric intensive care can focus his or her orientation on learning the pediatric specific aspects of critical care. The orientation program for this individual can be designed to allow credit for knowledge and skills previously learned. The experienced staff nurse who switches from the well-baby nursery to the NICU will need to focus on the critical care aspects of newborns since he or she already has a knowledge base about well infants and common concerns such as thermoregulation and hypoglycemia.

Ongoing Staff Development

While unit managers are responsible for documenting competency (i.e., validating the skill/knowledge), the individual employee must obtain the necessary ongoing education. The needed education is often obtained through continuing education programs offered by professional organizations and/or staff development programs offered by employing institutions. Maintaining individual competence is a professional obligation of every nurse. This requirement is clearly spelled out in the American Nurses Association's Code of Ethics for Nurses, which states, "The nurse is responsible and accountable for individual nursing practice . . ." (ANA, 2001, p. 4).

Professional Certification

Voluntary certification is an excellent mechanism for staff nurses to document their ongoing competence in nursing and to advance their careers. In addition to measuring specialty knowledge, these national certification examinations require documentation of ongoing education to maintain the nurse's certification. A recent study of 19,000 certified nurses suggests that certified nurses make fewer errors in patient care, have fewer adverse events, are more effective in interpersonal skills, and have more confidence in their ability to identify patient complications (Trossman, 2000). The variety of professional certification available for staff nurses is provided in Table 9-6.

Table 9–6 Specialty Certification Options For Staff Nurses

Specialty Area of Practice	Testing Agency	Credential Used by Certified Nurses
Low-risk newborn nursing	National Certification Corporation for the Obstetric, Gynecologic & Neonatal Nursing Specialties (NCC)	RNC
Neonatal intensive care nursing		
Maternal–newborn nursing		
Inpatient obstetrical nursing		
Critical care nursing (adult, pediatric, or neonatal)	American Association of Critical-Care Nurses Certifying Corporation (AACN)	CCRN
Emergency nursing	Board of Certification for Emergency Nursing (BCEN)	CEN
Flight nurse		CERN
Infusion therapy	Infusion Nurses Certification Corporation (INCC)	CRNI
Cardiac rehabilitation nursing	American Nurses Credentialing Center (ANCC)	RN, BC
College health nursing		
Community health nursing		
General nursing practice		
Gerontological nursing		
Home health nursing		
Informatics		
Medical–surgical nursing		
Nursing continuing education/ staff development		
Pediatric nursing		
Perinatal nursing		
Psychiatric–mental health		
School nurse		
Nursing administration		RN, CNA, BC

(continued)

Table 9–6   (continued)

Specialty Area of Practice	Testing Agency	Credential Used by Certified Nurses
Rehabilitation nursing	Association of Rehabilitation Nurses (ARA)	CRRN
Infection control	Certification Board of Infection Control & Epidemiology, Inc.	CIC
Nephrology nursing	Nephrology Nursing Certification Corporation (NNCC)	CNN
Dialysis nursing		CDN
Dermatology nursing	Dermatology Nursing Certification Board (DNCB)	DNC
Nurse massage therapy	National Certification Board for Therapeutic Massage & Bodywork	NMT
Addictions nursing	Center for Nursing Education & Testing	CARN
Ambulatory care nursing	American Nurses Credentialing Center in conjunction with American Association of Ambulatory Care Nurses	RN.Cm
Baromedical (hyperbaric) nursing	National Board of Diving & Hyperbaric Medical Technology	CHN
Childbirth education	Lamaze International	LCCE
Diabetes educator	National Certification Board for Diabetes Educators	CDE
Gastroenterology nursing	Certifying Board of Gastroenterology Nurses & Associates, Inc.	CGRN
Healthcare quality		CPHQ
HIV/AIDS nursing		ACRN
Holistic nursing		HNC
Hospice and palliative nursing		CHPN
Lactation consultant	International Board of Lactation Consultant Examiners	IBCLC
Legal nurse consultant		LNCC
Long-term care		
Managed care nursing		CMCN
Neuroscience nursing		CNRN
Occupational health nursing		COHN, COHN-S
Occupational health case manager		COHN/CM, CPHN-S/CM
Oncology nursing		OCN, AOCN
Ophthalmic nursing		CRNO
Orthopedic nursing		ONC
Pain management	American Academy of Pain Management	FAAPM
Pediatric nursing	National Certification Board for Pediatric Nurse Practitioners & Associates	CPN
Pediatric oncology nursing		CPON
Perianesthesia nursing		CPAN, CAPA
Perioperative nursing		CNOR
Plastic and reconstructive surgical nursing		CPSN
RN First Assistant		CRNFA
School nursing		CSN
Urology nursing		CURN

Divergent Expectations of Competency

Students want to "do," faculty want students to "think and do," and employers want to know when a novice nurse can function independently in a safe and competent manner. Because there is so much to learn, students, faculty, new graduates, and health care employers need to recognize that teaching is not the sole responsibility of nursing faculty and that learning is not complete at the time of graduation. While both the new graduate and the employer are clearly concerned with competency, neither should be under the impression that the new graduate is finished learning nor ready to function independently at the time of graduation. In order to gain the knowledge, skill, and understanding needed to provide unsupervised, safe, competent care, the employer and new graduate share the responsibility for continued professional development.

Institutional Expectations of Competency

Registered nurses continue to graduate from three different program types. While educators understand the difference between graduates from each program, it is clear employers and consumers do not always discriminate between new nurses prepared in different programs. Institutional expectations of basic competency for new graduates are consistent. Employers are interested in knowing whether a new graduate has theoretical knowledge, clinical experience, and skill competence to perform safely and accurately. Employers are also interested in how much supervision the new graduate will need and how quickly the graduate will be able to move to independence. Each new staff nurse's capability to perform specified activities is assessed while completing an orientation. The orientation familiarizes the new nurse with workplace responsibilities before beginning patient care. The orientation process also emphasizes specific job-related aspects of personal safety and safety of others.

To better understand employer expectations of entry-level nurses, the National Council of State Boards of Nursing (NCSBN) conducts job analysis studies every 3 years (Smith & Crawford, 2002). The studies identify changes over time in the work environment, employment characteristics, and activities of newly licensed nurses. New graduates who hold a nursing position and work a minimum of 20 hours per week are surveyed at 3-month intervals 3 to 6 months after successfully passing the NCLEX examination.

Data from these studies are analyzed in relation to the frequency of performance, impact on maintaining patient safety, criticality of nursing activities performed, and the various settings where nursing activities were performed. Criticality refers to activities that cannot be delayed or omitted without a *substantial risk of unnecessary complications, impairment of function, or serious distress to patients.* Those tasks found to have the highest priority level according to the 2002 job analysis survey include:

- Identify and intervene in life-threatening situations
- Apply principles of infection control
- Determine if vital signs are abnormal
- Administer medication
- Assess client's discomfort level
- Identify abnormalities on cardiac monitor strip
- Evaluate effectiveness of medications
- Notify others of change in status
- Protect from injury
  (Smith and Crawford, 2002, p. 55)

According to the 2002 job analysis survey, those activities identified as most frequently performed include:

- Applying principles of infection control
- Documenting patient care
- Determining if vital signs are abnormal
- Evaluating effectiveness of medication
- Assessing discomfort or pain
- Listening to patient's/family's concerns
- Providing privacy
- Administering medications
  (Smith and Crawford, 2002, p. 17)

Health Care Team Expectations of Competency

Nurses work with a myriad of people within as well as outside of institutions. They work with other nurses; physicians; certified nurse's aides; pharmacists; social workers; individuals in clerical roles; pastoral professionals; dietitians; respiratory, physical, and occupational therapists; and others. All of these members of the health care team have expectations of the nursing staff. The nurse often plays a key role as a coordinator in communicating the various needs of the patient to the other members of the health care team. Communication skills and competency are crucial in successful implementation of the coordinator role.

One of the most discussed and written about relationships is that between nurses and physicians. The relationship between these two has evolved from the historical "handmaiden to the physician" to "colleague to physician." While the road has not always been an easy one and there are still a few miles to go, the changes to date have been significant and heartening. Institutions and organizations recognize the strength in physician and nurse teamwork creating an atmosphere of support (Baggs et al., 1997). It behooves the new graduate as well as all practicing nurses to be aware of the philosophy of their institution and to make sure it creates a milieu where all can work together. Successful adaptation requires that the nurse relies on the empowered self and on colleagues with similar goals. This reliance builds power through strong professional relationships, which steadfastly can withstand destructive conflict (Thomas, 2001). With these goals in mind, the teamwork of nurses and physicians will continue to evolve and be strengthened.

Patient Expectations of Competency

Patients expect competent, efficient care from all professional nurses regardless of their years of service. Research suggests that patients as well as nurses define a good nurse primarily by "actions directed at maintaining physical comfort, hygiene, and medical treatment" (Bjork, 1995, p. 6). Despite the clear public perception of what constitutes a "good nurse," the practical importance of physical care has received diminished attention by both nursing service and education. More and more nurses are delegating everyday patient care tasks (e.g., bathing, wound care, nutrition) to auxiliary personnel. Because nurses supervise those in auxiliary roles, the public continues to expect nurses to be competent and responsible caregivers. Furthermore, the public expects competence to be combined with ethical and honest nursing practice. A recent public opinion poll ranked nurses second with regard to honesty and ethics behind firefighters (Gallup Organization, 2001).

More than ever before, consumers are knowledgeable about health care and are eager to be directly involved with the care they receive. Television, radio, newspapers, and magazines regularly feature articles concerning the current status of the health care delivery system. As consumers become increasingly knowledgeable about the health care system, they also become more involved in their own health care. Informed patients have come to expect more from those who deliver health care.

Competency Issues Related to Errors in Health Care

Lifelong competency assessment and evaluation is integral to safe professional practice (LaDuke, 2002). For new graduates, errors in the delivery of care can be one of the most frightening aspects of clinical practice. According to the 1999 Institute of Medicine (IOM) comprehensive report on medical errors, 98,000 Americans die each year from preventable adverse events, and 7,000 of these deaths are due to medication errors. Factors associated with these errors included lack of centralized pharmacists, hospital occupancy rate, and the number of registered nurses (Bond, 2001). Staffing issues, orientation deficiencies, inappropriate perception of hazards, and motivational difficulties can also contribute to errors. While the cost of these errors is significant; the loss of public confidence cannot be measured.

There are many obstacles to decreasing the number of health care delivery errors. These include a lack of awareness that the problem exists, lack of legal protection, out-of-date information systems, inadequate resources for improvement, and a lack of understanding of systems-based approaches to error reduction. A root cause analysis of errors will help provide information about an error, thereby creating the opportunity to address the mistake and prevent future occurrences. As a response to an error, punishment can be appropriate but may not be an effective way to handle all situa-

Critical Thinking and Reflection

As the public holds all health care providers more accountable for care provided, it seems prudent that nurses pay attention to the patient's perception/expectation of what constitutes good nursing care. Discuss how the current nursing shortage and workplace demands will influence patient perceptions of nursing care. Do you view these perceptions as accurate? In either case, how will patient perceptions impact the care you provide patients?

tions. Many errors are due to multiple factors and systemwide changes are indicated to correct the situation.

Employers are beginning to recognize that an atmosphere of punishment contributes to errors rather than serving to decrease their occurrence. The JCAHO sought federal statutory protection of reported information to facilitate the study and reporting of medical errors. The Quality Interagency Coordination Task Force report to the President of the United States discussed the federal response to the IOM report and called for the establishment of locally directed error prevention systems. As more institutions take a no-blame approach to errors, there is hope for better reporting and understanding of how the errors occur.

The ideal environment for nurses is one that encourages recognition and acknowledgement of risks to the safety of individuals. A system for the initiation of actions to reduce risks, an internal reporting mechanism that focuses on processes and systems, and minimization of individual blame or retribution are key factors in the reduction of health care error.

Nurses must educate patients and family about their responsibility for safe, error-free care. Individual patients and their families are responsible for providing accurate and complete information about the medical

Research Application

Nurses in the mid-nineteenth and early twentieth centuries sought to distance themselves from the reputation of earlier health care providers/nurses such as prisoners who were drafted into service. The reputation of these providers characterized by the Charles Dickens' character Sarie Gamp hampered the growth and acceptance of nursing as a respectable, independent profession. Nurse leaders of the time instituted rigid guidelines for the recruitment and training of nurses. According to one advertisement, individuals were accepted into nursing only if over the age of 30, single, and plain looking (Kalish & Kalish, 1995). The nurse "reformers" of this time were successful in their beginning attempts to make nursing a "respectable" profession attracting women of character.

Just as early reformers sought change, so have nurse scientists of the twenty-first century. As nursing evolved from a practical occupation dominated by physicians and hospital-based control of education to an independent discipline, nurse scientists have sought acceptance for this transition through research and development of nursing theory. Consequently, the more nurses have sought to assert their independence, the more they have abandoned any study of practical skill development. There seems to be little interest in this type of investigation despite patients' continued insistence that nurses who provide physical comfort, hygiene, and medical treatment are the most valued.

Ida Torunn Bjork has done extensive research regarding nursing and practical skill development (Bjork, 1995, 1998, 1999; Bjork & Kirkevold, 1999). Dr. Bjork (1995) contends that the "patient's body has moved out of focus in nursing" (p. 6). She suggests that research indicates that, while patients consistently value nursing actions directed at maintaining physical comfort, hygiene, and medical treatment, recent evidence suggests nurses value these same activities but place greater value on interpersonal relations and the psychosocial aspects of care rather than practice skills. Bjork contends that a conflict exists between nursing service and nursing education. She asserts that practical preparedness has diminished with the movement of education from the hospital setting into the academic setting.

It is the belief of the authors of this textbook that nurses should be interested in preserving and developing nursing as a practice discipline. For this reason, this chapter is included in this textbook. While today's nurses and nurse scientists should value psychosocial aspects of care, it is also important to acknowledge and value the physical and technical elements of care. The recent emphasis on evidence-based care would seem to support this notion. It is time for nurses to define and differentiate the domain of nursing skills from simple practice skills of unlicensed personnel. Further, nurse scientists need to address the process for acquiring and maintaining these skills within the context of patient care. As long as nurses view technical skills as simply a set of sequenced motor movements, the learning, performance, and significance of skills will not be a topic of research for nursing. In her work, Bjork concludes that nurses need to adopt a broader conceptualization of practical skills that includes the dimension of skilled performance, caring intentions, and disciplined understanding.

history. They are also responsible for reporting perceived risks in their care and unexpected changes in the individual's condition. By providing feedback about the service needs and expectations, patients and their families can help the organization to better meet their needs. They are responsible for asking questions when they do not understand what they have been told about their care or what they are expected to do.

Competency and Physical Safety

Nurses often ask themselves how safe is the health care work environment. Moreover, many nurses are concerned that lack of safety can impact their health and well-being. Safety within health care organizations is monitored and regulated by the JCAHO and the Occupational Safety and Health Administration (OSHA). While these regulatory agencies monitor safety, individual safety is first and foremost the responsibility of individuals as is determined by the care they take in their professional practice.

There are many hazards in health care settings. Nurses are frequently exposed to chemicals and patients with contagious diseases. They run the risk of needle sticks and injury from improper body mechanics. Furthermore, the overall physical demand of the profession is a hazard nurses face daily. Nursing is also demanding psychologically. Nurses are expected to work long shifts and interact, lead, and/or care for a variety of people/patients with a wide range of needs. The work is hard, and the nurse must understand what measures can be taken to avoid dangerous exposure, prevent injury, and remain physically and emotionally safe.

Institutions are responsible for keeping their employees safe via education, training, support, and counseling. Many require employees to have appropriate immunizations prior to working. They also require yearly training and review of safety practices. A nurse who has a strong safety foundation is more likely to maintain a safe environment for patients, other staff, and visitors to the institution. Most institutions seek to ensure physical and biological safety through competency training programs that involve:

- Fire safety
- General safety
- Patient safety, quality, and sentinel events
- Infant safety
- Patient confidentiality
- Patient rights

- Ergonomics and back safety
- Hazardous material management
- Internal and external disaster preparedness
- Age-specific competencies
- Infection control

While the institution provides education and training programs, the individual nurse is ultimately responsible for (a) knowing and understanding risks and (b) taking proper care to avoid injury. A key component to the safety of the nurse is his or her understanding of institutional policies and procedures.

Workplace Violence

OSHA also addresses the issue of workplace violence. Today, more assaults occur in the health care and social services industries than in any other. For example, Bureau of Labor Statistics (BLS) data for 1992 showed health care and social service workers having the highest incidence of assault injuries (BLS, 1992). Almost two-thirds of the nonfatal assaults occurred in nursing homes, hospitals, and establishments providing residential care and other social services (Toscano, 1995). In 2000, the rate of nonfatal occupational injuries and illnesses in nurses was 13.9 per 100 full-time workers (U.S. Department of Labor, 2000).

Assaults against workers in the health care professions are not new. According to one study between 1980 and 1990, 106 occupational violence-related deaths occurred among the following health care workers: 27 pharmacists, 26 physicians, 18 registered nurses, 17 nurse's aides, and 18 health care workers in other occupational categories (Goodman, Jenkins, & Mercy. 1994). Using the National Traumatic Occupational Fatality database, the study reported that between 1983 and 1989, there were 69 registered nurses killed at work. Homicide was the leading cause of traumatic occupational death among employees in nursing homes and personal care facilities.

A 1989 report by Cannel and Hunter found that the nursing staff at a psychiatric hospital sustained 16 assaults per 100 employees per year. This rate, which includes any assault-related injuries, compares with 8.3 injuries of *all* types per 100 full-time workers in all industries and 14.2 per 100 full-time workers in the construction industry (U.S. Department of Labor, 1991). Of 121 psychiatric hospital workers sustaining 134 injuries, 43% involved lost time from work with 13% of those injured missing more than 21 days from work. In 2001, 11 fatal occupational injuries were reported (BLS, 2001).

Of greater concern is the likely underreporting of violence and a persistent perception within the health care industry that assaults are part of the job. Underreporting may reflect a lack of institutional reporting policies, employee beliefs that reporting will not benefit them, or employee fears that employers may deem assaults the result of employee negligence or poor job performance.

Health care and social service workers face an increased risk of work-related assaults stemming from several factors, including:

- The prevalence of handguns and other weapons—as high as 25%—among patients, their families, or friends.
- The increasing use of hospitals by police and the criminal justice systems for criminal holds and the care of acutely disturbed violent individuals.
- The increasing number of acute and chronically mentally ill patients now being released from hospitals without follow-up care, who now have the right to refuse medicine and who can no longer be hospitalized involuntarily unless they pose an immediate threat to themselves or others.
- The availability of drugs or money at hospitals, clinics, and pharmacies making them likely robbery targets.
- Situational and circumstantial factors such as unrestricted movement of the public in clinics and hospitals; the increasing presence of gang members, drug or alcohol abusers, trauma patients, or distraught family members; long waits in emergency or clinic areas, leading to patient frustration over an inability to obtain needed services promptly.
- Low staffing levels during times of specific increased activity such as meal times, visiting times, and when staff are transporting patients.
- Isolated work with patients during examinations or treatment.
- Solo work, often in remote locations, particularly in high-crime settings, with no back up or means of obtaining assistance such as communication devices or alarm systems.
- Lack of training of staff in recognizing and managing escalating hostile and assaultive behavior.
- Poorly lighted parking areas.

Terrorist Threats

Traditional safety competencies include internal and external disasters and management of hazardous materials. In the aftermath of the tragic events of September 11, 2001, the definitions of these competencies have changed. Management of hazardous materials has traditionally meant managing hazardous chemicals normally found in the health care agency. With the threat of terrorism, hazardous material has come to include any number of chemical or biological warfare agents. An internal disaster is defined by any condition that can disrupt internal operation; an external disaster is defined as any event that would bring a large number of patients to a facility. Both of these definitions take on new meaning in light of the September 11 terrorist attacks. These attacks point out that the United States is vulnerable to attack and likely to see more such attacks in the future. Events of September 11 clearly convinced U.S. citizens that there are people who are willing to die in order to kill Americans.

Health care providers and the general public became desperate to understand terrorism and bio chemical warfare. The television media, popular news journals, professional journals, and the Internet were quickly filled with information on terrorism and biochemical warfare. The information provided quickly made it apparent that most planning for an attack such as that of September 11 was at the local level and preparedness was poor (Moser, White, Lewis-Younger, & Garrett, 2001; Wetter, Daniell, & Treser, 2001). Local preparedness was found to be limited to resources currently in use (e.g., hospitals, EMS, law enforcement agencies, and private providers). Limiting these resources even further, the current nursing shortage contributes significantly to inadequate preparedness. While many of these facilities and agencies quickly sought to improve disaster preparedness, it is likely that in the event of an event of the magnitude of September 11 they will be quickly overwhelmed (Garrett, Magruder, & Molgard, 2000; Terriff & Tee, 2001; Wetter, Daniell, & Treser, 2001).

In response to the lack of preparedness, the Centers for Disease Control and Prevention (CDC) has developed strategic plans in the event of a domestic biochemical attack. These plans focus on planning, detection and surveillance, laboratory analysis, emergency response, and communication (CDC, 2000). Furthermore, the federal government has begun to stockpile pharmaceuticals essential for treatment in the event of biological warfare. While the military stockpiles are more adequate, they are not sufficient to meet civilian needs in the event of a large-scale attack (Khan, Morse, & Lillibridge, 2000).

Terrorist attacks using biologic agents present a unique concern with regard to warning and response.

If the attack goes as planned it is unlikely civilian population will be aware of exposure for hours or days. Once recognized, emergency response teams will serve to warn the public; simultaneously these individuals will most likely be the first to receive secondary exposure to the biologic agent. The response of these teams is likely to be furthered hindered by the abnormally large number of critically ill individuals, limited supplies, inadequate facilities, and poor planning (Henry, 2001; Macintyre et al., 2000; Siegelson, 2000). In the worst case scenerio, when the terrorist attack goes as planned, the inability of health care providers and other relief workers to respond in an effective manner would most likely lead to massive social and political disorder (Bardi, 1999).

There are a variety of means for the delivery of biological agents. The most likely delivery mode is aerosol, as a large number of lethal agents (e.g., anthrax, plague, smallpox, tularemia, and botulinum toxin) are most efficiently delivered in this manner. Water contamination is unlikely; however, secondary contamination via aerosol contact with an infected individual is possible with exposure to individuals infected with some agents (e.g.,

plague and smallpox) (Burrows & Renner, 1999). Smaller terrorist attacks are possible by contaminating food with such agents as botulinum, staphylococcus enterotoxin B, and cholera. Unfortunately, even small attacks, such as the mailed athrax attacks that followed September 11, are capable of causing serious social and economic disruption (Table 9–7).

A terrorist attack is also possible using chemical and radiological or nuclear weapons. Chemical weapons were used in the Tokyo subway by a religious cult in 1995. These weapons are capable of causing mass casualties, particularly if the terrorist group develops a means for widespread dispersal of the agent in a heavily populated region. Signs and symptoms of exposure to chemical weapons is dependent on the agent used but may include blister formation, bleeding, pulmonary symptoms (choking), incapacitation, nervous symptoms, and vomiting.

In the event of a nuclear attack such as that seen in Hiroshima and Nagasaki, widespread havoc can be expected. Sophisticated nuclear devices are not the only mechanism for release of radioactive material. Casualties and long-term contamination of large areas

Table 9–7   Summary of Selected Class A Biological Warfare Agents

Disease and Agent Type	Probable BW Route	Incubation (Days)	Signs and Symptoms (Incomplete)	Treatment of Mass Casualties	Prophylaxis	Vaccine
Anthrax: Spore-forming bacteria	Aerosol; no person to person	1–7 (or more)	Febrile, flulike; then severe respiratory distress	Ciprofloxacin or doxycycline	Ciprofloxacin or, if susceptible, doxycycline	Available, but short supply
Smallpox: Virus	Aerosol; then person to person	7–17	High fever, prostration; then rash and pustules	Supportive only	None	Available but short supply
Plague: Bacteria	Aerosol; then person to person	1–6	Fulminate pneumonia; then sepsis	Doxycycline or ciprofloxacin	Doxycycline or ciprofloxacin	Not now available
Botulism: Toxin from bacteria	Aerosol; no person to person	2 hours to 8	Bulbar nerve palsies; descending flaccid paralysis	Passive immunization (antitoxin); supportive care	Passive immunization (antitoxin)	Antitoxin in short supply
Tularemia: Bacteria	Aerosol; no person to person	1–14	Febrile, flulike; respiratory; sepsis	Doxycycline or ciprofloxacin	Doxycycline or ciprofloxacin	Not widely available and incomplete protection

Reprinted with permission: Kemp, C. http://www.baylor.edu/~Charles_Kemp/bioterror.htm (last update 1/25/2002).

are possible with the dispersal of radioactive material. The contaminated casualties themselves severely complicate the evacuation process of a contaminated area. Sources for dispersal of radioactive material could come from nuclear power plants, waste processing facilities, medical clinics, and industrial plants to name just a few. In addition, an attack on a nuclear generating plant may lead to a breach in containment such as that seen at Chernobyl or Three Mile Island.

The information provided above is overwhelming in and of itself. In light of this information most nurses and nursing students would agree that they have only novice levels of competence regarding disaster preparedness. In response, many nurse leaders and educators have sought to increase nursing's preparedness in the event of a national disaster. It is the responsibility of each nurse to seek out additional educational programs so as to ensure his or her own competence within this very new health care threat.

A successful career in nursing is built by developing and maintaining expertise in psychomotor, interpersonal, and critical thinking skills. Career planning should be an active process initiated during nursing school and repeated at regular intervals while the nurse becomes more proficient in his or her chosen clinical practice area. Clinical competence occurs on a continuum from novice to expert. Nursing students must master core scientific principles related to all aspects of care for graduation and to be deemed competent in their employment setting. The competent nurse is aware of the risks and areas of possible error in nursing and practices safely and effectively using clinical reasoning skills. Critical thinking and decision-making are essential aspects in achieving competency in the delivery of patient care. Lifelong learning is essential for nurses to maintain competency requirements. Nurses must understand the relationship between various requirements of skills competency and expectations for health care delivery in all environments.[1]

TRANSITION INTO PRACTICE

As baccalaureate nursing students prepare for practice, they wonder what type of practice they will have. They ask how their practice will be different from that of graduates of other types of RN educational programs. The National Council of State Boards of Nursing seeks to address these questions every 2 years through a job analysis survey. Amazingly, survey results of 1999 and 2001 are strikingly similar. The majority of newly licensed (within the first 6 months of practice) registered nurses, regardless of educational preparation report working in hospital settings. Less than 10% report working in either community-based facilities or long-term care. Furthermore, most (approximately 80%) work in medical–surgical and critical care settings. Of this data, the only significant difference between the 1999 survey (Hertz et al., 2000) and the 2001 survey (National Council of State Boards of Nursing, 2001)[2] was a significant drop in the number of graduates seeking employment in medical surgical settings. Other differences include greater numbers of BSN graduates report working in critical care and pediatric settings, while more ADN graduates reported working in long-term care and nursing home facilities.

As would be expected from this data, BSN and ADN graduates reported working most frequently with elderly and adult patients who are (a) acutely ill, (b) stable with chronic conditions, (c) unstable with chronic conditions, and (d) at the end of life. In the 2001 survey, statistically more graduates were found to be caring for newborns and adolescent patients.

In response to work role and administrative activities, respondents in the 2001 survey continue to report spending the greatest amount of time providing direct care. Baccalaureate graduates reported more involvement in administrative responsibilities. Other performance activities remained similar to those reported in the 1999 job analysis survey presented earlier in this chapter.

How will the growing shortage of nurses impact those who are newly licensed? Will the focus move toward administrative duties and will unlicensed assistive personnel take on a greater role in providing direct patient care? Will the definition of nursing change, and, if so, who will define nursing? Will nurses, administrators, politicians, or the general public decide what nurses do? As nurse leaders, baccalaureate graduates should become proactive in answering these and other questions.

[1]Adapted with permission from Charles Kemp (Web site http://www.baylor.edu/~Charles_Kemp/bioterror.htm). The reader is referred to his Web site for more extensive information concerning terrorist threat.

[2]Reprinted and used by permission of the National Council of State Boards of Nursing Inc. (NCSBN). Copyright © 2002 National Council of State Boards of Nursing (NCSBN).

KEY POINTS

1. While the graduate nurse may possess many nursing skills, he or she is usually required to (a) learn additional skills or competencies, (b) adapt existing skills to the uniqueness of the specialty population, and (c) gain proficiency in the ability to perform skills.
2. Career planning requires self-assessment and goal setting. Career goals should be identified early in a nurse's career but many nurses fail to do so.
3. Learning is about making neurologic, cognitive, social, and experiential connections.
4. Professional nurses are responsible for maintaining competency in their area of practice.
5. A number of professional organizations have sought to define skills essential to patient care. In addition, employing institutions have expected levels of competence for novice nurses. Moreover, patients expect competence from nurses who provide their care.
6. Nurses and other health care providers are making errors. Factors associated with these errors included lack of centralized pharmacists, hospital occupancy rate, and the number of registered nurses. Staffing issues, orientation deficiencies, inappropriate perception of hazards, and motivational difficulties are also contributing to errors.
7. Nurses are concerned that lack of safety can impact their health and well-being. Safety within health care organizations is monitored and regulated by the Joint Commission on Accreditation of Healthcare Organizations (JCAHO) and Occupational Safety and Health Administration (OSHA).
8. In additional to traditional threats to safety, nurse's safety is now also dependent on knowledge of workplace violence, biological hazards, and terrorist threats.

EXPLORE MediaLink

Critical thinking questions, essay questions, key terms, web links, activities, NCLEX review questions, and more interactive resources can be found on the Companion Website at www.prenhall.com/haynes. Click on Chapter 9 to select activities for this chapter.

REFERENCES

Alspach, J. G. (1984). Designing a competency-based orientation for critical care nurses. *Heart & Lung, 13*(6), 655–662.

American Association of Colleges of Nursing. (1998). *Essentials of baccalaureate education for professional nursing practice.* Washington, DC: Author.

American Nurses Association. (1998). *Standards of clinical nursing practice* (2nd ed.). Washington, DC: Author.

American Nurses Association. (2000). *Working paper on continued professional competence: Nursing's agenda for the 21st century.* Washington, DC: American Nurses Association.

American Nurses Association. (2001). *Code for nurses with interpretive statements.* Washington, DC: Author.

Baggs, J. G., Schmitt, M. H., Mushlin, A. I., Eldredge, D. H., Oakes, D., & Hutson, A. D. (1997). Nurse–physician collaboration and satisfaction with the decision-making process in three critical care units. *American Journal of Critical Care, 6*(5), 393–399.

Bardi, J. (1999). Aftermath of a hypothetical smallpox disaster. *Emerging Infectious Diseases, 5*(4), 547–551.

Benner, P. (1984). *From novice to expert: Excellence and power in clinical nursing practice.* Menlo Park, CA: Addison-Wesley Publishers.

Bjork, I. T. (1995). Neglected conflicts in the discipline of nursing: Perception of the importance and value of practical skill. *Journal of Advanced Nursing, 22*(1), 6–12.

Bjork, I. T. (1998). Practical skill development in new nurses. *Nursing Inquiry, 6,* 34–47.

Bjork, I. T. (1999). What constitutes a nursing skill? *Western Journal of Nursing Research, 21*(1), 51–70.

Bjork, I. T., & Kirkevold, M. (1999). Issues in nurses' practical skill development in the clinical setting. *Journal of Nursing Care Quality, 14*(1), 72–84.

Bloom, R. S., Cropley, C., & AHA/AAP Neonatal Resuscitation Steering Committee. (2000). *Textbook of neonatal resuscitation.* Dallas, TX: American Academy of Pediatrics/American Heart Association.

Bond, C. A., Raehl, C. L., & Franke, T. (2001). Medication errors in United States hospitals. *Pharmacotherapy, 21*(9), 1023–1036.

Burrows, W. D., & Renner, S. E. (1999). Biological warfare agents as threats to potable water. *Environmental Health Perspectives, 107*(12), 975–984.

Centers for Disease Control and Prevention. (2000). Biological and chemical terrorism: Strategic plan for preparedness and response. *Morbidity and Mortality Weekly Report, 49*(RR-4), 1–14.

Chaisson, S. F. (1995). Role of the CNS in developing a competency-based orientation program. *Clinical Nurse Specialist, 9*(1), 32–37.

Cross, P. (1999). *Learning is about making connections.* The Cross Papers. Mission Viejo, CA: League for Innovation in the Community College.

Dewey, J. (1967). *Democracy and education* (originally published in 1916). New York: Free Press.

Diamond, M., & Hopson, J. (1998). *Magic trees of the mind.* New York: Dutton.

DiMauro, N. M. (2000). Continuous professional development. *Journal of Continuing Education in Nursing, 31*(2), 59–62.

Donner, G. J., & Wheeler, M. M. (2001). Career planning and development for nurses: The time has come. *International Nursing Review, 48,* 79–85.

Dunn, S. V., Lawson, D., Robertson, S., Underwood, M., Clark, R., Valentine, T., Walker, N., Wilson-Row, C., Crowder, K., & Herewane, D. (2000). The development of competency standards for specialist critical care nurses. *Journal of Advanced Nursing, 31*(2), 339–346.

Ehrlich, T. (1996). Forward. In B. Jacoby & Associated (Eds.), *Service learning in higher education: Concepts and practices.* San Francisco: Jossey-Bass.

Fey, M. K., & Miltner, R. S. (2000). A competency-based orientation program for new graduate nurses. *Journal of Nursing Administration, 30*(3), 126–132.

Gallup Organization. (2001, November). *Press release 11205.* Honesty and Ethical Standards of Professionals.

Garrett, L. C., Magruder, C., & Molgard, C. A. (2000). Taking the terror out of bioterrorism: Planning for a bioterrorist event from a local perspective. *Journal of Public Health Management Practice, 6*(4), 1–7.

Goodman, R. A., Jenkins, E. L., & Mercy, J. A. (1994). Workplace-related homicide among health care workers in the United States. *Journal of the American Medical Association 272,* 1686–1688.

Gunn, I. P. (1999). Regulation of health care professionals: Part 2: Validation of continued competence. *CRNA: The Clinical Forum for Nurse Anesthetists, 10*(3), 135–141.

Henry, L. (2001). Inhalation anthrax: Threat clinical presentation, and treatment. *Journal of the American Academy of Nurse Practitioners, 13*(4), 164–168.

Institute of Medicine. (1999). *To err is human: Building a better health system.* Washington, DC: National Academic Press.

Jeffrey, Y. (2000). Using competencies to promote a learning environment in intensive care. *Nursing in Critical Care, 5*(4), 194–198.

Kalish, P. A., & Kalish, B. J. (1995). *The advance of American nursing.* Boston: Little, Brown and Company.

Khan, A. S., Morse, S., & Lillibridge, S. (2000). Public health preparedness for biological terrorism in the USA. *The Lancet, 356*(9236), 1179–1182.

Kleinknecht, M. K., & Hefferin, E. A. (1982). Assisting nurses toward professional growth: A career development model. *Journal of Nursing Administration, 12,* 30–36.

Knowles, M. S. (1980). *The modern practice of adult education: From pedagogy to androgogy.* Chicago, IL: Follet.

LaDuke, S. (2002). Beyond the psychomotor realm. *Nursing Management, 33*(3), 41–42.

Luttrell, M. F., Lenburg, C. A., Scherubel, J. C., Jacob, S. R., & Koch, R. W. (1999). Competency outcomes for learning and performance assessment. *Nursing and Health Care Perspectives, 20*(3), 134–141.

Macintyre, A. G., Christopher, G. W., Eitzen, E., Gum, R., Weir, S., DeAtley, C., et al. (2000). Weapons of mass destruction events with contaminated casualties: Effective planning for health care facilities. *Journal of the American Medical Association, 283*(2), 242–249.

Marrone, S. R. (1999). Designing a competency-based nursing practice model in a multicultural setting. *Journal for Nurses in Staff Development, 15*(2), 56–62.

Mikos-Schild, S. (1999). Competency-based orientation. *Today's Surgical Nurse, 21*(3), 14–19.

Miller, E., Flynn, J. M., & Umadac, J. (1998). Assessing, developing and maintaining staff's competency in times of restructuring. *Journal of Nursing Care Quality, 12*(6), 9–17.

Moser, R., White, G. L., Lewis-Younger, C. R., & Garrett, L. C. (2001). Preparing for expected bioterrorism attacks. *Military Medicine, 166*(5), 369–374.

Nash, J. M. (1997, February 3). Fertile minds. *Time,* 48–56.

National Council of State Boards of Nursing. (2001). *2001 RN practice analysis update.* Chicago, IL: Author.

National Institutes of Health Clinical Center Nursing Department. (1995). *Nursing standards.* Rockville, MD: National Institutes of Health.

Neary, M. (2001). Responsive assessment: Assessing student nurses' clinical competence. *Nurse Education Today, 21*(1), 3–17.

O'Grady, T., & O'Brien, A. (1992). A guide to competency-based orientation: Develop your own program. *Journal of Nursing Staff Development, 8*(3), 128–133.

O'Halloran, V. E. (1996). Maintaining career marketability as a professional nurse. *Nursing Forum, 31*(4), 29–33.

Pew Health Professions Commission. (1998). *Strengthening consumer protection: Priorities for health care workforce regulation: Report of the Pew Health Professions Commission.* San Francisco, CA: Pew Health Professions Commission.

Ramsden, P. (1992). *Learning to teach in higher education.* London: Routledge.

Schmalenberg, C., & Kramer, M. (1979). *Coping with reality shock: The voices of experience.* Wakefield, MA: Nursing Resources, Inc.

Shugars, D. A., O'Neil, E. H., & Bader, J. D. (Eds.). (1991). *Healthy America: Practitioners for 2005, an agenda for action for U. S. health professional schools.* San Francisco, CA: The Pew Health Professions Commission.

Siegelson, H. J. (2000). Aftermath . . . Hospitals are on the front lines after acts of terrorism. Are you prepared? *Health Facilities Management, 13*(1), 24–28.

Smith, J., & Crawford, L. (2002). NCSBN Report Brief Volume 1 Report of Findings from the 2001 RN Practice Analysis Update Chicago, Illinois. National Council of State Boards of Nursing, Inc.

Staab, S., Granneman, S., & Page-Reahr, T. (1996). Examining competency-based orientation implementation. *Journal of Nursing Staff Development, 12*(3), 139–143.

Stewart, S. L., & Vitello-Cicciu, K. M. (1989). Designing a competency-based orientation program for the care of cardiac surgery patients. *Journal of Cardiovascular Nursing, 3*(3), 34–41.

Terriff, C. M., & Tee, A. M. (2001). Citywide pharmaceutical preparation for bioterrorism. *American Journal of Hospital Systems Pharmacies, 58*(3), 233–237.

Thomas, S. P. (2001). Climbing out of the crab bucket: Strategies for resolving conflict among nurses. In N. L. Chaska (Ed.), *The nursing profession: Tomorrow and beyond.* Thousand Oaks, CA: Sage Publications.

Toscano, G. (1995). Workplace violence: An analysis of Bureau of Labor Statistics data. *Occupational Medicine State of the Art Reviews, 11*(2), 227–235.

Trossman, S. (2000, January–February). Certified nurses report fewer adverse events: Survey links certification with improved health care. *The American Nurse,* 1, 9.

U.S. Department of Labor, Bureau of Labor Statistics (1991). *Survey of occupational injuries and illnesses.* Washington, DC: Author.

U.S. Department of Labor, Bureau of Labor Statistics. (1992). *Survey of occupational injuries and illnesses.* Washington, DC: Author.

U.S. Department of Labor, Bureau of Labor Statistics. (2000). *Workplace injuries and illnesses in 2000.* Washington, DC: Author.

U.S. Department of Labor, Bureau of Labor Statistics. (2001). *2001 Census of fatal occupational injuries data.* Washington, DC: Author.

Weinstein, C. E., & Mayer, R. E. (1985). The teaching of learning strategies. In M. C. Wittrock (Ed.), *Handbook of research on teaching.* New York: Macmillan.

Weinstein, S. M. (2000), Certification and credentialing to define competency-based practice. *Journal of Intravenous Nursing, 23*(1), 21–28.

Wetter, D. C., Daniell, W. E., & Treser, C. D. (2001). Hospital preparedness for victims of chemical or biological terrorism. *American Journal of Public Health, 91*(5), 710–716.

Whittaker, S., Carson, W., & Smolenski, M. C. (2000). Assuring continued competence. *Online Journal of Issues in Nursing.* Available http://www.nursingworld.org/ojin/to.

Wigens, L., & Westwood, S. (2000). Issues surrounding educational preparation for intensive care nursing in the 21st century. *Intensive and Critical Care Nursing, 16,* 221–227.

SUGGESTED READINGS

AACN Certification Corporation. (2001). *CCRN—certification for adult, pediatric and neonatal critical-care nurses.* Aliso Viejo, CA: Author.

Cashman, S., & Baldor, R. (2001). Bioterrorism and war: Ensuring public health. *Medscape Family Medicine, 1*(2).

Chaska, N. L. (Ed.). (2001). *The nursing profession: Tomorrow and beyond.* Thousand Oaks, CA: Sage Publications.

Disch, J. M. (2001). Creating healthy work environments for nursing practice. In N. L. Chaska (Ed.), *The nursing profession: Tomorrow and beyond.* Thousand Oaks, CA: Sage Publications.

Long, A. E. (2002). Crisis and recovery: Lessons in readiness—on bioterrorism's front lines. *Healthplan, 43*(1), 20–24.

Hager, M. (Ed.). (2001). *Enhancing interactions between nursing and medicine.* New York: Josiah Macy, Jr. Foundation.

Wigens, L., & Westwood, S. (2000). Issues surrounding educational preparartion for intensive care nursing in the 21st century. *Intensive and Critical Care Nursing, 16,* 221–227.

Unit 3

Issues Impacting Nursing Practice

10

Cultural Diversity in Health Care

NANCY WHITE
FAYE HUMMEL
DIANE PETERS
JUDITH M. RICHTER

> *The process of cultural competence has the ability to promote and transcend the notable differences among the cultures and focus on the commonalities of health and well-being.*
>
> *Rick Zoucha, 2001*

LEARNING OBJECTIVES

AT THE COMPLETION OF THIS CHAPTER, THE READER WILL BE ABLE TO:

➤ Explain factors influencing global health.

➤ Describe issues in global health and human rights.

➤ Identify ethnic, gender, and age disparities in health status among U.S. citizens.

➤ Describe clinical situations in which patients have experienced cultural pain as a result of inappropriate care.

➤ Identify Leininger's principles used in gathering information about cultural beliefs and values.

➤ Compare leading theories of transcultural nursing.

➤ Identify the rationale for using a transcultural theory to provide nursing care.

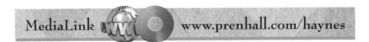

MediaLink   www.prenhall.com/haynes

Additional online resources including NCLEX review questions, critical thinking questions, and real-world activities for this chapter can be found on the Companion Website at www.prenhall.com/haynes.

The response to illness and the accepted means for expressing discomfort are learned behaviors passed from generation to generation. The transcultural nurse becomes familiar with these expressions and is able to respond appropriately. If health care providers do not have the knowledge and skills necessary to interpret the expressions, the patient may experience cultural pain.

The concept of **cultural pain** was introduced by Leininger (1995) to explain the result of culturally inappropriate care. Cultural pain occurs if hurtful or offensive acts or words are used that demonstrate lack of understanding by the nurse about the cultural needs of the patient (Leininger, 1997). The offender is often unaware that the words or actions were offensive. A frequent source of cultural pain is the breaking of cultural taboos and rituals that have been learned and practiced within a culture. For instance, it is customary to ask patients to undress for physical examinations or admission to a hospital unit. This practice would cause cultural pain for the person who, according to his or her own cultural practice, is forbidden to be fully undressed. On the other hand, actions that recognize and respect the unique cultural identity of the person provide the individual with **cultural safety** (Polaschek, 1998).

It may be difficult to identify cultural pain as it can result in silence or withdrawal by patients to protect themselves from further discomfort. After interacting with the patient, the nurse may be able to recognize clues by paying careful attention to what the individual says, or does not say, along with changes in body language. Other signs of cultural pain include avoidance, restlessness, or expressions of anger, which may be recognized by changes in voice or mannerisms exhibited by the patient or family members (Leininger, 1997). The family members may make protective gestures in an attempt to shield the patient from what may be felt as further assault or infliction of pain. Through the use of transcultural nursing knowledge, nurses will be able to learn appropriate ways to touch, to talk with, and to care for patients in order to prevent cultural pain.

Global Health Care

Our globe is becoming increasingly smaller. At the turn of the millennium, we are beginning to see ourselves as citizens of the world rather than from a specific geographical location within which we live and work. This worldview is being incorporated into contemporary nursing practice today. Nursing leaders around the world recognize the importance of global communica-

tion and cooperation to meet the health care needs of people across the globe. The interconnected nature of our world is reflected in the universal goal of professional nursing to promote and protect the health of humans, as individuals in families, communities, and societies. To meet this goal, nurses need (a) to consider demographic, technologic, socioeconomic, and political changes within local, regional, and global contexts and (b) to understand how these cultural changes influence health.

Global Demographics

During the twentieth century, the earth sustained an unprecedented increase in its human population, growing from a total of about 1.7 billion people in 1900 to over 6.1 billion in 2000. Ninety six percent of this increase occurred in the developing regions of Africa, Asia, and Latin America (U.S. Bureau of the Census, 1999).

International migration, in addition to fertility and mortality, has had a substantial impact on population growth rates. In the last 20 years, international migration has typically been from less developed, third world countries, to more developed, industrialized regions. International migrants from poor countries travel to areas across the globe seeking economic and social security. For example, migrant workers stream into the United States from many Latin American countries seeking economic opportunities. During the 1990s, the largest movements of populations across international boundaries involved **refugees**—people displaced because of war and disaster. Further, there has been a progressive decline in fertility levels, particularly in the world's developing nations, decreasing from an average of over six children in the 1950s to just over three births on average. As a result of improvements in child survival and decreases in adult mortality, global life expectancy at birth has increased from 47 years in the early 1950s to 63 years in 1998. This increased longevity has resulted in global population growth and contributed to a shifting global age structure characterized by a greater proportion of elderly and higher ratios of elderly dependent populations to working-age populations (U.S. Bureau of the Census, 1999).

The proportion of the world's population age 65 and older is currently 7%, and this figure is projected to more than double over the next 50 years (Sen & Bonita, 2000). As a result of the rapid rise in the elderly population living in less developed countries, over two-thirds of the world's population over 65 will be living in low-income regions by 2025. This aging world population implies greater elderly support burdens that will challenge not only health care systems but also pension plans, elder care, and other social support systems worldwide (U.S. Bureau of the Census, 1999).

Countries across the globe are becoming more urbanized. In 1975, just under 40% of humanity lived in urban areas. By 2025, it is projected that nearly 60% of the world population will be urban residents. Shifts from predominantly rural, agricultural economies to more urban, service-oriented economics will change national and regional production and consumption patterns. About two-thirds of the world's urban populations currently live in the world's less affluent regions (U.S. Bureau of the Census, 1999). Urban communities are comprised of a multiplicity of lifestyles, values, concerns, and philosophies. Cities are home to a wide range of cultures and ethnic groups who have come from many places. In contrast, rural areas tend to be more homogeneous and share similar values, beliefs, and practices.

Impacting significantly on culture care of population is religion. There have been immense global shifts in religious populations between 1900 and 2000. Christianity spread to become the first truly global faith in terms of geography and remained the most prevalent religion, although membership worldwide slipped from 32.2% to 31.2% by 2000. Second-ranking Islam expanded from 12.3% to 19.6% of the religious population. The numbers of nonreligious and atheists, negligible in 1900, soared to 18.9% by 1970 but declined to 15.2% since the collapse of European communism. Hinduism increased slightly to 13.4%, whereas Buddhism dropped somewhat to 5.9%. Chinese and other folk faiths fell from 30.8% in 1900 to 10.2% in 2000. Judaism declined from eight-tenths of 1% in 1900 to two-tenths of 1% the world's population in 2000 (Kurian, Johnson, & Barrett, 2001).

Globalization: Economic and Social Change

Globalization is a process in which societies are networked together, creating a world system in which diverse people, economies, cultures, and political processes are increasingly subjected to international influences. The result is a world linked by business interests, professional collaborations, and mutual interdependence of diverse peoples. People are made aware of the impact of these influences in their everyday lives (Midgeley, 1997). Globalization impacts every aspect of communities worldwide albeit social, economic, cultural, political, and environmental. For some, global-

ization has created new opportunities for economic and social development. Globalization, viewed by many as an economic concept, has been made possible through advances in technology and communication, which focuses on trade, markets, and exchange rates. Unfortunately, the benefits of globalization have not been evenly distributed in all communities or nations. An unprecedented increase of social and economic inequalities across the globe has occurred as the capital and power in the hands of a few privileged nations has increased (Navarro, 1998). These inequalities have resulted in the inability of poor countries to effectively negotiate with rich countries to determine their own futures. Multinational corporations have been allowed to exploit human labor, local economies, and natural resources under the guise of free trade and business.

Just as globalization is studied as an economic concept, it is also an important concept to be explored from a cultural perspective. **Economic globalization** involves the investment of capital for the creation of profits from a number of geographical locations across the globe. In contrast, **cultural globalization** has a single origin, almost exclusively the United States. In this phenomenon, described as "McDonaldization," familiar icons of American culture such as hamburgers, Levis, and Coca-Cola, have achieved international status. There is a push for everyone to join the global culture that is reflected in the way one dresses, eats, works, plays, and speaks. Unfortunately, this dominant cultural message to the rest of the world is a gross simplification of the American culture (Ife, 1998).

Global Health

There is an interrelationship between globalization and health as evidenced by the "microbial unification" of the world. As a consequence of human activity, the biological and physical environment of the planet is changing at an unprecedented rate. These changes have and will continue to impact human health and well-being (Woodward, Hales, Litidamu, Phillips, & Martin, 2000). The World Health Organization (WHO) considers social, economic, and political issues essential determinants of a society's health. Prior to globalization, the transmission of epidemics was limited to neighboring borders. However, economic globalization and the exchange of goods and people across borders have contributed to the spread of disease and health risks (Berlinguer, 1999). For example, increased opportunities for the transmission of emerging and resurging infectious diseases as well as exposure to substances from other countries such as food, tobacco, weapons, and banned drugs have created significant health risks. A reported one million people travel between developing and developed countries each week, thus contributing to the potential spread of infection. According to the WHO, in 1998 alone, communicable diseases caused the death of 13 million people worldwide, mainly in the poorest countries. Even though infectious diseases primarily affect people in developing countries, all nations, even the richest, are susceptible to the scourge of infection (WHO, 2000).

In the past 20 years, 30 new diseases have been identified including HIV/AIDS, SARS, and hepatitis C; several diseases considered eradicated have resurfaced (WHO, 2000). International travel, densely populated cities, inadequate sanitary conditions and unsafe water, human-induced ecosystem changes, international migration, resistant strains of microorganisms, and globalization of the world's food supply have contributed to the growing problem of infectious diseases (Keigher & Lowery, 1998). According to a 1997 report by the WHO, the 10 leading causes of death worldwide were

- Pneumonia and upper respiratory diseases
- Diarrheal diseases
- Tuberculosis
- Malaria
- Hepatitis B
- HIV/AIDS
- Measles
- Neonatal tetanus
- Whooping cough
- Intestinal worm diseases

Children are particularly at risk for infectious disease. Seven of 10 deaths in children under 5 occur in poor countries and are attributed to five preventable conditions—pneumonia, diarrheal diseases, malaria, measles, and malnutrition. These conditions are exacerbated by poverty (Sen & Bonita, 2000). Mortality in children under the age of 5 is considered a useful index of the overall climate governing healthy child development. Of the 11.2 million annual deaths in children under 5 years, less than 1% takes place in developed countries comprising North America, Western Europe, Japan, Australia, and New Zealand (U.S. Bureau of the Census, 1999).

Traditionally, mothers, across all cultural and socioeconomic boundaries, assume responsibility for the health and welfare of all family members, particularly their children. Female literacy is an important variable influencing health outcomes. Female literacy promotes healthy families and households as well as appropriate use of health services, particularly in relation to childbearing and child rearing (Robinson & Wharrad, 2000). Women with secondary education are more likely to use contraception than women with little or no schooling (U.S. Bureau of the Census, 1999). High birth rates result in large families who often lack adequate resources to feed and support themselves. In addition, high birth rates increase the potential for anemia, infection, and gynecological problems among the mothers. Knowledge creates an environment for mothers to make better decisions that optimize available resources and health outcomes for their families.

As a consequence of human activity, the biological and physical environment of our planet is changing at an unprecedented rate. These changes have and will continue to impact the human health and well-being (Woodward et al., 2000). The world's poor populations are exposed to environmental health risks such as fertilizers and pesticides, toxic fuels and waste, traffic, and a wide range of pollutants, without proper protection and education. Personal vulnerability is greatest where society's capacity to regulate business of strong economic markets is limited because governments are weak (Barten, 1994).

Compared to individuals living in disadvantaged regions, individuals in affluent societies consume many

Critical Thinking and Reflection

The globalization of infectious disease is such that an outbreak in one country is a potential concern for the whole world. The recent outbreak of SARS in Asia is one example. What are the implications for people in the United States where infectious diseases account for minimal mortality? What is the role of nursing in addressing potential stereotyping of immigrants with infectious disease?

times the resources of individuals living in developing countries. The one billion people residing in industrialized countries use 10 times the resources and produce 10 times the waste per capita than do the four billion people residing in developing countries (Benatar, 1998). The global ecosystem cannot support such affluent consumption by so many. Massive changes must be instituted; the future of occupational and environmental health will depend on the development of global policy and local grass roots intervention.

Disparities in Health and Human Rights

People in lower socioeconomic groups are the people who have the largest burden of disease and the fewest resources to deal with these problems (Darnton-Hill & Coyne, 1998). The variance between the developed and developing countries in environmental and occupational health and safety hazards, as well as standards for food, drugs, and medical devices, creates a serious health risk for everyone.

Despite global progress in social and economic development, the end of the twentieth century marked a widening gap in health and human rights at the global level. Multinational companies, free trade zones, free trade agreements, and the export of hazards from rich to poor countries all directly impact the health and safety of workers in developing nations. As the world economy becomes more integrated and industrial production expands into poor nations, workers in these nations face greater risk for morbidity and mortality related to workplace exposures (Frumkin, 1999). The increasing health and human rights inequities across the globe represent a fundamental health problem.

The gap between the rich and poor both among and within developed and developing countries is growing. The share of global incomes obtained by the poorest 20% of the world's population decreased dramatically from 2.5% in 1960 to 1.3% in 1990 (Darnton-Hill & Coyne, 1998). More than one-fifth of the world's population lives in extreme poverty. In 1960, the income of the richest 20% of the world's population was 30 times greater than that of the poorest 20%; by the early 1990s it was more than 60 times greater (American's Vital Interest in Global Health, 1997).

Life expectancy at birth, a measure of overall mortality, is expected to increase by 2025 to 69 years in less developed countries as compared to 79 years in the world's most affluent regions (U.S. Bureau of the Census, 1999). Despite unprecedented progress in world health and an increase in life expectancy since the 1950s of more than 25 years in most countries, the world's poorest people still suffer a heavy burden of largely avoidable disease and death. Much of this can be blamed on poverty (Sen & Bonita, 2000), which is both a direct and indirect cause of poor health. Almost a third of all children are undernourished, and up to 2.5 billion people lack regular access to essential drugs (America's Vital Interest in Global Health, 1997). In addition, poverty forces many urban dwellers to live in overcrowded and unhygienic conditions, without clean water and sanitation, where emerging and resurgent infectious diseases breed.

The United States is a nation of immigrants, thus connecting Americans with peoples all around the world. In 1997, the United States had the highest level of foreign-born residents (8.5%) since 1910 (Keigher & Lowery, 1998).

U.S. Health Care

Government administered national health programs providing universal access to health care by all citizens is evident in most developed countries (Shi & Singh, 2001). In stark contrast to other developed countries, the U.S. health care system actually consists of both government-managed programs, Medicare and Medicaid, and privately insured programs including fee-for-service and managed care plans. Consequently, access to health care is restricted, based on having health insurance, government or private, or one's ability to

---

Critical Thinking and Reflection

As a nation of immigrants, the United States is a nation with great cultural diversity. How is this cultural diversity similar to global diversity? What are the implications of the population diversity on economics, power, and health care for individuals of this nation? What are the implications for you as a nurse giving care to patients from a variety of cultures?

pay for services out of pocket. As a result, 16.1% of the U.S. population, or 43.4 million individuals, are uninsured (Shi & Singh, 2001). Ethnic minorities and other at-risk cultural groups such as the elderly, children, and the chronically ill are overrepresented among those who are uninsured, underinsured, and otherwise underserved among U.S. citizens. An examination of demographic trends with respect to ethnic minorities and other cultural groups will provide some insight as to the extent of the problem.

U.S. Demographic Trends[1]

Census data currently indicate increasing numbers of ethnic minorities, a trend that is expected to continue. The four most prominent minority groups in the United States are African-Americans, Hispanic-Americans, Asian-Americans and Pacific Islanders, and Native Americans and Alaska Natives. The Asian-Americans and Pacific Islanders (AAPIs) represent 29 Asian countries and 20 Pacific Island cultures found in the Far East, Southeast Asia, India, and the Pacific Islands (Shi & Singh, 2001). Current Census data (U.S. Bureau of the Census, 2001) indicate that AAPIs comprise 4.1% of the total U.S. population and are the fastest-growing ethnic minority in the United States. This group is expected to make up 10.7% of the U.S. population by 2050 (Kuo & Porter, 1998).

Hispanic-Americans are a culturally diverse group whose origins are from Mexico (63%). Central and South America (14%), Puerto Rico (11%), Cuba (5%), and other Hispanic subgroups (8%) (Pousada, 1995). Current census data places the Hispanic population at 12.5% of the U.S. total (U.S. Bureau of the Census, 2001). With a 60% increase since 1990, the growth in numbers of Hispanic-Americans is outpacing the growth of the total U.S. population. Their numbers now equal those of African-Americans, formerly the largest minority group. The Hispanic population is expected to reach 88 million by 2050 and comprise nearly one in four U.S. citizens. They are also among the youngest groups of Americans (average age 26 years); however, the elderly Hispanic population is expected to increase by 400% over the next decade as the pre-elderly age into the elderly ranks (Pousada, 1995; Frey, 1995). The current percentage of the U.S. population identified as African-Americans is 12.8%.

The numbers of African-Americans continue to increase, but at less dramatic rates than Hispanics and Asians and currently total 34.7 million (U.S. Bureau of the Census, 2001).

Native Americans and Alaska Natives (NA/AN) represent 0.9% of the U.S. population and are a predominantly young population, growing at a rate of 2.7% per year. Among the poorest U.S. citizens, many NA/AN live in deplorable health conditions both on reservations and in urban centers, and their health status remains poor compared to the general population (Shi & Singh, 2001). Indian Health Services, a federal agency in operation since 1955, is solely responsible for providing health services to Native Americans and Alaska Natives in 500 federally recognized tribes (U.S. Department of Health and Human Services, 2001). Despite the initiation of this unique service and the considerable expansion of health services provided, the NA/AN remain medically underserved.

Ethnic/Cultural Disparities in U.S. Health Care

The increase in minorities reported in the census data exceeded all predictions made prior to actual data collection. One of the most significant findings from the 2000 Census data is that 1 in 10 Americans is foreign born (U.S. Bureau of the Census, 2001). Globalization and diversification are now integral aspects of life in the United States and the American culture. These demographic trends underscore the problems of unequal access to health care and the result of such disparities in health outcomes. A review of the *Healthy People 2000* Progress Reports posted on the Department of Health and Human Services Web site indicates that neither the goals of *Healthy People 2000* nor the elimination of existing health disparities were achieved by 2000. Race, gender, and age issues continue to contribute to health disparities in the United States.

RACIAL HEALTH DISPARITIES

The infant death rate and incidence of low birthweight live births among African-Americans is still more than double that of whites. Hypertension affects one in four African-Americans while its prevalence among whites is 1 in 10 (Rosella, Regan-Kubinski, & Albrecht, 1994). The death rate for all cancers is 30% higher for African-

[1]In the United States, the term used to differentiate ethnic groups is somewhat variable. U.S. Census data refers to Blacks and Hispanics, while social scientists often use ethnic descriptors such as African-American or Mexican-American. Throughout this chapter, the authors will use the term used by social scientists, African-American.

Americans than for whites (U.S. Department of Health and Human Services, 2001). The death rate from HIV/AIDS for African-Americans is more than seven times that for whites (U.S. Department of Health and Human Services, 2001).

Diabetes morbidity rates for Latinos are nearly twice that of non-Hispanic whites. Latinos also have a higher rate of tuberculosis, hypertension, and obesity than non-Hispanic whites. Native Americans and Alaska Natives have an infant death rate double that of whites. They have higher rates of diabetes and disproportionately high death rates from injuries and suicide. According to the *Healthy People 2000* Progress Report, the problems of obesity and cirrhosis deaths worsened rather than improved from 1990 to 2000 (U.S. Department of Health and Human Services, 2001).

The health status of AAPIs is represented in a bipolar distribution—overall, they are among the healthiest population groups in the United States, but several subgroups represent some of the lowest levels of education, income, and health status. U.S. smoking rates are reported to be lowest among AAPIs; however, 92% of Laotians and 71% of Cambodians are smokers (Shi & Singh, 2001). Korean-American men have a higher incidence of stomach and liver cancer compared to whites. Women of Vietnamese origin experience cervical cancer at a fivefold increase over white women. New cases of hepatitis and tuberculosis are also higher for AAPIs than for whites (U.S. Department of Health and Human Services, 2001).

GENDER HEALTH DISPARITIES

The life expectancy of women exceeds that of men by six years. Men demonstrate higher death rates for each of the 10 leading causes of death, although the gap between men and women has narrowed (U.S. Department of Health and Human Services, 2001). Between 1980 and 1997 the death rate for men decreased from 745.3 to 573.8, while for women the rate decreased from 411.1 to 358.0 per 100,000. In fact, the death rate for women as a result of malignant neoplasm increased from 107.7 per 100,000 in 1980 to 110.1 per 100,000 in 1993 (Shi & Singh, 2001). This increase may reflect the increased smoking incidence by women 20 to 25 years earlier.

Insurance coverage for women places them at a disadvantage because women are more likely than men to work part time, receive lower pay, and experience interruptions in their work life (e.g., maternity leave)—all of which contribute to reduction in continuous health insurance coverage (Shi & Singh, 2001). Contraceptive services are poorly funded in the United States, requiring women to bear the majority of the cost themselves. Women are at greater risk for Alzheimer's disease and twice as likely as men to be diagnosed with major depression (U.S. Department of Health and Human Services, 2001). The prevalence of obesity in all adult females has increased to 37% since 1980 and the proportion of total AIDS cases among women has increased to 20% from 7% in 1985. Finally, U.S. teen pregnancy rates remain among the highest in developed countries (U.S. Department of Health and Human Services, 2001).

AGE HEALTH DISPARITIES

Issues associated with age health disparities relate to young and old populations. Despite improvements in the rate of motor vehicle accident deaths among youth, motor vehicle crashes remain the leading cause of death along with unintentional injuries, homicides, and suicides. Cigarette smoking among 12 to 17 year olds declined from 23% to 20% between 1988 and 1997; however, the proportion of young African-Americans who smoke increased during that time from 13% to 23%. One-half of all new HIV infections are diagnosed in persons under 25 years of age (U.S. Department of Health and Human Services, 2001). Alcohol use by youth has declined, but not to the target level identified by *Healthy People 2000*, while the prevalence of overweight young people has increased. The prevalence of chlamydia, a sexually transmitted disease, has increased.

Decreasing federal support for Medicaid programs has resulted in an increase in the number of uninsured children. Estimates from 1993 indicate that 13% or 9.4 million children in the United States are without health

---

Critical Thinking and Reflection

Why are health outcomes better for Whites than for other ethnic groups? How does education and income influence health status?

Why are the ethnic minority groups over represented among the uninsured? What are the implications for you as a nurse?

insurance (Shi & Singh, 2001). This represents an increase of more than 800,000 for that year. Federal and state initiatives are trying to correct this inequity by developing new programs to insure children. However, difficulties getting children signed up have caused these programs to fall short of anticipated goals. Vaccination rates for children vary along racial and socioeconomic lines, with white children and those above the poverty level achieving higher rates of immunizations compared to other ethnic groups and those below the poverty level (Shi & Singh, 2001).

There are presently 33 million Americans aged 65 and older—a number that will grow to 77 million as the "baby boomer" generation ages. Rates of hospitalization due to hip fractures have increased for all people aged 65 and over. Improvements in screenings for older women have been demonstrated in mammography, clinical breast exams, and Pap tests between 1987 and 1993 (U.S. Department of Health and Human Services, 2001). Despite improved screening efforts, primary care providers recommend health screening less frequently to older women than to their younger patients (Blair & White, 1998). Mortality rates increased for cancer (7%), chronic obstructive pulmonary disease (22%), and diabetes (30.5%) between 1987 and 1993 for older adults. To compound the problem, there is a substantial shortage of geriatric specialists, and this shortage is even more severe in rural and low-income areas.

The previous sections have demonstrated significant disparities in U.S. health care along the lines of race, gender, and age. The *Healthy People 2000* Progress Reports indicate that while many of the disparity gaps are narrowing, many inequities in health outcomes remain. In addition, there are several disadvantaged groups whose health care service and health outcomes are considered less than adequate. These include the uninsured and underinsured, rural Americans, the homeless, and those suffering from HIV/AIDS and mental illness. Each of these groups represents a population underserved by the U.S. health care system.

Disparities in the Health Care System Workforce and Nursing Education

The lack of multicultural diversity among the health care workforce has contributed to undesirable health outcomes by fueling cultural incompetence (Rosella, Regan-Kubinski, & Albrecht, 1994). A workforce that represents the dominant culture tends to think **ethno-centrically**—believing that their own values and beliefs

are the best—and fail to recognize or address health care needs that may have a cultural basis. The nursing profession has a moral responsibility to correct health care disparities and to develop cultural sensitivity among the workforce caring for multicultural patients.

Despite significant changes in demographic trends, the composition of the RN workforce has changed very little; Hispanic and African-American minorities remain underrepresented in nursing schools and in the workforce (Goba, 2001). The U.S. Department of Health and Human Services (1996) estimates that 28% of the U.S. population are members of a racial/ethnic minority; yet only 10% of the RN workforce is represented by minorities. Although Hispanics represent nearly 13% of the population, only 1.6% of the RN workforce is Hispanic (Chwedyk, 2001). In addition to insufficient numbers of Hispanic nurses in the workforce, very few are represented among doctorally prepared nurses or in academic settings.

Current data indicate that African-Americans constitute 4% of nursing students, Asian/Pacific Islanders 3.4%, Hispanics 1.6%, and Native American/Alaska Natives 0.5% of students (Goba, 2001). Compared to medical, dentistry, and pharmacy school enrollments, nursing schools have the highest percentage of white, non-Hispanic students. Minorities demonstrate higher dropout and failure rates among nursing students. Goba (2001) found that minority students reported being treated differently by faculty; some related negative faculty comments. Such unfriendly learning environments contribute to feelings of noninclusion and fear of failure.

In response to cultural issues such as these, 15 members of the American Nurses Association (ANA) ad hoc minority nurse committee chartered the National Association of Hispanic Nurses (NAHN). This group now addresses special issues and problems unique to Hispanic nurses from a culturally sensitive perspective (Chwedyk, 2001). Similar beginnings are noted for the National Black Nurses Association (NBNA).

Key Concepts in Culturally Sensitive Care

The term **culture** has also been defined from many different perspectives. For example, Leininger (1997) defined culture as the lifeways of an individual or group with reference to values, beliefs, norms, patterns, and practices that are learned, shared, and transmitted intergenerationally. Purnell and Paulanka (1998) defined culture as "the totality of socially transmitted behavioral patterns, arts, beliefs, values, customs, life-ways, and all other products of human work and thought characteristics of a population of people that guide their worldview and decision-making" (p. 2). Culture includes those qualities, unique to a particular group, that are passed down from generation to generation. The family thus becomes an important unit for transmitting the key aspects of culture over time. Culture is learned through and is represented by the language, customs, rituals, and symbols that create noticeable differences among groups of people. For example, burial rituals may be very different from one culture to the next. These differences are generally a source of great pride, but may also be a source of friction and animosity between people. It is helpful to gain a respect for cultural diversity so that we can learn from and provide culturally sensitive care. Nurses can learn about cultural differences by listening carefully and observing nonverbal behavior.

Cross-cultural is an anthropological term that describes the ability to perceive and understand differences between people of varying cultures. Donnelly (2000) suggested that cultural misunderstandings and language differences can lead to ethical dilemmas in cross-cultural nursing. The nurse may actually violate the values and beliefs of another without intending to. The nurse can harm a person from another culture by invading his or her personal space. It is imperative that nurses demonstrate care and compassion when trying to understand the health care needs of people from diverse cultures. The most important skill the nurse can utilize in the understanding and care of others is to listen.

The term **transcultural** is defined as "across all world cultures, whether a nation or not" (Leininger, 1991, p. 29). Leininger (1995) developed the term *transcultural nursing* to describe a nursing focus on "comparative human care, health and well being in different environmental contexts and cultures" (p. 26). The field of transcultural nursing was conceptualized as a comparative field of study and practice. Leininger is also credited with developing ethnonursing, a research process that uses a qualitative research approach to identify values and beliefs characteristic of a particular culture (Leininger, 1991, 1995). This is accomplished through the nurse's asking open-ended questions. Transcultural nursing principles and theory empower the nurse to discover the caring practices of people from many different cultures worldwide. Transcultural theory has led to (a) an increased understanding of universal aspects of caring behaviors and (b) a discovery of important diverse aspects of many varying cultures. Students who are interested in learning more about cultures that have been studied with a transcultural approach are

directed to the latest edition of *Transcultural Nursing* (2002) by Dr. Leininger. Leininger (1996) believes that health care practitioners are faced with diverse moral, ethical, spiritual, and political issues that influence culturally competent care. She believes that transcultural nursing provides an essential framework for all aspects of patient care. The framework is important because it allows the nurse to provide care that is culturally competent. The nurse moves beyond an approach that recognizes mind–body interaction to an approach that values cultural influences.

Another key concept for nurses to understand is **multiculturalism**, a belief that many different cultures exist in the world, and this diversity should be understood and valued in order to provide culturally sensitive care. This concept takes nurses beyond uniculturalism—the belief that there is one dominant cultural perspective that governs the world. Viewing a situation from a unicultural perspective is considered ethnocentrism and carries an assumption that one's own beliefs and behaviors are superior to the beliefs and behaviors of others (Leininger, 1995). This unicultural approach can lead to care that is not culturally congruent. The care provider may not be sensitive to the unique cultural needs of the patient. The patient's health condition may actually be compromised with care that does not recognize unique cultural differences.

Theoretical Perspectives in Culture Care

There are a variety of ways for health care practitioners to learn about cultural diversity to gain cultural competence. One way to begin developing cultural competence is to acquire knowledge. This can be accomplished through formal course work or through continuing education. Another is to increase awareness and sensitivity of cultural aspects in oneself and others. Travel and immersion in other cultures can provide rich opportunities for increasing cultural sensitivity. Behaviors that accommodate a multicultural perspective have the benefit of improving health care for all (Stoy, 2000). Behaviors that demonstrate respect for the other and caring will build trust and rapport. A trusting environment is more likely to promote healing.

Different theoretical perspectives exist for understanding culture-specific health care needs. These varying perspectives help the nurse to make culturally competent nursing decisions and actions in health care. The nurse learns about the patient's cultural values and beliefs by completing a cultural assessment. Information gained from the assessment will provide direction for nursing actions.

Culhane-Pera and Vawter (1998) examined heath care professionals' perceptions regarding an ethical dilemma that had been presented to an ethics committee at a major hospital prior to the survey time. The researchers presented the ethical conflict of a particular patient and family at seven different medical conferences in a two-part sequence. The patient presented had a ruptured thyroid cyst compressing the trachea, emergently intubated, and was from the Hmong culture. The first part of the case study presented the medical information of the patient. The second part of the case study presented the cultural information of the patient and family. After the first part of the presentation, the audience who agreed to participate answered a demographic questionnaire and then reviewed and agreed or disagreed with 10 statements presented to them, designed to assess their ethnorelativity and their ethnocentricity. The researchers then presented the second part of the case study, after which the participants answered a second questionnaire, which elicited their agreement or disagreement (on a Likert scale of 1 to 6) with the statements made by the original ethics committee members.

There were 156 questionnaires out of 192 attendees at the seven conferences, for an 81% return rate. Of those participants, 9% were nurses. After the first part of the case study, 57% of the respondents indicated that they would extubate the patient, while 43% would not at that point. After the

second part of the case was presented, 75% of the respondents indicated they would extubate the patient. Reasons given to extubate after the first part of the presentation ranged from "patient autonomy" (45%) to "miscellaneous" (4%). After the second part of the case study, the percentage of respondents who indicated they would extubate with patient autonomy being the reason rose to 59%. Reasons given for not extubating ranged from "taking other actions" (30%) to "medical–legal reasons" (2.5%). After the second part of the case study, the reasons for not extubating and taking other actions dropped to 10% of the response reasons. In addition, the responders who stated they would not extubate the patient both before and after the cultural information were more likely to agree with the ethnocentric statements than those that stated they would extubate the patient.

Conclusions drawn from this study indicated that there can be differences in beliefs of the healthcare professionals regarding the best course of action in the care of the patient, which can lead to ethical conflict. There is some association with gender, profession, and age—women, nurses, and those over 30 years of age were more likely to agree with the ethnorelative statements, leading the researchers to believe that women, nurses, and family physicians are trained and socialized to a greater degree in respecting patients' wishes.

PURNELL

Purnell (Purnell & Paulanka, 1998) developed a model (Box 10–1) for cultural competence that provides a framework for learning the important characteristics of culture as applied to a health care setting. Twelve domains are considered essential to understanding the ethnocultural characteristics of individuals, families, and groups and may be used to guide cultural assessment. These domains include: overview or concepts related to the country of origin, family roles and structure, communication, workforce issues, nutrition, biocultural ecology, high-risk health behaviors, pregnancy and child-rearing practices, spirituality, death rituals, health care practices, and health care practitioners (Purnell & Paulanka, 1998). The authors present a framework for collecting health information from individuals of diverse cultures in a non-

judgmental way. This model provides a structure that helps the practitioner to assess cultural domains. The practitioner analyzes the information gathered in a cultural assessment and makes treatment decisions based on this analysis. The quality of patients' health care experiences can be improved through this approach.

GIGER AND DAVIDHIZAR

Giger and Davidhizar introduced a Transcultural Assessment Model in 1991 as a response to a need for a useful assessment tool for evaluating the influence of culture on health and illness behaviors. An advantage of this model is that it allows the practitioner to complete a comprehensive assessment in a short period of time. The model guides the nurse in understanding key phenomena

Box 10-1   Domains of Cultural Assessment

PURNELL MODEL	GIGER AND DAVIDHIZER MODEL
Country of Origin	Space
Family Roles and Structure	Social Organization
Communication	Communication
Workforce Issues	Time Perception
Nutrition	Biologic Variations
Biocultural Ecology	Environmental Control
High-risk Health Behaviors	
Pregnancy and Childrearing Practices	
Spirituality	
Death Rituals	
Health Care Practices	
Health Care Practitioners	

related to the cultural background of the individual and can be applied to a variety of different clinical settings.

Enculturation refers to learned patterns of social behavior that occur through socialization. Most people learn behaviors and values in the family setting. The patient's relationship with his or her family is an important aspect of a thorough cultural assessment (Davidhizar, Bechtel, & Giger, 1998). In contrast, acculturation refers to the "process by which an individual or group from culture A learns how to take on behaviors, values, and lifeways of culture B" (Leininger, 1995, p. 72). Acculturation has also been referred to as assimilation. The process of assimilation occurs as a person from a given culture loses cultural identity to acquire a new one. It is important to recognize that this process may cause distress and conflict (Spector, 2000).

The six assessment domains that are considered important in the Giger and Davidhizar model are: communication, space, social organization, time, environmental control, and biological variations (Giger & Davidhizar, 1991). Communication, the first domain, and culture are closely interconnected. Communication conveys and preserves culture. Communication skills may be an asset, or when used inappropriately they may be a deterrent, in the assessment and planning of health care. Nurses ask questions and expect prompt responses from patients without respect to the communication patterns characteristic of the patient's culture. It is important to recognize that the response time and patterns between sender and receiver vary among cultures. Awareness of nonverbal behavioral assessment becomes particularly important when the patient is from a different culture (Davidhizar et al., 1998). For example, mak-

ing direct eye contact is not appropriate in all cultures. In fact, it may actually be a sign of disrespect. Space and spatial behavior also vary from culture to culture. The expectation in the Western culture is that three to six feet is the appropriate distance for most social encounters (Giger & Davidhizar, 1991), while in the Latino culture touch is considered an appropriate part of communication. Thus, it is important to provide an explanation to the patient before intruding on his or her personal space.

Beliefs and values about time perception also vary. The Navajo's present-time orientation makes obtaining a health history difficult because past events may be perceived as unrelated to the present health condition (Plawecki, Sanchez, & Plawecki, 1994). Environmental control is another important consideration in planning health care. Individuals may believe they are in control of their own lives or conversely believe that outside influences largely control behavior. A person might believe that fate controls his or her health. In addition to the cultural phenomena described previously, Giger and Davidhizar (1991) recognize the importance of including biological variations as part of a cultural assessment. Biological variations such as growth and development patterns, skin and hair physiology, anatomical features, and disease prevalence should be incorporated in a cultural health assessment (Davidhizar et al., 1998).

SPECTOR

Spector (1996, 2000) offers another perspective in understanding health and illness. Spector developed a model of Heritage Consistency (Figure 10-1). The Concept of Heritage Consistency was originally developed by Estes and Zitzow in 1980 to describe the extent "to which one's lifestyle reflects his or her respective tribal culture." The purpose of the Spector model, which is based on this early work, is to determine the extent to which a "person's lifestyle reflects his or her traditional culture, whether European, Asian, African or Hispanic" (Spector, 2000, p. 78). The nurse can use the model to learn the extent to which patients retain elements of their cultural heritage in daily life. The key components of the model are socialization, culture, religion, and ethnicity.

Each of these aspects are united within the person and related to each other. The practitioner uses the Heritage Consistency model to determine cultural differences in health beliefs and practices. Factors influencing heritage consistency include (a) environment in which the individual was raised and educated, (b) involvement of extended family members, and (c) pride about one's heritage (Spector, 2000). When the practitioner uses the Heritage Consistency Model, there will be increased

Figure 10–1 Model of Heritage Consistency

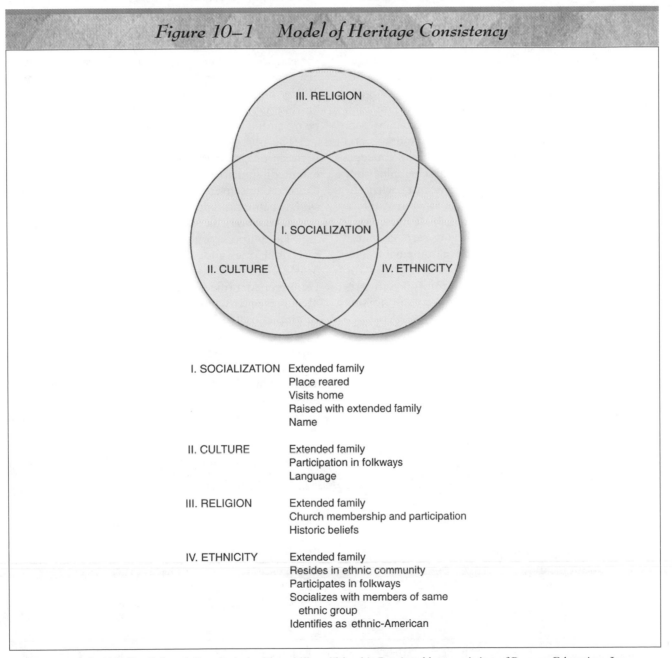

I. SOCIALIZATION	Extended family
	Place reared
	Visits home
	Raised with extended family
	Name
II. CULTURE	Extended family
	Participation in folkways
	Language
III. RELIGION	Extended family
	Church membership and participation
	Historic beliefs
IV. ETHNICITY	Extended family
	Resides in ethnic community
	Participates in folkways
	Socializes with members of same ethnic group
	Identifies as ethnic-American

Source: Spector, R. (2000). *Cultural diversity in health and illness* (5th ed.). Reprinted by permission of Pearson Education, Inc. Upper Saddle River, NJ.

knowledge about the patient's culture, and culturally congruent care is more likely to occur.

ANDREWS AND BOYLE

Andrews and Boyle (1999) developed an assessment tool (Box 10–2) to assist practitioners in gathering information to provide culturally congruent care. These authors believe that people are cultural beings, and therefore all nursing care should be considered transcultural. The cultural assessment process proposed by Andrews and Boyle include analysis of "cultural affiliations, values orientation, cultural sanctions and restrictions, communication, health-related beliefs and practices, nutrition, socioeconomic considerations, organizations providing cultural support, education, religion, cultural aspects of disease incidence, biocultural variations and developmental considerations across the lifespan" (p. 24). Andrews and Boyle effectively apply transcultural nursing concepts to important health conditions. For example, they provide five helpful strategies for dealing with the patient in pain: "identifying personal attributes; establishing an open relationship; establishing nurse competence; assessing pain; and clarifying responsibility" (p. 291). The authors also use a developmental framework to describe transcultural concepts across the lifespan. They incorporate a community-based perspective in applying transcultural concepts in nursing care delivery in diverse settings.

LEININGER'S THEORY OF CULTURE CARE DIVERSITY AND UNIVERSALITY

The theory of culture care, defined below, and the field of transcultural nursing were developed in the mid-1950s and early 1960s. As a clinical nurse specialist working with disturbed children, Leininger discovered the importance of culture in the care of children from varied backgrounds (Leininger, 1970, 1985). She pursued her doctorate in anthropology and later became the first nurse anthropologist. For more information on her life and work see the latest edition (2001) of her book *Transcultural Nursing.*

Leininger (1991) defined culture care as learned and transmitted values and beliefs that assist or enable individuals or groups to maintain their well being, and health, to improve their condition or to deal with illness, handicaps, or death. She envisioned culture care, the essence of nursing—as essential for survival, recovery from illness, growth, and well-being (Leininger, 1991). Furthermore, Leininger (1993) has stated that "caring is essential to curing and healing, for there can be no curing without caring" (p. 16).

The nurse may expect to find many differences between diverse cultures, but may be surprised at the extent of similarities or universalities. The theory of Culture Care Diversity and Universality was developed as the theoretical and research base for explaining the cultural phenomena associated with transcultural nursing. The purpose of this theory is to discover human care similarities and differences; while the goal is to provide culturally competent care (Leininger, 1991). Leininger identified "Major Universal Culture Care Meanings and Actions" from research findings on 87 cultures (Box 10–3). In Leininger's research of cultures worldwide, she discovered respect to be the most important care concept in all cultures. By becoming thoroughly familiar with cultural differences and similarities in health care needs of those being cared for, the nurse is able to provide culturally congruent care. In other words, when the nurse listens to the patient and

---

Box 10–2   Cultural Assessment

1. Cultural Affiliations or Contacts
2. Values Orientation
3. Cultural Sanctions and Restrictions
4. Communication
5. Health-related Beliefs and Practices
6. Nutrition
7. Socioeconomic Considerations
8. Organizations Providing Cultural Support
9. Educational Background
10. Religious Affiliation
11. Cultural Aspects of Disease Incidence
12. Biocultural Variations
13. Developmental Considerations

Summarized from Andrews, M. M., & Boyle, J. S. (1999). Transcultural nursing assessment guide. In M. M. Andrews & J. S. Boyle (Eds.), *Transcultural concepts in nursing care* (3rd ed.) (pp. 539–544). Reprinted with permission from Lippincott, Williams & Wilkins, Philadelpia, PA.

demonstrates respect for his or her requests for specific nursing intervention, then the care that is delivered will more likely be compatible with the patient's cultural background.

There are certain major concepts in transcultural nursing that are important for the nurse to integrate as he or she prepares to utilize this important theory. Culturally congruent care involves the application of culturally based knowledge in creative and meaningful ways in order to provide health care that is both satisfying and beneficial to members of diverse cultures. As the nurse prepares to gain an understanding of another culture, emic and etic views guide the nurse to discover important information (Leininger, 1991). *Emic* refers to an insider perspective of the culture. An example would be a patient in the intensive care unit who is Mexican-American holding the belief that the presence of family will speed recovery. *Etic* refers to the perspective from someone outside of the culture who has some knowledge of cultural beliefs and values. Using the same example, an Anglo-American nurse in the intensive care unit might have knowledge about the importance of family visits and could facilitate family visitation around the clock. In contrast, failure to have this knowledge or to incorporate it into the plan of care could create cultural clashes between the patient's family and the nursing staff.

Two other key concepts that are related to the emic and etic view are generic and professional care. Generic care involves traditional as well as folk practices that cultures have used over long periods of time as their basic primary care practice. Professional care is taught in formal programs of study (Leininger, 1991). As the nurse develops a relationship with the patient, he or she will learn examples of generic care practices that are valued in the culture of the patient and may integrate some of these practices with health care that is offered.

There are several general tenets and predictive hunches that enabled Leininger to discover and develop her theory (Leininger, 1991, 1995). She predicted that both diversities and universals affecting health care were present in all cultures, regardless of time or geographic area. Second, she believed that generic and professional care practices might not be the same worldwide. Third, Leininger knew that research was needed to discover culture care meanings, expressions, and practices in all cultures to establish meaningful care that was both holistic and professional. Fourth, Leininger predicted that in order for nurses to assist those from diverse and similar cultures, three dominant nursing decisions and actions would be essential to create a new direction in nursing practice. These three decisions and modes of action are (a) culture care preservation or maintenance, (b) culture care accommodation or negotiation, and (c)

Critical Thinking and Reflection

If you were providing care for a person who was from a culture you were not familiar with, how would you provide care that is culturally competent?

Describe the steps you would take. What nursing interventions would you provide to recognize an emic perspective of patient care?

culture care restructuring or repatterning. Finally, Leininger predicted that if culturally congruent care was used in explicit and knowing ways with patients, there would be many health-promoting benefits to the recipients of care (Leininger, 1991, 1995).

Other guiding principles for providing culturally congruent care include the patient's worldview and social structure. This would include spiritual or religious beliefs, kinship ties, economics, technologies, and specific cultural historical values. Additionally, environmental context greatly influences care, healing, and health practices. Caring, as explained in Chapter 6, is the essence and primary focus of the nursing profession and, as such, should address the needs of all members of the patient population, regardless of cultural background. A transcultural perspective addresses this need by guiding the nurse to understand the comparative values, beliefs, and practices of different cultures in order to provide safe, meaningful, and culturally congruent care (Leininger, 1995).

The Sunrise Model (Figure 10–2) was developed by Madeleine Leininger as a guide for researchers and clinicians to obtain a comprehensive picture of the experience of people from a transcultural perspective. Nurses may focus on the components most pertinent to the patient and the health care situation and begin anywhere in the model. The model allows the nurse to focus on similarities and differences of caring behaviors in different cultures and can be used with individuals, families, and groups.

One key principle guiding nursing practice is that nurses must understand the unique nature of their own culture in order to understand people from other cultures. The transcultural nursing perspective allows the nurse to enter the patient's world, as much as is possible, from an outsider's perspective. It is critically important to know oneself with regard to one's biases and prejudices so that the nurse can provide culturally congruent, meaningful, and reflective care to someone of another culture (Leininger, 2000).

Cultural Assessment

Leininger (1991) and other transcultural nurses have contributed knowledge to help nurses understand differing perspectives that influence patient response to care. By asking patients to share views and beliefs relevant to the cultural and social structure dimensions within the Sunrise Model, the nurse can acquire greater understanding of cultural similarities and differences

that can influence health care. It may take several encounters with each patient for the nurse to establish the rapport needed to learn the patient's cultural values.

Most clinical situations in current health care settings allow only for an abbreviated assessment. In settings where an extensive interview is unrealistic, nurses are encouraged to investigate shorter alternative formats. Almost all clinical situations allow at least a few minutes to ask the patient or family member about their most important beliefs and to try to respect those beliefs and incorporate them into the plan of care (Table 10–1). One important consideration during a cultural assessment is the determination of the patient's/family's level of acculturation. The nurse will want to know how long they have lived in the United States and to what degree they have assimilated values and beliefs from the dominant culture. Before sharing such personal information, patients need to feel comfortable talking with the nurse. It may take several interactions before the patient is willing to discuss what may be perceived as personal questions. It is important for the nurse to sit down, show genuine interest, and listen to responses. Interruptions in gathering information or assessments done on the run will likely result in minimal information sharing.

Although there are several commonalities among persons of the same culture, the nurse should remember to investigate and consider individual differences. It is important to avoid stereotyping the expected culture care values and meanings solely because a person is a member of a certain cultural group.

Leininger (1995) offers eight principles for consideration when doing a cultural assessment:

1. Study the Sunrise Model before the interaction.
2. Know your own culture.
3. Discover and remain aware of your own biases and prejudices.
4. Be aware of the possibility that the patient may be a member of a subculture or special group such as the homeless or deaf.
5. Explain to patient the purpose of the cultural assessment is to help the patient.
6. Show a genuine interest in the patient, sharing with them your desire to learn about their lifeways.
7. Give attention to gender differences, communication styles, interpersonal relationships, and use of personal space.
8. Maintain a holistic or total view of the patient's world (context) as the information is shared.

Figure 10–2 The Sunrise Model

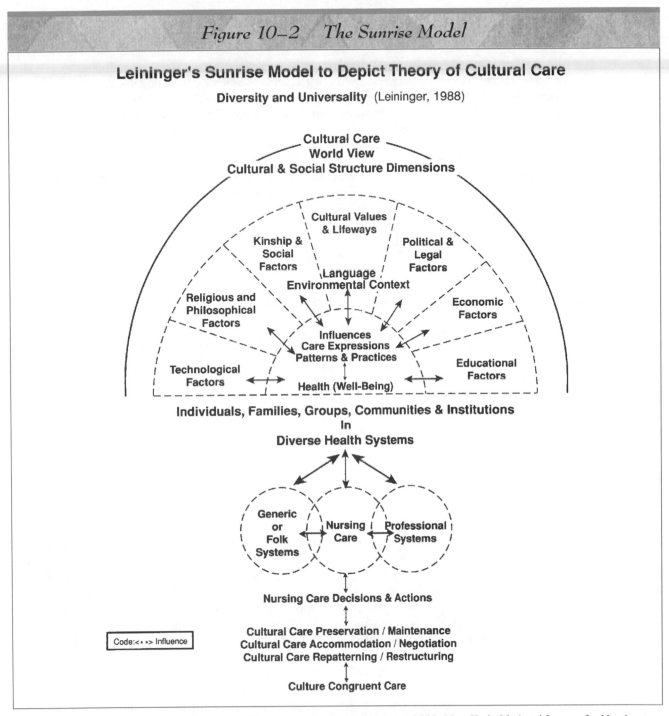

Leininger's Sunrise Model to Depict Theory of Cultural Care

Diversity and Universality (Leininger, 1988)

From *Culture care diversity and universality: A theory for nursing* by M. Leininger, 1991. New York: National League for Nursing. Reprinted with permission.

Nursing Decisions and Actions

After becoming familiar with a patient's culture care values and specific health needs the nurse can begin to establish a plan of care with the patient and family. In areas where the patient's health beliefs and lifeways do not interfere with health and well being, the nurse should encourage the preservation or maintenance of those culture care values. For example,

Table 10–1   Leininger's Short Culturalogic Assessment Guide

Phase I	Record observations of what you see, hear, or experience with patients (includes dress and appearance, body condition features, language, mannerisms and general behavior, attitudes, and cultural features).
Phase II	Listen to and learn from the patient about cultural values, beliefs, and daily (nightly) practices related to care and health in the patient's environmental context. Give attention to generic (home or folk) practices and professional nursing practices.
Phase III	Identify and document recurrent patient patterns and narratives (stories) with patient meanings of what has been seen, heard, or experienced.
Phase IV	Synthesize themes and patterns of care derived from the information obtained in phases I, II, and III.
Phase V	Develop a culturally based patient–nurse care plan as a co-participant for decisions and actions for culturally congruent care.

From Leininger, M. *Transcultural nursing: Concept, theories, research & practice.* Copyright © 1995 by McGraw-Hill, Inc. Reprinted by permission of McGraw-Hill, Inc.

handwashing before meal preparation would be a value to encourage.

If some of the culture care values are less likely to contribute to health and well-being, the nurse can encourage accommodation to some modifications in health practices. For example, in nutrition counseling, a nursing action would be a negotiation of tolerable adaptations to potentially harmful practices such as using low-fat options when available. Education about health benefits will enhance the patient's willingness to try the new behavior. The nurse, however, needs to remain cognizant of factors in the patient's life that may limit his or her ability to modify behaviors. Limited income, ethnic food preferences, or housing arrangements could all impact the patient's accommodation to a particular health program.

When the patient's health is threatened by specific detrimental practices, the nurse seeks to assist, support, and facilitate the individual in reordering or changing their life ways for a new health care pattern geared toward result in a more beneficial health outcome. Leininger (1991) refers to this nursing action as the process of repatterning. This action must be performed with respect and acknowledgment of the patient's self-determination and ultimate control in the situation.

It is through the combination of all these nursing actions and decisions that the nurse is able to help the patient make healthy choices. If the individual does not wish to make changes in health practices, the nurse should refrain from criticism that may result in negative treatment or attitudes toward the patient.

In order to provide safe and effective care, the nurse must first recognize the significance of his or her own cultural orientation to interpreting the responses of the patient and family experiencing the illness and treatment. Figure 10–3 provides a continuum of cultural competence beginning with cultural blindness and progressing developmentally to the level of advanced practice transcultural nurse.

Depending on their own cultural background and attitudes developed during formative years, nurses may practice at varying points along the continuum. Cultural blindness results from ethnocentrism related to one's own culture without regard for how other cultures might be similar or different in their beliefs about health, illness, or other significant life events. The first step to progress beyond blindness involves knowledge and understanding of variation between one's own culture and that of the patient. The nurse must be willing to receive the new knowledge and engage in an attitude change away from ethnocentrism. At this point, the nurse develops a beginning level of sensitivity and awareness. Awareness is the first step toward a more responsive approach to individuals of a different culture.

Cultural openness includes both cognitive and emotional receptivity with the goal of seeking common ground upon which to build patient–nurse relationships (Wenger, 1999). Reflection and cultural self-assessment are necessary in order to achieve openness to new or different ideas. Recognizing that differences exist is not the same as being willing to respect and honor those differences and to incorporate them into care.

Cultural openness occurs when the nurse begins to learn about the lifeways and beliefs of other people including peers, staff, and patients. Ideally, nurses have opportunities to begin building mutual respect as they learn to interact with all patients and families in a non-judgmental way. The assumption that there is only one

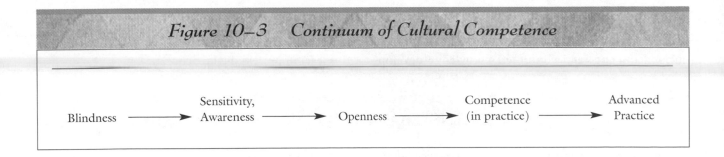

Figure 10–3   Continuum of Cultural Competence

Blindness ——→ Sensitivity, Awareness ——→ Openness ——→ Competence (in practice) ——→ Advanced Practice

way to view any situation results in poor communication and lack of understanding. It is not easy to change one's own perspective to include different approaches. The simple gesture of asking patients about themselves and their values lets them know you are interested in respecting those values.

Cultural competence is the deliberate and creative use of transcultural nursing knowledge and skills to assist or facilitate individuals and groups in maintaining their well being, recovering from illness, or facing a disability or death (Leininger, 1991). This level of skill is reached through self-evaluation and the desire to learn about other cultures. Nurses cannot learn everything about every culture but they can seek to understand culture care values and practices important to the cultural groups most frequently encountered in their clinical setting. With this insight comes acceptance that there are many ways to respond to health and illness. There are many opportunities in everyday practice to honor differences in belief systems without compromising care. The culturally competent nurse is self-assured, open to new ideas, and skilled at communicating this acceptance to patients so they feel comfortable sharing their beliefs. By simply asking the patient, "How can I best care for you?" or "What kind of care is important to you?" and then listening carefully to responses and

observing their nonverbal cues, nurses can begin dialogue necessary to incorporate culture care values into practice.

As this approach to care becomes internalized, nurses who wish to achieve the advanced practice level in transcultural nursing strive to learn more. Certification in transcultural nursing is achieved by taking both oral and written examinations after graduate-level preparation and experiences. Several universities such as the University of Northern Colorado, Keane University in New Jersey, Augsburg College in Minnesota, and Duquesne University in Pennsylvania offer graduate-level courses in transcultural nursing. Courses may be taken individually, for certificate, or master's/PhD degree in some programs. The Transcultural Nursing Society's (TCNS) Web page includes information and contacts for such courses. Some are offered in a summer condensed format, online, or in traditional academic year format.

Graduate nurses may obtain more information about the organization, research with a variety of cultural groups, and opportunities to meet other like-minded nurses by joining the Transcultural Nursing Society. Membership includes subscription to the TCNS scholarly journal. There is a tremendous need

Critical Thinking and Reflection

The Patient Self-Determination Act of 1990 is a federal law enacted to protect the rights of individuals to make their own decisions regarding medical treatment. The right to make autonomous decisions relating to the continuation, withholding, or withdrawing of life-prolonging treatment is at the very heart of the act (Braun, Pietsch, & Blanchette, 2000). However, the desire for autonomy may be viewed primarily as an Anglo-American, middle/upper-class value and may have little relevance for ethnic minorities. Describe some of the values of other ethnic groups. How might these influence end-of-life decisions? How could you learn about these values? What are the implications for you as a nurse providing end-of-life care to patients from different cultures?

for transcultural nurses who are not only competent in their own practice but who can help others develop these skills. Through staff education, research in transcultural nursing, and continued knowledge development, nurses can begin to make a difference in care for all patients. Formal coursework, reading, and certification in transcultural nursing are necessary to achieve this level of professional practice.

TRANSITION INTO PRACTICE

The nature of globalization and the interconnectedness among continents and nations have created a need for all citizens to demonstrate an awareness of the inequities which exist between nations and between citizens within nations. We can only begin to solve problems when we fully understand the roots of the problem. The events involving the attack on the World Trade Center have further emphasized the necessity for cultural understanding and sensitivity by all world citizens.

Providers are faced with the dilemma of how to provide care to an increasingly diverse population of immigrants, elderly, and low-income patients. Nurses are in the position to take a leadership role within the health care profession toward the achievement of cultural competence. We are challenged to provide quality health care in a culturally sensitive manner and to avoid causing cultural pain of our patients. In her "Founder's Focus" to members of the Transcultural Nursing Society, Leininger (1999) reflects on strangers who nurses encounter in everyday situations:

> Who is this stranger I am expected to care for or relate to in beneficial ways? Where does this stranger come from and what does he (she) believe, value, and live by? In what ways can I help this stranger in meaningful ways? . . . As one enters the stranger's world, one soon discovers that beings can be understood with an open mind and a sincere desire to learn from strangers . . . through transcultural nursing practices; the nurse discovers that a stranger can become a friend and no longer an unknown human being. Indeed, a stranger is a friend who needs to be respected, understood, and cared for in special ways by nurses and other health personnel.

To begin to understand and respect someone from another culture, students and nurses new to the profession must begin to examine their own beliefs and values. The nurse needs to be open to the unexpected and show genuine interest in the patient's values and beliefs. From this point, they can begin to develop a theoretical approach or personal philosophy toward cultural competence in nursing care. This chapter provides students and new nurses with the knowledge base necessary for practicing at the level of cultural competence. This process requires continual openness, education, and professional development. However, the motivation to achieve mastery over the content and desire to practice cultural competence comes from one's aspiration to move from stranger to friend.

KEY POINTS

1. Globalization is a process in which societies are networked together, creating a world system in which diverse people, economies, cultures, and political processes are increasingly subjected to international influences.

2. There is an unprecedented increase of social and economic inequalities across the globe which has resulted in the inability of poor countries to effectively negotiate with rich countries to determine their own futures.

3. Ethnic minorities and other at-risk cultural groups such as the elderly, children, and the chronically ill are over-represented among those who are uninsured, underinsured, and otherwise underserved among U.S. citizens.

4. Cultural pain occurs if hurtful or offensive acts or words are used that demonstrate lack of understanding by the nurse about the cultural needs of the patient (Leininger, 1997).

5. There are a variety of theoretical perspectives, which help the nurse to make culturally competent nursing decisions and actions in health care.

6. Transcultural nursing developed by Dr. Leininger enables nurses to provide culturally competent care

through discovering the caring practices of people from many different cultures worldwide.

7. The Sunrise Model developed by Leininger serves as a guide for researchers and clinicians to obtain a comprehensive picture of the experience of people from a transcultural perspective.

8. By asking patients to share views and beliefs relevant to the cultural and social structure dimensions within the Sunrise Model, the nurse can acquire greater understanding of cultural similarities and differences that can influence health care.

EXPLORE MediaLink

Critical thinking questions, essay questions, key terms, web links, activities, NCLEX review questions, and more interactive resources can be found on the Companion Website at www.prenhall.com/haynes. Click on Chapter 10 to select activities for this chapter.

REFERENCES

Andrews, M., & Boyle, J. (1999). *Transcultural concepts in nursing care* (3rd ed.). Philadelphia, PA: Lippincott.

Barten, F. (1994). Health in a city environment. *World Health, 47*(3), 24–25.

Benatar, S. R. (1998). Global disparities in health and human rights: A critical commentary. *American Journal of Public Health, 88*(2), 295–300.

Berlinguer, G. (1999). Globalization and global health. *International Journal of Health Services, 29*(3), 579–595.

Blair, K., & White, N. (1998). Are older women offered adequate health care? *Journal of Gerontological Nursing, 24*(10), 39–44.

Braun, K., Pietsch, J., & Blanchette, P. (2000). An introduction to culture and its influence on end-of-life decision-making. In K. Braun, J. Pietsch, & P. Blanchette (Eds.), *Cultural issues in end-of-life decision-making* (pp. 1–9). Thousand Oaks, CA: Sage Publications.

Chwedyk, P. (2001, Winter). 25 and counting. *Minority Nurse,* 34–37.

Culhane-Pera, K. A., & Vawter, A. (1998). A study of health-care professionals' perspectives about a cross-cultural ethical conflict involving a Hmong patient and her family. *Journal of Clinical Ethics, 9*(2), 179–190.

Darnton-Hill, I., & Coyne, E. T. (1998). Feast and famine: Socioeconomic disparities in global nutrition and health. *Public Health Nutrition, 1*(1), 23–31.

Davidhizar, R., Bechtel, G., & Giger, J. (1998) A model to enhance culturally competent care. *Hospital Topics: Research and Perspectives on Healthcare, 76*(1), 22–26.

Donnelly, P. (2000). Ethics and cross-cultural nursing. *Journal of Transcultural Nursing, 11*(2), 119–126.

Estes, G., & Zitzow, D. (1980). *Heritage consistency as a consideration in counseling Native Americans.* Paper read at the National Indian Education Association convention, Dallas, TX, November.

Frey, W. (1995). Elderly demographic profiles of U. S. states: Impacts of "new elderly births," migration and immigration. *The Gerontologist, 35*(6), 761–770.

Frumkin, H. (1999). Across the water and down the ladder: Occupational health in the global economy. *Occupational Medicine: State of the Art Reviews, 14*(3), 637–663.

Giger, J., & Davidhizar, R. (1991). *Transcultural nursing* (2nd ed.). St. Louis, MO: Mosby.

Goba, M. (2001, Winter). Mixed messages: Are nursing programs doing enough to make minority students feel welcome? *Minority Nurse,* 46–47.

Ife, J. (1998). Globalization, internationalism, and community services: Implications for policy and practice. *Journal of Applied Social Sciences, 23*(1), 43–55.

Keigher, S. M., & Lowery, C. T. (1998). The sickening implications of globalization. *Health & Social Work, 23*(2), 153–158.

Kuo, J., & Porter, K. (1998). Health status of Asian Americans: United States, 1992–94. *Advance data from vital and health statistics.* Hyattsville, MD: National Center for Health Statistics, No. 298, 1–3.

Kurian, G. T., Johnson, T. M., & Barrett, D. B. (2001). *World Christian encyclopedia: A comparative survey of churches and religions AD30–AD2200.* New York: Oxford University Press.

Leininger, M. (1970). *Nursing and anthropology: Two worlds to blend.* New York: John Wiley & Sons.

Leininger, M. (1985). *Qualitative research methods in nursing.* Orlando, FL: Grune & Stratton.

Leininger, M. (1991). *Culture care diversity and universality: A theory of nursing.* New York: National League of Nursing Press.

Leininger, M. (1993). Assumptive premises of the theory. In C. Reynolds & M. Leininger (Eds.), *Culture care diversity and universality theory* (pp. 16–30). Thousand Oaks, CA: Sage.

Leininger, M. (1995). *Trancultural nursing: Concepts, theories, research and practices* (2nd ed.). New York: McGraw-Hill.

Leininger, M. (1996). Major directions for transcultural nursing: A journey into the 21st century. *Journal of Transcultural Nursing, 7*(2), 28–31.

Leininger, M. (1997). Understanding cultural pain for improved health care. *Journal of Transcultural Nursing, 9*(1), 32–35.

Leininger, M. (2000). Founder's focus: Transcultural nursing is discovery of self and the world of others. *Journal of Transcultural Nursing, 11*(4), 312–313.

Leininger, M. (2002). *Transcultural nursing: Concepts, theories, research and practices* (3rd ed.). New York: McGraw-Hill.

Midgeley, J. (1997). *Social welfare in global context.* Thousand Oaks, CA: Sage Publications.

Mitty, E. (2001). Ethnicity and end-of-life decision-making. *Reflections on Nursing Leadership, 27*(1), 28–31, 46.

Navarro, V. (1998). Whose globalization? *American Journal of Public Health, 88*(5), 742–743.

Plawecki, H., Sanchez, T., & Plawecki, J. (1994). Cultural aspects of caring for Navajo Indian clients. *Journal of Holistic Nursing, 12*(3), 291–306.

Polaschek, N. (1998). Cultural safety: A new concept in nursing people of different ethnicities. *Journal of Advanced Nursing, 27,* 452–457.

Pousada, L. (1995). Hispanic-American elders: Implications for health care providers. *Clinics in Geriatric Medicine, 11*(1), 39–52.

Purnell, L., & Paulanka, B. (1998). *Transcultural health care* (3rd ed). Norwalk, CT: Appleton & Lange.

Robinson, J., & Wharrad, H. (2000). Invisible nursing: Exploring health outcomes at a global level. Relationships between infant and under-5 mortality rates and the distribution of health professionals, GNP per capita, and female literacy. *Journal of Advanced Nursing, 32*(1), 28–40.

Rosella, J., Regan-Kubinski, M., & Albrecht, S. (1994). The need for nulticultural diversity among health professionals. *Nursing & Health Care, 15*(5), 242–246.

Sen, K., & Bonita, R. (2000). Global health status: Two steps forward, one step back. *Lancet, 356*(9229), 577–582.

Shi, L., & Singh, D. (2001). *Delivering health care in America: A systems approach* (2nd ed.). Gaithersburg, MD: Aspen Publishers, Inc.

Spector, R. (1996). *Cultural diversity in health and illness* (4th ed.). Stamford, CT: Appleton & Lange.

Spector, R. (2000). *Cultural diversity in health and illness* (5th ed.). Upper Saddle River, NJ: Prentice Hall.

Stoy, D. (2000). Developing intercultural competence: An action plan for health educators. *Journal of Health Education, 31*(1), 16–19.

U.S. Bureau of the Census. (2001). U. S. Government Printing Office, Washington, DC: Author.

U.S. Bureau of the Census Report WP/98, World Population Profile: 1998, (1999). U. S. Government Printing Office, Washington, DC: Author.

U.S. Department of Health and Human Services. (2001). *Healthy people 2000*, Washington DC: Author.

U.S. Department of Health and Human Services. (1996). National sample survey of registered nurses. Health Resources & Services Administration, Division of Nursing.

U.S. Department of Health and Human Services. (1998, May 20). *Healthy people progress reviews.* Washington, DC: Author.

Wenger, A. (1999). Cultural openness: Intrinsic to human care. *Journal of Transcultural Nursing, 10*(1), 10.

Woodward, A., Hales, S., Litidamu, N., Phillips, D., Martin, J. (2000). Protecting human health in a changing world: the role of social and economic development. *Bulletin of the World Health Organization, 78*(9), 1148–1155.

World Health Organization. (2000). *World health report 2000.* Geneva, Switzerland: Author.

World Health Organization. (1997). Health briefs. *Escherichia coli* and food poisoning. *World Health, 50* (1), 29.

SUGGESTED READINGS

Dupree, C. (2000). The attitudes of black Americans toward advance directives. *Journal of Transcultural Nursing, 11*(1), 12–18.

Farrell, M. (1998). Trends in the global healthcare environment: The developed countries. *Contemporary Nurse, 7*(4), 180–189.

Giger, J., & Davidhizar, R. (1999). *Transcultural nursing* (3rd ed.). St. Louis, MO: Mosby.

Mouton, C. (2000). Cultural and religious issues for African Americans. In K. Braun, J. Pietsch, & P. Blanchette (Eds.), *Cultural issues in end-of-life decision-making* (pp. 71–82). Thousand Oaks, CA: Sage Publications.

Talamantes, M., Gomez, C., & Braun, K. (2000). Advance directives and end-of-life care: The Hispanic perspective. In K. Braun, J. Pietsch, & P. Blanchette (Eds.), *Cultural issues in end-of-life decision-making* (pp. 83–100). Thousand Oaks, CA: Sage Publications.

11

Spirituality

LINDA F. GARNER

"I stress the difference between providing care that is spiritual and spiritual care. Care that is spiritual may contain no direct references to God, scripture, or anything religious, but the care is performed as part of a ministry of service and as such the nurse is reflecting God's presence and love to the patient in need.

Verna Benner Carson, 2001

LEARNING OBJECTIVES

AT THE COMPLETION OF THIS CHAPTER, THE READER WILL BE ABLE TO:

- ➤ Define spirituality.
- ➤ Explain how spirituality impacted the development of nursing.
- ➤ Discuss the relationship of spirituality to current nursing practice.
- ➤ Discuss spiritual needs of patients and of the nurse as an individual.
- ➤ Assess spiritual needs.
- ➤ Describe interventions for providing spiritual care.
- ➤ Explain the importance of spiritual health for the caregiver.

MediaLink www.prenhall.com/haynes

Additional online resources including NCLEX review questions, critical thinking questions, and real-world activities for this chapter can be found on the Companion Website at www.prenhall.com/haynes.

*N*ursing is distinguished from other health care professions by its holistic or mind–body–spirit approach to providing health care for persons, families, and communities. Spirituality is a "cornerstone" for holistic nursing practice (Nagai-Jacobson & Burkhardt, 1989). The origins of nursing as a profession were strongly influenced by the religious community. Hospitals and schools of nursing emphasized established institutional religious practices. The development of technology and the emphasis on scientific study led nursing away from spiritual-based care and the accompanying religious practices. Early in the twentieth century, secularism became a predominant societal theme, though nurses continued to focus on providing care for the whole person. There was no mention of spirituality in schools of nursing, and nurses were no longer required to participate in institutional religious practices. In fact, any reference to spiritual needs was considered an invasion of the patient's privacy. In the last 20 years, health care providers have developed a resurgent interest in spirituality. There is increasing emphasis with regard to nursing's distinct focus on the wholeness of the individual. **Wholeness** refers to a focus on mind–body–spirit as a unified concept. This new focus on spirituality has integrated concepts from Eastern and Western religious doctrine.

Characteristics of Spirituality

Spirit is often thought of as a transcendent energy that elevates one from the humdrum of daily life and helps to give meaning and direction to one's life. The word *spirit* is derived from the Latin root for breath. The Greek and Hebrew words for spirit also stem from the root meaning wind or breath (Stuart, Deckro, & Mandle, 1989). Some authors view spirituality as a unifying or vital principle of a person that integrates all other dimensions of the human being (Burkhardt, 1989). In a broad sense, spirituality is a manifestation of the spirit just as physiology is one manifestation of the body and emotions are one manifestation of the mind (Heriot, 1992).

Several definitions of **spirituality** have been proposed in the nursing literature. Spirituality is a process, a journey, a personal transcendence, a quest for meaning and purpose, or a relationship or connection with God, a Higher Power, or the Universe. Terms associated with spirituality fall into five dimensions/categories, which include spirit, spirituality, spiritual dimension, spiritual well-being, and spiritual needs (Burkhardt, 1989). Burkhardt discusses the **spiritual dimension** as a common bond between individuals and God, a higher power, a deity, or a force that transcends all other dimensions. **Spiritual well-being** as a process of transcendence and interconnectedness between oneself, a deity, and others. **Spiritual needs** are described as the deepest requirements for self; factors that are necessary for a relationship with a higher being. Spirituality has been defined as an unfolding mystery that reveals meaning and purpose in life; inner strength, which manifests joy, peace, and awareness; and harmonious interconnectedness, which focuses on relationships with self, other, divinity, universe or higher power, and environment. (Burkhardt, 1989)

Other nursing scholars view spirituality as being manifested through patterns of connectedness that transcend everyday experience and endow the ordinary with extraordinary meaning. This connectedness or relatedness may be experienced **intrapersonally** (as a connectedness with oneself), **interpersonally** (in the context of others and the natural environment), and **transpersonally** (referring to a sense of relatedness to the unseen, God, or power greater than self) (Reed, 1992). Spirituality has further been defined as the ability to understand, which is brought on by a sense of relatedness to dimensions that transcend self. This relatedness includes a connectedness with self, others, the environment, and God or a higher power (Reed, 1992). Reed (1992) developed a paradigm for spirituality research that includes self-transcendence, contextual worldview, and the connectedness of spirituality to human development. Spirituality refers to developing meaning through a sense of relatedness to dimensions that transcend self. Carson describes spirituality in terms of a theistic worldview in which spirituality is experienced in an individual's heart. **Theism** emphasizes forgiving and practicing kindness, patience, gentleness, and forbearance in dealing with others. The spirit is viewed as the core of the individual and impacts all other dimensions of the person (Carson, 2000).

A number of common themes describing spirituality emerge from the literature. Spirituality has been viewed as: (a) a source for creating meaning and purpose in life (Ellison, 1983; Highfield & Cason, 1983; Howden, 1992; Miller, 1985); (b) an integrative energy (Ellison, 1983; Goddard, 1995; Howden, 1992); (c) harmonious interconnectedness with self, others, nature, and/or an Ultimate Other (Highfield & Cason, 1983; Howden, 1992; Nagai-Jacobson & Burkhardt, 1989); (d) the inner essence of a person (Nagai-Jacobson & Burkhardt, 1989); (e) an integrating factor (Burkhardt, 1989); and (f) transcendence

Table 11–1 Definitions Related to Spirituality

Term	Brief Definition/Description
Meaning and purpose in life	The reason for being
Integrative energy	Force empowering individual to make decisions and be a productive person
Connectedness	Feeling a part of the world around the person/relationship with deity and others
Transcendence	Ability or power to rise above oneself, particularly relationship with higher being
Theism	Worldview including the belief in a supreme being or higher power
Interconnectedness	Relationship with deity, others, and self; process of transcendence
Contextual worldview	Person and environment interact to transform challenges and conflicts into energy for innovative change
Religiosity	Being religious; excessive devotion to religion

(Howden, 1992; Miller, 1985; Reed, 1992). In this chapter, the following definition of spirituality is used.

> Spirituality is a person's inner resources and values that guide and give meaning to life. It is the inner core of the individual that permeates all aspects of the person: physical, psychological, and social. Spirituality involves relationship with self, others, and God/Higher Power. It is manifested through creative expressions, familiar rituals, meaningful work, and religious practices and beliefs (Garner, McGuire, Snow, Gray, & Wright, 2002, p. 372).

This definition was developed for use by researchers. It encompasses the essence of spirituality. Brief definitions of terms as related to spirituality are presented in Table 11–1.

Differentiating Spirituality from Religion

Spirituality is often confused with **religiosity** (Emblen, 1992), defined in the *Random House Unabridged Dictionary* (1993) as: (a) the quality of being religious; piety; devoutness; and (b) affected or excessive devotion to religion (p. 1628). Spirituality is a much broader concept than religiosity; which can be expressed with or without association to religious customs (Wright, 1998). It is an umbrella concept, which encompasses religion and the needs of the human spirit (Heriot, 1992). The relationship between spirituality and religion has also been described as the spirit having "greater depth and breadth than the limitations of religion, and is an integral part of every individual's char-

acter and personality which can ultimately affect the individual's response to episodes of health and illness" (Oldnall, 1996, p. 142). Spirituality is a way of life, permeating "to the very core of our human *being*, affecting the way we perceive the world around us, the way we feel about that world, and the choices we make based on our perceptions and sensations" (Kurtz & Ketcham, 1992, p. 68). Although spirituality does not equate to religion, it is a "slippery task" to distinguish spirituality from religion (Kurtz & Ketcham, 1992, p. 68). The spiritual see religion as rigid, while the religious see the spiritual as sloppy: religion connotes boundaries while spirituality seems haphazard and ill-defined. "The vocabulary of religion emphasized the *solid*; the language of spirituality suggest the *fluid*" (Kurtz & Ketcham, 1992, p. 23). Spirituality does not require connectedness to a religious institution or formal doctrine. Religion defines reality and provides a sense of significance and connection to a larger whole or entity.

"Religion and spirituality therefore are not synonymous. **Religion** refers to an external, formal system of beliefs, whereas spirituality is concerned more with a personal interpretation of life and the inner resources of people" (Heriot, 1992, p. 23). Each individual manifests spirituality in a variety of ways that include but are not limited to religious practices. Individuals are comprised of three components: biological, psychosocial, and spiritual (Beland & Parson, 1975). The biological component includes the five senses and world consciousness. The second component, psychosocial, focuses on the intellect, emotion, will, and moral sense and encompasses the soul, self-consciousness, and self-identify. The third component, spiritual, cannot be defined scientifically. Spiritual includes a conscious awareness and relationship with a higher power. The **spirit** is the core of the individual; the psyche lies between the spirit and the physical body. There is a dynamic interaction between each component. Life experiences, either positive or negative, impact each of these components while they in turn impact the individual's perception of and reaction to these experiences (Beland & Passos, 1975). Bayly (1969) suggests that the spirit "is the real person, the part of us nobody can see, the part that doesn't die . . . it's the inside you . . ." (p. 47).

Historical Development of Spirituality and Nursing

Although spirituality has not always been at the forefront of clinical concerns, it has always been closely tied to nursing and healing practices. In ancient times, priests were healers as well as spiritual leaders; illness was believed to be the work of gods or spirits. To maintain health, one had either to appease the gods or remove evil spirits. The words health and healing originate from an old Anglo-Saxon word meaning "hale or whole—sound in body, mind, and spirit" (Stewart & Austin, 1962, p. 4). Gods and goddesses were believed to have specific skills in healing or maintaining health. Fortuna, Jupiter's nurse, was prayed to for hygiene in the public baths. It was further believed that Apollo's (the god of health) anger was expressed through plagues and epidemics. His son Aesculapius, god of medicine and surgery, was considered to be a skilled healer and was worshipped for healing. Hygeia, daughter of Aesculapius, was the goddess of health (Donahue, 1996).

The religious community, specifically Christianity, influenced the development of hospitals and care of the sick and injured. Ministering to the sick was considered the duty of all Christians during the first and second centuries. During the early Christian era (1–500), the Christian church incorporated the care of the sick, the poor, and the suffering as a part of its responsibility. Wealthy women of influence became known as deaconesses and provided physical and spiritual care to those in need (Donahue, 1996). The religious establishment, as a result of St. Benedict's rule, which declared that every monastery should have a hospital, developed the first hospitals to provide care for those who were ill. Later, hospitals were built outside monasteries and named *Hotel Dieu*, meaning "House of God" (Kalisch & Kalisch, 1995).

Organized nursing also developed from the religious community. Religious orders, influenced by St.

Augustine, decreed that nursing should be a part of the duties of each member of the orders. The Sisters of Charity, founded by St. Vincent de Paul, provided a stabilizing influence for nursing during the "Dark Age of Nursing," the period of time that nursing was considered to be an undesirable job for respectable women. During this time, nurses who were not members of religious orders and were considered to be persons of questionable moral character. During the Crusades, military orders of nurses were organized to care for the sick and injured in their midst. The religious influence of the time helped to add a caring component to the role of the nurse (Kalisch & Kalisch, 1995).

The Christian era prompted the use of the terms vocation and profession. **Vocation** was originally defined a divine call or summons to some form of religious or charitable service. **Profession** meant that the individual had openly professed faith in the new religion and as a rule had made a vow dedicating his or her life sometimes to meditation and study, but more often to active works of charity. Gradually, the meaning of both vocation and profession was broadened to include a wide variety of secular occupations, the latter usually restricted to those requiring advanced study and higher ethical standards. The terms have also retained some of their earlier meaning, implying a higher motive than that of simply making a living (Stewart & Austin, 1962). Stewart and Austin suggest that nursing requires a three-sided preparation (Figure 11–1) that includes science, art, and spirit as integral components of the nurse's role, which is constantly expanding.

Nursing education was also strongly influenced by the religious community. Pastor Theodur Fliedner laid the groundwork for modern professional nursing education when he established a hospital and training school for nurses at Kaiserwerth in Germany. It was here that Florence Nightingale received her training (Kalisch & Kalisch, 1995). Florence Nightingale's belief that nursing was a calling of God is well known (Dossey, 2000). Nightingale laid the foundation for the profession of nursing with her views of good nursing practice and nursing education (Nightingale, 1859). She emphasized the importance of (a) scientific methods and (b) good or moral conduct. She viewed spirituality as a developmental process. Nightingale was conscious of God and believed that being one with God and one with man provided motivation for behavior. She emphasized compassion and caring as well as scientific study. Nightingale practiced prayer as a process of linking the outward personal self with the inner divine spirit. Moral and ethical conduct was central to her view of nursing. Nursing was a spiritual process to

Figure 11–1   Framework of Modern Nursing

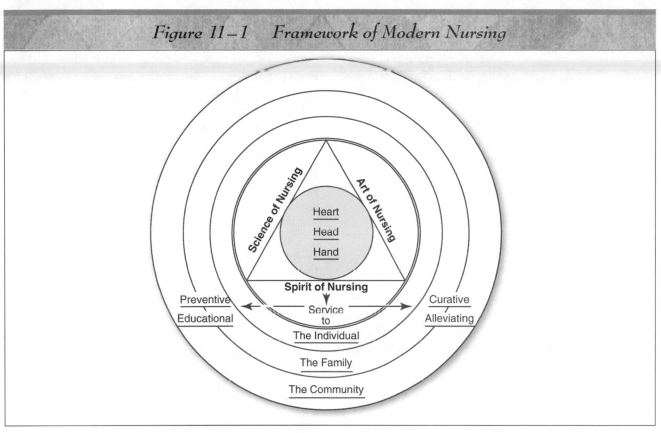

Reprinted with permission: Stewart, I. M., & Austin, A. L. (1962). *A history of nursing from ancient to modern time: A world view* (5th ed.). New York: GP Putnam & Sons.

Nightingale involving the divine laws of nature (Macrae, 2001).

As technology advanced and the emphasis on the scientific aspects of nursing increased, the pendulum began to swing away from a spiritual and religious focus. During most of the twentieth century, nursing as a profession directed its efforts toward developing a scientific basis for practice. Secularism became the accepted philosophy during the 1960s with spiritual aspects of care receiving little or no attention. Although nursing continued to claim a focus on the whole person, nurses were taught to minister to physical, social, and psychological needs; spiritual needs were ignored. This emphasis began to change in the late 1970s when publications dealing with spirituality began to appear. Contemporary nursing now emphasizes spiritual needs as well as the traditional physical, psychological, and social needs. Science is recognizing the impact of spirituality on health. In the past 20 years, a growing body of research has been published documenting the impact of spirituality on health, both physical and mental. Studies that have provided evidence supporting the relationship of spirituality and health as valuable to:

- Surviving heart surgery
- Preventing high blood pressure
- Improving immune functioning
- Recovering from depression
- Reducing length of hospital stays
- Predicting longer lives
- Expanding the life span

(National Institute for Healthcare Research, 2002)

Contemporary Views of Spirituality

The emphasis of spirituality has changed from a religious expression to include self-awareness and relationship with the world. The nurse needs to recognize that each individual interprets the meaning and expression of spirituality in ways that are personally significant. In order to develop a comprehensive view of spirituality, the nurse should understand the patient's values and beliefs. The nurse also needs to recognize that the relationship of spirituality and religion varies from individual to individual. Many people meet spiritual needs through a specific religion or religious framework. Religious development and practice may not parallel spiritual development. For example, a person may follow particular religious practices, but may not internalize the meaning behind the practices. Religious and spiritual beliefs may assume greater importance during illness than in times of health. The nurse needs to understand the patient's needs and preferences, and provide care that allows for individual expression of spirituality.

Western Perspective of Spirituality

Western worldview or perspective of spirituality includes beliefs that come from both Judeo-Christian and Muslim belief systems. These worldviews see the spirit as that part of a person that equips the person to experience meaningful relationships with God or Deity. God is the ultimate being in most religious beliefs, although differing religions use various terms for God. Christianity and Islam are the largest religions in the world today and are among the fastest-growing religions. They, as well as Judaism, hold a belief in one God as an ultimate power or being. This belief in a higher being or higher power is held by most societies.[1] Relationships with God are governed by the individual's spirituality. Spirituality also influences relationships with others and with one's own self through or because of forgiveness, love, and trust. Each component of the individual influences each other part; likewise, the whole influences interactions with others, with the environment, with self, and with God. These vertical and horizontal relationships are presented diagramatically in Figure 11–2.

Western religions believe the individual was created to serve God and to do God's will. The worth of the individual is deemphasized. Family is an important part of life; relationships with family are an extension of one's relationship with God.

Religious beliefs are an important consideration in providing nursing care. Each Western religion has specific beliefs that may impact the individual's response to illness or compliance with care regimens. Examples of these beliefs include periods of fasting that are practiced by Muslims, Jews, and some Christian groups. As a rule, individuals who are ill, pregnant women, and small children may be exempt from fasting. Other practices involve special ceremonies or prayer for those who are ill. Individuals may have physical representations of their religion (e.g., a rosary, crosses, medals, or jewelry). Beliefs differ concerning holy writings. For example, strict Muslims may believe that the Koran should not be touched by anyone who is not a Muslim.

Secularism is also a common Western worldview. It became a permanent force in Western culture through technical and scientific advances, particularly in the twentieth century. In its purest form, secularism does not consider spirituality as important and rejects religion as worthy of consideration. Any knowledge that cannot be demonstrated or proved by scientific inquiry is considered to be invalid or inferior.

Eastern Perspective

The Eastern worldview or religions regard the spirit as reality and the physical being as illusion. The concept of connectedness or being at one with the universe is a pervasive thought. Most Eastern religions believe that the spirit is the real person. Spirits are present in all animate beings and in inanimate objects. Unity and balance are emphasized. Yin and yang represent the life forces that are present in everything and must be balanced. Physical desires and needs may be denied and most certainly are secondary to the need for harmony. Meditation is a path often employed to aid the individual to find peace or harmony. Religious beliefs vary among the specific religions (e.g., Buddhism, Confusianism, Taoism, Shintoism, Hinduism, and spiritualism). In general, these religions range from atheis-

---

Critical Thinking and Reflection

What values of the nursing profession come from Judeo-Christian beliefs? What values come from Muslim or Eastern religious beliefs? What values are not related to spirituality? How do these values blend? How do they create conflicts for the nurse?

---

[1]While it is recognized that each individual holds personal beliefs about God or a higher power, in this chapter the term *God* is used to refer to the ultimate being or higher power.

Figure 11–2   The Person's Spiritual Interrelatedness

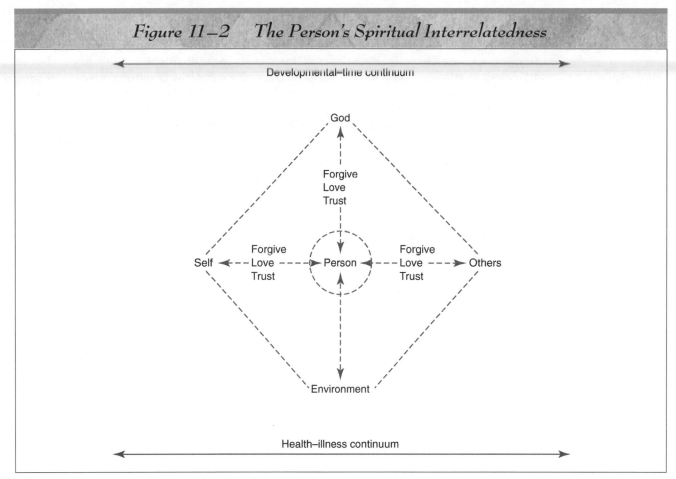

Redrawn by permission of Ruth I. Stoll. © Ruth I. Stoll, 1987.

tic to polytheistic. The focus is not as much the worship of one particular deity as in finding the path to harmony with the world. The beliefs of Native Americans tend to be consistent with this worldview. Spiritual practices may include prayer, burning incense, offering food or other items to a deity, and meditation. Yoga and meditation, two practices which originated in Eastern religions, have now found wide acceptance among people of other beliefs.

Expression of Spirituality

While each individual expresses spirituality in different ways, there are common spiritual needs that have been identified. Beland and Passos (1975) discussed the spiritual needs of forgiveness—from God, self, and others; love, not based on conditions, but unconditional love from God, self, and others; hope—looking toward the future; trust—faith in someone outside of self; and

meaning and purpose in life. Fish and Shelly (1978) state that spiritual needs have been a concern of nursing throughout history but that spiritual needs either have been classified as primarily religious practices or are considered vague and difficult to define. Fish and Shelly also discuss the needs of meaning and purpose, love and relatedness, and forgiveness.

Relationship with God or a Divine Being or Connectedness

The need for a relationship with God or a divine being is a foremost concern many individuals recognize. Other individuals would define this need as a relationship with the cosmos or the universe by finding harmony and oneness with the surrounding world. This need unifies all of the other identified spiritual needs and gives direction to the individual's life. In times of crisis, whether illness or trauma, the relationship with God may be disrupted by feelings of anger or guilt.

Some individuals may question God's role in the situation or may feel isolated from God. For other individuals, life circumstances in which they find themselves may precipitate examination of, or a greater desire for, a relationship with God that previously may not have been part of their day-to-day lives. The status of one's relationship with God is reflected in relationships with others and with self, a fact that is especially important to providers of direct patient care. The person who is ill or injured may feel isolated or alienated from God and require assistance in maintaining or developing a meaningful relationship with God. Another person may view the illness or injury as one's karma and feel powerless to change anything in the situation. In this case, the suffering that results may be the vehicle by which the person can learn to accept what is happening and be brought closer to acceptance. The nurse can use therapeutic communication to listen as the patient expresses feelings of abandonment and isolation. The nurse can aid the patient to (a) clarify or reinforce their relationship with God and/or (b) help the patient seek peace.

Need for Meaning and Purpose

The need for meaning or purpose is a critical spiritual need. All individuals need to have a meaning or purpose in life. Meaning and purpose have been identified as an essential element for survival. The search for meaning is a primary force in life (Frankel, 1971). Stressful events that have no meaning are difficult to handle. When a patient can attach meaning, he or she is more likely to grow, recover, and continue life. Joyce Travelbee stated that "the purpose of nursing is to assist an individual, family, or community to prevent or cope with the experience of illness and suffering and, if necessary, to find meaning in these experiences" (Travelbee, 1971, p. 16). The nurse can help the patient find meaning by accepting the patient's feelings and allowing them to talk while the nurse listens. Listening can be one of the most beneficial nursing interventions in assisting the patient to process and find meaning in a situation.

Values and Forgiveness

Values make up another area of spiritual need. One could argue whether religious beliefs determine values or values influence religious beliefs. For many people, religious beliefs determine their values or, at least, have a major impact on the formation of values. Spirituality may be manifested by religious beliefs that provide a framework for the standards that guide actions in daily life. While values are determined by the individual, they are influenced by family, peers, society, culture, and religion. Actions and behaviors, in turn, are determined by the individual's values. Conflicting values present challenges as an individual is deciding on a course of action. The nurse can provide spiritual care by assisting the individual to clarify values. The value of maintaining life may conflict with that of providing comfort and relieving pain. The nurse can assist the individual and family to determine which course will be followed. The nurse may experience the same conflicts as the patient. As a result, the nurse may also need to clarify his or her own personal values.

Forgiveness is another spiritual need that should be included in the realm of nursing care. Forgiveness involves resolving feelings of guilt, which are common in individuals who experience health crises. Guilt may be caused by lifestyle behaviors (e.g., not exercising, not following prescribed medical regimen, drinking while driving, or leaving hazardous materials within the reach of a child). Chronic illness may also precipitate feelings of guilt. Our society emphasizes productivity; however, the chronically ill may not be able to function as society expects. Illness is acceptable as long as the person seeks care, follows the regimen, and recovers quickly. The individual with a chronic condition who is not able to recover as expected may have feelings of guilt as a result. The nurse can play a critical role in assisting the individual to resolve these feelings and find forgiveness of self by actively listening and encouraging communication. Another area of forgiveness is forgiving others. Often, relationships with family members or others involve guilt either because of past experiences or because of present behaviors. The nurse can encourage the patient to discuss feelings and seek or give forgiveness. The last area of forgiveness is forgiveness from God. Some believe that illness or tragedy can be punishment because of sin; these individuals may need to find forgiveness before recovery can begin. The nurse can help the patient to clarify beliefs. The nurse may either assist the patient in this process by encouraging communication or refer the patient to clergy.

Love, Belonging, and Hope

Love and belonging are also spiritual needs. Some would argue that they are social rather than spiritual needs, while others would consider a relationship with God as encompassing the need for love and belonging. Love and belonging are related to spirituality and are needs that must be considered. Individuals need to be accepted as persons of worth and dignity. Not all individuals have had the life experiences that were needed to develop a positive self-concept. Individuals need to be accepted unconditionally in order to develop a sense of self-worth necessary for health. This type of relationship is a reflection of the individual's relationship with a higher power. Nurses can reflect this type of relationship through caring, nonjudgmental interactions with patients.

Hope, a vital spiritual need, is the characteristic that allows the individual to cope with crisis in a positive way and provides an opportunity for personal growth in the situation. Hope can be defined as a positive anticipation of a future good. It assists the individual in overcoming obstacles and engaging in tasks necessary for recuperation. Hope is a dynamic force that arises from the individual's faith, from relationships with others, from feeling needed, and from having something to accomplish. Religious beliefs are a prime source of hope for many people. The nurse may also find that the patient's anticipation changes as the situation or health status changes. The nurse must, however, encourage hope in the patient and not damage that optimism by an uncaring attitude. The nurse should nurture the patient's faith even though it may appear to be unrealistic. To do so, the nurse may need to reexamine personal interpretation of the situation and look at it from the patient's perspective. What the nurse may consider false hope could be the force that aids the patient to continue working toward recovery. Although complete recovery may not be possible physically, that work will help to provide a quality of life that would be impossible for the patient without hope.

Spirituality and Health

Spirituality is a vital contributor to overall individual health. The spirit is the core of the individual and as such influences all aspects of an individual's life. Health is one area impacted by the person's spirituality. It is not unusual to identify someone who survived a major illness or trauma in the face of insurmountable odds when the recovery cannot be explained by scientific rationale. On the other hand, persons may die when there is no identifiable reason, such as the individual who mystifies the surgeon by dying after a successful surgery. Another example is the individual who had frequent episodes of tonsillitis as a child until the physician said the next episode would require a tonsillectomy. The individual then never had another case of tonsillitis although that incident was over 30 years ago. Just as the physical and psychological domains influence each other, (e.g., anxiety causing a headache or a positive experience making one forget a toothache), so also the spiritual influences physical and emotional well-being. Frequently, the individual who has spiritual needs met functions on a higher level emotionally. This in turn enables the person to maintain physical health. On the other hand, the individual who is in touch with personal spirituality approaches illness or injury with an attitude that facilitates recovery or successful adaptation to disability. For an individual to maintain optimum health, there must be health in all aspects of the person's life.

Factors Influencing Spiritual Well-Being

Spiritual well-being, defined as "personal expressions of connectedness with self, others, higher power, all life, nature, and the universe that transcend and empower the self" (Johnson, Maas, & Moorhead, 2000, p. 407), depends on an individual's ability to fulfill spiritual needs. There are many factors that impact the ability of the individual to meet spiritual needs. The age of the individual is one factor that influences spiritual needs. Fowler (1974), drawing on work by Piaget, Kohlberg, and Erikson, described stages of spiritual development of the individual across the life span. Piaget is known for his theory of cognitive or intellectual development. Kohlberg is known for his stages of moral judgment. Erikson is known for his theory of psychosocial development. Borrowing from these theorists, stages for the development of spiritual well being are presented. An infant needs to be loved and to have basic physical and emotional needs met. Love provides the foundation for the development of trust and faith in later life. A child begins by imitating parents and accepting beliefs and values without questioning. The existence of God or a deity is accepted, and the meaning of good versus bad progresses as a conscience develops. Experiences as well as maturation shape the individual. Adolescents may experience spiritual dissonance as they begin to question beliefs of others and experience contradictions between religious authority and personal experiences. Adults continue to develop their concepts of a deity and the impact of spirituality. As aging occurs, the elderly begin to reflect on their lives, and many rely on their spirituality to provide guidance and comfort as physical health and abilities decline. Others may develop increased spiritual needs if life goals are unfulfilled. Religious beliefs impact how an individual handles approaching death. Nurses need to consider the

Nursing focuses on caring for the whole person. What have you observed in your experience that illustrates the relationship of spirituality to the health of the individual? How would you prioritize nursing care while considering both physical and spiritual needs? Life-threatening needs should come first. Is there a situation in which spiritual needs would have priority over life-threatening physical needs? What part should a person's religious beliefs play in determining priorities of care?

---

developmental stage of the person when planning developmentally appropriate spiritual interventions.

Culture has a profound influence on a person's spirituality and on the expression of spirituality. Culture must be considered when providing spiritual care. Religion is only one aspect of culture influencing spirituality. Behaviors acceptable to express spirituality are also defined by the person's culture. Some cultures permit open and uninhibited expressions or spirituality while others are closed and private. Worldviews and specific beliefs also shape a person's spirituality. Eastern religions and Native Americans view the world from a spiritual framework, with little, if any, emphasis on the physical. The Western world emphasizes the physical, sometimes to the exclusion of the spiritual. Individual religions also vary in specific beliefs that guide the person's spirituality and expression of it (Carson, 1989).

The relationship (a) between males and females and (b) foods that are commonly eaten are two examples of cultural practices that can have a major impact on health care and may be dictated by religious beliefs. Some cultures and religions emphasize modesty for women to the point of not allowing male health care providers to treat female patients. Some religions have strict beliefs regarding foods that are acceptable to eat and those that are forbidden. The nurse needs to be familiar with the beliefs of the common religions of patients frequently encountered. Spiritual care requires sensitivity to the beliefs of each patient; however, knowledge of all specific religious beliefs is not essential or realistic. If the nurse is not familiar with a particular religion and its specific beliefs, references can be consulted as questions about religious practices are assessed. The nurse needs to remember that not all individuals of the same religion believe the same things or practice their faith in the same way. Beliefs and practices in all religious groups range from strict adherence to tenets to free interpretation and/or individual disregard for tenets. Nurses who ignore customs and practices that are important to the patients or who make assumptions based on inadequate information can offend patients.

Few patients are offended by sincere inquiry to determine areas of need and concern.

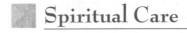

Spiritual Care

Assessment of Spirituality

Assessing spirituality is a challenge in the nurse's busy workworld. Time constraints may prohibit a thorough assessment that would be ideal and a detailed spiritual assessment may not be realistic in every setting. Interventions may need to be instituted before assessment is complete. The nurse should be attuned to the fact that spiritual assessment requires the assessment of the total person. For example, data collected regarding the individual's psychological status—such as emotions, attitudes, affect, feelings, and behaviors—contribute essential information. Often, information can be observed while the nurse is performing other assessments or procedures. The individual's social relationships add to the pool of data. To obtain this information the nurse might ask whether the patient has visitors and, if so, who they are. Many times spiritual support will be visible during crisis, either by the pastor, priest, rabbi, or others of the congregation who gather to aid the individual.

Observations about the individual are equally important. Are religious objects, such as a crucifix or rosary, present? Does the person have religious literature, such as a Bible, Koran (sometimes called Quron), or religious literature present? Does the patient pray before eating? Behaviors and practices such as these contribute to the data pool.

Including spiritual needs in history taking or when interviewing the patient or family provides additional information about the person's spirituality. Many consider spiritual matters to be personal and private; therefore, they may not be comfortable talking about religion or spirituality. Others may not hold religious beliefs. One approach to data collection includes yes and no questions such as "Is religion important to you?" If the answer is "yes," an open-ended question, such as "Tell me how religion is important to you.", will encourage the person to explain how religion may be important. If the answer is "no," the nurse will know that this is an area that the person may not value or may not wish to discuss. A negative response does not mean that the individual has no spiritual needs. It adds to the challenge of assessing and providing care.

Timing of history taking concerning spirituality needs to be considered. A nurse will have better results if the interview is initiated after establishing a good rapport with the patient. Rapport usually requires more than one contact with the patient, although sometimes a bond can be established very quickly. Also, spirituality may not be the first area that needs to be assessed. Priorities are usually established, with physical needs first, psychosocial next, then spiritual. Nurses do need to be aware that spiritual needs might be the first priority for some patients followed by needs in other areas. Consideration of areas to be discussed during the con-

versation must be prioritized. Nurses may find that they postpone topics that are not as comfortable to discuss (e.g., sexuality, elimination, and spirituality). Most nurses understand that spirituality does not mix with these other highly personal topics.

Once the proper timing has been established to assess spiritual needs, the nurse can use an assessment tool to give direction and define areas that should be covered. Guidelines established by Ruth Stoll for assessing the patient's spiritual well-being have been widely accepted. Stoll (1979) outlines four areas to be considered. These areas include one's concept of God or deity, one's religious practices, one's source of hope and strength, and the relationship of one's beliefs to the situation they find themselves in at the time. Examples of questions in each of these categories are listed in Box 11–1. Other tools with similar questions can be substituted. The nurse must individualize the spiritual assessment. Asking about religious practices can be an excellent beginning for a new admission to an inpatient or residential setting, while source of hope and strength

---

Box 11–1   Areas of Spiritual Assessment

Guidelines for Spiritual Assessment

To Determine Patient's Concept of God or Deity
- Is religion or God significant to you? If yes, can you describe how?
- Is prayer helpful to you? What happens when you pray?
- Does a god or deity function in your personal life? If yes, can you describe how?
- How would you describe your god or what you worship?

To Determine Patient's Sources of Hope and Strength
- Who is the most important person to you?
- To whom do you turn when you need help? Are they available? In what ways do they help?
- What is your source of strength and hope?
- What helps you the most when you feel afraid to ask for special help?

To Determine Patient's Religious Practices
- Do you feel your faith (or your religion) is helpful to you? If yes, would you tell me how?
- Are there any religious practices that are important to you?
- Has being sick made any difference in your practice of praying? Your religious practices?
- What religious books or symbols are helpful to you?

Relation Between Spiritual Beliefs and Health
- What has bothered you most about being sick (or in what is happening to you)?
- What do you think is going to happen to you?
- Has being sick (or what has happened to you) made any difference in your feelings about God or the practice of your faith?
- Is there anything that is especially frightening or meaningful to you now?

Adapted from Stoll (1979).

Box 11–2   Spiritual Assessment Tool

To facilitate the healing process in clients/patients, families, significant others, and yourself, the following reflective questions assist in assessing, evaluating, and increasing awareness of the spiritual process in yourself and others.

Meaning and Purpose

These questions assess a person's ability to seek meaning and fulfillment in life, manifest hope, and accept ambiguity and uncertainty.

- What gives your life meaning?
- Do you have a sense of purpose in life?
- Does your illness interfere with your life goals?
- Why do you want to get well?
- How hopeful are you about obtaining a better degree of health?
- Do you feel that you have a responsibility in maintaining your health?
- Will you be able to make changes in your life to maintain your health?
- Are you motivated to get well?
- What is the most important or powerful thing in your life?

Inner Strengths

These questions assess a person's ability to manifest joy and recognize strengths, choices, goals, and faith.

- What brings you joy and peace in your life?
- What can you do to feel alive and full of spirit?
- What traits do you like about yourself?
- What are your personal strengths?
- What choices are available to you to enhance your healing?
- What life goals have you set for yourself?
- Do you think that stress in any way caused your illness?
- How aware were you of your body before you became sick?
- What do you believe in?
- Is faith important in your life?
- How has your illness influenced your faith?
- Does faith play a role in regaining your health?
- Do you use relaxation or imagery skills?
- Do you meditate?
- Do you pray?
- What is your prayer?

- How are your prayers answered?
- Do you have a sense of belonging in this world?

Interconnections

These questions assess a person's positive self-concept, self-esteem, and sense of self; sense of belonging in the world with others; capacity to pursue personal interest; and ability to demonstrate love of self and self-forgiveness.

- How do you feel about yourself right now?
- How do you feel when you have a true sense of yourself?
- Do you pursue things of personal interest?
- What do you do to show love for yourself?
- Can you forgive yourself?
- What do you do to heal your spirit?

These questions assess a person's ability to connect in life-giving ways with family, friends, and social groups and to engage in the forgiveness of others.

- Who are the significant people in your life?
- Do you have friends or family in town who are available to help you?
- Who are the people to whom you are closest?
- Do you belong to any groups?
- Can you ask people for help when you need it?
- Can you share your feelings with others?
- What are some of the most loving things that others have done for you?
- What are the loving things that you do for other people?
- Are you able to forgive others?

These questions assess a person's capacity for finding meaning in worship or religious activities and a connectedness with a divinity or universe.

- Is worship important to you?
- What do you consider the most significant act of worship in your life?
- Do you participate in any religious activities?
- Do you believe in God or a higher power?
- Do you think that prayer is powerful?
- Have you ever tried to empty your mind of all thoughts to see what the experience might be like?

Box 11–2 (continued)

These questions assess a person's ability to experience a sense of connection with all of life and nature, an awareness of the effects of the environment on life and well-being, and a capacity or concern for the health of the environment.

- Do you ever feel at some level a connection with the world or universe?
- How does your environment have an impact on your state of well-being?
- What are your environmental stressors at work and at home?

- Do you incorporate strategies to reduce your environmental stressors?
- Do you have any concerns for the state of your immediate environment?
- Are you involved with environmental issues such as recycling environmental resources at home, work, or in your community?
- Are you concerned about the survival of the planet?

Reprinted from Guzzetta, A., & Dossey, B. M. (1992). *Cardiovascular Nursing Practice* (p. 9). Copyright 1992, with permission from Elsevier Science.

might be more appropriate to a long-term or terminally ill patient. Burkhardt has developed another assessment tool to be used to assess spirituality. This tool is found in Box 11–2. Howden developed a spiritual assessment scale that may also give insight into the individual's perceptions related to spirituality (Table 11–2) (Dossey, Keegan, & Guzzetta, 2000).

Recognizing Spiritual Concerns

Nursing has a mandate to consider spirituality in planning patient care. Definitions of nursing consider the human individual as a physical, psychological, social, and spiritual being. Holistic care implies that the spiritual is included as well. The Joint Commission on Accreditation of Healthcare Organizations (JCAHO) requires patient care plans include spiritual needs. The North American Nursing Diagnosis Association (NANDA International, 2003) has identified nursing diagnoses that are applicable to spirituality. Spiritual Distress and Risk for Spiritual Distress are commonly used nursing diagnoses for patients in many situations. Etiology may be related to a variety of factors in the patient's situation. Feelings of hopelessness or helplessness can lead to spiritual distress. Challenges to an individual's belief system or views of deity create spiritual distress, as does separation from religious practices. Potential for enhanced spiritual well-being is also a legitimate area of nursing concern. The nurse can assist growth and provide support for the patient. Other nursing diagnoses such as Hopelessness and Dysfunctional Grieving are directly related to the person's spirituality (NANDA International, 2003).

Nursing Care to Enhance Spiritual Well-Being

The nurse has many resources to use in providing spiritual care to patients. The foremost resource is the nurse's therapeutic use of self. Listening can be the single most important intervention in helping to meet spiritual needs. Often, the patient needs to be able to express feelings without fear of criticism or being told what to do about their problems. Good communication skills are essential to a complete assessment of the spiritual domain. Communication barriers can prevent the nurse or the patient from expressing the necessary information. Stumbling blocks to listening include the nurse's own values and beliefs when the patient holds differing values and beliefs. The nurse must be able to put personal values aside in order to be able to remain nonjudgmental in dealing with the patient so as to hear the intended message accurately. Preconceptions about an individual from another culture or religious belief may not be accurate and will hinder hearing the intended message. Word meanings present another barrier, particularly in the spiritual domain. Many words commonly used by some in discussing religious beliefs may not be understood by others or may be used to mean something different. For example, the term *Christian* is used by some to mean a personal relationship with Jesus Christ, while others may mean that they come from a background associated with Christian beliefs instead of another major world religion. Often, the busy schedule reflected in the nurse's priorities present a hindrance to listening when time is short and tasks are many.

Table 11–2   Spirituality Assessment Scale

DIRECTIONS: Please indicate your response by circling the appropriate letters indicating how you respond to the statements.

MARK:

SA if you STRONGLY AGREE
A if you AGREE
AM if you AGREE MORE than DISAGREE
DM if you DISAGREE MORE than AGREE
D if you DISAGREE
SD if you STRONGLY DISAGREE

There is no "right" or "wrong" answer. Please respond to what you think or how you feel at this point in time.

1. I have a general sense of belonging.	SA	A	AM	DM	D	SD
2. I am able to forgive people who have done me wrong.	SA	A	AM	DM	D	SD
3. I have the ability to rise above or go beyond a physical or psychological condition.	SA	A	AM	DM	D	SD
4. I am concerned about destruction of the environment.	SA	A	AM	DM	D	SD
5. I have experienced moments of peace in a devastating event.	SA	A	AM	DM	D	SD
6. I feel a kinship to other people.	SA	A	AM	DM	D	SD
7. I feel a connection to all of life.	SA	A	AM	DM	D	SD
8. I rely on an inner strength in hard times.	SA	A	AM	DM	D	SD
9. I enjoy being of service to others.	SA	A	AM	DM	D	SD
10. I can go to a spiritual dimension within myself for guidance.	SA	A	AM	DM	D	SD
11. I have the ability to rise above or go beyond a body change or body loss.	SA	A	AM	DM	D	SD
12. I have a sense of harmony or inner peace.	SA	A	AM	DM	D	SD
13. I have the ability for self-healing.	SA	A	AM	DM	D	SD
14. I have an inner strength.	SA	A	AM	DM	D	SD
15. The boundaries of my universe extend beyond usual ideas of what space and time are thought to be.	SA	A	AM	DM	D	SD
16. I feel good about myself.	SA	A	AM	DM	D	SD
17. I have a sense of balance in my life.	SA	A	AM	DM	D	SD
18. There is fulfillment in my life.	SA	A	AM	DM	D	SD
19. I feel a responsibility to preserve the planet.	SA	A	AM	DM	D	SD
20. The meaning I have found for my life provides a sense of peace.	SA	A	AM	DM	D	SD
21. Even when I feel discouraged, I trust that life is good.	SA	A	AM	DM	D	SD
22. My life has meaning and purpose.	SA	A	AM	DM	D	SD
23. My innerness or an inner resource helps me deal with uncertainty in life.	SA	A	AM	DM	D	SD
24. I have discovered my own strength in times of struggle.	SA	A	AM	DM	D	SD
25. Reconciling relationships is important to me.	SA	A	AM	DM	D	SD
26. I feel a part of the community in which I live.	SA	A	AM	DM	D	SD
27. My inner strength is related to belief in a Higher Power or Supreme Being.	SA	A	AM	DM	D	SD
28. I have goals and aims for my life.	SA	A	AM	DM	D	SD

Printed with permission. Copyright © 1992, Judy W. Howden.

Problem: Vance defined spirituality as "an interconnection with God or god being, that enables a human being to transcend the circumstances at hand and give purpose and meaning to life" (Vance, 2001, p. 265). Most studies focused on the relationship between nurses' attitudes and spiritual care practices have investigated oncology and mental health nurses. This study was designed to survey nurses in general practice (Vance, 2001).

Methods: A descriptive correlational assessment surveyed acute care nurses' spirituality and the spiritual care they delivered to their patients. A proportionate, stratified, random sample of RNs who provided direct patient care in critical care, medical–surgical, women's health, and behavioral health nursing units at a large community teaching hospital in a large midwestern city were studied. Two instruments, the Spiritual Well-Being Scale and the Spiritual Involvement and Beliefs Scale, were used to measure both the metaphysical and the existential dimension of spirituality within a person's life. Both instruments have demonstrated validity and reliability. The investigator developed the Spiritual Care Practice Questionnaire used to determine spiritual practices of nurses. It was reviewed for content validity and test–retest reliability. All of the instruments demonstrated acceptable validity and reliability for use.

Results: A positive significant ($p = 0.05$) correlation was found between spirituality and nursing assessment and interventions. Nurses who scored higher in their personal attitudes toward spirituality also scored higher in their spiritual practices. There was no correlation to the number of barriers they perceived to providing spiritual care. Only 34.6% of the respondents provided spiritual care at a level predetermined to the ideal for nursing practice. Barriers to providing spiritual care were identified. The greatest barrier perceived was lack of time, followed by insufficient education related to spirituality and spiritual care. The third most common barrier was the belief that spiritual matters are private and should not be addressed by the nurse. A negative correlation was found between assessment and intervention to barriers perceived by nurses. Nurses who scored higher in providing care perceived fewer barriers to the delivery of spiritual care.

Conclusion: Nurses surveyed considered themselves to be spiritual; however, only about 25% provided adequate spiritual care to their patients. The greatest barrier to providing care was identified as lack of time. Other barriers included lack of educational preparation, lack of confidence, differences in faith between the nurse and patient, and confusion between proselytizing and spiritual care.

Basic and continuing education concerning providing spiritual care would help nurses in this area. Further studies are still needed to assess the gap between assessing spiritual needs and carrying out interventions. Study is also needed to determine patients' perceptions of how well their spiritual needs are being met.

Anxiety is yet another obstacle. An anxious nurse will miss many cues from the patient since the focus is on the "nervous nurse" rather than on the patient. The nurse must be willing to take time to communicate with the patient when anxiety is decreased.

EMPATHY AND TOUCH

Empathy, defined as "the ability to understand what a person is feeling and to communicate that understanding to him while remaining objective enough to see why he feels as he does and to be able to assist him" (Fish & Shelly, 1978, p. 88), is a nursing quality that promotes spiritual care. Empathy is more than sympathy; it implies use of both emotions and reasoning based on assessment of the patient. This capability enables the nurse to communicate caring for the patient, understanding of the patient's needs, and ability to assist in fulfillment of the needs (Shelly, 2000). In order to have empathy, the nurse must first recognize their own values, and then see the situation as the patient does. This may be difficult when the nurse is caring for a patient from a different culture, religion, or value system. Nursing care, however, cannot be based on the nurse's values, but must focus on the values of the patient. Next, the nurse must put aside personal values and remain nonjudgmental in the situation. Finally, the nurse must postpone meeting personal needs and focus on meeting the patient's needs.

The use of touch is an effective intervention in meeting spiritual needs. Holding the patient's hand or touching the forearm or shoulder communicates understanding and caring. Words are not always needed; in fact, words may be a hindrance rather than help in many situations. The nurse needs to be aware of the cultural meaning of touch to the patient and consider how touch could be interpreted. Some cultures do not allow touching in public, while others are very demonstrative. In our modern society, touch can be interpreted as a sexual advance if it is used improperly. Asking the patient's permission to hold the hand or to give a hug will help to eliminate a misunderstanding. Sometimes a compassionate hand is the intervention needed to communicate caring to the patient (Shelly, 2000).

PRAYER AND SCRIPTURE

Prayer is an essential element of spirituality to most individuals and is an intervention the nurse can use effectively. First, the nurse should carefully assess the situation and determine the patient's real concerns. Then, the nurse needs to determine if the patient has a need for prayer. The prayer must be based on the patient's need, not the nurse's. Prayer should not be used as a pat answer or a magic remedy for the patient's problems. Knowledge of the patient's religious practices will help direct the nurse in determining how to pray with the patient. If the nurse does not know how the patient is accustomed to praying, it is appropriate to ask if the patient would like to pray together with the nurse. It is not appropriate to assume that everyone will pray in the same manner. If the patient desires prayer, the nurse can ask if praying as the nurse is accustomed is acceptable. This recognizes that the patient may pray in a manner different from the nurse. Prayer should be a short, simple statement of God's ability to meet the patient in his situation, recognizing the patient's hopes, fears, and needs (Fish & Shelly, 1978).

Use of scripture is another strategy the nurse can use in meeting spiritual needs. One must consider the religious beliefs of the patient. The Bible is one source of comfort for those of a Judeo-Christian heritage. Others may appreciate the Bible as literature and find comfort in passages such as Psalms, while other faiths may also accept the Bible as authoritative. The nurse may use other sacred writings as long as that practice is acceptable to the patient's belief system. For example, strict Muslims believe that the Koran is not truly the Koran if it has been translated into a language other than its original language of Arabic and that those not of Islam faith should not be allowed to touch the Koran. Persons of other faiths may have scriptures they allow the nurse to share with them. Care must be taken that the nurse does not give the appearance of proselytizing when using scripture. The nurse must also evaluate whether the passage to be shared is appropriate to the patient's situation. One way of not offending the patient when using scripture is to ask if the nurse may share something that has been personally helpful in a time of crisis. Another approach to the use of scripture is to ask if the patient has a favorite passage that could be read by the nurse. Other religious books and literature may also provide the patient comfort.

INTERDISCIPLINARY SUPPORT

Referral to a chaplain, pastor, rabbi, imam, or another member of the clergy is a common intervention. The chaplain or cleric has the same focus on ministering to the whole person but approaches meeting needs from the perspective of theology and pastoral care. For many nurses, the most comfortable approach for meeting spiritual needs is to refer the patient to the chaplain or his own minister. However, the minister or chaplain may not be available when the patient needs to talk or find support. Some patients may believe that only the pastoral care person is qualified to deal with the spiritual needs, while other patients find it refreshing and meaningful that nurses and other health care professionals are concerned about spirituality and take the time to include spiritual needs in their priorities. Many religious groups have special provisions for ministering to the ill and appreciate being notified when members need assistance. Some patients may feel slighted if their personal minister does not call while they are ill. The nurse should discuss whether a cleric needs to be notified about the patient's situation. The hospital chaplain can assist the nurse in determining if other clergy need to be consulted to provide more personalized care.

INTERVENTION AND OUTCOMES

Nursing Interventions Classification (NIC) includes a multitude of interventions aimed toward the nursing diagnosis of Spiritual Distress, which is defined as "impaired ability to experience and integrate meaning and purpose in life through a person's connectedness with self, others, art, music, literature, nature, or power greater than oneself" (NANDA International, 2003). Interventions that may be used for the nursing diagnosis Spiritual Distress also include Anticipatory Guidance and Emotional Support (McCloskey & Bulechek, 2000). Facilitating the patient's work toward grieving, resolving guilt, and coping effectively are other means of assisting in meeting spiritual needs. Counseling and crisis intervention are additional interventions that may be needed in some situations. Supporting the patient in decision-making and providing values clarification help the patient to define spiritual needs and to determine the best ways of meeting them. Providing spiritual support and spiritual growth facilitation are other interventions the nurse can use to contribute to the patient's welfare. Active listening and presence, the act of "being there" for the patient when needed, are vital interventions of the nurse. In some situations, broader interventions, such as family support or caregiver support, are needed. Enhancing religious rituals by encouraging or allowing their performance in an acute care or residential setting may be a critical link for the individual experiencing spiritual distress when separated from familiar surroundings and practices. Encouraging hope and communicating acceptance and self-esteem will also assist the individual for meet spiritual needs (McCloskey & Bulechek, 2000).

Outcomes that result from spiritual care directed at alleviating spiritual distress include hope and spiritual well-being. For some patients, dignified dying is the successful end of spiritual care, providing the patient with an optimal quality of life as long as possible. Hope is another valued result of successful nursing intervention. The nurse has a vital role in assisting the individual to continue to hope during illness or crisis. Participation in spiritual rites, meditation, prayer, and spiritual readings are outcomes the patient may be able to accomplish. Expressions of faith, hope, meaning and purpose, and love are among outcomes of spiritual care (Johnson, Maas, & Moorhead, 2000). The patient benefits when the nurse is sensitive to individual religious practices and expressions of spirituality. An example of this is the family of a child who was scheduled to be discharged from the hospital. The mother was most upset when she learned that the child could not leave the hospital because a special ceremony had to be performed for the child that day. The nurse assessed the situation and determined that the ceremony could be performed anywhere but involved burning incense. Fire regulations forbade holding the ceremony in the child's room. The nurse made arrangements for the child to be taken to the hospital chapel where candles were permitted. The family experienced the outcomes of expression of their faith and meaning and purpose as well as feeling the love of the nurse who aided them. Ideally, the patient will be able to feel connectedness with inner self as well as with others, thus enabling the sharing of thoughts, feelings, and beliefs.

Evaluation of spiritual care may be difficult in situations where the patient's physical health deteriorates or the patient dies. The nurse must remember that spiritual health is not the same as physical health. An individual who is terminally ill may experience spiritual needs but may also attain a high level of spiritual health. Individuals whose religious beliefs include life after death spent with God may view the end of life as the ultimate spiritual health and look forward to the end of pain and suffering. Providing presence to the patient who is dying can be one of the most effective ways of providing spiritual care.

Providing spiritual care should also include the concerns of the patient's family. Patients who have long-term illnesses require care for a long period of time. Often, the family will be the primary caregivers. Such care can exhaust the caregivers, who often experience their own spiritual needs. Questions of meaning and purpose, potential (or actual) loss of relationships, feelings of guilt, and loss of hope can affect the caregivers as well as the patient. The nurse must be alert to situations when interventions for the family are needed. The same principles of assessment and intervention will apply to families as well as to individuals.

Critical Thinking and Reflection

As a nurse who must assess and provide care to the whole person, how comfortable are you in providing spiritual care? How would you approach a patient who obviously has spiritual needs? Do you feel that providing such care is within the realm of your capabilities or would you refer spiritual care to the chaplain or other clergy? How would you go about planning the needed care and ensuring that the patient receives that care? How would you provide care to a patient whose religious beliefs were different from yours?

What personal resources do you have to maintain your own spiritual health? In light of long hours and heavy workloads, what measures can you take to maintain spiritual, mental, and physical health? How can you prevent burnout and continue to give quality care? How can the chaplain be a resource to you and other nurses in maintaining personal spiritual health?

The Nurse's Need for Spiritual Health

The need for spiritual health is as important to the nurse as to the patient. Just as a nurse who is not physically healthy will have difficulty providing care to patients, the nurse who is not spiritually healthy will have difficulty providing care for spiritual needs. The nurse must find ways to receive care and refreshment to continue to give. It has been said that one can give only as much as one receives. Therefore, it may be important that the nurse remains in good spiritual health in order to provide the spiritual care that patients need and deserve. Regular attention to one's own spiritual needs can enable the nurse to continue providing the level of care needed by patients.

Some nurses may not feel comfortable dealing with spiritual needs. That discomfort, however, does not excuse the nurse from providing needed care. Any nurse is qualified to listen and use therapeutic communication, the foundation of spiritual care. As in situations of physical needs when the nurse is confronted with a diagnosis or problem that is not one of the nurse's expertise, the nurse needs to find a resource who can provide the needed care rather than ignore the need of the patient. The nurse is not expected to be an expert in all areas, but is expected to assess and find the appropriate resource to provide holistic care to the patient.

TRANSITION INTO PRACTICE

Mr. Brown was admitted a week ago following an automobile accident that occurred when his family was returning home from a family vacation. He and his two sons were sleeping while his wife drove. The accident occurred when Mrs. Brown fell asleep. Mrs. Brown was uninjured. Mr. Brown sustained fractures of both legs and pelvis as well as other injuries, but is recovering. The 13-year-old son was killed. The 10-year-old son sustained a head injury, including a skull fracture and multiple lacerations requiring over 50 stitches across his head, and is still unconscious in the intensive care unit (ICU). You are assigned to care for Mr. Brown. He asked you to help put up pictures of the wrecked van on his wall. The pictures show the van from all sides, including a rear view in which the 13-year-old son's effects can be seen. You notice that Mr. Brown has a Bible on his overbed table. A urinal is sitting on the Bible. On the first day you care for Mr. Brown, he only talks about the van and asks that the pictures be put on his wall. On the second day he talks about the younger son, saying that he needs to get the son back in school in "a couple of days." He does not talk about the older son except that you overhear him on the telephone saying, "Yeah, about the time you start to like them, they leave you." He refused to talk to the social worker and ordered her out of the room because he "doesn't have any problems." His wife immediately left the room to apologize to the social worker. His chart reflects good physical assessment but nothing about his psychosocial/spiritual status.

How would you approach Mr. Brown's spiritual care? What needs can you assess in this situation? Do you agree with his statement that he does not have any problems? How would you plan interventions to meet his needs when he does not recognize or admit to having needs?

The first approach would be the use of an accepting attitude and therapeutic communication. A statement such as "It must be difficult to lose a child" can provide an opening to Mr. Brown to share his feelings at this point. Another opening statement is "I don't know how I would feel if I lost a child." Either statement allows for a variety of responses. While Mr. Brown appears to be in denial, he may be feeling anger—toward himself (for not driving), his wife (for falling asleep), his son (for dying), and God (for allowing this to happen).

Another essential approach would be consultation with the chaplain. The chaplain is trained to deal with situations of denial, anger, and questioning and will have time required to be a sounding board for Mr. Brown. Even though the chaplain may be of another faith than Mr. Brown, the chaplain will be able to assess needs that he has and secure the needed resources to meet the needs. The chaplain is also a good resource for the nurse to discuss personal feelings about caring for Mr. Brown and provide support for the nursing staff as they attempt to plan care appropriate to his needs.

KEY POINTS

1. Spirituality is the core of the individual and is made up of inner resources and values that give meaning to life.
2. The individual's spirituality influences and is influenced by the physical, psychological, and social aspects of the person.
3. Spiritual care and physical care are integral parts of providing quality care to patients.
4. Spiritual needs include a relationship with God/Higher Power, meaning and purpose, love and belonging, hope, forgiveness, and values.
5. Spiritual needs impact the health of the individual as much as physical, psychological, or social needs.

6. Assessment of the patient to determine spiritual needs occurs in an environment of a good rapport with the patient.
7. Assessment of the physical and emotional aspects of the individual contributes to spiritual assessment.
8. Therapeutic use of self and listening are key elements of spiritual care.
9. Other interventions for spiritual care include prayer, scripture, and referral to clergy.
10. The nurse should be spiritually healthy to be able to provide the best spiritual care to others.

EXPLORE MediaLink

Critical thinking questions, essay questions, key terms, web links, activities, NCLEX review questions, and more interactive resources can be found on the Companion Website at www.prenhall.com/haynes. Click on Chapter 11 to select activities for this chapter.

REFERENCES

Bayly, J. (1969). *View from a hearse*. Elgin, IL: David C. Cook Publishing Co.

Beland, I. L., & Passos, J. Y. (1975). *Clinical nursing: Pathophysiological and psychosocial approaches*. New York: Macmillan.

Burkhardt, M. A. (1989). Spirituality: An analysis of the concept. *Holistic Nursing Practice, 3*(3), 69–77.

Carson, V. B. (1989). *Spiritual dimensions of nursing practice*. Philadelphia, PA: W. B. Saunders Company.

Carson, V. B. (2000). *Mental health nursing: The nurse–patient journey*. Philadelphia, PA: W. B. Saunders.

Carson, V. B. (2001). *Reflections from Verna Benner Carson*. College Park, MD: University of Maryland School of Nursing.

Donahue, M. P. (1996). *Nursing the finest art: An illustrated history* (2nd ed.). St. Louis, MO: Mosby.

Dossey, B. M. (2000). *Florence Nightingale: Mystic, visionary, healer*. Springhouse, PA: Springhouse Corporation.

Dossey, B. M., Keegan, L., & Guzzetta, C. E. (2000). *Holistic nursing: A handbook for practice*. Gaithersburg, MD: Aspen.

Ellison, C. W. (1983). Spiritual well-being: Conceptualization and measurement. *Journal of Psychology, 11*, 330–340.

Emblen, J. (1992). Religion and spirituality according to current use in nursing literature. *Journal of Professional Nursing, 8*(1), 41–47.

Fish, S., & Shelly, J. A. (1978). *Spiritual care: The nurse's role*. Downers Grove, IL: InterVarsity Press.

Fowler, J. W. (1974). Toward a development perspective on faith. *Religion Education, 69*, 207–219.

Frankel, V. E. (1971). *Man's search for meaning.* New York: Washington Square Press.

Garner, L. F., McGuire, A., Snow, D. M., Gray, J., & Wright, K. (2002). Spirituality from the baccalaureate nursing student perspective: Comparisons of a private religious university and a state university. *Christian Higher Education, 1,* 371–384.

Goddard, N. C. (1995). "Spirituality as integrative energy": A philosophical analysis as requisite precursor to holistic nursing practice. *Journal of Advanced Nursing, 22,* 808–815.

Highfield, M. F., & Cason, C. (1983). Spiritual needs of patients: Are they recognized? *Cancer Nursing, 6*(3), 187–192.

Heriot, C. S. (1992). Spirituality and aging. *Holistic Nursing Practice, 7*(1), 22–31.

Howden, J. W. (1992). *Development and psychometric characteristics of the spirituality assessment scale.* Denton, TX: Texas Woman's University.

Johnson, M., Maas, M., & Moorhead, S. (Eds.), *Nursing outcomes classification (NOC)* (2nd ed.). St. Louis, MO: Mosby.

Kalisch, P. A., & Kalisch, B. J. (1995). *The advance of American nursing.* Boston: Little, Brown and Company.

Kurtz, E., & Ketcham, K. (1992). *The spirituality of imperfection: Storytelling and the journey to wholeness.* New York: Bantam Books.

Macrae, J. A. (2001). *Nursing as a spiritual practice.* New York: Springer.

McCloskey, J. C., & Bulechek, G. M. (Eds.), *Nursing interventions classification (NIC)* (3rd ed.). St. Louis, MO: Mosby.

Miller, J. F. (1985). Assessment of loneliness and spiritual well-being in chronically ill and healthy adults. *Journal of Professional Nursing, 1*(2), 79–85.

Nagai-Jacobson, M. G., & Burkhardt, M. A. (1989). Spirituality: Cornerstone of holistic nursing practice. *Holistic Nursing Practice, 3*(3), 18–26.

International Center for the Integration of Health & Spirituality. National Institute for Healthcare Research (NIHR). (2002). *Top 10 research studies on spirituality and health in the mid-late 1990s.* Rockville, MD: Author.

Nightingale, F. (1859). *Notes on nursing: What it is, and what it is not.* London: Harrison and Sons.

NANDA, International (2003). *Nursing diagnoses: Definitions & classification 2001–2002.* Philadelphia, PA: Author.

Oldnall, A. (1996). A critical analysis of nursing: Meeting the spiritual needs of patients. *Journal of Advanced Nursing, 23*(1), 138–144.

Random House, (1993). *Random House unabridged dictionary* (2nd ed.). New York: Random House.

Reed, P. G. (1992). An emerging paradigm for the investigation of spirituality in nursing. *Research in Nursing & Health, 15,* 349–357.

Shelly, J. A. (2000). *Spiritual care: A guide for caregivers.* Downers Grove, IL: InterVarsity Press.

Stewart, I. M., & Austin, A. L. (1962). *A history of nursing: From ancient to modern times a world view.* New York: G. P. Putnam's Sons.

Stoll, R. (1979). Guidelines for spiritual assessment. *American Journal of Nursing, 79*(9), 1574–1577.

Stuart, E. M., Deckro, J. P., & Mandle, C. L. (1989). Spirituality in health and healing: A clinical program. *Holistic Nursing Practice, 3*(3), 35–44.

Travelbee, J. (1971). *Interpersonal aspects of nursing* (2nd ed.). Philadelphia, PA: F. A. Davis.

Vance, D. L. (2001). Nurses' attitudes towards spirituality and patient care. *MEDSURG Nursing 10*(5), 264–268, 278.

Wright, K. (1998). Professional, ethical, and legal implications for spiritual care in nursing. *Image: Journal of Nursing Scholarship, 30*(1), 81–83.

SUGGESTED READINGS

Bright, M. A. (2002). *Holistic health and healing.* Philadelphia, PA: F. A. Davis.

Dossey, L. (1993). *Healing words: The power of prayer and the practice of medicine.* San Francisco: HarperCollins.

Dossey, L. (1996). *Prayer is good medicine: How to reap the benefits of prayer.* San Francisco: HarperCollins.

Frisch, N. C., Dossey, B. M., Guzzetta, C. E., & Quinn, J. A. (2000). *AHNA standards of holistic nursing practice: Guidelines for caring and healing.* Gaithersburg, MD: Aspen.

Henry, G. C. (1998). *Christianity and the images of science.* Macon, GA: Smyth & Helwys.

Puchalski, C. M. (2001). The role of spirituality in health care. *BUMC Proceedings, 14,* 352–357.

Shelly, J. A., & Miller, A. B. (1999). *Called to care.* Downers Grove, IL: InterVarsity Press.

Taylor, E. J. (2002). *Spiritual care: Nursing theory, research and practice.* Upper Saddle River, NJ: Prentice Hall.

Westberg, G. E., & McNamara, J. W. (1990). *The parish nurse: Providing a minister of health for your congregation.* Minneapolis, MN: Augsburg Fortress.

Wilt, D. L., & Smucker, C. J. (2002). *Nursing the spirit: The art and science of applying spiritual care.* Washington, DC: American Nurses Association.

12

Evidence-Based Practice and Nursing Research

Lisa Sams
Barbara Ritzert

> " To move evidence from the "book to the bedside," information from evidence-based guidelines must be integrated into daily patient care processes, and information must be readily available and observable for practitioners. "
>
> Titler, 2001

LEARNING OBJECTIVES

At the completion of this chapter, the reader will be able to:

➤ Identify the essential characteristics of evidence-based practice.

➤ Discuss the steps to beginning an evidence-based approach to clinical practice.

➤ Define evidence-based practice.

➤ Distinguish between the traditional approach to answering clinical questions and an evidence-based approach to addressing clinical questions.

➤ Delineate the barriers to using evidence.

➤ Identify strategies that research has shown to be effective in helping clinicians incorporate and change their practice.

MediaLink   www.prenhall.com/haynes

Additional online resources including NCLEX review questions, critical thinking questions, and real-world activities for this chapter can be found on the Companion Website at www.prenhall.com/haynes.

For decades, professional nurses have arrived at work every day fully embracing their commitment to the mission of providing optimal patient care to each and every patient they encounter. Providing care in a managed care environment has challenged nurses to reframe this mission to include the delivery of optimal health care in a cost-conscious manner, using available resources. This approach has necessitated close examination of health care practices so as to ensure that patient care interventions are based on sound clinical judgment and scientific evidence rather than the limitations of tradition, organizational culture, and ritualistic practices. The rising cost of health care has stimulated the need to ground clinical decisions using a systematic determination of which patient care interventions are clinically effective and, when evidence supports, economically efficient. In order to respond to this demand, practice must be continuously examined, evaluated, clarified, and refined through systematic evaluation of best practices from a plethora of information sources available to the practitioner. Evidence methodology will free the clinician from unnecessary searches and reviews because these methods focus on sources that will most directly aid patient-problem clinical decision-making.

Evidence-based practice is characterized as an approach to care in which clinical decision-making is based on the clinician's critical appraisal of available relevant research. This type of practice emphasizes the patient's role in the decision-making process (Sackett, Rosenberg, Gray, Haynes, & Richardson, 1996). On the surface this appears to be a logical approach to patient care; however, evidence-based practice is indeed countercultural because clinician preference is deemphasized (Dooks, 2001; Soukup, 2000). Instead, clinical decision-making incorporates patient preferences into the triad with consideration of the evidence and clinical circumstances (Guyatt & Drummond, 2001).

Evidence-based practice as a formalized methodology can trace its origins to Canada and the United Kingdom. In the 1970s, Archie Cochrane, a British epidemiologist, challenged physicians to learn how to apply research rather than rely on habits and opinions to guide their practice. In a now famous speech, he "awarded" a wooden spoon to the specialty in medicine that applied research least in practice, obstetrics and gynecology. He was vocal about medical education's reliance on authority with little value placed on current research as a constantly renewing source of knowledge to guide care.

Today, the result of that lightning strike by Dr. Cochran is the Cochrane Collaborative. The Cochran Collaborative is an international and virtual organization with practice specialty groups that systematically appraise studies and report findings in easy-to-use two-page abstracts that busy clinicians can readily access from the Cochrane Web site. The fuel for much of the change occurring within medical and nursing education and health care decision-making in general has come from the Cochrane movement.

As expected, this paradigm shift has generated a flurry of controversy in the literature over what constitutes "best available evidence" (Colyer & Kamath, 1999; Goode & Piedalue, 1999). Considerable confusion still exists about the intent of "best evidence." Not only have some physicians labeled it "cookbook medicine," but also many who believe in the need to appraise and apply quality research feel that evidence methodology values only randomized controlled trials as the legitimate research and, therefore, the only research that has value in clinical decision-making. However, exclusive reliance on randomized controlled trials is no longer seen as the only study design useful in supporting clinical decisions (Sackett, Straus, Richardson, Rosenberg, & Haynes, 2000).

It is important to remember that when Cochrane launched his wake-up call there was no methodology for categorizing or grading any of the millions of published studies. It was impossible to compare studies and make recommendations based on strength of the evidence because that methodology did not exist. Beginning the transition to more systematic methods with classification and use of randomized controls was a logical starting point.

During the past decade, evidence-based practice has gradually been embraced as a positive direction in multidisciplinary circles of health care. Criteria to determine best evidence has expanded to include multiple sources of data to appropriately address the clinical question at hand (Jennings, 2000; Stetler et al., 1998; Tanner, 1999). Despite the gradual adoption of the terminology of some of the methods, a single unifying definition of evidence-based practice is lacking. A recent review of the literature points to two definitions for evidence-based medicine and seven definitions for evidence-based practice in nursing (Table 12–1). The one underlying commonality is use of research in practice (Jennings & Loan, 2001).

The overall goal of evidence-based practice is to improve patient outcomes. This can be accomplished by bridging the gap between research and clinical care, reducing variations in individual practice, replacing questionable practice with proven effective practice, and ultimately improving quality while reducing costs (Deaton, 2001; Rosenfeld et al., 2000).

Historically, answers to clinical questions in nursing were sought in a textbook, an isolated journal article, consultation with another nurse on the unit, the nurse manager, or perhaps a clinical nursing instructor (Kessenich, Guyatt, & DiCenso, 1997; Stotts, 1999). Using evidence-based practice, nurses seek a more in-depth analysis, which requires critical thinking skills, a working knowledge of research evaluation, documented standards of care, and the ability to determine applicability of documentation or data to the patient issue or the population at hand (Table 12–2).

Beginning an Evidence-Based Approach to Clinical Practice

Evidence-based practice provides a systematic approach to implementation of the concepts in any practice setting (Greenlaugh, 1997). This type of practice requires that the nurse:

- Formulate a problem statement reflecting the clinical question or patient care issue.
- Investigate and identify the best evidence available to answer the question.
- Appraise the evidence critically to assess validity, reliability, and clinical applicability.
- Implement or apply the results of the critical appraisal in the clinical setting.
- Evaluate the results of the practice decision in terms of patient outcome or clinical performance.

Focusing Clinical Questions

Evidence-based practice begins with a precise definition of a clinical problem or issue to be addressed; clinicians structure a clinical question in order to find the best answer that evidence can provide. There are two types of questions that the clinician needs to learn how to structure in order to begin the process of using the evidence. The questions are described as either background or foreground questions.

Background questions help the clinician identify basic facts about a problem. For example, "What are the most common pathogens identified in nosocomial pneumonia for patients on ventilators?" The answer to this question provides basic information to understand a clinical situation. **Foreground questions**, on the other hand, are outcome-based questions. Learning to effectively structure this type of question is the starting point for the clinician to clearly define the problem in question and then to find answers more efficiently.

Sackett et al. (2000) delineate the questions further by showing how the level of the clinician's experience affects the type of question most frequently used. Background questions are most often used by less experienced clinicians in order to build their knowledge base in basic principles related to patient problems, whereas more experienced clinicians focus on the outcomes of their interventions a larger percentage of the time. The questions are a developmental approach to clinical decision-making and effective use of the evidence. For example, if the background question on nosocomial pneumonia in ventilator patients is expanded to a foreground question about a specific patient (e.g., Mrs. Jones, a 75-year-old patient with Alzheimer's disease), the question might be "In elderly patients diagnosed with Alzheimer's disease who are confused, is the nursing intervention of increased surveillance as effective as use of siderails as a treatment intervention to decrease patient falls?"

Properly constructed questions include four essential elements: (a) the patient or problem, (b) the link between the proposed issue and current intervention, (c) an alternative intervention if known, and (d) the desired outcome for the patient (Greenlaugh, 1997). When properly formulated, this question will focus the literature review or scope of search to retrieve the needed information. For example, "In women who are diagnosed with preterm labor and cervical changes, are those women who are treated with bed rest and

---

Critical Thinking and Reflection

How will increasing your competence in structuring clinical questions improve your ability to use the evidence? Develop background and foreground questions to initiate a search with the Cochrane Abstracts. Select a clinical problem you have recently confronted (for example, a patient with respiratory disease and another co-morbid diagnosis) and define both types of questions to guide your search for an abstract. If a Cochrane Review does not exist for this problem, what are your next steps?

Table 12-1　Definitions of Evidence-Based Practice

Evidence-Based Medicine	Evidence-Based Practice as Defined in Nursing Literature	Commonalities and Differences
"Evidence-based medicine deemphasizes intuition, unsystematic clinical experience, and pathophysiologic rationale as sufficient grounds for clinical decision making and stresses the examination of evidence from clinical research" (Evidence-Based Medicine Working Group [EBMWG], 1992, p. 2420).	"Uses research findings derived chiefly from randomized controlled clinical trials or other experimental designs to evaluate specific interventions" (Gerrish & Clayton, 1998, p. 58).	• Specific reference to randomized controlled trials (RCTs) and interventions. • Congruent with the Cochrane framework.
"Evidence-based medicine is the conscientious, explicit, and judicious use of current best evidence in making decisions about the care of individual patients. The practice of evidence-based medicine means integrating individual clinical expertise with the best available external clinical evidence from systematic research" (Sackett, Rosenberg, Gray, Haynes, & Richardson, 1996, p. 71).	"Evidence-based clinical practice involves the synthesis of knowledge from research, retrospective or current chart review, quality improvement and risk data, international, national, and local standards, infection control data, pathophysiology, cost effectiveness analysis, benchmarking data, patient preferences, and clinical expertise" (Goode & Piedalue, 1999, p. 15).	• Expands what qualifies as evidence beyond research. • Inclusion of pathophysiology is a notable departure from the EBMWG (1992) definition that deemphasized pathophysiology as evidence.
	"Evidence-based nursing practice is the conscientious, explicit, and judicious use of theory-derived, research-based information in making decisions about care delivery to individuals or groups of patients and in consideration of individuals' needs and preference" (Ingersoll, 2000, p. 152).	• Expands Sackett and colleagues' concept of evidence to include information from theory and research. • Includes consideration of patients' preferences.

Adapted with permission from Jennings & Loan (2001).

tocolytics more likely to experience increased gestation than women who are treated with tocolytics alone but allowed bathroom privileges?" If the clinician is also interested in knowing about the effects of bed rest on the mother, a second question could be formulated: "In women who are treated with bed rest and tocolytics, is the outcome of increased gestation likely to compensate for the maternal effects from prolonged bed rest?"

Identify the Best Evidence Available

Evidence may be obtained from a variety of studies ranked in terms of reliability, validity, and clinical effec-tiveness. Traditionally, the medical community has ranked the randomized controlled trial (RCT) as the "gold standard" for clinical research because of its ability to establish controls on other factors that could affect the outcomes or findings. The most rigorously designed and implemented RCTs provide a higher degree of confidence in their findings than even other RCTs that are not as rigorously structured.

Concealment is an example of how bias can be presented or introduced into a study. For example, does everyone know who is receiving an intervention, or is only the patient unaware, or are the patient and the researcher both unaware? Critical appraisal, using evi-

Table 12-2   Definitions of Evidence-Based Nursing

Source	Definition
Kessenich, Guyatt, & DiCenso, 1997, p. 26	"Evidence-based nursing involves skills of problem definition, searching, evaluation and the application of original research literature . . . [it] is a- . . . philosophy of learning that guides students to develop skills in problem definition, location, and evaluation of research to assist them in clinical decision-making throughout their professional education and practice."
Stetler et al., 1998, pp. 48–49	"Evidence-based nursing de-emphasizes ritual, isolated, and unsystematic clinical experiences, ungrounded opinions, and tradition as a basis for nursing practices, and stresses instead the use of research findings and, as appropriate, quality improvement data, other operational and evaluation data, the consensus of recognized experts, and affirmed experience to substantiate practice."
Stevens & Pugh, 1999, p. 155	"Evidence-based nursing [is] practice that relies on information generated from results of scientific research."

Source: Reprinted with permission from Jennings & Loan (2001).

dence methods, helps the clinician recognize elements in the study where bias is introduced. Lack of concealment is just one example.

Not all questions of clinical importance are interventional in nature; therefore, RCTs may not be the appropriate method of applied research. For example, if the researcher wants to look at neonatal outcomes of males who were exposed to certain toxins in the work environment, a cohort study design would be used. The investigator would select an unexposed group of males and an exposed group. Each group would be followed and evaluated for differences in neonatal outcomes. Another study design, the case control, is begun by first identifying the outcome, whereas the cohort study begins by looking at the exposure. Case control studies help look at problems that tend to develop over time or are rare in occurrence (Guyatt & Drummond, 2001). Learning how to evaluate the strength of the study design, whether it is an interventional, trial, or observational study is essential if the clinician is going to decide which evidence merits use in practice.

Stetler et al. (1998) provides a scale rating the quality of different levels of evidence with the meta-analysis of controlled studies at the highest level, followed in descending level of evidence by individual experimental studies, quasi-experimental studies, nonexperimental studies (comparative, descriptive, or qualitative studies), program evaluation, and expert opinions as the lowest level of acceptable evidence. However, the overall basis for nursing practice described by Stetler et al. (1998) includes evidence-

based practice methods (research findings, performance data, consensus recommendations of recognized experts, affirmed experience) in conjunction with philosophical/conceptual guidelines for practice, regulatory basis for practice, and traditional basis for practice.

There are a number of rating scales in use that provide a frame of reference for selecting a study design and therefore the level of control that the design provides regarding the question under investigation. The rating scale is a quick reference for the clinician as well as a means for standardizing the way clinicians communicate about types of studies. For example, if the clinician wanted to know whether one form of skin preparation over another was more effective for IV insertion with immunocompromised patients, a one case descriptive study from one hospital is not a good basis for making changes in clinical practice. On the other hand, if the clinician were able to access a **meta-analysis** (a statistical method of combining the results of similar studies to look at the results when all of the studies have been combined) of several RCTs on the issue the synthesis of the meta-analysis would have more value in decision-making about the best form of skin preparation to use in immunocompromised patients.

Goode and Piedaluc (1999) expand the repertoire of acceptable sources of evidence-based data to include synthesis of information from valid and current research as the pinnacle of evidence, with connecting or supportive evidence from a variety of nonresearch resources to further clarify or strengthen the evidence.

Additional sources identified are (a) retrospective or concurrent chart review; (b) quality improvement and risk data; (c) international, national, and local standards; (d) infection control data; (e) pathophysiology; (f) cost-effectiveness analysis; (g) benchmarking data; (h) patient preferences; and (i) clinical expertise. The additional sources provide evidence in the form of supporting data to assist overall decision-making in effective patient care.

Searching for the Evidence

Searching for the answers to focused clinical questions can be time consuming and even frustrating to the uninitiated. Although all clinicians should have basic search skills, clinicians who practice evidence-based clinical decision-making also know that the health science librarian is a key member of the care team. In fact, some centers have librarians round with the residents and nurses in order to support the clinical questions in real time. McMaster University in Canada has pioneered these strategies, and the work of Ann McKibbon offers a helpful resource for searching the literature (McKibbon, Eady, & Marks, 1999).

Effective search strategies lay the foundation for an evidence-based practice. Because the volume of information sources is too large for anyone to find useful, McKibbon et al. (1999) offer a five-source strategy to approach maintaining clinically helpful information. This strategy includes:

- Textbooks
- Journal subscriptions
- Personal collection
- MEDLINE or other large database services
- Internet connection

Textbooks, no less than two years out of date when published, provide a good resource for "established" knowledge such as anatomy, developmental milestones, and incubation periods of diseases (McKibbon et al., 1999). Textbooks can be a good resource for many questions posed by clinicians.

Journal subscriptions are an investment in knowledge growth, when selected wisely, to support the clinician's specific purpose. Studies have shown that the number of articles in the leading journals that are directly useful in clinical practice is less than 20% (Geyman, Deyo, & Ramsey, 2000). In an effort to address this gap for clinicians, secondary journals are now available. These secondary journals provide abstracts and commentaries on published studies for quick reference. When a study is relevant to the clinician's daily work, the clinician should obtain a copy of the full text in order to critically appraise it before making substantial change in practice. Secondary journals to address the clinical practice gap include the *ACP Journal Club, Evidence-Based Nursing, Evidence-Based Mental Health*, and *Evidence-Based Health Policy and Management* (McKibbon et al., 1999).

Personal collections are another way to maintain ongoing knowledge development. Computers and the Internet have made maintaining a collection much easier. Sigma Theta Tau provides a service that allows clinicians to enter clinical preference and obtain weekly updates of studies published in specified topic areas.

With over 25,000 health care journals now in print, clinicians need to use research systems such as MEDLINE and CINAHL to make retrieval possible. MEDLINE is operated by the National Library of Medicine and contains over 4,000 journals in its database. The National Library of Medicine provides free access to MEDLINE. Also within the National Library of Medicine is Gateway, a site that allows the clinician to access project records for health services research and the development of clinical practice guidelines.

The CINAHL database is smaller than MEDLINE, with about 600 journals, and is specific to nursing and allied health literature. McKibbon et al. (1999) describe this database as much more complete than others because it provides enhancement over the traditional biographic information (e.g., full text of articles and other resources such as clinical practice guidelines).

EMBASE (Excerta Medica) is another resource that contains over 3,800 journals that focus on biomedical and pharmacological articles. Clinicians looking for information on drug-related studies, human medicine research, and European health care material will find EMBASE a good source (McKibbon et al., 1999). Without Internet access the clinician cannot gain essential information from any of these databases or obtain systematic reviews from the Cochran Collaboration or guidelines from the National Guideline Clearing House.

The Cochrane databases provide a collection of carefully catalogued clinical trials meeting specific criteria for reliability and validity as a source of evidence-based practice. The Cochrane Collaboration is a group of international institutions and scholars that maintain a systematic review of randomized clinical trials. Included in the review are descriptions of the research evidence and evaluation of the validity or the research findings to provide a concise source of information to clinicians to assist with clinical judgments. This information is not intended to dictate clinical protocols, but is provided as a piece of evidence taken into consideration along with the many other factors contributing to clinical patient decision-making strategies (Callister & Hobbins-Garbett, 2000).

Familiarity with search strategies or techniques enables one to streamline the search without compromising the breadth of available literature. Often, the best place to start with an electronic database search is to select the appropriate Medical Subject Heading or "MeSH" term used to identify the primary area of interest, and then narrow the search to include only review articles, meta-analysis, or practice guideline articles. Most databases will have a pull-down menu of available MeSH terms to choose from in identifying search criteria. Familiarity with Boolean search terms such as *and*, *or*, and *not* will assist with further refinement of the search to include or exclude subset topics associated with the area of interest. For example, to research our question regarding best practice associated with preterm labor, use of tocolytics, and bed rest, one would start with the MeSH term *preterm labor*. The search would then be refined with the connector "and" to include the terms *tocolytics* and *bed rest*. Online databases also provide numerous options to limit the search such as specific years of publication, types of subjects, types of articles (i.e., meta-analysis, review), and types of studies (i.e., randomized controlled trials, case-controlled studies). Most databases provide an online tutorial for the user; however, structure time in training with a health science librarian is essential to build a foundation in the complex process of searching the literature. Clinicians who are skilled in use of evidence methodologies rely on the expertise of the health science librarian to assist their more involved searches.

Critical Analysis of Literature

Following data retrieval, critical analysis of appropriateness of research design, validity, reliability, and applicability of the data to a particular clinical question is the next step in developing evidence-based practice (Stotts, 1999). **Internal validity** refers to the degree to which the study results can be attributed to the action of the independent variable versus other extraneous factors. **External validity** describes the degree to which the results can be generalized outside of the study population to a target population. Initial evaluation of validity is usually based on the study design used in describing clinical practice. The higher the degree of control in the research design, the greater degree of validity. The randomized clinical trial provides the highest degree of control where subjects are randomly assigned to an intervention group or a control group for concurrent study. The least controlled study with the least validity would be a case study or case report, which does not include randomization or study of a control group.

Reliability refers to the ability of the study measurements to be replicated and achieve the same outcome on a repeated basis. Applicability of the data to a particular clinical question addresses the appropriateness of the match between the study design and population to the clinical query at issue (Greenlaugh, 1997). Were the study patients similar to the population of patients of concern, and can the results be applied to local expectations and resources for patient care to improve patient outcomes (Deaton, 2001; Stotts, 1999)?

In the *Users Guide to the Medical Literature*, Guyatt and Drummond (2001) outline three key prompts that should be asked when critically appraising any study. These are:

1. Are the results valid?
2. What are the results?
3. How can the results be applied to patient care?

Within each of the three questions are imbedded subquestions that reflect the nature of the study. The subquestions for studies about therapy will differ from the subquestions about diagnosis and so on. This approach of structured questioning is one of the hallmark signs of evidence methodology—it is systematic. Without a systematic approach to appraisal, the clinician is unlikely to identify flaws that may affect the decision (a) to apply study findings or (b) understand other factors that may bring value to their practice. Learning the basic skills of evidence-based critical appraisal requires a commitment to knowledge acquisition. This skill represents the beginning of the lifelong learning described by Sackett in his early writing about evidence-based practice.

Systematic reviews are another important tool for the clinician. A systematic review is a study of other studies. The review begins with a systematic method similar to the one described above. The difference is that criteria are established before the review begins. The investigators define the clinical question to be reviewed, then undertakes an exhaustive search of the literature under that question. In a Cochrane systematic review, the team searches well beyond MEDLINE and other databases to include hand searches within the literature for studies, which have not been catalogued. Researchers whose studies were not published are interviewed if the research was completed, and the findings are available privately from the researcher. These important steps are taken to offset the documented publication bias for successful finding versus unsuccessful finding. When the review team has accumulated all of the literature, it is first reviewed according to the predetermined criteria for inclusion into the study. If a study does not meet the criteria, it is not reviewed.

All of the information about the review process is available to the clinician on the first page of the Cochran summary, where the methodology is described in brief sentences. Each Cochrane abstract includes the following framework, making the abstract a clinically useful tool:

- Background
- Objectives
- Search strategy
- Selection criteria
- Data collection and analysis
- Results
- Review conclusions

Systematic review may also contain a meta-analysis (Box 12–1). This provides "an analysis of analyses where pooled results of several studies provide a systematic quantitative review of the data" (Conn & Armer, 1994, p. 6).

Application and Implementation

Nursing practice, as well as care provided by other providers, is often based on habits or local opinion rather than evidence. This practice creates inconsistencies in care provided. Inconsistencies in practice have been one of the main driving forces that have led regu-

lators and consumers to demand quality improvement. These inconsistencies, also called variations, confuse patients and family members, which results in stress for the patient and family members and frustration among the health care givers.

How does the clinical care team begin to apply evidence related to a specific type of patient problem? Is "raw searching and appraising" the only answer? Fortunately, no. Creation of an interdisciplinary evidence-based practice team to evaluate the appropriateness of the literature and develop practice recommendations serves dual purposes of achieving collaboration with other disciplines, as well as building consensus to implement recommended changes in practice. Based on the review of current data in the literature, as well as collateral sources of evidence-based practice information (i.e., benchmarking data, cost-effective analysis, pathophysiology, chart review, quality improvement/ risk management data, standards of care, and patient preferences), a systematic plan to implement target areas of change in clinical practice to improve patient outcomes can be initiated.

Establishing a clinical guideline is an example of this type of project on a patient care unit. Guidelines are one of the tools that aid clinical decision-making and provide the method to control unnecessary variations. Ideally, the clinical team will have resources that are more refined than piles of individual studies. This is not always possible because systematic reviews, meta-analysis, and national evidence-based guidelines are not always available on the clinical problem under discussion. However, if this is a clinical team's first effort at

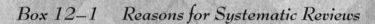

Box 12–1   Reasons for Systematic Reviews

A systematic review accomplishes the following:

1. Reduces large quantities of information into a manageable form.
2. Integrates existing information for decisions about clinical care, economic decisions, future research design, and policy formation.
3. Increases efficiency in time between research and clinical implementation.
4. Establishes generalizability across participants, across settings, and treatment variations and different study designs.
5. Assesses consistency and explains inconsistencies of relationships across studies.
6. Increases power in suggesting the cause and effect relationship.
7. Reduces bias from random and systematic error improving true reflection of reality.
8. Provides better continuous updates of new evidence.

Reprinted from Stevens, K. R., & Ledbetter, C. A. (2000) *Seminars in Perioperative Nursing*, Volume 9, Basics of Evidence-Based Practice, Part I: The Nature of the Evidence, pp. 91–97. Copyright 2000, with permission from Elsevier Science.

guideline development, it would be wise to begin with a clinical problem for which these higher-level resources exist.

Guyatt and Drummond (2001) offer four questions to keep in mind when evaluating the guideline or systematic review as a resource for a practice setting, or as a basis for an organization's guideline or pathway. These include:

- Did the recommendations consider all relevant patient groups, management options, and possible outcomes?
- Is there a systematic review of evidence linking options to outcomes for each relevant question?
- Is there an appropriate specification of values or preferences associated with outcomes?
- Do the authors indicate the strength of their recommendations? (Is there an evidence table?) (p. 185)

It is not uncommon for a clinical group to undertake a project such as a pathway or guideline and not use a systematic approach to produce their document. The lack of a systematic evaluation leaves the interpretation of various studies open to individual opinions and thus undermines the intent of an evidence-based document to guide clinical care. For an example of a national guideline that meets all four questions outlined above, the reader is referred to the American College of Cardiology and American Heart Association Guidelines for Management of Patients with Acute Myocardial Infarction (Ryan et al., 1996).

Evidence methodology helps the clinicians recognize the difference between opinion and evidence-based practice. This recognition is the first step toward evidence-based care as opposed to a traditional form of clinical decision-making that relies heavily on expert opinion. Often, many of the documents that come from national organizations rely primarily on expert opinion. It is important for clinicians to use the evidence methods questions that have been outlined here in order to evaluate information that is labeled "guidelines" or "standards." References alone do not provide reassurance that the document is based on anything other than opinion.

Evaluation

Outcomes as a result of evidence-based practice are determined by several factors including (a) quality of the clinical evidence on which practice is based and (b) successful communication and implementation of a change or modification in a clinical intervention or standard. Lack of communication, lack of an organized approach to a change in practice, or resistance from providers may interfere with anticipated outcomes of evidence-based practice (Goode & Piedalue, 1999). Evaluation, therefore, should address traditional practices, as well as process, impact, and outcome criteria following the recommended improvement in practice (Green & Kreuter, 1999; McKenzie & Smeltzer, 2001).

Process evaluation refers to the measurement of parameters specific to the process of investigating and implementing evidence-based practice. Was the review of evidence-based practice resources regarding a particular issue overwhelming, resulting in a limited assessment? Was there adequate communication and dissemination of information of what constitutes evidence-based practice? Were the procedures to implement a particular evidence-based practice approach organized and system friendly?

Impact evaluation focuses on the immediate, observable effects related to implementation of evidence-based practice. What is the acceptance level of the staff implementing evidence-based practice? Has clinical practice actually changed as a result of implementation of evidence-based practice recommendations, or is the revised standard in place but the practice remains the same? Has the change in practice resulted in time conservation, or has it added steps, requiring additional time to complete the procedure?

Outcome evaluation measures the overall result of the change in practice. Is there a reduction in the incidence of intravenous site infections as a result of a

---

Critical Thinking and Reflection

Imagine you have worked on the medical–surgical unit for less than a year and now you are part of the group that is preparing a guideline for management of asthma. Where will you begin to gather evidence when you are assigned to work on a guideline development committee? Use your understanding of the levels of studies and how to evaluate guidelines to outline an approach that will make the work more efficient. Access the National Guideline Clearinghouse and search for guidelines that may support your work, and evaluate the guideline for how the evidence was appraised and whether the strength of the evidence is clearly stated.

change in dressing technique? Is the recurrence of preterm labor treated with tocolytics increased in the patient on strict bed rest or the patient with bathroom privileges? Is the change in practice beneficial from a cost-conscious point of view?

The move for an outcome orientation to care is changing the face of how care is rendered, measured, and reimbursed. Outcome orientation is much more than measuring the length of stay, although this data is helpful. Outcome orientation looks for the effectiveness of interventions on the patient's outcomes. Outcome orientation takes into consideration multiple variables and also links with the evidence methods. The following formula describes these variables:

$$\text{Outcomes} = \frac{f\,(\text{baseline patient clinical characteristics and demographics-psychosocial})}{\text{Treatment and setting}}$$

"This formula indicates that clinical outcomes are the result of several factors which can be classified as risk factors (baseline status, clinical status, and demographic/psychological characteristics) and treatment characteristics (treatment and setting)" (Kane, 1997, p. 7).

The formula also points to the importance of adjusting for the risks that are inherent in some of the variables. Without this adjustment, comparisons between interventions and patient types will not be equitable, and erroneous conclusions may be drawn. This model can also draw the connection for the use of evidence methods and measuring outcomes.

Earlier in this chapter, discussions for structuring clinical questions were addressed as the first step for finding answers about the management of patient problems. Kane's (1997) outcome model can be used to show the connection between structuring of the clinical question and the outcomes. Using the earlier examples about nosocomial pneumonia for ventilator patients, the example can be expanded to the next logical step for clinical quality management. The question is revised from one that was designed to help identify the best treatment option to one that will now help measure (and therefore evaluate) the outcomes of the care. For example:

- *Sample foreground question.* In elderly patients diagnosed with Alzeheimer's disease who are con-

fused, is the nursing intervention of increased surveillance as effective as use of siderails as a treatment intervention to decrease patient falls?"

- *Extending the question to review the outcomes.* In elderly patients in a long-term care facility who are diagnosed with dementia, did the outcomes of those who had increased surveillance by registered nurses versus use of siderails only have less falls during the 12 month period of 2003?

This question becomes a quality improvement measure that will yield further data to guide clinical decision-making. Evidence-based practice can be the vehicle to outcomes management if the outcomes are tracked and the data used in conjunction with evolving research findings. This combination will be a renewing source of improvement to benefit all patients.

Barriers to Adoption of Evidence-Based Practice

Organizational Culture

If evidence-based practice is good for the patient and good for the clinician, why is it not integrated into every clinical care unit? Studies have looked at barriers to this use of evidence, and the findings are summarized in Table 12–3. The barriers fall into two general categories, clinician and environmental barriers.

A consistent finding among all studies that seek to determine barriers to the implementation of evidenced-based care includes reliance on routine or usual care (Newman, Papadopoulos, & Sigsworth, 1998; Nolan et al., 1998; Parahoo, 2000; Thompson, Bell, & Prevost, 1999). This reliance on routines is likely to be the biggest barrier for clinicians who are working to develop evidence methods within their clinical areas. Changing these routines means the culture is being challenged, and this is very threatening.

Clinicians developing evidence-based practice will be more successful if they are working in the context of an environment supporting evidence-based concepts

---

Critical Thinking and Reflection

Transition to an evidence-based practice approach to clinical care requires a change in practice for individuals. How will knowledge of change theory and stages of change facilitate adoption of evidence-based practice in your clinical setting?

French (1999) describes a particular obstetrical unit in which 5% of the patients experienced perinatal loss; however, there were no provisions for bereavement support services. Studies available in the literature at the time supported and clearly extolled the benefits of bereavement interventions; however, the cultural climate of the caregivers was such that such interventions were believed to actually have negative consequences on their unique patient population. It was therefore decided by the staff to engage in a qualitative study in their unit to explore the patients', nurses', and physicians' experience with a therapeutic relationship providing bereavement support measures described in the literature. Using an open-ended questionnaire, a group of patients experiencing perinatal loss were interviewed at their post-

partum visit. The interviews concluded in fact that patients perceived the interventions, as well as the staff, to be helpful. Through the study they were also able to isolate the cultural barriers among the medical and nursing staff that were thought to be obstacles to adopting bereavement interventions. As a result, both medical and nursing staff participated in established bereavement support programs for perinatal loss, instituting a formalized bereavement program in their unit.

In certain settings, randomized controlled studies are not feasible, nor are they the desired method of study. In this circumstance, a qualitative study was initiated with a positive outcome in patient care and a leap forward in unit culture.

(Colyer & Kamath, 1999; McSherry & Proctor-Childs, 2000; Rambur, 1999). The overall success of an evidence-based practice approach is directly proportional to the depth and breadth of support in various leadership tiers from the patient unit to the executive board of the organization. As one would anticipate, early involvement of representatives at all levels will generate an infusion of financial, philosophical, and operational support for this approach to patient care. Potential barriers to evidence-based practice are (a) lack of education about evidence-based practice concepts, (b) lack of relevant nursing research, (c) tradition, (d) perceived threat to power or control, (e) local customs and opinions, (f) economic dissonance, (g) lack of information technology resources, (h) resistance to change, (i) insufficient infrastructure to support the change process, (j)

impaired communication processes, (k) perceived lack of time, and (l) lack of training to interpret research findings (Gennaro, Hodnett, & Kearney, 2001; Hunt, 2001; Kessenich et al., 1997; Rosenfeld et al., 2000).

Strategies to Help Clinicians Change

Many studies, hundreds in fact, have looked at strategies to help bring evidenced-based changes into the clinician's daily work. In 1999, the University of York published a review titled "Effective Health Care: Getting Evidence into Practice." This article provided a systematic review of over 400 selected studies that provide helpful insights into strategies that work and those that do not work. The resounding message about the strategies themselves is that passive dissemination alone

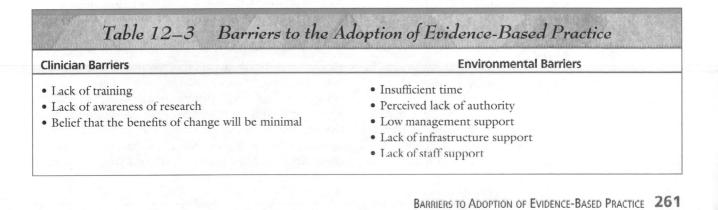

Table 12–3   Barriers to the Adoption of Evidence-Based Practice

Clinician Barriers	Environmental Barriers
• Lack of training • Lack of awareness of research • Belief that the benefits of change will be minimal	• Insufficient time • Perceived lack of authority • Low management support • Lack of infrastructure support • Lack of staff support

What potential barriers to adoption of evidence-based practice have you observed in the clinical setting? What advantage will you have as a new graduate in facilitating adoption of evidence-based practice initiatives?

does not work: "The naïve assumption that when research information is made available it is somehow accessed by practitioners, appraised and then applied in practice is now largely discredited" (University of York, 1999, p. 2). Passive dissemination includes printed materials (e.g., guidelines) and activities (e.g., lectures). These findings are summarized below:

- While individual beliefs, attitudes, and knowledge influence professional behavior, other factors including the organizational, economic, and community environments of the practitioner are also important.
- Any attempt to bring about change should first involve a "diagnostic analysis" to identify factors likely to influence the proposed change. Choice of dissemination and implementation interventions should be guided by the "diagnostic analysis and informed by knowledge of relevant research."
- A range of interventions has been shown to be effective in changing professional behavior in some circumstances. Multifaceted interventions targeting different barriers to change are more likely to be effective than single interventions.
- Successful strategies to change practice need to be adequately resourced and require people with appropriate knowledge and skills.
- Any systematic approach to changing professional practice should include plans to monitor and evaluate, and to maintain and reinforce the change (University of York, 1999).

Supporting Evidence-Based Practice Through Nursing Research

Nurturing Research in the Practice Environment

Health care finance in the United States is largely driven by outcome-oriented health care delivery systems. Escalating costs, disparities in allocation of resources, and a continuing decline in reimbursement for health care services from third-party payers have contributed to the demand for outcome-oriented care (Rambur, 1999). Prior to engaging in a health care initiative, consumers and financiers want to know what outcome is anticipated and what evidence is available to support certain practices that will result in the desired outcome (Myer, 1999; Sheinfeld Gorin, 1998; Soukup, 2000; Tanner, 1999). Valid studies measuring interventions for specific groups of patients have become the normative standard in allocation of funding and resource management.

Until recently, there has been limited availability and development of research studies to support many of the interventions in nursing practice (Kessenich et al., 1997; Manton, 1998). Studies have also validated that even if there is research available regarding clinical practice interventions, it is largely ignored by practicing nurses (Hunt, 2001; Rodgers, 2000). Collaborative practice research can accelerate the development of an accessible body of knowledge for nursing, as well as benefit overall patient care by generating enthusiasm for an evidence-based culture with a comprehensive approach to clinical practice. Collaborative research also serves to generate enthusiasm from a variety of health care resources, thus broadening the scope of expertise and extending the base of potential funding resources (Hockenberry-Eaton, Barrera, & Kline, 1998). The clinical staff nurse is often the best resource in identifying essential questions that will ultimately make a difference at the bedside. In collaboration, researchers provide expertise in study methodologies and data analysis. Nurse educators and health care administrators have access to information support services and personnel to gather data.

During the past 20 years, nursing literature has struggled with an acceptable avenue for integrating research into practice, and evidence-based practice brings us one step closer to achieving a realistic approach to this conundrum while promoting innovative practice strategies. In traditional settings for clinical nursing care, evidence-based practice will serve to translate research findings into real-world, practical application strategies at the patient's bedside. How much more exciting it would be to translate research finding to primary prevention strategies. As professional nurses embrace health promotion strategies and engage individuals in their home, social, and work environments, what a difference we can make before individuals reach nurses in our clinical environments.

Through evidence-based practice, we have the opportunity to combine current research, clinical judgment, and patient preferences to create a new standard for true collaboration and innovation in health care. We will then be equipped to proceed forward doing the things we ought to do, instead of looking backward at things left undone, which we ought to have done.

TRANSITION INTO PRACTICE

Is Policy or Evidence Driving the Practice?

This is not an esoteric question. Nurses daily confront the need to determine what is driving decisions about care. One example from the professional literature is a case study for analyzing the driving forces. What would you change in the following scenario?

> A dying patient is admitted to the hospital for supportive care and prescribed a nitroglycerin intravenous drip to control cardiac pain. He is transferred within the clinical setting twice to conform with the organization's policy, which requires that patients receiving nitroglycerin via IV drip to be admitted to the intensive care unit (ICU). His first move is out of the ICU because unit policy dictates that only patients eligible for full resuscitation efforts are admitted to the ICU. He never receives the medication because staff believed they were caught between an organization policy that said nitroglycerin drips must be administered in the ICU, but an ICU policy that precluded admitting patients that would not be resuscitated. The patient dies without having received relief from cardiac pain (Hansten & Washburn, 1999, p. 39).

When care is driven by evidence, the desired outcome is the basis for questioning and decision-making. The model for evidence-based decision-making appears in Figures 12–1 and 12–2.

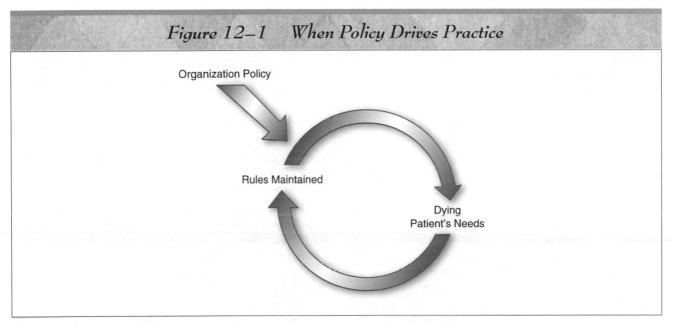

Figure 12–1   When Policy Drives Practice

Organization Policy

Rules Maintained

Dying Patient's Needs

Figure 12–2   Evidence-Driven Clinical Unit

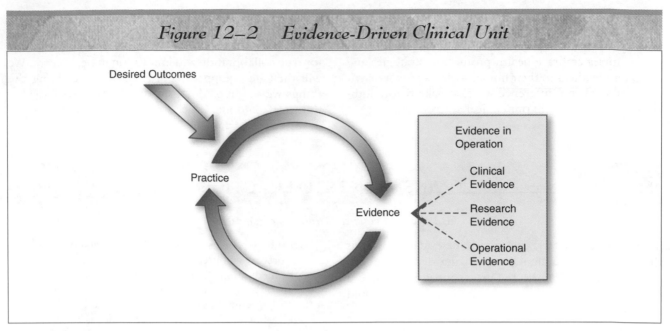

Copyright Clinical Linkages, Inc. 2000.

In this case, the desired outcome was a peaceful death wherein cardiac pain was controlled. **Clinical evidence** for a dying patient focuses on how effectively comfort is maintained. **Research evidence** for pain management is clear, and yet in this case evidence-based care was not used. With policy-driven clinical practice, **operational evidence** provides the basis for care. In this case the operational evidence, or the policy for nitroglycerin infusion, and the process used to support the policy rather than the patient were the driving forces. It is operational issues that present barriers to use of evidence, and for this patient an inability to attain the desired goal: death without cardiac pain (Hansten & Washburn, 1999).

If a patient problem–centered evidence-based approach had been used, staff would have questioned the purpose of the existing policy. The nurses caring for this patient would have questioned the policy and asked, "Was it designed for terminal patients?" Obviously, it was not; therefore, use of the policy should not have applied. Clearer analysis of the situation would have focused on the desired outcome, a death without cardiac pain. Use of evidence-based practice begins by asking patient problem–centered questions. Unfortunately for this man, the habits and routines within practice drove the outcomes.

KEY POINTS

1. The rising cost of health care has stimulated the need to ground clinical decisions using a systematic determination of which patient care interventions are clinically effective and, when evidence supports, economically efficient. In order to respond to this demand, practice must be continuously examined, evaluated, clarified, and refined through systematic evaluation of best practices from a plethora of information sources available to the practitioner.

2. Despite the gradual adoption of the terminology for the methods to establish best practice, a single unifying definition of evidence-based practice is lacking; however, the one underlying commonality for all definitions is research.

3. The goal of evidence-based practice is to improve patient care.

4. Evidence-based practice requires the nurse to focus clinical questions, identify the best evidence avail-

able, structure the evidence, critically analyze the literature, apply the information to the clinical situation, and evaluate the outcomes.

5. There are clinician and environment barriers to the adoption of evidence-based practice.

6. Until recently, there has been limited availability and development of research studies to support many of the interventions in nursing practice. Even when there is research available regarding clinical practice interventions, it is largely ignored by practicing nurses.

7. Evidence-based practice will serve to translate research findings into real-world, practical application strategies at the patient's bedside.

8. Through evidence-based practice, nurses have the opportunity to combine current research, clinical judgment, and patient preferences to create a new standard for true collaboration and innovation in health care. Nurses will then be equipped to proceed forward doing the things they ought to do, instead of looking backward at things that were left undone, which ought to have been done.

EXPLORE 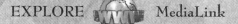 MediaLink

Critical thinking questions, essay questions, key terms, web links, activities, NCLEX review questions, and more interactive resources can be found on the Companion Website at www.prenhall.com/haynes. Click on Chapter 12 to select activities for this chapter.

REFERENCES

Callister, L., & Hobbins-Garbett, D. (2000). Cochrane pregnancy and childbirth database: Resource for evidence-based practice. *Journal of Obstetric, Gynecologic & Neonatal Nursing, 29*(2), 123–128.

Colyer, H., & Kamath, P. (1999). Evidence-based practice. A philosophical and political analysis: Some matters for consideration by professional practitioners. *Journal of Advanced Nursing, 29*(1), 188–193.

Conn, V., & Armer, J. (1994). A public health nurse's guide to reading meta-analysis research reports. *Public Health Nurse, 11*(3), 163–167.

Deaton, C. (2001). Outcomes measurement and evidence-based nursing practice. *Journal of Cardiovascular Nursing, 15*(2), 83–86.

Dooks, P. (2001). Diffusion of pain management research into nursing practice. *Cancer Nursing, 24*(2), 99–103.

Evidence-Based Medicine Working Group (EBMWG). (1992). Evidence-based medicine: A new approach to teaching the practice of medicine. *Journal of the American Medical Association, 268*(17), 2420–2425.

French, P. (1999). The development of evidence-based nursing. *Journal of Advanced Nursing, 29*(1), 72–87.

Geyman, J., Deyo, R., & Ramsey, S. (2000). *Evidence-based clinical practice: Concepts and approaches.* Boston: Butterworth-Heinemann.

Gennaro, S., Hodnett, E., & Kearney, M. (2001). Making evidence-based practice a reality in your institution. *American Journal of Maternal Child Nursing, 26*(5), 236–244.

Gerrish, K., & Clayton, J. (1998). Improving clinical effectiveness through an evidence-based approach: Meeting the challenge for nursing in the United Kingdom. *Nursing Administration Quarterly, 22*(4), 55–65.

Goode, C., & Piedalue, F. (1999). Evidence-based clinical practice. *Journal of Nursing Administration, 29*(6), 15–21.

Green, L., & Kreuter, M. (1999). *Health promotion planning: An educational and ecological approach* (3rd ed.). Mountain View, CA: Mayfield.

Greenlaugh, T. (1997). *How to read a paper: The basics of evidence based medicine.* London: BMJ Publishers.

Guyatt, G., & Drummond, R. (2001). *User's guide to the medical literature: A manual for evidence-based clinical practice.* Washington, DC: American Medical Association.

Hansten, R., & Washburn, M. (1999). Individual and organizational accountability for development of critical thinking. *Journal of Nursing Administration, 29*(11), 39–45.

Hockenberry-Eaton, M., Barrera, P., & Kline, N. (1998). Evidence-based practice: A role for nurse practitioners. *Journal of Pediatric Health Care, 12*, 338–339.

Hunt, J. (2001). Research into practice: The foundation for evidence-based care. *Cancer Nursing, 24*(2), 78–87.

Ingersoll, G. I. (2000). Op-ed. Evidence-based nursing: What it is and what it isn't. *Nursing Outlook, 48*(4), 151–152.

Jennings, B. (2000). Evidence-based practice: The road best traveled? *Research in Nursing & Health, 23*, 343–345.

Jennings, B., & Loan, L. (2001). Misconceptions among nurses about evidence-based practice. *Journal of Nursing Scholarship, 33*(2), 121–127.

Kane, R. (1997). *Understanding health care outcomes research.* Gaithersburg, MD: Aspen.

Kessenich, C., Guyatt, G., & DiCenso, A. (1997). Teaching nursing students evidence-based nursing. *Nurse Educator, 22*(6), 25–29.

Manton, A. (1998). Validating what we do: A word about evidence-based practice. *Journal of Emergency Nursing, 24*(1), 1–3.

McKibbon, A., Eady, A., & Marks, S. (1999). *PDQ: Evidence-based principles and practice.* London: B. C. Decker.

McSherry, R., & Proctor-Childs, T. (2000). Working out a strategy for evidence-based practice. *Nursing Times, 96*(3), 40–41.

McKenzie, J., & Smeltzer, J. (2001). *Planning, implementing, and evaluating health promotion programs* (3rd ed.). Boston: Allyn and Bacon.

Myer, S. (1999). Outcomes-based education in a critical care nursing course. *Critical Care Nursing Clinics of North America, 11*(2), 283–290.

Newman, M., Papadopoulos, I., & Sigsworth, J. (1998). Barriers to evidence-based practice. *Intensive and Critical Care Nursing, 14,* 231–238.

Nolan, M., Morgan, L., Curran, M., Clayton, J., Gerrish, K., & Parker, K. (1998). Evidence-based care: Can we overcome the barriers? *British Journal of Nursing, 7*(20), 1273–1278.

Parahoo, K. (2000). Barriers to, and facilitators of, research utilization among nurses in Northern Ireland. *Journal of Advanced Nursing, 31*(1), 89–91.

Rambur, B. (1999). Fostering evidence-based practice in nursing education. *Journal of Professional Nursing, 15*(5), 270–274.

Rodgers, S. (2000). The extent of nursing research utilization in general medical and surgical wards. *Journal of Advanced Nursing, 32*(1), 182–193.

Rosenfeld, P., Duthie, E., Bier, J., Bowar-Ferres, S., Fulmer, T., Iervolino, L., et al. (2000). Engaging staff nurses in evidence-based research to identify nursing practice problems and solutions. *Applied Nursing Research, 13*(4), 197–203.

Ryan, T. J., Anderson, J. L., Antman, E. M., Braniff, B. A., Brooks, N. H., Califf, R. M., et al. (1996). ACC/AHA guidelines for management of patients with acute myocardial infarction. A report of the American College of Cardiology/American Heart Association Task Force. *Journal of the American College of Cardiology, 28*(5), 1328–1428.

Sackett, D. L., Rosenberg, W. M., Gray, J. M., Haynes, R. B., & Richardson, W. S. (1996). Evidence based medicine: What it is and what it isn't. *British Medical Journal, 312,* 71–72.

Sackett, D., Straus, S., Richardson, W. S., Rosenberg, W., & Haynes, B. (2000). *Evidence-based medicine: How to practice and teach EBM* (2nd ed.). Edinburgh: Churchill-Livingstone.

Sheinfeld Gorin, S. (1998). Health promotion and education. In S. Sheinfeld Gorin & J. Arnold (Eds.), *Health promotion handbook.* St. Louis, MO: Mosby.

Soukup, M. (2000). The center for advanced nursing practice evidence-based practice model. *Nursing Clinics of North America, 35*(2), 301–309.

Stetler, C., Brunnell, M., Giuliano, K., Morsi, D., Prince, L., & Newell-Stokes, V. (1998). Evidence-based practice and the role of nursing leadership. *Journal of Nursing Administration, 28*(7/8), 45–53.

Stevens, K. R., & Ledbetter, C. A. (2000). Basics of evidence-based practice. Part I: The nature of the evidence. *Seminars in Perioperative Nursing, 9*(3), 91–97.

Stevens, K. R., & Pugh, J. A. (1999). Evidence-based practice and perioperative nursing. *Seminars in Perioperative Nursing, 8*(3), 155–159.

Stotts, N. (1999). Evidence-based practice what is it and how is it used in wound care? *Nursing Clinics of North America, 34*(4), 955–963.

Tanner, C. (1999). Evidence-based practice; research and critical thinking. *Journal of Nursing Education, 38*(3), 99.

Thompson, P., Bell, P., & Prevost, S. (1999). Overcoming barriers to research-based practice. *MEDSURG Nursing, 8*(1), 59–63.

Titler, M. G. (2001). Research utilization and evidence-based practice. In N. L. Chaska (ed.), The nursing profession: Tomorrow and beyond (pp. 423–437). Thousand Oaks, CA: Sage.

University of York. (1999). Effective health care: Getting evidence into practice. *Effective Healthcare, 5*(1), 1–16.

SUGGESTED READINGS

Dickersin, K., & Manheimer, E. (1998). The Cochrane Collaboration: Evaluation of health care and services using systematic reviews of the results of randomized controlled trials. *Clinical Obstetrics and Gynecology, 41*(2), 315–331.

Giacomini, M. K., & Cook, D. J. (2000). Users' guides to the medical literature. XXIII. Qualitative research in health care. A: Are the results of the study valid? *Journal of the American Medical Association, 284*(3), 357–362.

Giacomini, M. K., & Cook, D. J. (2000). Users' guide to the medical literature. XXIII. Qualitative research in health care. B: What are the results and how do they help me care for my patients? *Journal of the American Medical Association, 284*(4), 478–482.

Goode, C. (2000). What constitutes the "evidence" in evidence-based practice? *Applied Nursing Research, 13*(4), 222–225.

Lohr, K. N., & Carey, T. S. (1999). Assessing "best evidence": Issues in grading the quality of studies for systematic reviews. *Joint Commission Journal on Quality Improvement, 25*(10), 539–544.

13

Health Promotion

MELANIE MCEWEN

"To insure good health eat lightly, breathe deeply, live moderately, cultivate cheerfulness and maintain an interest in life.

William Louden (Zuck, 1997)

LEARNING OBJECTIVES

AT THE COMPLETION OF THIS CHAPTER, THE READER WILL BE ABLE TO:

➤ Discuss patterns of morbidity and mortality among Americans of various age groups.

➤ Explain the purpose of *Healthy People 2010* and relate how it can be used in nursing practice.

➤ Explain the Health Promotion Model and give examples of how it can be applied in nursing.

➤ Discuss risk factors for the leading cause of death and propose strategies to reduce mortality.

➤ Suggest interventions that can be used to promote health.

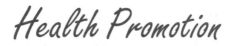

MediaLink   www.prenhall.com/haynes

Additional online resources including NCLEX review questions, critical thinking questions, and real-world activities for this chapter can be found on the Companion Website at www.prenhall.com/haynes.

*H*ealth promotion refers to those activities or actions related to encouraging individual lifestyles or personal choices that positively influence health. Physical activity and fitness, nutrition, and substance (tobacco, alcohol, etc.) use and abuse are examples of controllable behaviors or actions that will ultimately affect health (U.S. Department of Health and Human Services [DHHS], 2000a). In their practice, all nurses should be prepared for opportunities to assist patients (whether individual, families, groups, or communities) by providing information, counseling, advocacy, referral, or other interventions that will allow the patient to make informed choices to promote health.

Along with the care of the sick in and across all health environments and poplulation-based health care, the *Essentials* (1998) documents identifies health promotion as a fundamental aspect of nursing practice. Health promotion and illness prevention encompasses those interventions, such as counseling, screening, immunization, or education, that directly impact health to enhance wellness and/or prevent acute or chronic disease or disability. Health care providers have recognized for some time that for a disease (i.e., cancer or diabetes) or health problem (i.e., pregnancy or accidental injury) to occur, the host must be susceptible. This susceptibility may be termed **risk**.

In many cases, there are several characteristics that will increase an individual's risk; these are termed **risk factors**. For some illnesses, there may be only one or two risk factors. For example, a nonimmunized child being in contact with a child who has the virus may cause measles. In other cases, there may be a number of risk factors that work together or separately to affect a person's susceptibility. For example, teenage pregnancy is attributable to a complex interaction between a number of causative and contributing factors, including a lack of knowledge about sexuality and pregnancy prevention, lack of easily accessible contraception, peer pressure, low self-esteem, social patterns where teen mothers are more likely to be children of teen mothers, use of alcohol or other drugs, and so on.

Initially, general health promotion strategies such as health risk appraisal, promotion of exercise and physical fitness, improving nutrition, and reduction or elimination of harmful substances are described in the discussion of "health promotion." As positive health practices and potential threats to health are identified, nurses can assist individuals, families, and groups by developing plans and programs to promote health and prevent illness.

This chapter will present an overview of the many aspects of health promotion and risk reduction that are important for nurses to understand. Patterns of health for various groups, and examples of strategies to equip nurses to assist patients in identifying and reducing potentially harmful risk factors and in promoting health will be presented. Nurses practicing in all areas should learn and remain informed about actual and potential health problems and threats that are commonly encountered in the population they serve. They should be aware of risk factors and be prepared to offer education, counseling, and/or referral to patients to address these factors and thereby promote health. Strategies for obtaining and maintaining up-to-date health promotion information will be provided.

Indicators of Health

Leading causes of death in the United States are listed in Table 13–1. As depicted in the table, heart disease, cancer, cerebrovascular disease, and chronic obstructive pulmonary disease (COPD) are the leading four causes of death for Americans. But, as will be discussed later in the chapter, the leading causes of death change dramatically based on such factors as age and gender.

Risk factors for these causes of mortality have been identified, and measures to remove or moderate many

---

Critical Thinking and Reflection

Identify some of your risk factors based on age, gender, family history, socioeconomic status, lifestyle choices, and other factors described in this chapter. Identify possible risk factors in family members and friends. Make a list of what can be done to reduce the threat of your identified risk factors and develop a plan to reduce or eliminate at least one. Obtain a copy of *Healthy People 2010*. Review the priority areas and select those that are most applicable to your practice. Study the objectives and determine what actions you can take to help meet the objective in your practice.

Table 13–1　Ten Leading Causes of Death in the United States—1998

Cause of Death	Percentage of All Deaths
Diseases of the heart	31.0
Malignant neoplasms	23.2
Cerebrovascular diseases	6.8
COPD and allied conditions	4.8
Accidents and adverse effects	4.2
Pneumonia and influenza	3.9
Diabetes	2.8
Suicide	1.3
Kidney disease	1.1
Liver disease	1.1
All other causes	19.8

Source: National Center for Health Statistics (2000). *Health United States: 2000.* Hyattsville, MD: USDHHS/NCHS.

of them can be taken. For example, tobacco use, particularly cigarette smoking, is a risk factor strongly associated with each of the four leading causes of death. Indeed, according to McGinnis and Foege (1993), tobacco is implicated in almost 20% of deaths in the United States each year, totaling approximately 400,000 individuals. Additionally, diet and activity patterns are deemed to account for 14% of deaths (about 300,000/year). This is followed by alcohol, which contributes to about 5% of all deaths, as alcohol is associated with a significant percentage of accidents, suicides, and homicides, as well as chronic liver disease. Table 13–2 depicts the relationship between various risk factors and the 10 leading causes of death.

Overview of Health Promotion and Illness Prevention

Health promotion and illness prevention activities are aimed at protecting persons from disease and its consequences. In a classic discussion of disease prevention, Leavell and Clark (1965) presented the concepts of primary, secondary, and tertiary prevention, in which:

- **Primary prevention** activities prevent a problem before it occurs (e.g., immunizations to prevent disease).
- **Secondary prevention** activities provide early detection and intervention (e.g., screening for sexually transmitted diseases).

- **Tertiary prevention** activities correct a disease state and prevent it from further deteriorating (e.g., teaching insulin administration in the home).

As practiced today, most health services have little to do with health promotion and disease prevention, because they primarily focus on "cure" and illness management. As stated by Lamarche (1995) and others (Evans & Stoddard, 1994; Torrens, 1999), there is no convincing evidence that the amount of money expended for health care improves health. The real determinants of health are preventative efforts and include the provision of education, housing, food, a minimum decent income, and a safe social and physical environment. A large proportion of the gross domestic product in the United States—close to one-seventh—is spent on health care or "cure" for individuals. This focus on cure may divert money from needed resources and services that do determine health promotion strategies for tobacco, alcohol, and drug use and other public health interventions such as immunizations, clean water, and air quality (Evans & Stoddard, 1994; National Center for Health Statistics [NCHS], 2000).

Continuing overexpansion of the current health care system may be detrimental to health by preventing significant expenditures on education and other efforts that could positively impact health. Managed care organizations (MCOs), which focus on prevention, have begun to show that the rate of increase in health care costs has slowed for persons receiving these services (Shine, 1995; Torrens & Williams, 1999). Prevention programs for those enrolled in MCOs may help reduce costs. Reductions in health care spending

Table 13–2   Relationship Between Risk Factors and 10 Leading Causes of Death

Cause of Death	Smoking	High-Fat, Low-Fiber Diet	Sedentary Lifestyle	High Blood Pressure	Elevated Cholesterol	Obesity	Diabetes	Alcohol Abuse
Heart disease	X	X	X	X	X	X	X	X
Cancer	X	X	X			X		X
Stroke	X	X		X	X	X		
COPD	X							
Unintentional injury	X							X
Pneumonia and influenza	X							
Diabetes		X	X			X	X	
Suicide								X
Kidney disease	X			X	X	X	X	X
Liver disease								X

Who pays for health care services for the uninsured, poor, and other vulnerable populations? Discuss the moral/ethical implication of the growing uninsured/underinsured population in the United States. Do you see this as a national economic crisis?

What national and local efforts are being implemented to address health care needs of this population? What activities do you and your school of nursing engage in that support health care for vulnerable populations?

focusing on "cure" could allow investments in adequate housing, jobs, nutrition, and safe workplaces and other environments. This will ultimately reduce disparities in health and enhance health and quality of life for all Americans. To reduce the need for "cure," though, more attention needs to be directed toward reducing preventable, costly health problems, such as lung cancer, teenage pregnancy, or AIDS. Nurses can play an important role in this process.

Healthy People 2010

Healthy People: The Surgeon General's Report on Health Promotion and Disease Prevention was initially published in 1979 as a national prevention initiative of the U.S. Department of Health and Human Services (DHHS, 2000a). The 1979 version included a set of five goals (reduce mortality among four different age groups—infants, children, adolescents, and adults—and increase independence among older adults).

An updated version, *Healthy People 2000*, was published in 1989. *Healthy People 2000* contained three board goals:

- Increase the span of healthy life for Americans.
- Reduce health disparities among Americans.
- Achieve access to preventive services for all Americans (DHHS, 1989).

Healthy People 2000 was developed to provide direction for individuals to change personal behaviors, and for organizations and communities to use to improve health through health promotion. It was organized under the broad categories of health promotion, health protection, and preventive services. The document contained more than 300 objectives organized into 22 priority areas. Although only a portion of the objectives set forth in *Healthy People 2000* were met, the initiative was extremely successful in raising public and professional awareness of health behaviors and health promotional activities. The objectives were used by states, local health departments, and private-sector health care

workers to (a) determine the relative health of their community and (b) set goals for the future.

A third edition, *Healthy People 2010*, was introduced in January 2000. It expands on the objectives of *Healthy People 2000*. A broadened scientific base and improved surveillance and data systems were emphasized. There is also a heightened awareness of preventive health services, which is reflective of changes in demographics, science, technology, and disease. *Healthy People 2010* lists two broad goals:

Goal 1: Increase quality and years of healthy life.
Goal 2: Eliminate health disparities.

Goal 1 moves beyond the idea of increasing life expectancy to incorporate the concept of "health-related quality-of-life." **Health-related quality-of-life** (HRQOL) is a concept of health that includes aspects of both physical and mental health and their determinants, and measures functional status and well-being. By integrating mental and physical health concepts, it provides a way to expand the definition of health beyond simply being the opposite of the negative concepts of disease and death (DHHS, 2000a).

Implications for Nursing

In *Healthy People 2010*, some 467 objectives are divided into 28 focus areas (Box 13–1). The objectives may be used as a framework to guide health promotion activities in schools, clinics, worksites, and so forth, as well as for community-wide initiatives (DHHS, 2000a). All health care practitioners should review *Healthy People 2010* objectives, focusing on those areas relevant to their practice. Whenever possible, objectives should be incorporated into programs, events, and publications, and should be used as a framework to promote healthy individuals, families, groups, and communities.

Progress toward achieving the goals of *Healthy People 2010* focus on positively impacting health through:

- Increased physical activity
- Weight management

Box 13–1 Healthy People 2010 *Focus Areas*

1. Access to quality health services
2. Arthritis, osteoporosis, and chronic back conditions
3. Cancer
4. Chronic kidney disease
5. Diabetes
6. Disability and secondary conditions
7. Educational and community-based programs
8. Environmental health
9. Family planning and sexual health
10. Food safety
11. Health communication
12. Heart disease and stroke
13. HIV
14. Immunizations and infectious diseases
15. Injury and violence prevention
16. Maternal, infant, and child health
17. Medical product safety
18. Mental health and metal disorders
19. Nutrition
20. Occupational safety and health
21. Oral health
22. Physical activity and fitness
23. Public health infrastructure
24. Respiratory diseases
25. Sexually transmitted diseases
26. Substance abuse
27. Tobacco use
28. Vision and hearing

- Reduction in tobacco and other substance abuse
- Responsible sexual behavior
- Promotion of mental health
- Reduction in injury and violence
- Improvements in environmental quality
- Greater access to immunizations and health care

These indicators are intended to help all Americans understand the importance of health promotion and disease prevention and to encourage participation for improving health in the next decade.

The Health Promotion Model

Since Nightingale's time, nurses have recognized the need to impact health through interventions aimed at reducing risk and preventing illness. This notion received increasing emphasis in the discipline during the 1970s and into the 1980s. In the early 1980s, noted scholar Nola Pender first presented the Health Promotion Model (HPM). The HPM was proposed as a framework for integrating nursing and behavioral science perspectives that influence health behaviors. The model was used as a guide to explore the bio/psycho/social processes that motivate individuals to engage in behaviors directed toward health enhancement. The model was modified slightly in the late 1980s, and then again in 1996, and has been used extensively as a framework for research aimed at predicting health promoting lifestyles (Pender, 1996).

The three major concepts of the HPM are (a) individual characteristics and experiences, including prior related behavior and personal factors; (b) behavior-

Research Application

The Health Promotion Model

Lucas, Orshan, and Cook (2000) used Pender's Health Promotion Model to investigate the role that certain cognitive-perceptual factors (i.e., health self-determinism, learned helplessness, self-esteem, and perceived health) and modifying factors (i.e., age, race, marital status, education, and income) play in older women's health-promoting behaviors. Their study involved conducting several surveys on a convenience sample of 107 older women (mean age 76.7). Health promoting behaviors examined by the researchers included health responsibility, physical activity, nutrition, spiritual growth, interpersonal relations, and stress management.

Using canonical correlations, the researchers determined that age, marital status, race, education, self-esteem, perceived health, and health self-determinism contributed to health-promoting behaviors of physical activity, nutrition, spiritual growth, and interpersonal relations. Benefits noted among those engaging in health promotional behaviors were better psychological well-being, coping with issues of aging, social interaction, improved function, and management of existing health problems.

One significant internal barrier identified by the study was perceived physical difficulties with health-promoting behaviors. External barriers included lack of support from others and structural barriers.

The researchers concluded that nurses should establish partnerships with older women to foster health promotion. Interventions should include: clarification of the women's goals, motivations, and perceived barriers to achieving goals, and identification of ways to enhance health promotion knowledge and resources to overcome barriers.

specific cognitions and affect such as perceived benefits of action, perceived barriers to action, perceived self-efficacy, activity-related affect, interpersonal influences, and situational influences; and (c) behavioral outcomes such as commitment to a plan of action, immediate competing demands and preferences, and health-promoting behavior (Pender, Murdaugh & Parson, 2002). According to the model, the behavior outcome of "health promoting behavior" results from a commitment to a plan of action that is set in place by behavior-specific cognitions and affect. These behavior-specific cognitions will have been influenced by individual characteristics and experiences, such as prior related behavior and personal factors. Figure 13–1 shows the HPM.

Health promotion services are essential for improving health everywhere. People of all ages can benefit from health promotion care, which should be delivered at sites where people spend much of their time (e.g., schools and worksites). Using the model, nurses can develop and execute health-promoting interventions focusing on individuals, groups, and families in schools, nursing centers, occupational health settings, and the community at large. Nurses should work toward empowerment for self-care and enhancing patients' capacity for self-care through education and development. The focus of nurses should also help reduce barriers or modify situational influences that interfere with health.

Health Promotion Across the Lifespan

As mentioned earlier, causes of morbidity and mortality vary considerably based on age, gender, race/ethnic group, and socioeconomic status, as well as on other factors. Age and gender are typically considered the most relevant factors that impact health status. This section presents an overview of health indicators, risks, and health promotion strategies for children, adolescents, women, men, and elders.

Health Promotion for Children

PATTERNS OF CHILDHOOD MORBIDITY AND MORTALITY AMONG CHILDREN

As discussed, the leading causes of death in the United States are heart disease, cancer, and stroke. The leading causes of death are very different for infants, children, and adolescents as shown in Table 13–3. Indeed, for infants, congenital anomalies are the leading cause of death; problems related to birth comprise the four leading causes of death. This changes dramatically after the first year of life; accidents account for most deaths of children and adolescents. The other common causes of death among children and adolescents are homicide and cancer, although congenital anomalies still contribute to many deaths in these age groups.

The leading causes of acute illness in children are respiratory conditions; other infective and parasitic diseases, such as viral infections, intestinal viruses, and acute ear infections; and injuries. The most common chronic conditions in children are respiratory conditions, including asthma, allergic rhinitis, chronic sinusitis and chronic bronchitis, and skin conditions. Musculoskeletal conditions, vision, speech, and hearing impairments are identified in many children (NCHS, 2000).

Respiratory conditions contribute to the most time lost from school, accounting for more that 50% of days absent. Viral infections, ear infections,

Figure 13–1   The Health Promotion Model

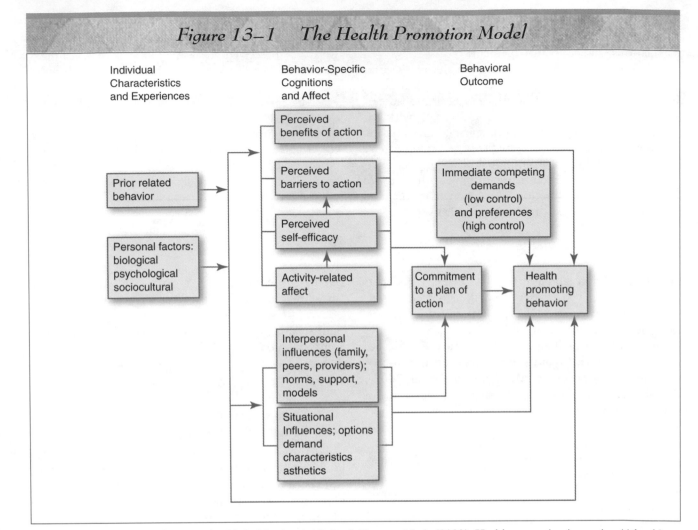

Reprinted with permission from Pender, N. J., Murdaugh, C. L., & Parsons, M. A. (2002). Health promotion in nursing (4th ed.), p. 60. Upper Saddle River, NJ: Prentice Hall.

injuries, and digestive complaints are also common reasons for school absenteeism. Children younger than 5 years see physicians more than any other age group until age 65, averaging 6.9 physician contacts each year. In contrast, children and adolescents 5 to 17 years have about 3.5 physician contacts per year (NCHS, 2000).

HEALTH PROMOTION STRATEGIES FOR CHILDREN

To prevent, detect, and minimize disease, disability, and death in infants and children, a number of issues relating to health should be assessed and appropriate interventions developed and implemented when problems or potential problems are identified. Strategies for health promotion include routine infant screenings (height and weight, head circumference, phenylketonurea [PKU], hemoglobin, thyroxine [T_4] or thyroid-stimulating hormone [TSH], and lead), immunizations, instruction on proper diet and exercise, and routine dental care.

To reduce threats from the leading cause of death (accidents), counseling for all parents and care providers should include ways to minimize risks. Motor vehicle accidents, drowning, burns, and suffocation are the leading causes of accidental death in children, and motor vehicle accidents are the greatest danger to life and health. Head injury from cycling and other sports is another leading cause of child death and disability. Unfortunately, although studies have shown that helmets reduce the risk of head injuries in biking accidents by 85%, fewer than 5% of children wear helmets when

Table 13–3 Leading Causes of Death and Percentage for Children

Less than 1 Year	Children 1–4 Years	Children 5–14 Years
Congenital anomalies (21%)	Accidents (37%)	Accidents (41.7%)
Short gestation and low birth weight (11%)	Congenital anomalies (10.7%)	Cancer (13%)
Perinatal complications (11%)	Homicide (7.6%)	Homicide (6%)
Sudden infant death syndrome (SIDS) and respiratory distress syndrome (7%)	Cancer (7%)	Congenital anomalies (5%)

Source: National Center for Health Statistics (2000). *Health United States: 2000.* Hyattsville, MD: USDHHS/NCHS.

riding (Centers for Disease Control and Prevention [CDC], 1995a). Box 13–2 provides a list of topics to include in health education and counseling for childhood injury prevention.

Immunizations against a number of communicable diseases are available and recommended for all infants and children. The immunization schedule is quite complex and regulated by state law. Children receiving immunizations should be properly screened. Parents should be educated regarding identification and management of possible side effects.

The importance of good nutrition, plenty of physical activity and exercise, and adequate sleep and rest are areas that should be stressed in health promotion of infants and children. Finally, it is vital to promote dental health care. This includes hygiene as well as routine visits to dentists and dental hygienists for preventative care and to treat caries.

Health Promotion for Adolescents

Because as a group adolescents are very healthy, they are often overlooked with regard to health, health promotion, and risk reduction. This is unfortunate as many poor health practices, including smoking, substance use, and potentially detrimental activities (e.g., early, unprotected sex; driving habits) are commonly initiated during the adolescent years. Health care providers who routinely work with this group should be aware of potential health threats and therefore seek opportunities to conduct health teaching and other interventions designed to prevent problems.

PATTERNS OF MORBIDITY AND MORTALITY AMONG ADOLESCENTS

The leading causes of death for adolescents and young adults, ages 13 to 25 are: accidents (43.6%), homicide (18%), and suicide (13.5%) (DHHS/NCHS, 2001). Motor vehicle injuries and firearm-related injuries are the two leading causes of death among adolescents 10 to 19 years of age, accounting for 55% of all deaths and 75% of all injuries. Motor vehicle traffic death rates increase markedly with age, with the greatest increase occurring between ages 15 and 16 years (DHHS/NCHS, 2001).

Box 13–2 Recommended Areas for Health Education for Childhood Injury Prevention

- Child safety seats (all children should be restrained in motor vehicles at ALL times)
- Bicycle helmet use
- Smoke detectors, flame retardant sleepwear
- Hot water temperature (less than 120°F)
- Window/stair guards, pool fence
- Safe storage of drugs, toxic substances, firearms, and matches
- Syrup of ipecac, poison control phone number
- Cardiopulmonary resuscitation (CPR) training for parents and caretakers

The most common reasons for hospitalization of adolescents are injuries, such as fractures, sprains, and strains; open wounds; and contusions. Asthma, upper respiratory conditions, abdominal or gastrointestinal conditions, sexually transmitted diseases (STDs), and urinary tract infections are also common reasons for seeking health care. STDs are the most commonly reported infectious diseases among adolescents; chlamydia and gonorrhea are the most prevalent STDs.

There are a number of health risks commonly identified among adolescents. For example, approximately one-half of all high school students report that they have been sexually active; 66% of 12th grade female and 64% of 12th grade males report that they have had intercourse. More than 33% of high school students report that they have smoked in the previous 30 days, and 17% report smoking frequently. Finally, about one-half of all high school students report alcohol use in the previous 30 days (DHHS/NCHS, 2001).

HEALTH PROMOTION STRATEGIES FOR ADOLESCENTS

Adolescents have lower rates of health care utilization than others despite the health problems mentioned. Despite this lack of utilization, they are particularly in need of health education and counseling. Maturation and puberty is an important topic for adolescent health. Both girls and boys need to understand the physical changes that take place during puberty. They also need to be taught how to appropriately manage sexual issues they will face. Prevention of substance use, including a strong emphasis on anti-smoking education, is essential at this age, as it is estimated that well over 90% of those who ever start smoking do so by age 17 (DHHS, 2000a).

Vehicle safety education and education to reduce violence are very important issues in promoting the health of adolescents. Violence is a growing concern. Risk factors associated with violence include:

- Low socioeconomic status
- Involvement with gangs, drug use, and drug dealing
- Access to guns
- Media exposure to violence
- Community exposure to violence

Other factors include alcohol and drug use, peer pressure, poor impulse control, and a history of family violence. Box 13–3 presents a list of strategies nurses can use to help prevent teen violence.

Health Promotion for Women

PATTERNS OF MORBIDITY AND MORTALITY AMONG WOMEN

The leading causes of death are quite different between women and men, and vary considerably with age (Table 13–4 and Table 13–5). In addition to health problems related to cancer, heart disease, and stroke, which are common to both men and women, women have significant health issues related to reproduction. More women than men are hospitalized each year in the United States, largely due to issues pertaining to childbirth and gynecologic issues. Cesarean delivery is the most prevalent surgical procedure experienced by women, and hysterectomy is the second most common.

There are other significant differences in patterns of morbidity. For example, women experience depression at two to three times the rate of men. Also, women are more likely than men to be disabled from chronic conditions. Further, women are more prone to arthritis, asthma, ulcers, and colitis, and slightly more likely to be hypertensive. Because of these factors, women have more frequent contact with health care providers and are more likely to attain preventative health care.

HEALTH PROMOTION STRATEGIES FOR WOMEN

Family planning is a significant issue that relates to health promotion. Indeed, it is estimated that about half of all pregnancies among American women are unintended, either mistimed or unwanted (DHHS, 2000a). There are several reasons for this, including

---

Box 13–3   *Nursing Strategies to Prevent Teen Violence*

Teach conflict resolution strategies.
Provide training in social skills and peer education.
Support regulation of access to weapons and weaponless schools.
Support regulation of access to alcohol, drugs, and tobacco.
Advocate appropriate punishment in schools for violation of rules.
Support and maintain dress codes at schools.

Table 13–4   Leading Causes of Death and Percentage for Women

25–44 Years	45–64 Years	65+ Years
Cancer (26.0%)	Cancer (41.8%)	Heart disease (34.8%)
Accidents (15.4%)	Heart disease (20.2%)	Cancer (19.2%)
Heart disease (11.0%)	Stroke (4.6%)	Stroke (9.2%)
Suicide (5.5%)	COPD (4.5%)	COPD (5.0%)
HIV/AIDS (5.4%)	Diabetes (4.0%)	Pneumonia/influenza (4.9%)

Source: National Center for Health Statistics (2000). *Health United States: 2000*. Hyattsville, MD: USDHHS/NCHS.

lack of knowledge, failure to translate knowledge into behavior, and lack of family planning services and information. Family planning services provide health care and counseling that allow women to make informed choices about whether and when to become pregnant, and how to care for themselves during and following a pregnancy. Women also need to be informed on contraception options, including the effectiveness and positive and negative consequences of each option.

Prenatal care has been recognized as being vitally important in reducing infant and maternal mortality. Comprehensive prenatal care can help reduce the risk of low-birth-weight infants and other complications, and can help ensure that both the infant and mother will be as healthy as possible. Prenatal care should include:

- Ongoing risk assessment
- Individualized care based on identified problems or potential problems
- Nutritional counseling
- Education to reduce or eliminate unhealthy habits
- Stress reduction
- Social support services as needed
- General health education

Other important health issues for women include unique cancers (breast and gynecologic) and osteoporosis. Breast cancer is one of the most commonly diagnosed cancers among women and the second leading cause of cancer deaths. Women should be aware of the risk factors for breast cancer, which include:

- Age (over 50)
- Personal or family history
- First pregnancy after age 30
- Having had no children
- Menarche before age 12
- Menopause after age 50
- Postmenopausal
- Obesity
- A personal history of ovarian or endometrial cancer (American Cancer Society, 2002)

The stage of the breast cancer will strongly influence mortality; therefore, early detection is critical. Detection is promoted by breast self-examination (BSE), examination by a trained clinician, and mammography. Other, more advanced technologies (e.g., ultrasound) are becoming increasingly common. Box

Table 13–5   Leading Causes of Death and Percentage for Men

25–44 Years	45–64 Years	65+ Years
Accidents (23.4%)	Cancer (30.5%)	Heart disease (34.1%)
Heart disease (23.4%)	Heart disease (30.2%)	Cancer (25.2%)
Suicide (11.3%)	Accidents (5.6%)	Stroke (6.4%)
Cancer (11.2%)	Stroke (3.6%)	COPD (6.2%)
HIV/AIDS (7.5%)	Liver disease (3.5%)	Pneumonia/influenza (4.5%)

Source: National Center for Health Statistics (2000). *Health United States: 2000*. Hyattsville, MD: USDHHS/NCHS.

Box 13–4   Guidelines for Screening for Breast Cancer

- All women should be taught how to perform BSE and encouraged to practice it monthly.
- All women 20 to 39 should have a breast examination performed by a health professional at least every 3 years, and annually after age 40.
- All women 40 to 49 should have a screening mammogram every 1 to 2 years, and women 50 years and older should have screening mammograms every year.
- High-risk women should have annual mammograms beginning at 35 years of age.
- Any palpable breast lump, even if not detected on a mammogram, should be carefully evaluated.

13–4 outlines breast cancer screening guidelines proposed by the American Cancer Society (2002).

Cancers of the cervix, ovary, and endometrium are relative common and successfully treatable if caught early. Frequency, risk factors, and common symptoms of these cancers are found in Table 13–6. To identify women with gynecologic cancers, there are several recommendations. First, a Pap test should be performed annually for all sexually active women. After a woman has had three or more consecutive "normal" examina-

tions, the Pap test may be performed less frequently, at the discretion of the health care provider and patient. Women who experience postmenopausal bleeding or other atypical discharge should be evaluated immediately. Finally, women who experience abnormal abdominal or pelvic discomfort that persists should seek health care.

Osteoporosis is a common bone disease characterized by decreased bone mass, which leads to increased skeletal fragility and subsequently increases the ten-

Table 13–6   Frequency, Risk Factors, and Symptoms Associated with Endometrial, Ovarian, and Cervical Cancer

Type of Cancer	Frequency	Risk Factors	Symptoms
Endometrial	• Most frequent form of gynecology cancer • Occurs in postmenopausal women • Average age at diagnosis is 58 years	• Nulliparity • Late menopause • Early menarche • Obesity • Family history of breast cancer, pelvic irradiation, and endometrial hyperplasia	• Abnormal vaginal bleeding • Enlarged uterus
Ovarian	• Quite rare but most deadly of the cancers of the reproductive organs • Death rate attributable to delayed diagnosis	• Family history of ovarian cancer • Nulliparity • Older age at the first pregnancy • Fewer pregnancies • Personal history of breast, endometrial, or colorectal cancer	• Symptoms rare until advanced stages are reached
Cervical	• One of the most common cancers in women • Invasive cervical carcinoma most common in women 40–45 • African-American women have dramatically higher incidences of invasive cancer than do white females	• Early age at first intercourse • Multiple sexual partners • Positive test for human papillomavirus • History of tobacco use	• Vaginal bleeding or discharge, often associated with douching or intercourse

dency to fracture. Although osteoporosis concerns both men and women, women are particularly at risk. Indeed, osteoporosis affects about 50% of women older than 45 years, and 90% of women older than 75. Over half of all women will have fractures related to osteoporosis. The most common sites of fractures are the vertebral column, upper femur, distal radius, and proximal humerus. The most serious fractures are hip fractures, which affect about 250,000 Americans each year. It is estimated that about one-third of women and 17% of men will experience a hip fracture by the time they reach 90 years of age (DHHS, 2000a). Osteoporosis is also associated with back pain, kyphosis, and loss of height.

Risk factors for osteoporosis include age; family history; inadequate calcium and vitamin D, and excessive protein and phosphate in the diet; decreased activity; sedentary lifestyle; use of alcohol and caffeine; smoking; medications such as corticosteroids; excess thyroid replacement; long-term heparin therapy; chemotherapy; and radiation therapy. At greatest risk for osteoporosis-related fractures are women who are older, white or Asian, and slender, and who have had early onset menopause or had their ovaries removed.

Preventative measures to reduce osteoporosis include maintaining physical activity, increased calcium intake, maintaining adequate vitamin D intake, and avoiding excess meat and phosphoric acid–containing beverages. Premenopausal women should be taught the benefits of calcium supplementation and encouraged to do weight-bearing exercises regularly.

Health Promotion for Men

PATTERNS OF MORBIDITY AND MORTALITY AMONG MEN

In developed countries, life expectancy for men consistently lags behind life expectancy for women. Although the gender gap has closed somewhat in recent years, it is still around 6 years, as males born in 1996 will live an average of 73 years compared with females born in the same year who will live an average of 79.1 years (McFalls, 1998). This discrepancy has been attributed to several factors. First, males lead females in mortality rates in each of the leading causes of death. Also, men are about seven times as likely to die from AIDS as women, and men are more than four times as likely to die from suicide and homicide than women. Furthermore, men are two to three times more likely to die from accidents and twice as likely to die of heart disease (Morgan, 2001). Death

resulting from such causes as homicide, AIDS, and accidents tend to impact younger men, which, in turn, impacts the average life expectancy of men. The leading cause of mortality of men from three different groups is listed in Table 13–5.

Although they die earlier, men are, for the most part, healthier than women. The incidence for acute conditions, including digestive system conditions and respiratory conditions, is higher for women than for men. The only exception is for injuries, which are considerably more common in men. Likewise, chronic conditions tend to affect women more than men for several conditions (i.e., ulcers, arthritis, and colitis). Other chronic conditions, such as gout, ischemic heart disease, and vertebral disk disorders, are more common in men (Morgan, 2001). Because of their relatively good health, and because of the lack of reproductive health problems common to women, men are considerably less likely than women to seek health care, and subsequently, they are also less likely to use preventative health care. Men should be encouraged to seek preventative health care.

HEALTH PROMOTION STRATEGIES FOR MEN

For the most part, men's specific health promotion needs reflect the general health promotion issues described in this chapter. Two distinctive issues are discussed in this section, however, as they apply only to men (prostate cancer) or predominantly to men (violence).

Prostate cancer is the most common type of cancer, other than skin cancer, found in American men. Each year there are almost 200,000 new cases diagnosed, and about 31,500 deaths from prostate cancer. Risk factors include: (a) age—more than 80% of all cases are found in men over the age of 65; (b) race—African-American men are almost twice as likely as white men to get prostate cancer; (c) family history; and (d) diet—a high-fat diet may contribute to prostate cancer. Prostate cancer, if caught at an early stage, is very treatable. Indeed, if the cancer is found before it has spread outside the prostate, the 5-year survival rate is 100%, and if the cancer has spread to tissues near the prostate, the survival rate is 94%. If the cancer has spread to other parts of the body, however, the survival rate is only around 31% (American Cancer Society, 2002).

In screening for prostate cancer, the American Cancer Society (2002) recommends that beginning at age 50, all men should be offered annually both the prostate-specific antigen (PSA) blood test and a digital rectal examination. Men in high-risk groups, African-Americans, and men with close family members who have had prostate cancer at a young age should begin testing at 45 years of age. Men should receive information regarding possible risks and benefits for early diagnosis and treatment of prostate cancer. If the digital rectal examination or a high PSA level suggests cancer, the next step should be an ultrasound test and a biopsy.

Violence is a very significant health threat to men. According to the CDC, the United States ranks first in the industrial world in deaths due to violence. Murder and suicide together claim the lives of over 50,000 individuals each year, and an additional 2.2 million are injured in violent assaults (CDC, 1995b). Homicide claimed the lives of almost 20,000 people in 1997.

Homicide is the second leading cause of death among men aged 15 to 24 and the leading cause of death among black males aged 15 to 34 years (NCHS, 2000). At greatest risk for homicide are young people, particularly African-American and Hispanic males (CDC/NCIPC, 2000).

Suicide is the eighth leading cause of death for all Americans, accounting for 30,500 deaths in 1997. At greatest risk are white males, who account for 72% of all suicides across the age spectrum. In addition, 83% of suicides among people aged 65 and older are male (CDC/NCIPC, 2000).

Violence has been termed a public health epidemic and efforts should be made by all health care professionals, including nurses, to prevent violence whenever possible. Nurses can help the prevention of violence through promotion of optimal parenting and family wellness. Also, education is important and should begin with instructing children in grade schools regarding nonviolent methods of conflict resolution.

Health professionals should increase their awareness of violence among their patients and facilitate case detection and provision for early treatment. Nurses can advocate community responsibility in educating citizens about the problems of violence, its potential causes, and services that are needed to address it. Nurses are professionally responsible for reporting injuries caused by violence and can be involved with local social service agencies for referral and follow-up. In addition, nurses can provide referrals to professional counseling services and self-help groups.

Health Promotion for Older Adults

PATTERNS OF MORBIDITY AND MORTALITY AMONG OLDER ADULTS

As of 1995, a 65-year-old American can expect to live an average of 18 more years, and a 75-year-old can expect to live an average of 11 more years (DHHS, 2000b). As mentioned in Table 13–1, the leading causes of death are heart disease, cancer, and stroke, which combined account for about 60% of all deaths. There is, however, some variation based on age, even among older adults. For example, for those 65 to 74 years old, the leading causes of death are cancer, heart disease, COPD, stroke, and pneumonia, but that changes for those 75 to 84 years old, when heart disease overtakes cancer.

Chronic diseases are common with aging and almost 80% of Americans 70 years of age and older report that they have at least one chronic condition. The most common chronic conditions are arthritis, hypertension, heart disease, and hearing and vision difficulties. Other disabling conditions are orthopedic impairment, chronic sinusitis, cataracts, and diabetes (NCHS, 2000; DHHS, 2000a).

People 65 years of age and older are the major consumers of inpatient care in the United States. Hospitalizations increase with age, and people 85 years of age and older have more than twice the rate of hospital discharges than those 65 to 74 years old (NCHS, 2000). Rates of ambulatory care increase with age, and people 75 years of age and older have the highest rate of physician visits, with 6.5 visits per person. The major reasons for ambulatory care visits are routine chronic problems, acute problems, and presurgery or postsurgery follow-up.

HEALTH PROMOTION STRATEGIES FOR OLDER ADULTS

There are many ways to promote the health of older adults, and only a few will be discussed here. One important factor in promoting the health of elders involves nutritional assessment and teaching. Malnutrition is quite common in older adults, particularly in those living alone (McEwen & Davis, 2001). Reasons for this include loneliness, depression, grief, anxiety, inability to prepare meals, inability to buy food, and dental problems. Nurses who routinely care for older adults should assess the patient's diet and be prepared to intervene with education and possibly referral to a community agency, such as Meals on Wheels.

Vision and hearing problems are very common among older adults and can contribute significantly to lowering quality of life. For example, about 20% of those over age 70 have visual impairments, which cause activity limitation and disability, and place elders at greater risk of falls and other injuries. The main causes

Explore health promotion versus disease treatment with an older individual you know. Do you believe lifelong health habits have influenced the individual's current quality of health? Do health promotion strategies need to be implemented? What resources are needed to implement a health promotion plan? What barriers will prevent the implementation of a health promotion plan?

of visual impairment are cataracts, glaucoma, macular degeneration, and diabetic retinopathy. Treatment is available for cataracts, glaucoma, and diabetic retinopathy. Macular degeneration should be assessed frequently for worsening, as there is no treatment available. Older Americans should be screened regularly for vision problems and managed appropriately (NCHS, 2000).

Hearing impairment affects 33% of those 65 and older, and hearing loss may contribute to social isolation, depression, and/or an exacerbation of coexisting psychiatric problems. Older adults with hearing problems should be encouraged to see an otolaryngologist and an audiologist for evaluation and management.

Prevention of accidents is important in older people. Accidents are caused by poor vision, poor mobility, loss of muscle strength and flexibility, medications and alcohol, chronic diseases, and dementia (Walker, 1998). Safety issues and related health instruction may focus on protection from falls, because falls and related injures contribute to other health problems including fractures of the hip, femur, humerus, wrist, and ribs. To prevent accidents, elders should be encouraged to do the following:

- Remove all loose rugs.
- Install handrails in the bathroom and wherever else needed.
- Use a nonskid mat in the tub or shower.
- Check stairs for stability.
- Eliminate clutter.
- Avoid slippery floors.

Elders should also be instructed to lower hot water temperatures, install and maintain smoke detectors, and increase artificial lighting in all rooms.

Other areas for assessment and intervention include mental and cognitive functioning. Indeed, depression is one of the most prevalent conditions among older adults. Risk factors for depression among older adults include death or severe disability of a spouse, physical illness, educational attainment less than high school, impaired functional status, and alcohol consumption. Older adults who experience depression should be offered counseling and medication as appropriate.

Finally, immunizations are not just for children. Those over age 65 years should receive a single dose of pneumoccocal polysaccharide vaccine and an annual vaccination against influenza. Tetanus vaccination may be necessary for those who sustain cuts and other injuries.

Strategies for Health Promotion and Risk Reduction

Nurses should be aware of the risk factors that contribute to disease and disability and know how to address these factors to reduce or even eliminate them. Screening for early identification of a disease or health problem is one way to reduce risk. This section outlines principles for screening and presents suggestions of strategies for health promotion and risk reduction for the leading causes of death.

Screening

The purpose of **screening** is to identify risk factors and disease in their earliest stages. In order for the information from screening tests to be useful, certain guidelines must be followed. Principles for screening are shown in Box 13–5 (DHHS/Office of Disease Prevention and Health Promotion [ODPHP], 1994).

As explained above, whenever screening is offered there must be some method for referral and follow-up for those who test positive for whatever condition is being assessed. Nurses are often in a position to perform screening tests and must be prepared to offer appropriate education and counseling for patients whose test results are either positive or negative. In

Box 13–5 Principles for Screening

- The condition must have a significant effect on the quality and quantity of life.
- Acceptable methods of treatment must be available.
- The condition must have an asymptomatic period during which detection and treatment significantly reduce morbidity or mortality.
- Treatment in the asymptomatic phase must yield a therapeutic result superior to that obtained by delaying treatment until symptoms appear.
- Tests that are acceptable to patients must be available, at a reasonable cost, to detect the condition in the asymptomatic period.
- The incidence of the condition must be sufficient to justify the cost of the screening.
- The screening test performed must be reliable and valid (i.e., the tests should have good "sensitivity" and "specificity").
- Methods for follow-up tracking for patient referrals should be available.
- Patients should be clearly informed of the potential cost and morbidity of necessary follow-up testing and treatment.

addition, if an individual tests positive, the nurse should be prepared for referral and follow-up care. Finally, there should be a mechanism to re-test patients if the original test is suspect.

Risk Reduction Strategies for Leading Causes of Death in Adults

HEART DISEASE AND STROKE

As discussed earlier and presented in Table 13–1, heart disease and stroke are the number one and number three leading causes of death, respectively, in the United States each year. Indeed, each year as many as 1.1 million Americans will have a heart attack, and almost half a million will die from heart disease. It is important to note that although heart disease is associated with aging, about 5% of all heart attacks occur in people under age 40, and 45% occur in people under age 65. The lifetime risk of developing coronary heart disease (CHD) after age 40 is 49% for men and 32% for women (American Heart Association, 2000). Strokes, the leading cause of serious disability in the United States, afflict more than 500,000 Americans each year. Risk factors associated with heart disease and strokes are listed in Box 13–6.

Box 13–6 Risk Factors for Heart Disease and Stroke

- Smoking significantly increases the risk of both heart disease and stroke.
- Hypertension is a major risk factor in heart disease and the most important risk factor in stroke.
- Hypercholesterolemia with low HDL causes narrowing in the arterial walls and increases the possibly of occlusion.
- Diabetes is linked with increased risk of both heart disease and stroke.
- Obesity increases the risk of heart disease, particularly if the individual is more than 30% above ideal body weight.
- Aging steadily increases the risk of heart disease and stroke increase steadily with age.
- Men have three to four times greater risk of heart disease than premenopausal women; after menopause, women's rate of heart disease increases sharply.
- Risks increase if a parent or sibling has had a heart attack or stroke or died of heart disease before age 55.

Several tools for assessment of an individual's risk of heart disease are available. Most of these also describe how risks can be lowered or managed. For example, the American Heart Association's Health Risk Assessment assesses the potential threat of heart attack based on such factors as age, gender, family history, blood cholesterol level, blood pressure, and lifestyle habits including smoking and diet. Nurses and others may use these tools as part of a comprehensive program that includes health teaching and counseling on nutrition, exercise, and smoking cessation if applicable, to lower risk for all individuals.

CANCER

Cancer, as has been discussed, is the second leading cause of death in the United States overall and the leading cause of death among some age groups (all adults 45 to 64 and women 25 to 44). The American Cancer Society estimates that 1.2 million new cancer cases are diagnosed each year, resulting in about 552,000 deaths or 1,500 people each day. It should be noted that these figures do not include basal cell and squamous cell skin cancers. Skin cancers are more common than cancers of any other organ, with over 1.3 million cases of basal cell and squamous cell skin cancer diagnosed each year (American Cancer Society, 2002).

Nearly 80% of all cancers are diagnosed in people age 55 and older. Overall, men have about a 1 in 2 lifetime risk of developing cancer; for women, the risk is about 1 in 3. The chance of an individual getting certain cancers will vary greatly depending on one's risk factors. For example, male smokers have a 20-fold risk of developing lung cancer compared with nonsmokers; women who have a first-degree family history of breast cancer have a 2-fold increased risk of developing breast cancer compared with women who do not (American Cancer Society, 2002).

In men, cancer deaths are most commonly caused by cancer of the lung and bronchus (90,100 deaths/year), cancer of the colon/rectum (31,700 deaths/year), and cancer of the prostate (31,500 deaths/year). In women, cancer deaths are most commonly caused by cancer of the lung and bronchus (67,300 deaths/year), breast cancer (40,200 deaths/year), cancer of the colon/rectum (29,000 deaths/year), and cancers of the genital tract (i.e., uterus/cervix/ovary) (25,900 deaths/year) (American Cancer Society, 2002).

Cancer prevention efforts focus on changing behaviors and lifestyle factors such as avoiding tobacco and reducing alcohol consumption. Indeed,

it is estimated that about 172,000 cancer deaths are caused by tobacco use, and about 19,000 cancer deaths may be related to excessive alcohol use (American Cancer Society, 2002). About one-third of cancer deaths will be related to nutrition, physical activity, and other lifestyle factors. Most skin cancers can be prevented by protection from the sun's rays. Other cancers are related to STDs. For example, the hepatitis B virus increases risk of liver cancer, human papillomavirus (HPV) is the primary cause of cervical cancer, and HIV increases the risk of lymphoma and Kaposi's sarcoma.

Regular screening can result in detection of cancers of the breast, colon/rectum, cervix, prostate, testes, oral cavity, and skin at stages when treatment is more likely to be successful. Early detection and treatment of cancer has resulted in improved survival rates for most cancers, and nurses should be aware of risk factors and counsel patients accordingly.

DIABETES

Diabetes is one of the leading causes of death and disability in the United States, contributing to 200,000 to 250,000 deaths each year. Additionally, diabetes is associated with many severe illnesses and conditions including blindness, heart disease, stroke, kidney failure, nerve damage, amputations, and birth defects in babies born to women with diabetes.

Approximately 15.7 million Americans have diabetes, and it is estimated that about a third are not aware of it. Each year almost 800,000 people are diagnosed with diabetes. Ninety to ninety-five percent of people with diabetes have Type 2 diabetes, which usually develops in adults over the age of 40. Type 2 diabetes is nearing epidemic proportions in the United States due to the increased number of older Americans and a greater prevalence of obesity and sedentary lifestyles. The remaining 5% to 10% represent individuals with Type 1 diabetes, which most often develops in children and young adults. In addition, gestational diabetes develops in 2% to 5% of all pregnancies, but disappears when the pregnancy is over. Women who have had gestational diabetes are at increased risk for developing Type 2 diabetes later in life (American Diabetes Association, 2000).

Risk factors for Type 2 diabetes include: obesity (about 80% of people with Type 2 diabetes are overweight), increasing age, family history, and/or being a member of certain minority groups. African Americans and Hispanics are at increased risk for developing diabetes. The prevalence of Type 2 diabetes is particularly high among Native Americans—almost 50% of members of certain tribes are known to be diabetic, and there is an overall prevalence of greater than 12% among all Native Americans (American Diabetes Association, 2000).

All adults should be taught the warning signs of diabetes. These include:

- Frequent urination
- Unusual thirst
- Extreme hunger
- Unusual weight loss
- Extreme fatigue
- Irritability
- Frequent infections
- Blurred vision
- Cuts/bruises that are slow to heal
- Tingling/numbness in the hands or feet
- Recurring skin, gum, or bladder infections

Those at risk should be encouraged to reduce and maintain weight; to eat a healthy, balanced diet; to exercise regularly; and to be screened periodically.

Health Promotion Interventions for Nursing Practice

As identified in the *Essentials* (1998) document health promotion, risk reduction, and disease prevention have been identified core knowledge to the education of the professional nurse. As in all other cases, when applying the nursing process to health promotion and illness prevention, nurses begin with assessment. In addition to the individual physical, functional, and cognitive assessments, which are routinely accomplished, an assessment of behaviors and habits that influence health is also important. An understanding of the patient's health beliefs and knowledge, as well as health habits (both positive and negative), will assist in planning appropriate interventions.

Health promotion interventions should be both general and specific. They should be targeted toward the needs of the particular individual, family, group, or population seeking or needing care. General interventions include assessment of health risks and health habits, promotion of physical activity and fitness, health education regarding good nutrition practices, and the importance of weight control. Nutrition counseling should include information on how to lower fat and cholesterol intake, and to ensure sufficient vitamins, minerals, and fiber.

Health education should strongly discourage the use of tobacco; health care providers should supply recommendations or referrals for smoking cessation. Other health promotional activities include encouraging breast self-examination (BSE) and testicular self-examination (TSE) in men, and screening for hypertension, hypercholesterolemia, occult blood in stools, and diabetes as appropriate, based on age, gender, race/ethnicity, and identified risk factors. Health teaching should provide data on risk factors and signs and symptoms for the most common health problems, such as certain cancers, heart disease and stroke, and diabetes. Finally, additional measures include: stressing the use of sunscreen and avoiding overexposure to the sun; explaining safety measures, such as seatbelt use and home smoke detectors; advocating "safer" sexual practices including use of condoms; and promoting good mental health.

Guidelines to facilitate health promotional behaviors and practices for nurses were presented In the Nursing Intervention Project (McCloskey & Bulechek, 2000). Among others, these include:

- Target high-risk groups and age ranges that would benefit most from education.
- Identify internal or external factors that may enhance or impaired motivation for healthful behavior.
- Determine current health knowledge and lifestyle behaviors of individuals, families, or target groups.
- Assist individuals, families, and communities in clarifying health beliefs and values.
- Prioritize learner needs based on patient preference, skills of the nurse, resources available, and likelihood of successful goal attainment.
- Avoid use of fear or scare techniques as strategies to motivate people to change health or lifestyle behaviors.
- Emphasize immediate or short-term positive health benefits rather than long-term benefits.
- Teach strategies that can be used to resist unhealthful behavior or risk-taking.
- Determine family, peer, and community support for behaviors conducive to health.
- Use social and family support systems to enhance effectiveness of lifestyle or health behavior modification.

Each year, the American Cancer Society (ACS) publishes a summary of existing recommendations for early detection of cancer. These updates include emerging issues related to cancer detection along with relevant screening methods. These guidelines provided by the American Cancer Society (Table 13–7) are based on cumulative data and research findings and are periodically updated. They provide a wealth of information that can be used by nurses for ongoing health promotion education.

The guidelines developed by the ACS cover many of the most common types of cancer (i.e., breast, colorectal, and prostate) for which screening has been shown to be effective in improving survival rates by encouraging early detection and treatment. Similar guidelines are published for prevention and early detection of many chronic health problems including hypertension, heart disease, diabetes, and AIDS.

Guidelines that address screening recommendations are not static, however. As new information becomes available, recommendations change. In addition, different groups or organizations may have somewhat differing views on when or even if a particular screening test should be used. For example, the effectiveness of widespread use of mammography has recently been questioned with respect to improving mortality rates, and the debate is still ongoing. Nurses should diligently follow new developments and changes in recommendations and alter education accordingly.

In addition to the ACS, other organizations and groups that publish guidelines for early detection of disease include the American Heart Association, the American Diabetes Association, and the U.S. Preventive Services Task Force.

Table 13–7 American Cancer Society Recommendations for the Early Detection of Cancer in Average-Risk, Asymptomatic People

Cancer Site	Population	Test or Procedure	Frequency
Breast	Women, age 20+	Breast self-examination	Monthly, starting at age 20.
		Clinical breast examination	Every 3 years, ages 20–39.
		Mammography	Annual, starting at age 40.[a]
Colorectal	Men and women, age 50+	Fecal occult blood test (FOBT) and flexible sigmoidoscopy[b]	Annual FOBT and flexible sigmoidoscopy every 5 years, starting at age 50.
		or	
		Flexible sigmoidoscopy	Every 5 years, starting at age 50.
		or	
		FOBT	Annual, starting at age 50.
		or	
		Colonoscopy	Colonoscopy every 10 years, staring at age 50.
		or	
		Double-contrast barium enema (DCBE)	DCBE every 5 years, staring at age 50
Prostate	Men, age 50+	Digital rectal examination (DRE) and prostate-specific antigen (PSA) test	The PSA test and the DRE should be offered annually, starting at age 50, for men who have a life expectancy of at least 10 years.[c]

(continued)

Table 13–7 (continued) table and key points.

Table 13–7 (continued)

Cancer Site	Population	Test or Procedure	Frequency
Cervix	Women, age 18+	Pap test and pelvic examination	All women who are, or have been, sexually active, or have reached age 18 should have an annual Pap test and pelvic examination. After a woman has had three or more consecutive satisfactory normal annual examinations, the Pap test may be performed less frequently at discretion of the physician.
Cancer-related check-up	Men and women, age 20+	The cancer-related check-up should include examination for cancers of the thyroid, testicles, ovaries, lymph nodes, oral cavity, and skin, as well as health counseling about tobacco, sun exposure, diet and nutrition, risk factors, sexual practices, and environmental and occupational exposures.	Examinations every 3 years from ages 20 to 39 years and annually after age 40.

[a]Beginning at age 40, annual clinical breast examination should be performed prior to mammography.
[b]Flexible sigmoidoscopy together with FOBT is preferred compared with FOBT or flexible sigmoidoscopy alone.
[c]Information should be provided to men about the benefits and limitations of testing.
Source: *Cancer Facts and Figures—2002*. Reprinted by the permission of the American Cancer Society, Inc.

KEY POINTS

1. Health promotion refers to activities or actions that increase health and well-being and maximize health potential. The focus of health promotion is on encouraging lifestyle choices to positively influence health.
2. All nurses should be prepared for opportunities to assist patients by providing information, counseling, advocacy, referral, or other interventions that will allow the patient to make informed choices to promote health.
3. Overall, the four leading causes of death in the United States are heart disease, cancer, cerebrovascular disease, and COPD; however, the leading causes of death change dramatically based on factors such as age and gender.
4. Disease prevention interventions are typically categorized as: primary prevention (activities that work to prevent a problem before it occurs), secondary prevention (activities that provide early detection and intervention), and tertiary prevention (activities to correct a disease state and prevent it from further deteriorating).
5. *Healthy People 2010*, the health objectives for the United States, list two broad goals: (a) increase quality and years of healthy life and (b) eliminate health disparities. In *Healthy People 2010*, 467 objectives are divided into 28 focus areas that may be used to guide health promotion activities in schools, clinics, and worksites as well as for community-wide initiatives.

6. The Health Promotion Model (HPM) helps nurses explore the bio/psycho/social processes that motivate individuals to engage in health-promoting behaviors and has been used extensively as a framework for research aimed at predicting health-promoting lifestyles and specific health behaviors.

7. Health promotion for infants and children includes routine screenings, immunizations, instruction on proper diet and exercise, routine dental care, and efforts to reduce morbidity and mortality from accidents.

8. Health promotion for adolescents should focus on understanding the physical changes that take place during adolescence and how to manage sexual issues. Prevention of substance use, including a strong emphasis on anti-smoking education, is essential for adolescents. Vehicle safety education and education to reduce violence are extremely important.

9. Health promotion for women should include family planning and prenatal care as well as addressing other health issues unique to women, including gynecological cancers and breast cancer. Also, depression and osteoporosis are significantly more common in women than men.

10. Health promotion needs specific for men include early detection of prostate cancer and prevention of violence. Prostate cancer is the second leading cause of cancer in men (after skin cancer) and is very treatable when caught early. Homicide is the second leading cause of death among men aged 15 to 24 and the leading cause of death among black males aged 15 to 34 and must be addressed.

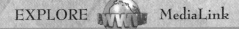

EXPLORE MediaLink

Critical thinking questions, essay questions, key terms, web links, activities, NCLEX review questions, and more interactive resources can be found on the Companion Website at www.prenhall.com/haynes. Click on Chapter 13 to select activities for this chapter.

REFERENCES

American Association of Colleges of Nursing. *The Essentials of Baccalaureate Education for Professional Nursing Practice*. (1998) Washington D.C.: Author.

American Cancer Society. (2002). *Cancer facts and figures 2002*. Atlanta: Author.

American Diabetes Association. (2000). *Basic diabetes information*. Alexandria, VA: Author.

American Heart Association. (2000). *Heart and stroke statistical update—2000*. Dallas, TX: Author.

Centers for Disease Control and Prevention (CDC). (1995a). Injury control recommendations: Bicycle helmets. *Morbidity and Mortality Weekly Report, 44*(RR-1), 1–17.

Centers for Disease Control and Prevention (CDC). (1995b). Suicide among children, adolescents and young adults: United States, 1980–1992. *Morbidity and Mortality Weekly Report, 44*(15), 289–291.

Centers for Disease Control and Prevention/National Center for Injury Prevention and Control (CDC/NCIPC). (2000). *Suicide in the United States*. Atlanta: Author.

Evans, R. G., & Stoddard, G. L. (1994). Providing health, consuming health care. In R. G. Evans, M. L. Baver, & T. R. Marmor (Eds.), *Why are some people healthy and others not? The determinants of health of populations* (pp. 27–64). Hawthorn, NY: Aldine de Gruyter.

Lamarche, P. A. (1995). Our health paradigm in peril. *Public Health Reports, 110*, 556–560.

Leavell, H. R., & Clark, E. G. (1965). *Preventative medicine for the doctor in his community: An epidemiologic approach* (2nd ed.). New York: McGraw-Hill.

Lucas, J. A, Orahan, S. A., & Cook, F. (2000). Determinants of health-promoting behavior among women ages 65 and above living in the community. *Scholarly Inquiry for Nursing Practice: An International Journal, 14*(1), 77–98.

McCloskey, J. C., & Bulechek, G. M. (2000). (Eds.), *Nursing interventions classification (NIC)* (2nd ed.). St. Louis, MO: Mosby.

McEwen, M., & Davis, L. (2001). Senior health. In M. A. Nies & M. McEwen (Eds.), *Community health nursing: Promoting the health of populations* (3rd ed.) (pp. 457–495). Philadelphia, PA: W. B. Saunders.

McFalls, J. A. (1998). Population: A lively introduction, part II. Mortality differences. *Population Bulletin, 53*(3), 1–44.

McGinnis, M. J., & Foege, W. (1993). Actual cause of death in the United States. *Journal of the American Medical Association, 270*, 2208.

Morgan, C. (2001). Men's health. In M. A. Nies & M. McEwen (Eds.), *Community health nursing: Promoting the health of populations* (3rd ed.) (pp. 382–408). Philadelphia, PA: W. B. Saunders.

National Center for Health Statistics. (2000). *Health United States: 2000*. Hyattsville, MD: USDHHS/NCHS.

Pender, N. J., Murdaugh, C. L., & Parson, M. A. (2002). *Health Promotion in Nursing Practice* (4th ed.). Upper Saddle River, NJ: Prentice Hall.

Shine, K. I. (1995). Informed joint decision-making. *Public Health Report, 110*, 555.

Torrens, P. R. (1999). Historical evolution and overview of health services in the United States. In S. J. Williams & P. R. Torrens (Eds.), *Introduction to health services* (5th ed.) (pp. 3–36). Albany, NY: Delmar Publishers.

Torrens, P. R., & Williams, S. J. (1999). Managed care: Restructuring the system. In S. J. Williams & P. R. Torrens (Eds.), *Introduction to health services* (5th ed.) (pp. 151–170). Albany, NY: Delmar Publishers.

U.S. Department of Health and Human Services. (1989). *Healthy people 2000.* Washington, DC: U.S. Government Printing Office.

U.S. Department of Health and Human Services. (2000a). *Healthy people 2010: Conference edition.* Washington, DC: U.S. Government Printing Office.

U.S. Department of Health and Human Services. (2000b). *Surveillance for selected public health indicators affecting older adults—United States—1999, 48*(8), 11–156.

U.S. Department of Health and Human Services/National Center for Health Statistics. (2001). *Health, United States, 2000 with adolescent health chartbook.* Hyattsville, MD: National Center for Health Statistics.

U.S. Department of Health and Human Services/Office of Disease Prevention Health Promotion. (1994). *Clinician's handbook of preventative services.* Washington, DC: U.S. Government Printing Office.

Walker, B. L. (1998). Preventing falls. *RN, 61*(5), 40.

SUGGESTED READINGS

American Cancer Society. (2002). *Cancer facts and figures 2002.* Atlanta: Author.

American Heart Association. (2000). *Heart and stroke statistical update—2000.* Dallas, TX: Author.

Centers for Disease Control and Prevention. (1999). Ten great public health achievements: United States, 1900–1999. *Morbidity and Mortality Weekly Reports, 48*(12), 241–243.

U.S. Department of Health and Human Services. (2000). *Healthy people 2010.* Washington, DC: U.S. Government Printing Office.

U.S. Department of Health and Human Services/Office of Disease Prevention Health Promotion. (1999). *Clinician's handbook of preventative services* (2nd ed.). Washington, DC: U.S. Government Printing Office.

14

Complementary and Alternative Therapies in Health Care

Marilyn Terrado
Jacquelin S. Neatherlin

> *We live in a time when there are more techniques for healing than ever before. The question we must ask is this: What is it, beyond or beneath those techniques, that really fosters the healing process?*
>
> *O. Carl Simonton, 1989*

LEARNING OBJECTIVES

AT THE COMPLETION OF THIS CHAPTER, THE READER WILL BE ABLE TO:

➤ Review the demographic trends and issues that contribute to increasing interest in complementary and alternative medicine (CAM) therapies.

➤ Discuss the dominant philosophical perspectives that shape the biomedical paradigm.

➤ Describe the five major domains of CAM defined by the National Center for Complementary and Alternative Medicine.

➤ Identify relevant market and public policy trends that influence costs and reimbursement for CAM therapies.

➤ Discuss how the nurse can integrate CAM therapies into professional practice.

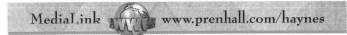
MediaLink www.prenhall.com/haynes

Additional online resources including NCLEX review questions, critical thinking questions, and real-world activities for this chapter can be found on the Companion Website at www.prenhall.com/haynes.

Nurses are facing broadening responsibilities for patient care as the health care landscape has changed, and consumers have found that traditional medical practices do not always offer an immediate or satisfactory cure. Many of these individuals are turning to complementary and alternative therapies for health promotion and healing. Consumers and health care providers alike are seeking to learn more about these therapies. Over 50% of physicians use or refer patients for complementary therapies (Jonas, 1998). Increasingly, medical and nursing schools are including Complementary and Alternative Medicine (CAM) content in electives or required courses (Wetzel, Eisenberg, & Kaptchuk, 1998). The *Essentials* (1998) document asserts that nurses need to develop an awareness of complementary modalities and their usefulness to promote health.

Even though information regarding CAM therapies is readily available, individuals may have difficulty making safe choices due to the large number of options and inconsistent quality of resources for making decisions. Without adequate supervision, CAM therapies combined with conventional treatment can result in unexpected and potentially dangerous outcomes. Nurses play a vital role in helping patients make wise and informed decisions about CAM use.

The increasing likelihood of CAM interventions in acute care settings, long-term care facilities, and the community generates exciting opportunities and challenges for nurses. As nurses increase their knowledge, keep abreast of relevant research, and become acquainted with practitioners in their communities, they can make a unique contribution to promote positive patient care outcomes. Using a holistic approach to nursing practice, this contribution will reflect a respect for the individual's ability to heal themselves.

This chapter defines various basic terms related to CAM (Table 14–1), discusses relevant philosophical paradigms, and reviews pertinent demographic and market trends. Public policies and regulations influencing CAM practice are addressed. Approaches and implications for integrating CAM into nursing practice are offered.

Changing Paradigms

The desired goal in conventional allopathic medicine has been "to cure the disease" or to relieve symptoms. This **paradigm**, or way of thinking, has prevailed for many years based on Cartesian dualism, which leads to reductionism. **Dualism** separates the material/physical body from the nonmaterial mind and spirit; the body and mind do not affect the physical body. A dualistic view does not recognize the impact of social, psychological, emotional, and spiritual influences on physical function. Conventional western medicine emphasizes the physical body; it reduces the body to the sum of its "physical" parts, which leads to **reductionism**. "Man as machine" is the common metaphor for understanding this reductionistic, **mechanistic** view of the human body. A machine is understood by knowing all the parts and how they fit and work together. Once the parts (i.e., anatomy) and the function (i.e., physiology) are

---

Table 14–1   *Common Definitions of Complementary and Alternative Medicine Terms*

Traditional/Ancestral	Health care practices tied to cultural, folk, or family-based traditions.
Allopathic medicine	Health care practices that focus on the biological mechanism of disease, primarily medications and surgery (synonymous terms include conventional, mainstream, Western, orthodox, biomedicine, and modern).
Alternative medicine	Originally defined as therapies not taught in U.S. medical schools, alternative also includes those treatments not offered by conventional providers. Some use the term alternative to imply the consumer has chosen to exclusively use a healing remedy outside conventional mainstream treatment practices.
Complementary medicine	Refers to alternative therapies that are used in combination with conventional treatment; these treatments are used as adjuncts to enhance conventional biomedical choices.
Integrative medicine	A term used to imply the selection of the best options available given the patient's condition and preferred mode of treatment. The treatment objective for integrative therapies is health and healing rather than disease and treatment.

Consider for a moment, what is the relationship between conventional, alternative, complementary, and integrative therapies? What is the difference between healing and curing? How do the various philosophies/paradigms fit with your view of healing?

understood, then malfunctions can be repaired (e.g., surgical intervention).

Conventional medicine has operated largely from this perspective. To cure, the physician identifies the malfunctioning or defective part, diagnoses what process went awry, and then makes repairs. Advances in technology and surgical procedures make it possible to replace once irreparable vital organs. Ongoing pharmaceutical and genetic research produce more powerful remedies for previously hopeless conditions. Required study in health care curricula of the human anatomy, physiology, and pathophysiology are a testament to this dualistic, reductionistic, mechanistic, biomedical approach to health care. The names of the more common clinical specialties reflect the emphasis on body "parts" (e.g., cardiology, pulmonary, neurology, or psychiatry). Even subspecialties, which focus on developmental stages (i.g., pediatric versus geriatric) or illness trajectories (i.g., acute versus chronic), generally operate within the prevailing paradigm; focus on "parts" and seek a "cure."

Although the patient may be "cured," the work of healing has at times yet to begin. The unique nature of healing evolves from the complexities of a largely invisible interaction within the whole of human experience. To say that nurses integrate the body, mind, and spirit is only another reductionistic exercise; integration still implies that there are "parts." Indeed, the mind is the body and vice versa. Research investigating the role of neuropeptides and receptors in the psychosomatic network lends credibility to the "mind–body" connection (Pert, Dreher, & Ruff, 1998).

Holistic care takes into account not only the familiar manifestations of the body–mind network such as psychological and emotional states, or social and environmental interactions, but also the dimension of "spirit." Holism, from the Greek *holos* meaning "whole," asserts that everything is greater than and different from the sum of its parts. An **organismic** or **holistic** view of health and healing acknowledge the "wholeness" and unique indefinable essence of the organism.

While there may appear to be shifting a paradigm in health care, the reality is that health care providers are simply revisiting an old paradigm that emphasizes healing and mutuality in the healing relationship. Fifty years ago, health care was simpler; there were fewer options. Neither the scope of surgical and pharmaceutical options nor assessment and screening technology was available. With little else to provide, caregivers offered themselves, their presence and intentions, as instruments of healing. Today's holistic practitioner contends that "intent" or "presence" remain an intrinsic, salient, and critical component of a holistic healing relationship. The holistic practitioner respects the patient as an equal partner and recognizes the essential role of individuals to heal themselves and maintain health.

Current Trends in Complementary and Alternative Medicine

Consumer Demand

There is growing consumer demand for CAM. Based on two telephone surveys conducted in 1990 and 1997, researchers from Harvard Medical School (Eisenberg et al., 1993, 1998) found that the number of Americans who used at least one CAM therapy had increased by 25%. The researchers attribute this rise to a larger proportion of the population seeking alternative therapies. Researchers also found that the total number of visits to CAM providers increased by almost 50% during this same period. Americans made nearly 650 million visits to CAM practitioners; this figure exceeds the total number of visits to U.S. primary care physicians. Of the 42% of respondents who used a CAM therapy, only 11% of this group did so under the supervision of a conventional primary health care provider. In both surveys, 40% of patients failed to tell their primary physicians about CAM therapies used. More recent studies of emergency room patients (Weiss, Takakuwa, & Ernst, 2001) and patients undergoing cardiac surgery (Liu et al., 2000) reiterate these findings.

Characteristics of the Typical Consumer

Individuals most commonly use CAM therapies to treat back pain, allergies, arthritis, insomnia, sprains/strains, headache, high blood pressure, digestive disorders, anxiety, and depression. The most frequently used common therapies (Eisenberg et al., 1998) include herbs, chiropractic, megavitamins, relaxation techniques, self-help groups, biofeedback, hypnosis, massage, acupuncture, guided imagery, spiritual healing, energy healing, and homeopathy. Table 14–2 offers a brief overview of common integrative therapies. Common botanical and nutritional supplements used are presented in Table 14–3. Dietary supplements used to improve overall general health are presented in Table 14–4.

Table 14–2   Common CAM Therapies

Therapy	Reported Action	Reported Clinical Conditions Treated	Concerns
Chiropractic therapy	Correction of spinal abnormalities	Low back pain, neck pain, and headaches	No significant concern; however, if during the assessment process the nurse determines the patient is engaged in chiropractic care that includes neck manipulation, this information should be noted and the patient advised of potential hazards.
Energy therapies			
Therapeutic Healing touch Reiki	Balance the body's energy using light or gentle touch	Decrease pain and anxiety, hasten wound healing, ease emotional distress, and decrease side effects of chemotherapy	No reported concern; thought to decrease pain and therefore increase mobility; may encroach on the patient's religious belief system.
Crystal therapy	Crystals and gems used with the belief that they are sources of energy and light	Decreasing pain, increasing circulation, enhancing meditation, and promoting emotional release and well-being	No reported concern or clinical efficacy.
Acupuncture and Acupressure	Simulate points to affect the body's energy system and bring balance	Acute and chronic musculoskeletal pain and other medical and emotional disorders including substance abuse	No reported perioperative concern. Efficacy of these therapies is well supported in the literature.
Massage	Manipulation of muscles and soft tissue to stimulate skin, nerves, blood, and lymph systems	Fulfills needs for touch; removes bodily toxins; increases mobility; corrects posture; decreases stress; and speeds recovery from injury	Massage is not recommended with certain cardiac and circulatory conditions and malignancies; direct massage is contraindicated when inflammation or edema is present; massage decreases pain, alleviates stiffness, and therefore promotes mobility; reduces anxiety, heart rate, and blood pressure and promotes relaxation.

Table 14–2 (continued)

Therapy	Reported Action	Reported Clinical Conditions Treated	Concerns
Aromatherapy	Application and are inhalation of oils used to activate healing energy	Boost the immune system, reduce stress, promote relaxation, hasten recovery and healing, stimulate circulation, promote digestion, reduce nausea after chemotherapy, act as a decongestant, anti-inflammatory, or antibacterial	Use of oils is unwise and should be avoided in individuals sensitive to scents (asthmatics); some oils may lower blood pressure or produce hypoglycemia.
Homeopathy	Small doses of diluted preparations that mimic symptoms of a disorder are used to heal or help the body heal itself	Relief from symptoms of multiple chronic illnesses	Insurance coverage is not available for homeopathic therapy.
Magnet therapy	Enhance blood flow to an affected area; activate electrical activity in the body thus releasing certain neurotrans-mitters	Decreases inflammation and pain; increases bone healing	Safe and easy to use; however, there is not a preponderance of scientific support for magnet therapy.
Imagery and relaxation	Increases release of endorphins and stimu-lates the immune system	Decreases severity of stress, fatigue, pain	Easy to learn, easy to implement; no reported concerns.
Hypnosis	Heightened susceptibility to suggestions	Asthma, decreases stress, smoking cessation, pain management	No reported concerns.
Laughter and humor	Strengthen immune system	Overall general health and well-being; decrease malignancy and infection	No reported concerns.
Biofeedback	Promote control over specific autonomic nervous system responses	Musculoskeletal rehabilitation, Raynaud's syndrome; autogenic training; attention deficit disorder	No reported concerns.
Reflexology—zone therapy	Body is divided into zones and stress, injury, and disease can impede the energy flow in these zones	Healing; pain management	No concern; however, patients with circulatory problems of the lower extremities, diabetes, renal calculi, and pacemakers should consult a physician before engaging in reflexology.

Sources: Lorenzi, E. A. (1999). Complementary/alternative therapies. So many choices. *Geriatric Nursing, 20*(3), 125–133; and Shua-Haim, J. R., & Ross, J. S. (1999). Alternative medicine in geriatrics: Competing with or complementing conventional medicine. *Clinical Geriatrics, 7*(6), 37–49.

Table 14–3   Common Botanicals/Nutritional Supplements Used

Botanical/Nutritional Supplement Used	Clinical Condition	Botanical/Nutritional Supplement Used	Clinical Condition
Gingko Biloba Vitamin E Phosphatidylserine L. Carnitine	Memory loss	St. John's Wort Kava Hops Valerian Passion Flower	Depression, anxiety, and/or insomnia
Glucosamine Sulfate Chondroitin MSM SAM-e	Osteoarthritis	Echinacea Colloidial Silver Olive Leaf Extract Vitamin C	Immunity
Shark Cartilage Fish Oil Garlic Flax Seed Oil Red Yeast Rice	Hypercholesteremia	Ginseng	Improve mental/physical performance
Hawthorne L. Carnitine Coenzyme Q10	Cardiovascular	Bilberry Saw Palmetto	Improve vision Treat benign prostatic hyperplasia
Mahuang Licorice Grape Seed Extract Quercetin Nettles MSN	Respiratory—allergy/asthma	Gotu Kola	Treat varicose veins

Sources: Blumenthal, M. (2000). Interaction between herbs and conventional drugs. Introductory consideration. *Herbalgram,* *49*(Summer 2000), 52–63; Blumenthal, M. (Ed.). (2000). *Integrative medicine access: Professional reference to conditions, herbs, and supplements.* Newton, MA: Integrative Medicine Communications: Author; and *The Complete German Commission & Monographs: Therapeutic Guide to Herbal Medicines.* (1998). Boston, MA: Integrative Medicine Communications: Author.

The major consumers of CAM are individuals between ages 25 and 49 and over age 65. Women rather than men are more likely to use CAM therapies. These consumers more often have some college education and earn annual incomes over $50,000. African-Americans are less likely to use CAM than are individuals from other cultural groups (Eisenberg et al., 1998). Astin (1998) found that individuals selected CAM therapies based on a congruence or agreement with personal values. CAM users in this study were better educated, suffered from poor health status or had multiple chronic conditions, held a holistic orientation toward health, and had experienced a transformational life experience that significantly affected their worldview. Kessler et al. (2001) found that the use of 20 CAM therapies ranging from acupuncture to yoga has increased in popularity since the 1960s. Further, the research findings indicated that among those individuals who have tried a CAM therapy, almost 50% are still using them 11 to 20 years later and that use of CAM therapies may be independent of gender, ethnic background, level of education, and regional and city/rural differences.

Table 14–4 Dietary Supplements Used to Improve Overall General Health

Multivitamins	Vitamin E
Used to improve overall general health; use of multivitamins is justified if natural sources of vitamins are determined to be inadequate.	Use to prevent cardiovascular disease and cancer; studies are under way to determine efficacy of supplement use. Short-term use (up to 4 months) has been found to present no risk; safety of long-term use has not been established.
Vitamin A/beta-carotene	**Vitamin K**
Diets rich in vitamin A and beta-carotene may lower risks of some types of cancer; there is a possible association between high intake of different forms of vitamin A and the development of osteoporosis; excess consumption may be associated with liver and bone damage.	Associated with decreased risk of hip fractures; no adverse effects are reported associated with the consumption of vitamin K supplements in humans or animals; patients on anticoagulant therapy should limit intake of foods high in vitamin K to assure therapeutic anticoagulation.
Vitamin C	**Calcium**
Diets high in vitamin C may decrease the risk for or help alleviate, clinical symptoms associated with coronary heart disease, cataracts, some common neurodegenerative diseases, and viral infections; potential though rare complications of excessive vitamin C intake include urinary problems, increased irorn absorption, diarrhea, and possible destruction of vitamin B_{12}.	Used to prevent and treat osteoporosis; individuals with a history of urolithiasis containing calcium-rich stones should consult their health care provider before taking calcium supplements.
Vitamin D	**Folic Acic**
Used to prevent and treat osteoporosis; individual daily requirement can be met with one glass of milk; excessive doses are associated with hypercalcemia.	Leads to reduced homeocysteine levels and thus reduces heart disease; no serious adverse reactions.

Adapted with permission: Haynes, L. C., Martin, J. H., & Endres, D. (2003). Nontraditional therapies and older adults: Effects of botanical, herbal, and nutritional supplements, *RN, 77*(5), 913–922.

Market Factors and Public Interest in CAM

There are several market factors fueling public interest. First, the increasing supply of CAM services and products coupled with economic conditions in the last 10 years have prompted consumers to shop around for health care rather than passively accept the constraints and restrictions of managed care. Second, aggressive marketing and corporate maneuvers to increase profit margins have transformed health care from a "service" to a business orientation. This transformation has engendered perceptions of an insurmountable maze of bureaucracy, excessive dependence on science and technology, and growing depersonalization between the provider and patient. Third, rapid technological development, advances in medical diagnosis and treatment techniques, complex pharmaceuticals, and genetic engineering have created illusions of "expressway cures" or "magic bullets," which do not always result in affordable or accessible care. One of the trade-offs is an underlying expectation for a rapid cure, which may be counterproductive to convalescence and healing. Fourth, the therapeutic milieu of the provider–patient relationship, which addresses less tangible spiritual and soothing aspects of healing, has been set aside in favor

Why are consumers seeking CAM? How have demographics and culture influenced health care?

How do these considerations and this information fit with your own background?

of high-tech interventions and increasing subspecialization among conventional practitioners. Finally, poor communication and perceptions of hasty, impersonal, and sometimes indifferent provider–patient relationships has increased consumer discontent.

Advances in information technology, wider accessibility and use of Internet communications, and burgeoning abundance of information and advertisement about CAM via the Internet and other media have also promoted CAM in the global marketplace. The capability of making online purchases of CAM services and products has eliminated the restrictions of time and space. Further, herbs and supplements are found not only in specialty, "organic" supermarkets, but also widely available in general markets and drug stores. Finally, consumers' interests in CAM have been fueled by their desire to take responsibility for their health. The expansion of health and fitness clubs/programs, focus on prevention and health maintenance activities, fear of adverse reactions from conventional therapies, and consumer interest groups are signs of this trend. Furthermore, environmental hazards such as use of pesticides/herbicides and development of genetically engineered food raise concerns about the potential and actual toxic effects on health and the environment among many individuals.

Public interest in CAM therapies has grown as Americans live longer and experience more chronic illnesses. Complementary and alternative therapies are often used to augment treatment of these chronic conditions (Astin, 1998; Gordon, 2001b). Researchers report that 42% of all CAM therapy use is attributed to existing chronic conditions when compared to 58% who ascribed to prevention and health maintenance (Eisenberg et al., 1998). Complementary and alternative therapies added to clinical specialization offer practitioners the unique opportunity to augment conventional therapies for treating patients with chronic illness. Technical advances in surgical procedures and pharmaceutical developments have done relatively little to cure chronic disease. Instead, they further complicate the labyrinth patients follow to seek and find the appropriate interventions. Patients interact not only with a primary care provider but also with numerous others (e.g., referred specialists, consultants, service providers, agencies, and facilities) in a health care system where coordination and communication can be limited.

Almost 100 million Americans suffer from at least one chronic condition; this number is projected to double by the year 2050 (Newcomer, 1997). In 1990, direct medical costs for persons with chronic conditions totaled approximately $425 billion; this figure is also expected to double by the year 2050. Combined with $234 billion spent indirect costs (e.g., loss of productivity), chronic conditions account for a large proportion of health care dollar expenditures. Furthermore, approximately 75% of Americans living with chronic conditions are younger than age 65. The long-term trajectory of chronic conditions and the rising numbers of Americans advancing into old age translates to a need for greater supervision by practitioners well grounded in both conventional and CAM treatment modalities (Centers for Disease Control and Prevention [CDC], 1999).

Domains of Complementary and Alternative Medicine Therapies

Alternative medicine therapies are complete systems of knowledge and practice that developed independent of and prior to conventional biomedicine (National Center for Complementary and Alternative Medicine [NCCAM], 2001a). NCCAM has defined five domains of complementary therapies (see Table 14–5). Many, if not most, of these are complex ancient healing systems steeped in traditions, which evolve from cultural origins. Examples of ancient systems evolving from an Eastern philosophy include traditional Oriental/ Chinese medicine, Native American healing, and Ayurveda (from India). Several systems that developed from the Western biomedical approaches of Europe and North America include homeopathy, osteopathy, and naturopathy. These systems, unlike conventional biomedicine, share a common belief in energy or a life

Table 14–5	NCCAM Categories of Complementary and Alternative Therapies
Biological-based therapies	Herbs, diets
Manipulative therapies	Therapeutic massage, chiropractic, osteopathy, movement therapies
Energy therapies	Reiki, acupuncture, therapeutic/healing touch
Mind–body interactions	Guided imagery, progressive relaxation, hypnosis, art, prayer, music, dance
Alternative systems of medical practice	Traditional Chinese medicine, Ayurveda, Native American healing

force as central to healing and understanding illness. Balancing and maintaining harmony of spirit, mind, and body are critical in the healing process. The patient is viewed as an active and essential participant, particularly in Eastern-based systems that integrate lifestyle interventions such as diet, exercise, meditation, sleep/rest, massage, and breathing techniques, as well as herbal preparations to restore balance and health.

Mind–Body Interventions

Mind–body interventions focus on strategies to use the mind, thoughts, and emotions to improve physical health. These interventions are helpful to reduce stress and promote the relaxation response. Mind–body interventions have been integrated extensively in the care of cancer patients with various symptoms including nausea, vomiting, anxiety, pain, and to reduce the number of cancer cells (Sherman & Simonton, 1998). Recent developments in the field of psychoneuroimmunology (Pert, 1997; Pert et al., 1998) are beginning to detail more fully the mind–body network. Findings show that "emotional expression generates balance in the neuropeptide-receptor network and a functional healing system" (Pert et al., 1998, p. 30). In other words, emotions influence healing.

Mind–body interventions encompass several strategies familiar to nurses and nursing practice including guided imagery, meditation, support groups, hypnosis, biofeedback, dance, art, music therapies, and prayer. The potential benefits of mind–body interventions on fibromyalgia and on cardiovascular disease are documented by several NCCAM research centers (NCCAM, 2001c). Prayer, also known as distant or nonlocal healing in the literature, is gaining interest in the media, the public, and academic circles. Ongoing empirical studies such as the Monitoring and Actualizing of Noetic Trainings (MANTRA) at Duke University (Horrigan, 1999) and ongoing academic discussions are being aimed at empirically analyzing the impact of nonlocal healing (Bird, 1988; Dossey, 1999; Targ, 1997). Furthermore, NCCAM researchers are currently investigating the effects of spiritual practices among (a) African-American women with breast cancer and (b) patients undergoing coronary artery bypass surgery (NCCAM, 2001).

Biological-Based Therapies

Biological-based therapies encompass a wide range of interventions including specialty diets (e.g., anti-cancer, anti-cardiovascular diets), dietary supplements, herbs (i.e., phytomedicine), and orthomolecular therapies (e.g., megavitamins and minerals). Examples of lesser-known therapies include chelation for individuals with coronary heart disease, shark cartilage therapy for cancer, and light therapy for those with seasonal affective disorder (SAD).

Manipulative and Body-Based Methods

Manipulative and body-based methods incorporate those modalities that use movement and/or physical manipulation (e.g., adjustment or pressure) of the body. In chiropractic care, misalignments of the spine are readjusted to relieve low back pain and other musculoskeletal conditions (Fugh-Berman, 1997). In contrast, therapeutic massage manipulates soft tissues to achieve similar goals. Other methods in this category of CAM target movement repatterning. The focus of these methods is also misalignment, though practitioners do not physically manipulate the body. Instead, patients are taught several strategies for posture adjustment and physical movement to improve symptoms and restore health.

Energy Therapies

Energy therapies address the healing potential of the human body's bioenergy field and the utility of external sources of electromagnetic energy to restore health. Energy-based therapies are grounded in a vitalistic or "energy" view of health and disease (Kaptchuk, 1996). Imbalances of vital energy are believed to account for disease; restoring energy balance and mobilization of energy are believed to maintain or regain health.

Therapeutic touch (TT) and healing touch (HT) are two energy-based therapies developed and used by nurses. These therapies are grounded in the ancient practice of "laying on of hands" with the intent to promote healing rather than curing. TT and HT are best known for alleviating pain and anxiety.

Energy-based therapies from Eastern traditions like Reiki (Japan) and qigong (China) have gained increasing popularity in this country. The efficacy of these therapies for treating neurodegenerative and cardiovascular disease is currently being examined at NCCAM-funded research centers. Finally, external sources of electromagnetic energy (e.g., application of electric currents and magnets) are reported to be useful in facilitating healing of nonuniting bone fractures (Gordon, 1996). Magnets have also been utilized for sports injuries, sprains, and muscle strains to restore the body's bio-electromagnetic balance.

The Complementary and Alternative Medicine Market Place

Economics of CAM

In 1997, it was estimated that over $27 billion was paid out of pocket for all CAM therapies, including professional services, vitamins, herbs, dietary supplements, books, and classes (Eisenberg et al., 1998). Exclusive of inflation, $21.2 billion was spent on professional services alone; an increase of almost 45% between 1990 and 1997. These conservative estimates rival or exceed out-of-pocket expenditures for hospitalizations and physician visits for that same time period.

Until recently, consumers paid all the costs incurred for CAM treatment modalities. Obstacles that have prevented third-party payment include (a) lack of proven efficacy; (b) economics; (c) lack of knowledge about CAM; (d) provider competition; and (e) lack of standards of practice (Pelletier, Krasner, & Haskell, 1997). The most common therapy reimbursed by health maintenance organizations (HMOs) is chiropractic (65% of all HMOs) followed by acupuncture (31%) and massage therapy (11%).

Consumers are beginning to demand that insurers and hospitals consider the benefits of incorporating CAM into their health plans and services. In 1996, the state of Washington required all health insurers to add coverage of CAM treatments to standard medical coverage. The California Health Care Association has

mandated CAM treatments be routinely available by 2005.

Health maintenance organizations are also recognizing the tidal wave of interest in CAM therapies. Landmark Healthcare's (1998) survey of HMO executives reports that while 33% of HMOs do not offer alternative care, all believed that there is a demand for these options. The driving force behind the growing inclusion of CAM treatment modalities is consumers' (individual members, employers, and groups) interest and state mandates.

Emergence of "CAM" Industry—Phytomedicine Market

The World Health Organization (WHO) estimates that 4 billion people, 80% of the world population, use herbal medicine, now known as **phytomedicine** (Sierpina, 2001; Springhouse, 2002). Terms related to phytomedicine include nutraceutical, phytochemical, and phytonutrient. **Nutraceutical** refers to particular chemical compounds in foods that have a pharmacological benefit such as amino acids, enzymes, minerals, vitamins, and other dietary supplements. **Phytochemical** emphasizes the plant source of disease-preventing compounds. Phytochemicals are "biologically active substances in plants that are responsible for giving them flavor, color, and natural disease resistance" (Balch & Balch, 1997, p. 7). For example, beta-carotene, a well-known carotenoid belonging to a class of compounds related to vitamin A, is found in sweet potatoes, carrots, and yams. This phytochemical is responsible for the orange-yellow color commonly associated with these root vegetables. Other phytochemicals currently under study for their possible role in preventing cancer include genistein, found in soybeans; indoles, present in cruciferous vegetables such as broccoli; and polyphenols, found in green tea. **Phytonutrient** is a term used synonymously with phytochemical, but focuses on plant nutrients useful to humans such as fiber in fruits and grains.

The phytomedicine industry in the United States is booming. Between 1990 and 1997, use of herbal remedies increased by 380%; megadose vitamin use increased by 130% (Eisenberg et al., 1998). Commercialization, mass marketing and distribution, and wide media attention, combined with unlimited and unrestricted public access, contribute to this growth. In contrast to 10 years ago, herbal products are available not only in specialty stores but also in local groceries, and can also be purchased via mail order and online.

Ever-increasing acceptance and use of herbal medicines has stimulated herbal research. Evidence from these studies has attracted interest from conventional and complementary health professionals, the general public, and manufacturers. Recent market statistics show that herb sales decreased by 15% in 2001 from almost $600 million to $510 million (Blumenthal, 2001). Media attention on research studies questioning the efficacy of some herbal claims as well as a more informed and discerning consumer may account for this trend.

Relevant Social and Health Policy

Dietary Supplements and Health Education Act of 1994

Congress passed the Dietary Supplements and Health Education Act (DSHEA) in 1994 as a response to the rapidly growing public consumption and increased interest in the benefits of nutrients and dietary supplements. The act was formulated to provide a framework for assuring safety through labeling of dietary supplements. With this legislation, Congress defined a new class of products, **dietary supplements**. These products are neither food nor drugs. According to the act, dietary supplements include one or more of the following "dietary ingredients": (a) a vitamin, (b) a mineral, (c) an herb or other botanical, (d) an amino acid, and (e) substances such as enzymes, organ tissues, glandular, and metabolites (U.S. Food and Drug Administration [FDA], 2001). These products must have information on labels that designates them as dietary supplements. Dietary supplements must have nutritional labels that list ingredients. Importantly, the labeling of dietary supplements cannot imply that the ingredients diagnose, prevent, treat, or cure a specific disease (FDA, 2000).

While provisions in the DSHEA facilitate consumer access to desired products, the relative leniency of the legislation signals alarm. Unlike new drug approval that requires disclosure of effectiveness, contraindications, and potential side effects, dietary supplements do not need FDA approval prior to being placed on the market. Manufacturers are responsible for determining that the product is safe and that there is substantiated evidence to support claims on product labels. Yet, it is not mandated that manufacturers disclose this information to either the FDA or interested consumers.

Of further concern, the FDA has yet to establish standards that delineate appropriate manufacturing practices that ensure purity, quality, strength, or com-

position of dietary supplements. Consequently, herbal remedies are not bound by strict FDA standards. The FDA does not require a consistent "standardized" amount of a "dietary ingredient" in dietary supplements across different manufacturers or even within one manufacturer's production batches. Thus, there is the potential for significant variation in the potency of products with each lot or batch. Unlike manufacturers of drugs, manufacturers and distributors of dietary supplements are not mandated to record, investigate, or otherwise inform the FDA of any reports of adverse effects related to a dietary supplement. Thus, consumers rely on reports from advocate groups or complaints from the public.

The FDA has not been successful in removing hazardous products from the marketplace or mandating appropriate warnings on labels (Haller & Benowitz, 2000; Talalay & Talalay, 2001; Winslow & Kroll, 1998). In 1997, despite several years of investigation and over 800 reports of adverse events associated with ephedra-containing products, the FDA was only recently able to issue official safety concerns. Herbal products derived from ephedra herbs, also called "ma huang," contain an amphetamine-like compound that stimulates the nervous system and heart. Consumers use ephedra-containing products to raise their energy level, improve performance, or lose weight. After reviewing reports of adverse effects associated with ephedra use, such as high blood pressure, insomnia, irregular heart rate, and stroke, and death among otherwise healthy young to middle-aged adults, the FDA proposed limitations on the daily intake of ephedra. The FDA also recommended that manufacturer labels warn against long-term use, adverse side effects, and contraindications (U.S. Department of Health and Human Services [DHHS], 1997). The dietary supplement industry, which realized annual sales over $1 billion for ephedra-containing products in 2000, successfully lobbied against the FDA proposal (Talalay & Talalay, 2001).

National Center for Complementary and Alternative Medicine

In response to growing public interest and increasing demand for alternative therapies, Congress established within the National Institutes of Health (NIH) the Office of Alternative Medicine (OAM) (OAM, 1992). In succeeding years, as alternative therapies became more popular and were used in combination with conventional biomedical treatments, practitioners and consumers alike began to use the term complementary. In

1998, the OAM was renamed National Center for Complementary and Alternative Medicine, expanding from a $2 million budget in FY1993 to almost $69 million in FY2000. The Center (a) sets standards for evaluating competency of CAM practitioners, (b) provides information about CAM to providers and consumers, (c) conducts and supports basic and clinical research, (d) initiates and funds research training on CAM, and (e) evaluates and promotes integration of effective therapies into mainstream care.

White House Commission on Complementary and Alternative Medicine Policy

The 1999 Omnibus legislation, which expanded the Office of Alternative Medicine to more than 20 Institutes and Centers of the NIH, also established the White House Commission on Complementary and Alternative Medicine Policy (WHCCAMP). The Commission's role was to offer recommendations for legislation and administrative action to the White House and Congress regarding CAM research, services, reimbursement, professional education, and public information (Gordon, 2001a). WHCCAMP presented its final report to the president on March 22, 2002 (WHCCAMP, 2002).

After various hearings and town hall meetings sponsored by the WHCCAMP, the Commission reached consensus on several items (Gordon, 2001a). Some are summarized below:

- Curricula of undergraduate, graduate, and continuing education programs of both CAM (e.g., homeopathy, massage therapy, acupuncture, etc.) and conventional professions (e.g., physicians, nurses, social workers, psychologists, etc.) should integrate content that promotes an understanding of both CAM and conventional principles and approaches.
- Board/certification exams should include CAM/conventional content along with requisite basic science and core clinical practice issues.
- Good manufacturing practices and truthful labeling for marketing should be guaranteed on all supplements, and a mechanism should be developed to identify, admonish, and prosecute those who violate these standards.
- Agencies or boards that regulate integrative and CAM practitioners should include representation by integrative practitioners.

- CAM therapies should emphasize the prominent role of self-care in healing.
- Research strategies should be developed that value the integrity and traditions behind CAM practices.
- Reliable and authoritative information about CAM should be disseminated to professionals and the public.
- CAM practices should have greater availability for everyone and not only for those who can afford them.
- Cultural diverse systems of health care and unique needs of traditional communities should be respected.

These recommendations were submitted as part of the final report. In addition, several recommendations were made to expand, coordinate, and increase research fundings (WHCCAMP, 2002).

Research Issues

A recurrent and contentious criticism of CAM is the lack of evidence-based support regarding efficacy (Abbot, 2000; Ernst, 1998; Ernst & White, 2000; Fontanarosa & Lundberg, 1998; Moylan, 2000). There is the prevailing assumption that conventional medicine is "scientific," while CAM is not. Critics of CAM research cite several flaws in design methodology that include (a) small sample sizes that are vulnerable to effects of confounding variables, (b) a preponderance of anecdotal case studies, (c) no controls to account for the placebo effect, (d) lack of randomization of subjects and standardized treatment protocols, and (e) absence of blind or double-blind methodology to reduce bias of researcher and subject. In short, empirical evidence based on a large sample size that is double blind and has a randomized controlled trial (RCT) is generally lacking in existing CAM research.

CAM advocates argue that these modalities do not fit into the scheme of empirical research methodologies (Dossey, 1995; Fugh-Berman, 1997; Hamilton & Bechtel, 1996; Nield-Anderson & Ameling, 2000). The editor of *Alternative Therapies in Health and Medicine* rejects the notion that CAM therapies can be validated by randomized control trials.

Many alternative interventions are unlike drugs and surgical procedures. Their action is affected by factors that cannot be specified, quantified, and controlled in double-blind designs. *Everything that counts cannot be counted* (emphasis is mine).

Matthees, Anatachoti, Kreitzer, Savik, Hertz, and Gross (2001) conducted a study to describe the use of complementary and alternative medicine (CAM) therapies in lung transplant recipients. The study further examined whether CAM therapies increased the recipients' quality of life, health status, and adherence to medical regimens when compared to nonusers of CAM therapies. The researchers used a conceptual model of quality of life related to transplant indicating that behavioral, personal, and environmental characteristics all influence the person's decision to use conventional and/or CAM therapies. The researchers also recognized that adherence to the chosen treatment(s) would mediate the impact of treatment, which included quality of life.

Lung and/or heart/lung transplant patients were surveyed regarding use of complementary therapies, adherence to therapy, and feelings regarding postoperative quality of life. Of the 145 surveys mailed 99 responses (68%) were received. Results indicated that 88 of 99 survey participants reported used of at least one CAM therapy. In addition, 70% reported using more than one nontraditional therapy.

CAM users and nonusers did not differ significantly in their medication adherence. Sixty-three percent of the patients were classified as having high adherence to their routine medication protocols following the transplant. Individuals using complementary therapies did not differ significantly from nonusers in their perception of quality of life. The researchers described patient use of CAM therapies as complimentary to the ongoing medical regimen, rather than as an alternative. Despite using the therapy as complimentary to the traditional treatment modality, only 63% of survey participant's patients had discussed the use of the complimentary therapy with their primary care provider.

In summary, the researchers emphasized the need for nurses and other health care providers to work with all patients, including long-term patients, to determine if CAM therapies are being used. The authors encouraged providers to become knowledgeable regarding complementary and alternative health care modalities and to provide sensitive counseling regarding safety issues so as to provide better care and offer an improved quality of life to the patient.

To subject alternative therapies to sterile, impersonal double blind conditions strip them of intrinsic qualities that are part of their power (Dossey, 1995, p. 7).

Alternative therapies such as traditional Chinese medicine, Ayurveda, homeopathy, and hand-mediated healing approaches like Reiki and therapeutic/healing touch have been particularly vulnerable to criticism. Therapeutic touch (TT), an approach best known among nurses, has been scrutinized in both medical and nursing literature (Easter, 1997; Meehan, 1998; Winsted-Fry & Kijek, 1999). In the absence of accurate, reliable, and consistent instruments to measure objective changes in the human "energy" field, existing studies of hand-mediated healing approaches such as TT have relied on proxy variables ranging from relief of symptoms (e.g., pain, anxiety, and stress) to changes in immune function. Other persistent methodological challenges for researchers in energy-based therapies include inconsistent protocols, differences between practitioners, and the inability to distinguish the impact of the "intent" or "presence" of the practitioner from the treatment.

There are those who believe that evidence-based studies should be the basis for deciding which CAM therapies will be incorporated into clinical practice. Third-party payers would then be more inclined to pay for these services (Gordon, 2001b).

To address the need for more rigorous empirical research, NCCAM has established 12 centers (see Table 14–6) to investigate alternative therapies for specialty areas or chronic conditions such as addictions, arthritis, cancer, cardiovascular disease, cardiovascular disease and aging in African-Americans, craniofacial disorders, neurological disorders, neurodegenerative diseases, chiropractic, and pediatrics. These centers will evaluate relevant therapies and provide databases of information for dissemination to the public (NCCAM, 2001c).

Table 14–6   NCCAM Research Centers

Location	Specialty
Minneapolis Medical Research Foundation	Addictions
Columbia College, College of Physicians and Surgeons	Aging and women's health
University of Maryland, School of Medicine	Arthritis
	Botanicals[a]
Purdue University West Lafayette	Age-related diseases
University of Illinois at Chicago	Women's health
University of California, Los Angeles	Dietary supplements
University of Arizona School of Pharmacy	Ayurvedic herbs
Johns Hopkins University	Cancer
University of Pennsylvania	
University of Michigan, Ann Arbor	Cardiovascular disease
Maharishi University of Management, Fairfield, IA	Cardiovascular disease and aging in African-Americans
Palmer Center for Chiropractic Research, Davenport, IA	Chiropractic
Kaiser Foundation Hospitals, Portland, OR	Craniofacial disorders
Oregon Health Sciences University, Portland	Neurological disorders
Emory University	Neurogenerative disorders
University of Arizona, Tuscon	Pediatrics

[a]Funded in collaboration with the Office of Dietary Supplements (ODS).

Four Centers for Dietary Supplement Research are funded by the collaborative efforts of the Office of Dietary Supplements (ODS) and NCCAM. The Centers study the potential hazards and health benefits of botanicals and dietary supplements. Research findings will help develop standards for popular herbal and dietary supplements. The Centers also focus on expanding the scientific knowledge base of the biological characteristics, mechanisms of action, and potential clinical application of botanicals and dietary supplements for specific diseases and conditions including osteoporosis, cardiovascular disease, and cancer. Some of the well-known and commonly used herbs or botanicals to be studied are black cohosh, red clover, dong quai, Asian ginseng, gingko, cranberry, licorice, valerian, soy, grapes, green tea, St. John's wort, ginger, turmeric, and boswellia.

Regulation of Complementary and Alternative Medicine Therapies

Regulations are imposed to protect the public's health, welfare, and safety, and to ensure the competency of health care providers. Regulations are designed to prevent unskilled or unlicensed practitioners from using

Critical Thinking and Reflection

What is the impact of the Dietary Supplement and Health Education Act? There is contentious debate about the efficacy of CAM therapies. Assume you are an advocate. What arguments would you advance in support of CAM? Assume you are an opponent. What arguments would you advance in opposition?

designated CAM treatment modality. Regulations are also intended to direct consumers to appropriately trained providers and shield the public from harmful treatments or advice. There are disparate perspectives motivating the need for regulation. One view argues that regulation serves to protect the "self-interest" or territory of practice for a specific professional group; public protection is a secondary gain (Cohen, 1998). The alternate view assumes that consumers are generally uninformed and thus unable to determine competency of practitioners without designated credentials afforded by regulation. This concern may be warranted considering the wide variation in state-to-state regulation of CAM practitioners. Another reason some professional groups support regulation is the belief that there is greater likelihood of third-party payment. (Milbank Memorial Fund, 1998).

The continuum of regulation ranges from registration, to certification, to licensure. The least restrictive, **registration**, allows for participation in an occupation provided the clinician is registered with a regulatory agency. Registration is generally applied to those occupations that have little or no threat to life, health, or safety of the public. A more restrictive form of registration, **certification**, is based on a practitioner's ability to meet standards set by a state agency or professional self-regulatory organization. Requirements may include education, experience, and/or passing an examination similar to that required for licensure. Professional organizations for various CAM therapies (e.g., yoga, craniosacral therapy, reflexology, healing touch, and guided imagery) have certification requirements for practitioners.

Licensure is the most rigorous level of regulation. **Licensure** restricts the scope of practice so that only licensed individuals may provide specific services. Licensure establishes the minimum standard for authority to practice. Licensure is controlled at the state level by licensing scheme, different laws, regulations, and processes for interpreting scope of practice (Cohen, 1998). The existence and scope of licensure for specific professional practices varies from state to state. Health professionals, including nurses, physicians, physical therapists, and chiropractors, are licensed based on educational preparation, and they have a clearly circumscribed scope of practice defined and regulated by state law.

Table 14–7 lists licensure status for several of the more popular CAM therapies including chiropractic, acupuncture, massage, homeopathy, and naturopathy. Only chiropractic is licensed in all states. State regulations for other CAM practitioners may vary by state. For acupressure, some states require physician referral or a record

of physician supervision, while others do not have such restrictions. Two states allow practice pending approval of the Board of Medical Examiners and five other states have introduced licensure legislation (Acupuncture and Oriental Medicine Alliance, 2001). Some states allow certain practitioners (e.g., physicians, dentists, chiropractors, osteopaths, and naturopaths) to perform acupuncture under their own license. Acupuncture, as well as naturopathy and chiropractic, have accrediting bodies recognized by the U.S. Department of Education (Milbank Memorial Fund, 1998). Training in acupuncture ranges from programs requiring 1,500 to 2,000 hours of practice to qualify for an acupuncture license in states where licensure exists, to programs such as UCLA Medical Acupuncture for Physicians program, which requires significantly fewer hours and two weeks of hands-on sessions (Sierpina, 2001).

A recurring concern in the nursing literature is the impact of CAM popularity on the nursing practice (Kreitzer & Jensen, 2000; Quinn, 2000). Nurses have provided massage, a fundamental skill, to alleviate pain, provide comfort, or enhance well-being in their patients. In recent years, massage therapists have gained licensure or certification in 26 states and Washington, D.C. Title protection, included in massage therapy practice acts of some states, prohibits noncertified individuals to use the "certified" title "massage therapist." Notably, title protection does not preclude nurses from providing massage to their patients. Concern arises when certification or licensure of CAM practitioners or specific state regulations threaten to restrict nurses from performing skills or implement clinical interventions basic to nursing practice. Thus, it is important that nurses monitor new or revised certification or licensure legislation that may impact nursing practice.

Role of the Nurse

Professional Development: Expanding Nursing's Knowledge of Complementary and Alternative Therapies

The nursing intervention classification system (Dochterman & Bulechek, 2004) include aroma therapy, music therapy, progressive muscle relaxation, guided imagery, massage, and therapeutic touch as independent nursing interventions. Other common therapies that nurses have incorporated into their clinical practice include relaxation techniques, meditation, healing touch, nutritional

Table 14–7 Licensure of CAM Modalities by State

State	Chiropractic	Acupuncture	Massage	Homeopathy	Naturopathy
Alabama	X	B	N		X
Alaska	X	X			X
Arizona	X	X		X	X
Arkansas	X	X	X		
California	X	X			P
Colorado	X	X			P
Connecticut	X	X	X	X	X
Delaware	X		X		
Washington, D.C.	X	X	X		X
Florida	X	X	X		X
Georgia	X	X			
Hawaii	X	X	X		X
Idaho	X	X			
Illinois	X	X			
Indiana	X	X			
Iowa	X	X	X		
Kansas	X	B			X
Kentucky	X	P			P
Louisiana	X	X	X		
Maine	X	X	X		X
Maryland	X	X	C		
Massachusetts	X	X	X		P
Michigan	X	B+P			
Minnesota	X	X			P
Mississippi	X				
Missouri	X	X	N		
Montana	X	X			X
Nebraska	X	X	X		
Nevada	X	X		X	
New Hampshire	X	X	X		X
New Jersey	X	X			P
New Mexico	X	X	X		
New York	X	X	X		
North Carolina	X	X	N		
North Dakota	X		X		
Ohio	X	X	X		
Oklahoma	X	P			
Oregon	X	X	X		X
Pennsylvania	X	X			
Rhode Island	X	X	X		
South Carolina	X	X	X		N
South Dakota	X				
Tennessee	X	X	X		N
Texas	X	X	R		
Utah	X	X	X		X
Vermont	X	X			N

(continued)

Table 14–7   (continued)

State	Chiropractic	Acupuncture	Massage	Homeopathy	Naturopathy
Virginia	X	X	C		
Washington	X	X	X		X
West Virginia	X	X	N		
Wisconsin	X	X	R		
Wyoming	X	P			

N, new legislation yet to be enacted; C, certification only; R, registration; P, licensing bill introduced, still pending; B, review by board of medical examiners.

counseling, yoga, reflexology, craniosacral therapy, and stress reduction strategies (Snyder & Lindquist, 2001). While some of these complementary approaches are familiar options in nursing practice, they have not been consistently included in basic nursing education programs nor addressed in graduate-level studies. In 1996, the OAM invited nursing and medical school educators in complementary and alternative medicine to make recommendations regarding the integration of content into curricula. Most nursing programs, particularly at the undergraduate level, already have a full curriculum; thus, CAM content is likely offered as an elective or interspersed in requisite courses. At the graduate level, more nursing schools are offering academic degrees or certificate programs in holistic nursing or complementary therapies (see Box 14–1).

Integrating CAM into Professional Nursing Practice

The American Holistic Nurses Association (AHNA) position statement (2001) to the White House Commission on Complementary and Alternative Medicine offered the following recommendations on the role of nurses in CAM:

- Identify the need for CAM interventions.
- Assist individuals in locating CAM providers.
- Educate, counsel, coach, or otherwise assist individuals to safely seek and use CAM.
- Coordinate the use of CAM among various providers participating in the patient's care.
- Evaluate the effectiveness and safe integration of therapies.

Nurses do not unanimously embrace CAM therapies either because they know little about them or because they are skeptical of their efficacy. Whether nurses accept CAM or not, they must recognize that patients are and will use these therapies with or without the health care provider's knowledge. Thus, an essential first step in integrating CAM into practice is to create an open, nonjudgmental line of communication that will invite the patient to share information about

Box 14–1   Schools Offering Academic Degrees or Certificate Programs in Holistic Nursing or Complementary Therapies

University of California at San Francisco
Beth-El College of Nursing in Colorado Springs, Colorado
Canyon College in Caldwell, Indiana
College of New Rochelle in New York
University of Minnesota's Center for Spirituality and Healing in Minneapolis
Rush University College of Nursing in Chicago, Illinois
New York University
Humboldt State University
Holistic Nursing Institute in Tucker, Georgia
Westbrook University–Online

their use of CAM options (Parkman, 2002). In one survey of nurse practitioners, only 10% reported regularly asking patients about the use of CAM modalities (Hayes & Alexander, 2000). This finding, combined with the significant proportion of patients who do not volunteer CAM-use information to their physician, is a concern since "complementary and alternative" does not mean safe and without danger.

The nurse needs to collaborate with all members of the health care team and maintain critical, ongoing communication with primary providers about patients who seek or use CAM modalities. To promote open communication, nurses need to establish credibility with patients by demonstrating familiarity with pertinent CAM approaches or knowledge of relevant consumer resources. While nurses are obliged to support the autonomy and self-determination of the patient, they are also legally accountable for the care they provide. It is crucial that nurses become more familiar with the complementary and alternative therapies their patients use. A solid knowledge base should be combined with information/referral sources, and the ability to advise patients who may not be aware of the benefits, risks, and limitations of specific therapies. It is not imperative that nurses become adept at performing a CAM technique; however, nurses should be informed practitioners (Parkman, 2002).

Professional nursing practice has traditionally assumed a comprehensive, if not holistic, approach to healing and caring. Notably, nurses have incorporated complementary or alternative modalities such as meditation, relaxation response, or guided imagery in acute, long-term, or community health settings for years. Some nurses have achieved Holistic Nurse certification through the American Holistic Nurses Association, while others have completed training programs and certification in Reiki, acupressure, aromatherapy, biofeedback, guided imagery, music therapy, meditation, therapeutic touch, or healing touch as initial steps toward expanding their practice. Although most nurses do not actively perform specific CAM modalities, growing numbers of nurses have established independent healing practices or regularly integrate one or more CAM approaches into their clinical settings.

Advising the Patient

Contemporary consumers are demanding the right to be involved and make informed choices. In making choices, the consumer needs to be advised that natural is not always safe. Ethically, practitioners need to be concerned when patients delay seeking or discontinue known effective care because CAM options are sought first (Schneiderman, 1998). Growing evidence about the direct toxic effects of unproven therapies, unknown doses, and adverse interactions between herbs and medications warrant scrutiny. Advising patients can be challenging because the safety and efficacy of some therapies or practices are not known, particularly in older population groups. Advising patients is complicated when they seek care from several unrelated providers who are unlikely to communicate.

There is a growing body of literature concerning the advice given to patients who seek or use complementary and alternative therapies (Eisenberg, 1997; NCCAM, 2001b; Novey, 2000; Sierpina, 2001). Advising should take into account the person's view, characteristics of the CAM modality used, expertise/credentials of the practitioner or reputation of the manufacturer, and availability/accessibility of treatment options. Table 14–8 offers the nurse an assessment guide for use when assisting the patient interested in CAM therapies.

Table 14–8	Guide for Assessing Patient Interest in Complementary and Alternative Medicine Therapies
Concern	**Questions to Ask**
Needs, preferences, expectations, or experiences of the patient	What are the patient's symptoms? Are these complaints related to a chronic or acute condition? Is the patient using a CAM modality to promote or maintain health? How do cultural views or the patient's view of symptoms influence health care practices?

(continued)

Table 14–8 (continued)

Concern	Questions to Ask
Characteristics of the modality or therapy	How does the therapy work?
	What conditions is it used for?
	What is known about its safety and efficacy specific to the patient's condition?
	What are the risks and benefits?
	What is the expected time frame to determine results?
	When will one know if it does not work?
	Under what conditions is it contraindicated?
	Is this modality compatible with current conventional therapy?
	What are the synergistic or antagonistic relationships, if any?
Expertise or experience of the CAM practitioner	What experience does the provider have with similar patients?
	If there is regulatory certification or licensure in the state, is the practitioner properly credentialed?
	How long has the practitioner been in practice?
	What type of patients does the CAM practitioner commonly serve?
	Does the CAM practitioner have experience with the type of patient you may refer?
	How often is there communication between the primary or other health care provider and the CAM practitioner?
	If the CAM practitioner is the primary provider, does the practitioner refer patients to a conventional practitioner?
Accessibility	Does the patient have a wide or narrow range of choices?
	Who or what are the CAM options in the local area?
	What are the costs?
	Is there reimbursement by a third-party payer or will this be an out-of-pocket expense for the patient?

TRANSITION INTO PRACTICE

Gaining an understanding of herb use is important because this is one area where consumers are likely to self-prescribe. Unrestricted (i.e., unsupervised) access to herbs is potentially dangerous, particularly if taken in adverse combinations with other herbs, over-the-counter (OTC) products, or prescribed medications. Eisenberg et al. (1998) report that 1 in 5 persons who take prescription medications also take herbal supplements or high-dose vitamins. The researchers emphasize that this places the patient at risk for adverse reactions, especially when patients do not inform their health care providers about dietary supplement and herb use. Compounding this problem are health care providers who avoid or omit asking about supplement use or who are unaware of potentially dangerous drug interactions.

Herbs are being used as drugs. However, unlike OTC and prescribed medications, herbal compounds (i.e., herb combination products) are not standardized. There are questions about the lack of stringent standards of quality for herbal products. Consumers may be misled or have misconceptions about "natural" or herbal, believing that this means products are risk free. Products may not be equal or equivalent across manufacturers or production lots; thus, it is even more difficult for consumers to make purchase decisions. Furthermore, herbal products may not contain insufficient concentrations of active ingredients to produce desired outcomes (Kuhn, 1999). Even worse, imported herbal products may have toxins from residues of the manufacturing process (Senior, 1998).

In an age when we tend to think, "If it works, more is better," the implications for nurses and other health care professionals advising patients are clear. What do we know about herbs and drug–herb combinations? More drug handbooks for nurses are including content about synergistic and antagonistic relationships between drugs and herbs. There is also an increasing number of handbooks available dedicated to herbal medicines. What herbs or drugs is the patient taking? What is the potential for abuse or misuse of herbals or other dietary and nutritional supplements?

Consumers should be cautioned about taking excess supplements. Herbs can be toxic. If the herb nutrient is taken as food, it is less likely toxic. The consumer needs to shift his notion from "more is better" to "less may be safer." Since there is insufficient evidence regarding herbal combinations, it is also advised to avoid regular use of a wide variety of herbs. Time is also an important factor. It may take longer for some herbs to be effective. For example, St. John's Wort, similar to well-known psychotropic drugs such as Prozac, may take several weeks before it is effective. On the other hand, there may be potentially toxic or harmful effects of long-term herb use such as Echinacea. This herb is commonly taken as an immune system booster; however, if taken longer than 2 to 3 weeks, it may interfere with the body's normal immune response. Consumers should work with a good resource and health care provider who is familiar with the herbs as well as prescribed medications. Finally, nurses should caution patients about self-diagnoses and self-prescribing with herbal products. What they do not know could hurt them.

KEY POINTS

1. Women, people between ages 25 and 40 and over age 65, residents of western states, middle-class people, well-educated people, those with incomes over $50,000, and non–African-Americans are major consumers of CAM.

2. A desire for simpler, more "natural," less toxic, and less costly interventions has fueled the interest in CAM.

3. Greater levels of excess disposable income, the transformation of health care to "big business," rapid technological advances leading to more expensive health care, indifferent patient–provider relationships, advances in information technology, and increased consumer responsibility have contributed to the growing demand for CAM options.

4. Five major domains of CAM as defined by the NCCAM are: alternative medical systems, mind–body interventions, biological-based therapies, manipulative and body-based therapies, and energy therapies.

5. Consumers are paying out of their own pocket for CAM services. More third-party payers (i.e., insurance companies and HMOs) are covering selected CAM therapies as an expanded benefit.

6. Congress established the White House Conference on Complementary and Alternative Medicine Policy (WHCCAMP) and the National Center for Complementary and Alternative Medicine (NCCAM) in response to the growing public interest and demand for CAM modalities.

7. The Dietary Supplement and Health Education Act of 1994 has precipitated growth of the dietary supplement (i.e., phytomedicine) industry, which includes megavitamins, nutritional supplements, and herbs.

8. Professional nurses can integrate CAM into their practice by (a) expanding their knowledge and clinical practice skills; (b) educating, counseling, and otherwise assisting patients to use CAM interventions safely; (c) facilitating more communication between patients and the various providers; and (d) evaluating the effectiveness and safe integration of therapies.

EXPLORE MediaLink

Critical thinking questions, essay questions, key terms, web links, activities, NCLEX review questions, and more interactive resources can be found on the Companion Website at www.prenhall.com/haynes. Click on Chapter 14 to select activities for this chapter.

REFERENCES

Abbot, N. C. (2000). Healing as a therapy for human disease: A systematic review. *Journal of Alternative and Complementary Medicine, 6*(2), 159–169.

American Association of Colleges of Nursing. The Essentials of Baccalaureate Education for Professional Practice (1998). Washington D.C.: Author.

Astin, J. (1998). Why patients use alternative medicine: Results of a national study. *Journal of the American Medical Association, 279*(19), 1548–1553.

Balch, J., & Balch, P. (1997). *Prescription for nutritional healing* (3rd ed.). Garden City Park, NY: Avery Publishing.

Bird, R. (1988). Positive therapeutic effects of intercessory prayer in a coronary care unit population. *Southern Medical Journal, 81*(7), 826–829.

Blumenthal, M. (2000). Interaction between herbs and conventional drugs. Introductory consideration. *Herbalgram, 49*(3), 52–63.

Blumenthal, M. (Ed.). (2000). *Integrative medicine access. Professional reference to conditions, herbs and supplements.* Newton, MA: Integrative Medicine Communications: Author.

Blumenthal, M. (2001). Herb sales down 15 percent in mainstream market. *Herbalgram, 51,* 69.

Centers for Disease Control and Prevention. (1999). *CDC FY1999 performance plan: Executive summary.* Atlanta: Author.

Cohen, M. (1998). *Complementary and alternative medicine: Legal boundaries and regulatory perspectives.* Baltimore: Johns Hopkins University Press.

The Complete German Commission & Monographs. Therapeutic Guide to Herbal Medicines. (1998). Boston: Integrative Medicine Communications: Author.

Dochterman, J., & Bulechek, G. (eds.) (2004). *Nursing Intervention Classification* (NIC) (4th ed.). St. Louis: Mosby.

Dossey, L. (1995). How should alternative therapies be evaluated? An examination of fundamentals. *Alternative Therapies in Health and Medicine, 1*(2), 6–10, 79–85.

Dossey, L. (1999). *Reinventing medicine: Beyond mind–body to a new era of healing.* San Francisco: Harper.

Easter, A. (1997). The state of research on the effects of therapeutic touch. *Journal of Holistic Nursing, 15*(2), 158–175.

Eisenberg, D. (1997). Advising patients who seek alternative medical therapies. *Annals of Internal Medicine, 127*(1), 61–69.

Eisenberg, D. (2001). Opening remarks and orientation. Presentation at Harvard Medical School Symposium, "Complementary and integrative medicine: Clinical update and implications for practice," February 11, 2001.

Eisenberg, D., Kessler, R., Foster, C., Norlock, F., Calkins, D., & Delbanco, T. (1993). Unconventional medicine in the United States: Prevalence, costs, and patterns of use. *New England Journal of Medicine, 328,* 246–253.

Eisenberg, D. M., Davis, R. B., Ettner, S. L., Appel, S., Wilkey, S., Van Rompay, M., & Kessler, R. C. (1998). Trends in alternative medicine use in the United States, 1990–1997: Results of a follow-up national survey. *Journal of the American Medical Association, 280*(18), 1569–1575.

Ernst, E. (1998). Harmless herbs? A review of recent literature. *American Journal of Medicine, 104,* 170–178.

Ernst, E., & White, A. (2000). Contradictory systematic reviews: Acupuncture for back pain. *Focus on Alternative and Complementary Therapies, 4,* 66–67.

Fontanarosa, P. B., & Lundberg, G. D. (1998). Alternative medicine meets science (Editorial). *Journal of the American Medical Association, 280*(18), 1618–1619.

Fugh-Berman, A. (1997). *Alternative medicine: What works.* Baltimore, MD: Williams & Wilkins.

Gordon, J. (1996). Alternative medicine and the family physician. *American Family Physician, 54*(7), 2205–2212.

Gordon, J. (2001a). Collaboration, consensus, and challenges: A progress report (White House Commission Report). *Alternative Therapies in Health and Medicine, 7*(3), 23–24.

Gordon, J. (2001b). *The White House Commission.* Presentation at Harvard Medical School Symposium, "Complementary and integrative medicine: Clinical update and implications for practice," February 13, 2001.

Haller, C. A., & Benowitz, N. L. (2000). Adverse cardiovascular and central nervous system events associated with dietary supplements containing ephedra alkaloids. *New England Journal of Medicine, 343*(25), 1833–1838.

Hamilton, D., & Bechtel, G. (1996). Research implications for alternative health therapies. *Nursing Forum, 31*(11), 6–10.

Hayes, K., & Alexander, I. (2000). Alternative therapies and nurse practitioners: Knowledge, professional experience, and personal use. *Holistic Nursing Practice, 14*(3), 49–58.

Haynes, L. C., Martin, J. H., & Endres, D. (2003) Nontraditional therapies and older adults: Effects of Botanical, herbal and nutritional supplements. *RN, 77*(5), 913–922.

Horrigan, B. (1999). Mitchell W. Krucoff: The MANTRA study project. *Alternative Therapies in Health and Medicine, 5*(3), 74–82.

Jonas, W. (1998). Alternative medicine and the conventional practitioner. *Journal of the American Medical Association, 279*(9), 708–710.

Kaptchuk, T. J. (1996). Historical context of the concept of vitalism in complementary and alternative medicine. In M. Micozzi (Ed.), *Fundamentals of complementary and alternative medicine* (pp. 35–48). New York: Churchill-Livingstone.

Kessler, R., Davis, R., Foster, D., Rompay, M., Walters, E., Wilkey, S., Kaptchuk, T., & Eisenberg, D. (2001). Long-term trends in the use of complementary and alternative medical therapies in the United States. *Annals of Internal Medicine, 135*(4), 262–268.

Kreitzer, M., & Jensen, D. (2000). Healing practices: Trends, challenges, and opportunities for nurses in acute and critical care. *AACN Clinical Issues, 11*(1), 7–16.

Kuhn, M. (1999). *Complementary therapies for health care providers.* Philadelphia, PA: Lippincott, Williams & Wilkins.

Landmark Healthcare. (1998). *The Landmark Report I: On public perceptions of alternative care.* Sacramento, CA: Author.

Liu, E., Turner, L., Lin, S., Klaus, L., Choi, L., Whitworth, J., Ting, W., & Oz, M. (2000). Use of alternative medicine by patients undergoing cardiac surgery. *Journal of Thoracic Cardiovascular Surgery, 120*(2), 335–341.

Lorenzi, E. A. (1999). Complementary/alternative therapies. So many choices. *Geriatric Nursing, 20*(3), 125–133.

Matthees, B. J., Anatachoti, P., Kreitzer, M. J., Savik, K., Hertz, M. I., & Gross, C. R. (2001). Use of complementary therapies, adherence, and quality of life in lung transplant recipients. *Heart & Lung, 30,* 258–268.

Meehan, T. C. (1998). Therapeutic touch as a nursing intervention. *Journal of Advanced Nursing, 28*(1), 117–125.

Milbank Memorial Fund. (1998). *Enhancing the accountability of alternative medicine.* New York: Milbank Memorial Fund.

Moylan, L. (2000). Alternative treatment modalities: The need for a rational response by the nursing profession. *Nursing Outlook, 48*(6), 259–261.

National Center for Complementary and Alternative Medicine. (2001a). *About NCCAM: General information.* Gaithersburg, MD: Author.

National Center for Complementary and Alternative Medicine. (2001b). *Information available at NCCAM.* Gaithersburg, MD: Author.

National Center for Complementary and Alternative Medicine. (2001c). *Overview of NCCAM Research Centers.* Gaithersburg, MD: Author.

Newcomer, R. (1997). *Trends monitoring in chronic care.* Princeton, NJ: Robert Wood Johnson Foundation.

Nield-Anderson, L., & Ameling, A. (2000). The empowering nature of Reiki as a complementary therapy. *Holistic Nursing Practice, 14*(3), 21–29.

Novey, D. (2000). *Clinician's complete reference guide to complementary and alternative medicine.* St. Louis, MO: Mosby.

Office of Alternative Medicine. (1992). *Alternative medicine: Expanding medical horizons—A report to the National Institutes of Health on Alternative Medical Systems and Practices in the United States.* (DHHS Publication no. 017-040-00537-7). Washington, DC: U.S. Government Printing Office.

Parkman, C. A. (2002). CAM therapies and nursing competency. *Journal for Nurses in Staff Development, 18*(March/April), 61–67.

Pelletier, K., Krasner, M., & Haskell, W. (1997). Current trends in the integration and reimbursement of complementary and alternative medicine by managed care, insurance carriers, and hospital providers. *American Journal of Health Promotion, 12*(2), 112–122.

Pert, C. (1997). *Molecules of emotion: Why you feel the way you feel.* New York: Scribner.

Pert, C., Dreher, H., & Ruff, M. (1998). The psychosomatic network: Foundations of mind–body medicine. *Alternative Therapies in Health and Medicine, 4*(4), 30–41.

Quinn, J. (2000). The self as healer: Reflections from a nurse's journey. *AACN Clinical Issues, 11*(1), 17–26.

Schneiderman, L. (1998). Medical ethics and alternative medicine. *Scientific Review of Alternative Medicine, 2*(1), 63–66.

Senior, K. (1998). Herbal medicine under scrutiny (science and medicine news). *Lancet, 352,* 1040.

Sherman, A., & Simonton, S. (1998). Psychological aspects of mind–body medicine: Promises and pitfalls from research with cancer patients. *Alternative Therapies in Health and Medicine, 4*(4), 50–67.

Shua-Haim, J. R., & Ross, J. S. (1999). Alternative medicine in geriatrics: Competing with or complementing conventional medicine. *Clinical Geriatrics, 7*(6), 37–49.

Sierpina, V. (2001). *Integrative health care: Complementary and alternative therapies for the whole person.* Philadelphia, PA: F. A. Davis.

Simonton, O. C. (1989). The harmony of health. In R. Carlson & B. Shield (Eds.), *Healers on healing* (pp. 48–52). New York: G. P. Putnam's Sons.

Snyder, M., & Lindquist, R. (2001). *Issues in complementary therapies: How we got to where we are. Online Journal of Issues in Nursing, 6*(2).

Springhouse (2002). *Nurse's handbook of alternative and complementary therapies.* Springhouse, PA: Author.

Talalay, P., & Talalay, P. (2001). The importance of using scientific principles in the development of medicinal agents from plants. *Academic Medicine, 76*(3), 238–247.

Targ, E. (1997). Evaluating distant healing: A research review. *Alternative Therapies in Health and Medicine, 3*(6), 74–78.

U.S. Department of Health and Human Services. (1997, June 2). FDA proposes safety measures for ephedrine dietary supplements. *U.S. Department of Health and Human Services News.* Washington, DC: Author.

U.S. Food & Drug Administration. (2000, January 5). *FDA finalizes rules for claims on dietary supplements. FDA talk paper.* U.S. Department of Health and Human Services. Washington, DC: Author.

U.S. Food & Drug Administration. (2001, January 3). *Overview of dietary supplements.* Center for Food Safety and Applied Nutrition. Washington, DC: Author.

Weiss, S., Takakawa, K., & Ernst, A. (2001). Use, understanding, and beliefs about complementary and alternative medicines among emergency department patients. *Academy of Emergency Medicine, 8*(1), 41–47.

Wetzel, M., Eisenberg, D., & Kaptchuk, T. (1998). Courses involving complementary and alternative medicine at U.S. medical school. *Journal of the American Medical Association, 280*(9), 784–787.

White House Commission on Complementary and Alternative Medicine Policy. (2002, March). Final report. Washington, DC: Author.

Winslow, L., & Kroll, D. (1998). Herbs as medicine. *Archives of Internal Medicine, 158*(20), 2192–2199.

Winsted-Fry, P., & Kijek, J. (1999). An integrative review and meta-analysis of therapeutic touch research. *Alternative Therapies in Health and Medicine, 5*(6), 58–67.

SUGGESTED READINGS

Ang-Lee, M., Moss, J., & Chun-Su, Y. (2001). Herbal medicines and perioperative care. *Journal of the American Medical Association, 286*(2), 208–216.

Carlson, R., & Shield, B. (1989). *Healers on healing.* New York: G. P. Putnam's Sons.

Dossey, B., Keegan, L., & Guzzetta, C. (2000). *Holistic nursing: Handbook for practice* (3rd ed.). Gaithersburg, MD: Aspen.

Ehling, D. (2001). Oriental medicine: An introduction. *Alternative Therapies in Health and Medicine, 7*(4), 71–82.

Fadiman, A. (1997). *The spirit catches you then you fall down: A Hmong child, her American doctors, and the collision of two cultures.* New York: Farrar, Strauss, Giroux.

Fontaine, K. L. (2000). *Healing practices: Alternative therapies for nursing.* Upper Saddle River, NJ: Prentice Hall.

Hufford, D. (1997). Ethics: Cultural diversity, folk medicine, and alternative medicine. *Alternative Therapies in Health and Medicine, 3*(4), 78–80.

Kiefer, D., Shah, S., Gardiner, P., & Wechkin, H. (2001). Finding information on herbal therapy: A guide to useful sources for clinicians. *Alternative Therapies in Health and Medicine, 7*(6), 74–78.

Kessler, R., Davis, R., Foster, D., Rompay, M., Walters, E., Wilkey, S., Kaptchuk, T., & Eisenberg, D. (2001). Long-term trends in the use of complementary and alternative medical therapies in the United States. *Annals of Internal Medicine, 135*(4), 262–268.

Unit 4

Health Care Delivery from an Economic, Political, and Legal Perspective

15

Economic Aspects of Health Care

Joan Carter
Jennie Echols
Leona D. Stoll

In a world of increased wealth and income, where our common heritage of knowledge has made the potential for satisfactory life so much greater than in earlier ages, the need for community has made the universal provision of high-level health care and education necessary.

Minsky, 1995

LEARNING OBJECTIVES

At the completion of this chapter, the reader will be able to:

➣ Explain how health care is financed.

➣ Analyze how cost containment impacts the quality of health care.

➣ Describe the fiscal differences between for-profit and not-for-profit health care agencies.

➣ Explain the relationship between standards of care, an institution's mission statement, and budgetary guidelines.

➣ Describe how cyber-care technologies enhance quality of care.

➣ Identify economic challenges facing nursing and the health care industry.

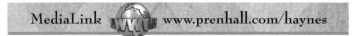

MediaLink   www.prenhall.com/haynes

Additional online resources including NCLEX review questions, critical thinking questions, and real-world activities for this chapter can be found on the Companion Website at www.prenhall.com/haynes.

$\mathcal{U}$nderstanding the economic aspects of health care is critical to the education of nurses, yet many schools of nursing fail to adequately prepare their graduates with this essential knowledge. In the current economic climate, knowledge of basic economics, health care issues, and reimbursement systems is as important to nursing practice as is any other skill in order for the nurse to offer quality care in an efficient, cost-effective manner. This chapter addresses economic trends and issues currently impacting health care in general and nursing in particular.

Economic Effects on Health Care

Economics is a social science that describes and analyzes how goods and services are produced, distributed, and consumed. A market-driven economy promotes competition for goods and services, which, in turn, influences the prices charged. As important as the principles of economics are to the welfare of a capitalist society, economics as the sole determinant for health care is dangerous. In the 1990s, economic pressures led to health care reform, which was designed to conserve financial resources. Nurses and patients in all practice settings experienced the economic consequences (e.g., restructuring, downsizing, and substitution) of health care reform. The consequences of economic reform have not all lead to positive patient outcomes. Since nurses have a special relationship with the public, represent an important symbol of quality in health care, and are the largest group of direct health care providers, they are in the best position to bring together quality care, patient advocacy, and sound economic practices (American Hospital Association, 2000).

Economic factors constrain the health care industry just as they do any other economically driven business. In simple terms, buyers purchase goods or services from sellers; in health care the buyer is the patient, and the seller is the health care provider. The resources (e.g., money or insurance) that the buyer has available to pay for the health care largely determines which services the individual can and/or will access.

Today's economic environment is quite complex. Most buyers (patients) have a limited supply of financial resources to dedicate to health care. In fact, most buyers do not directly pay the entire costs for the health care services offered by sellers (hospitals, physicians, nurses, etc.); rather, those costs are largely paid by a third party (e.g., an insurance company or government agency). The third party pays or reimburses the seller on behalf of the buyer. Because many patients and their families do not have the necessary means (money or insurance) to obtain health care, they may be forced to go without needed services.

Economic factors influence what health care services can be delivered in all health care settings. In the current economic environment, patients and especially third-party payers who largely foot the bill demand that health care costs be controlled. To meet this demand, health care providers have been forced to change the manner in which services are provided. An example of this type of change is evident in the evaluations and diagnostic procedures that are often performed before a patient is hospitalized in order to shorten the patient's length of stay in the hospital. On admission, a discharge plan is created that focuses on sending the patient home as quickly as possible. Discharging a patient at the earliest possible time minimizes the use of hospital resources, thus reducing costs.

Economic constraints also directly affect whether some individuals receive any health care at all. Individuals may not receive needed health care if (a) they lack health insurance, (b) their insurance coverage does not meet their needs, or (c) they lack financial resources to pay for the needed services. This is a very real problem in the United States. In 1998, the Bureau of the Census estimated that 43.3 million Americans had no health insurance at all. That number represented over 16% of the total population of the United States. Of persons with health insurance, over 70% were provided coverage by their employers, and almost 25% were provided health insurance through a governmental agency (such as Medicare, Medicaid, or the military). Even though employers provide health insurance many employees remain uninsured.

Even persons with health insurance may not be able to meet all their health care needs. Insurance companies and other third-party payers not only specify which services are or are not covered, but also what amount will be paid out of pocket and what deductibles are required of the patient. These costs and uncovered services cause many to forgo needed health care services. For example, some health care plans do not pay for the cost of prescription drugs, home-care, or long-term care services (e.g., Medicare covers hospital services, but does not pay for outpatient prescription drugs). Additionally, preventative care (e.g., immunizations or annual mammograms) is often reimbursed on a limited dollar basis or not covered at all. The end result is high out-of-pocket payments by the patient.

Economics has further effected health care in that insurance programs provided by employers have steadily declined as increased costs of health care have resulted in higher costs of health insurance coverage. Due to higher premium costs for health insurance, some employers have reduced or eliminated health benefits, limited the employee's choice of insurance, or passed more of the costs on to their employees. Additionally, many employers also limit their coverage to include only managed care options. **Managed care** options provide variety of strategies, systems, and mechanisms for monitoring and controlling the utilization of health services while maintaining satisfactory levels of quality health care.

In health care, unlike the traditional free-market system, consumers often have no control over the need for health care services. In a free-market system, the consumer can choose to delay purchase or even do without a service. Such an approach to health care could be detrimental, if not catastrophic. A consumer could make his or her condition worse or even suffer death by delaying treatment. A decision by a consumer to put off or forgo annual mammograms, for example, could be the difference between discovering breast cancer at an earlier, more treatable phase or discovering that same cancer at an advanced, untreatable stage.

Regardless of the source for and/or the urgency of the demand for services or availability of financial resources, health care providers must make enough money to stay in business. This means the provider must be able to pay personnel, maintain buildings and equipment, and pay for supplies, medications, goods, and other essential services. Unfortunately, cost containment in health care can potentially have an adverse effect on patient safety and quality of care. The challenge is to balance cost with quality of care.

To reduce labor costs, health care administrators have reduced the number of nurses on staff and substituted unlicensed personnel. The current literature suggests that this strategy is misguided. Nurse staffing levels are closely tied to a hospital's ability to provide cost-effective health care with successful outcomes to patients; a reduction in the registered nurse workforce can lead to unforeseen health care cost (e.g., increased length of stay, more errors, and even greater patient mortality). Inadequate staffing with registered nurses has been associated with adverse patient outcomes, according to a 7,400-page United States Department of Health and Human Services (DHHS) study completed in 2001. The study found inadequate staffing had led to an increased frequency of errors in providing health care. This increased error rate has caused the public to become concerned about their safety and well-being within the health care system. At some point, health care ceases to be cost effective when inad-

equate staffing (e.g., reduction in nursing staff levels) results in longer hospital stays, more complications, and adverse patient outcomes, including death.

Allocation and Access to Health Care Resources

Since health care resources are not unlimited, basic decisions (choices) must be made about how these limited or scarce resources will be allocated. For example, health care resources can be allocated to high-cost technology, but then fewer dollars will be available for preventative care (e.g., immunizations, mammograms, health teaching, etc.). With limited resources, health care providers and consumers are asking, "What types or combinations of health care do we choose? Should we concentrate on high-tech, crisis-oriented medical care or a prevention-oriented system emphasizing primary care and prevention of illness?"

Even though the health care industry continues to grow, the dominant economic health issue, now and in the foreseeable future, is likely to be cost and access to health care for the growing number of uninsured and underinsured Americans. Lack of access to health care largely results from a lack of insurance coverage. In 2000, the DHHS determined that 41 million Americans under the age of 65 had no health insurance at all. One reason for this shocking statistic is demonstrated by the many small companies nationwide that often cannot afford insurance coverage for their employees. Moreover, temporary and/or part-time workers in companies of all sizes are not generally eligible for the benefits that permanent full-time employees receive. Most of these temporary or part-time workers have no medical insurance coverage for themselves or their dependents. The unemployed and working poor simply cannot afford health insurance. Medicaid, originally created by Congress in 1965, was intended to improve access to health care for the poor. A study completed in 2000 by the DHHS determined that the poor, despite the availability of Medicaid, often lack a regular source of health care, do not use preventative health services, and often put off health care until conditions, even avoidable ones, lead to a critical event that requires hospitalization. The study also found that others fail to seek health care because they simply cannot afford to miss work since missed work means lost wages. Thus, cutting costs for preventive care or early treatment ends up costing more in the long run.

Lack of insurance also poses economic hardships for health care providers and the public. The uninsured and underinsured patients are unable to pay health care costs and create bad debt for health care providers. These unpaid costs are absorbed by patients and their insurers who do pay so that health care providers can continue to provide services. This practice is known as **cost-shifting**.

To shift costs, health care providers increase their charges to patients and private or public insurers who can afford to pay. This practice results in increases of insurance premiums, which makes health insurance even less affordable for individuals and/or employers. In response to "cost-shifting," some payers have restricted the amounts reimbursed to health care providers for services rendered. This action drastically reduces the provider's ability to cover or shift the costs of health care for the uninsured. Advocates for a national health insurance system cite unpaid health care and "cost-shifting" as one rationale for national health coverage for all citizens. Moreover, they express concern for individuals living in rural and inner city areas that are doubly burdened by lack of sufficient health care providers, specialists, new technologies, and facilities.

This "tug-of-war" over health resources raises the question, "Who should received health care?" Unfortunately, in the United States the answer largely depends on who has health insurance coverage to finance/purchase health care. That same question is answered differently in other parts of the world. In contrast to U.S. health care, most industrialized Western countries have a national health insurance system that provides financial access to some form of health care for all citizens. Great Britain, for example, illustrates a centralized, government-run, nationalized system. Most health care agencies (hospitals, clinics, etc.) are owned and operated by the British government. In the United States, federal or state funding provides some individuals with the "right" to health care through programs such as Medicaid and Medicare. The health care received, free of charge, in a Veterans Administration (VA) hospital is another example of an entitlement or right to health care provided to a specific group (i.e., veterans) by the federal government. While these are selected examples of government-supported health care in the United States, the entire population does not have a legally established right to health care.

▓ Health Care in the United States

Health care delivery for the middle-class, who are employed and insured, is generally devoid of any formal delivery system. These individuals and their families put together an informal group of services that meets their personal or family needs. The service is financed by personal, nongovernmental funds and health insurance plans. The care for this population of individuals tends to be an informal, uncoordinated collection of services. The individual and/or family seeks to access services that are convenient and meet the needs of the moment. While individuals seek to control costs, the system of care they use is poorly integrated and can be costly (Torrens, 2002). It is difficult to measure the cost effectiveness of health care outcomes for this population due to the fragmentation of services.

The health care delivery structure for the unemployed, uninsured, inner-city, and many minority populations is also fragmented and lacks a formal coordinated system. The individual or family usually avoids health services except those provided by local government agencies such as city or county hospitals and the local health department. The emergency room often serves as the point of entry to the rest of the health care system for these individuals (Torrens, 2002).

For those with the ability to pay, health care delivery is available from investor-owned, for-profit hospitals. Consumers witnessed the birth of these investor-owned hospitals in the 1960s. Although not-for-profit community hospitals are still the largest class of hospitals, investors expanded their ownership of community hospitals during the 1990s through the purchase of academic and teaching hospitals. The two largest for-profit hospital companies in the U.S. market are Hospital Corporation of America (HCA) and Tenet Health Care Corporation. While consumers may expect better services from these for-profit health care providers, it is not clear if there is a discernable qualitative difference in quality of care, patient satisfaction, and illness prevention provided by for-profit institutions as compared to not-for-profit institutions.

Expansion of investor ownership occurred primarily in the south and southwestern United States, where population growth was rising and the demand for health care services and competition for health care was intense. For-profit hospitals quickly responded to consumer health care needs as they had cash available to initiate capital changes for expanded or updated services. For-profit companies also responded to changing health care needs of communities as inpatient hospital care declined and outpatient services increased. This shifting focus led the for-profit corporation to construct ambulatory health care facilities (e.g., outpatient surgical centers and diagnostic imaging centers).

Just as with any other corporation, the for-profit health care enterprises are answerable to their stockholders, who expect a profit on their investment. The profits of investor-owned facilities have been impacted by the same economic factors that are currently impacting the entire health care industry. In addition, they are also impacted by local, state, and federal taxes. The Federation of American Hospitals, a powerful voice in Washington, D.C., has championed the needs of investor-owned health care agencies.

Paying for Health Care

Reimbursement strategies for health care services have changed dramatically over the past two decades. **Reimbursement**, the term used to indicate money received for services delivered, is essential to secure the financial stability of health care organizations and providers. Nurses need to understand how their employers are paid for the services rendered to patients since it is the balance between the cost of providing care and the payment received that determines the financial stability of an organization or provider.

In today's health care environment, the provider is not alone in assuming increased financial risks. During the past five years, consumers have been forced to bear greater responsibility for health care and the costs of insurance coverage. Employers are shifting a greater portion of the costs of insurance premiums to the employee as well as increasing deductibles and copayments. Medicare recipients are also paying increased premiums for Medicare Part B, medical insurance; they also have increased out-of-pocket expenses for Medicare Part A, hospital insurance.

From an economic point of view, the nurse must understand each method of reimbursement to fully understand the financial risks to health care providers. Table 15–1 shows the benefits and risks for the five common methods of reimbursement, which include:

- **Capitation**—A set amount of money received or paid out; it is based on membership rather than on services delivered and usually is expressed in units of per member per month (PMPM).
- **Fee-for-Service**—Providers are reimbursed for charges.
- **Per Diem Reimbursement**—Reimbursement of an institution, usually a hospital, is based on a set rate per day rather than on charges.
- **Per Case Reimbursement**—Reimbursement is at a fixed rate, usually based on a diagnosis or a procedure.
- **Diagnosis-Related Groups (DRGs)**—A form of per-case reimbursement, a prospective payment method, based on diagnosis-related groups that use similar resources.

Health care costs that are covered by third-party payment serves to reimburse health care providers for services rendered. Voluntary hospital groups and state medical societies organized early insurance providers in response to the economic and health care needs of consumers. The insurance industry has grown dramatically since its inception. The percentage of Americans covered by health insurance has risen from less than 20% at the end of World War II to over 70% in 2001 (Torrens, 2002).

Before the advent of health care insurance, individuals were fully responsible to make payment for their own health care. Between 1940 and 1950, health insurance became an accepted and expected benefit of employment; employers took on a large portion of the risk for payment of employee health care needs. A premium was paid to the insurance company, which then became responsible for reimbursing health care providers. The traditional indemnity insurance system maximized the consumer's ability to choose the provider and facility from which they would receive services. Providers were motivated to focus on customer satisfaction while providing services since reimbursement was based on services performed. As utilization grew, insurance companies periodically evaluated costs and charged higher premiums to the employer; initially, insurance companies did little to control health care costs.

Traditionally, Americans have been enmeshed in a fee-for-service method of reimbursement with insurance companies paying the bill. Health care analyst Kenneth Abramowitz (1991) described this traditional fee-for-service model as an unaffordable luxury that encouraged demand and inflated charges. Today many believe fee-for-service medicine can never contain costs. This belief led to the push for managed care in the 1990s.

With the enactment of the Social Security Amendments of 1983, the fee-for-service method of payment was transformed to the prospective payment method of reimbursement for older persons under Medicare. The advent of the diagnostic-related groups (DRGs) created a per-case method of reimbursement. This dramatic change influenced the length of stay phenomenon from one of increased reimbursement for longer lengths of stay to increased reimbursement for shorter lengths of stay. This phenomenon affected hospitals greatly in that the occupancy of hospitals was largely curtailed, units were closed, and there were large numbers of unoccupied beds.

Table 15–1   Common Methods of Reimbursement

Type of Reimbursement	Benefits	Risks
Capitation	• Providers obtain their money up front. • There is a known amount of money allowing budgeting of resources. by the provider.	• The provider assumes the entire financial risk. • There is always the potential for serious illness of any member creating additional costs that must be assumed • Enrollment of many persons with chronic illnesses will take additional time and money. • This form of reimbursement has the potential for encouraging underutilization of health care services.
Fee-for-Service	• The insurer assumes the financial risk; therefore, the provider has financial protection. • Usually entails less administrative work.	• There is no incentive for the provider to be cost effective.
Per Diem	• The provider knows the reimbursement amount and can plan accordingly.	• Managed care organizations (MCOs) usually negotiate discounted per rate with the provider. • The consumer may use extensive resources costing more than the per diem rate will cover.
Per Case	• The provider benefits financially if cases are managed effectively and efficiently. • The provider knows initially what the payment will be and can monitor accordingly.	• Complications and delays in treatment can be costly to the provider. • Providers must be able to quantify all costs for a specific procedure to determine if adequate reimbursement is received.
DRGs	• Location of the hospital, urban or rural, and wage levels are factored into the fixed price. • The provider has the opportunity to keep the revenue difference if the patient does not use all of the resources allocated under a certain DRG.	• Hospitals have a financial incentive to discharge patients early. • Severity of illness is not adequately factored into the fixed rate.

Rising Health Care Costs

The health care industry has become one of the largest industries in the United States. In 1999, health care expenditures in the United States totaled $1.2 trillion and represented a 5.6% increase in expenses in just one year. In 1996, 84% of persons under age 65 reported medical expenses averaging $1,900 per year; but that same year 96% of elderly persons reported medical expenses averaging $5,600 per year (National Center for Health Statistics, 2001).

Health care costs are rising at a higher rate than all other economic indicators used to measure the U.S.

economy. Estimates show that by 2030, 32% of the country's entire gross domestic product will be spent on health care services. Despite rising costs of health care and increased high-tech expenditures in acute care, there is little doubt that the net health of the nation has not improved. Some have argued that the longevity of Americans along with their good health is a result of (a) excellent sewage systems, (b) comprehensive immunization programs, and (c) available public health services rather than technologic advances, which generally serve the needs of a relatively small portion of the American public (Wilson & Porter-O'Grady, 1999).

The U.S. health care industry continues to focus on the high-intensity, high-tech needs of individuals who are sick. This focus is in part supported by the third-party financial reimbursement system. Most benefit plans pay to treat illness; few provide benefits to maintain health. This sickness-based health care payment model has led to the development of valuable and expensive, specialized technological advancements. These advances and specialization have resulted in expensive medical care, which "has become fragmented, organ based, procedure based, functional, and interventionist" (Wilson & Porter-O'Grady, 1999, p. 7).

As could be predicted, health care costs have increased at an alarming rate while the level of satisfaction with the current health care system has remained low. Other forces that have served to increase health care costs include:

- Inflation, both general and health care related
- Expectations of consumers
- Medically unnecessary and inappropriate care
- Ineffective services
- Excess capacity of hospitals and other providers
- Inefficient management of health care resources
- Malpractice insurance rates and defensive medical practice
- Antitrust regulation

While these forces have increased health care costs, hospital care remains the largest health care expense (32%) despite the push to reduce length of stay and contain costs. Health care expenditures can be further broken down into physical and clinical services (22%), drugs (9%), and other spending (29%) such as home care, dental care, durable medical supplies, and over-the-counter drugs. The 2002 PricewaterhouseCoopers report identified seven factors fueling rising health care costs:

- Drugs, medical devices, and other medical advances
- Rising provider expenses
- Inflation
- Increased demand
- Government mandates and regulation
- Impact of litigation
- Fraud, abuse, and other cost drivers

Comparison of the overall inflation rate, which is determined by the percentage change in the **consumer price index** (CPI) from one year to the next, with the inflation rate in medical care service costs indicates that the cost of medical care has out paced general inflation for the past 10 years (Feldstein, 1999).

The medical care services index has created concerns since U.S. consumers now spend approximately 14% of the **gross domestic product** (GDP) for health care. Economists define the GDP as the market value of all final goods and services produced domestically in a single year. This is the single most important measure of economic performance (Duffy, 1993). Of all the goods and services produced within the United States, nearly 14% or over $1 trillion is spent for health care in one year. This statistic is a cause for great concern. The most any other country spends is 10.6% of its GDP. Whether the United States should use another country's expenditures as its benchmark is debatable. There are many cultural and environmental factors that influence health in a country. The difference in spending is striking, as in the early 1990s when the United States was spending 50% more per capita on health care than Canada, Japan, and Germany; 60% more than Scandinavian countries; and 70% more than the United Kingdom (Mitsunaga, 1999).

The **medical care services index** is continuing to rise, causing renewed alarm. Escalating increase in the prescription drug index has been of particular concern. On the other hand, physician care services have remained stable. The income of physicians has not grown at nearly the same inflation rate as other medical care services measured during the past 10 years.

In 1998, the government conducted a study on prescription drug pricing. The House Government Reform and Oversight Committee concluded that pricing is and has been the real issue (*Congressional Record*, 1998). The report indicated that pharmaceutical manufacturers sell drugs to managed care companies, insurance companies, hospitals, and the federal government at discounted prices. To compensate for these low prices, drug manufacturers sell trade name drugs to retail pharmacies at dramatically higher prices. Thus, the average American without a prescription drug plan who buys drugs at a retail pharmacy pays higher prices.

Controlling Health Care Costs

As costs rose in the 1980s, consumers, employers, and politicians became increasingly alarmed at the cost of health care. Employers faced dramatic increases in health insurance premiums and the potential inability to continue providing health care benefits. For example, Sultz (1991) noted that the cost of auto workers' health benefits exceeded the cost of steel in an automobile. Officials in both the public and private sector were challenged to search for economically prudent avenues for providing health care benefits to employees (Winegar, 1996).

Laws Designed to Control Costs

The health care system in America can perhaps be described as a pluralistic system with multiple payers in a complex array of services. Politics has played a major role in the number and types of health care legislation proposed both now and in the past. Legislation that governs health care has been aimed at (a) consumer protection, (b) employment and hiring practices, (c) workplace safety, and (d) funding. Some of the laws are federal laws with federal enforcement, while others are regulated by state and local government agencies.

Prior to the 1930s, there was little social legislation that involved health care. In fact, the first social legislation passed by the U.S. Congress was the enactment of the Social Security Act of 1935. This legislation created the Old Age and Survivors Insurance (OASI) program, which provided retirement income benefits to workers ages 65 and older in commerce and industry. Gradually, Social Security benefits were extended to others.

Prior to 1966, funding of medical care was covered primarily by private insurance or paid from available out-of-pocket monies. Thirty years after Congress enacted the Social Security Act, the first social legislation to provide reimbursement for health care was passed, the Social Security Amendments Act of 1965. This act established funding for medical services of older persons (**Medicare**) and indigent individuals (**Medicaid**). The outcome of this funding was increased medical care for older persons and the poor. These programs provided payments to hospitals based on what the provider determined to be the costs of services provided. Reimbursement to physicians was paid as the usual, customary, and reasonable fee. The Medicare and Medicaid programs are two of the most important social programs enacted by the U.S. Congress in the hotly contested right versus privilege health care debate. This debate continues today. In 1972, Congress predicted that Medicare and Medicaid expenditures would exceed the predicted $240 billion cost anticipated during the first 25 years following implementation of the Act.

Both President Nixon in the early 1970s and President Carter in the late 1970s introduced cost-control programs aimed at keeping the escalating costs of health care in pace with the general rate of inflation. In 1971, because of high inflation, President Nixon placed the entire U.S. economy under a wage and price freeze (Feldstein, 1988). Nixon's agenda was known as the Economic Stabilization Program. For most products, the freeze was lifted after one year. Health care costs remained frozen until 1974. The following year physician and hospital expenditures increased 17.5% and 19.4%, respectively. In 1979, President Carter made cost containment within hospitals one of his highest priorities in a program known as the Voluntary Effort. Unfortunately, the American Medical Association and the various hospital associations garnered enough support to defeat the proposed legislation and stymied his efforts.

The enactment of the federal HMO Act of 1973 served to promote the growth of managed health care, which was designed to address escalating health care costs while maintaining positive health care outcomes (McCullough, 2001). This Act was designed to reduce health care costs by increasing competition in the health care market and promoting access to health care coverage for individuals without insurance or with only limited benefits. The HMO Act required that employers with more than 25 employees offer their employees a choice between traditional insurance and managed care health plans. The Act also encouraged the development of HMOs through grant funding. Further legislative action designed to halt escalating cost of health care are presented in Table 15–2.

One recent piece of legislation impacting health care providers and insurance companies is the Employee Retirement Income Security Act (ERISA). This broad-reaching law (a) establishes the rights of participants and (b) defines the requirements for disclosure of benefits and alternatives.

The most recent highly political debate regarding health care costs has been about patient rights, the ability

---

Critical Thinking and Reflection

A new drug has been prescribed for your patient on the day of discharge. How will you access the drug information? In what format will you educate the patient and/or family member about the drug?

Does the rising prescriptive drug index mean more persons are using prescription drugs or has the price of medications skyrocketed?

Table 15–2 Legislation of the U.S. Government Affecting Social Changes

Year	Title	Selected Coverage (not inclusive)
1935	Social Security Act of 1935	Established retirement benefits to commerce and industry workers, ages 65 and older. Funds are derived from payroll taxes assessed on employers and employees.
1965	Social Security Amendment Act of 1965—Title XVIII (Medicare) and XIX (Medicaid)	Established health care reimbursement at reasonable costs for the older person and for indigent persons. The Act included a 2% plus factor added to the reimbursable costs.
1972	The Social Security Amendment Act of 1972 (PL 92-603)	Established the concept of reimbursement at the lower of costs or charges. This Act also established the Professional Standards Review Organizations (PSROs).
1973	Health Maintenance Organization Act of 1973—Title XIII of the Public Health Service Act	Established federal funding for the expansion of health maintenance organizations (HMOs). It provided more than $364 million to not-for-profit groups to establish HMOs.
1974	The Health Planning and Resource Development Act of 1974	Established health system agencies and the procedures for the certificate of need (CON), which required hospitals to obtain approval from health planning agencies for capital expenditures above a stated amount. Many states have phased out the CON process because it has not proven to be successful in controlling hospital costs.
1981	The Omnibus Reconciliation Act of 1981	Provided for the: (a) phase out of the Health Planning Systems and the Health Systems Agencies (HSAs), (b) reduction of the nursing differential to 5%, and (c) restriction of freedom of choice for Medicare beneficiaries to providers who were deemed cost effective.
1982	The Tax Equity and Fiscal Responsibility Act	Established a limit on all inpatient hospital costs. The nursing differential was eliminated.
1983	The Social Security Amendments of 1983	Completely changed the reimbursement system for those caring for Medicare patients in that payment was based on a fixed price per diagnosis-related group (DRG) for inpatient hospital services.
1985	The Consolidated Omnibus Budget Reconciliation Act (COBRA) of 1985	Provides employees with the option of continuing group health insurance at their own expense for up to 18 months at the group rate. Requires that hospitals with emergency departments that participate in the Medicare program must treat all patients requiring emergency treatment or who are in labor.
1986	The Omnibus Budget Reconciliation Act (OBRA) of 1986	Provides the regulations for ambulatory surgery procedures payment criteria.
1987	The Omnibus Budget Reconciliation Act of 1987	Introduced over 100 Medicare and Medicaid provisions to reduce expenditures for the subsequent 2 years. Requires HMOs to provide supplemental coverage for up to 6 months if the HMO drops Medicare as insurance.
1990	The Omnibus Budget Reconciliation Act of 1990	Requires Medicare-contracting HMOs to comply with requirements imposed on hospitals and other providers to make Medicare beneficiaries aware of the right to have medical care subject to advanced directives (living wills).
1996	The Health Insurance Portability and Accountability Act (HIPAA)	Limits the use of preexisting conditions. Lowers the chance of losing existing coverage. Helps buy coverage if you lose your employer's plan.

Year	Title	Selected Coverage (not inclusive)

Table 15-2 (continued)

Year	Title	Selected Coverage (not inclusive)
1997	The Balanced Budget Act of 1997	Reduce Medicare spending by $115 billion over 5 years. Created the State Children's Health Insurance Program that provided $24 billion over 5 years to help states offer health insurance to underinsured children whose family income exceeds the Medicaid eligibility requirements but not enough to afford private insurance. Allows HMOs to determine whether nurse practitioners (NPs) should become provider panel members and be reimbursed. This is in contrast to a previous, more flexible law that included reimbursement for NPs.

to sue HMOs, and prescription drug costs, especially for the elderly. Political campaigns often address health care reform as an important issue but limited actual reform is enacted. Other current legislative issues include:

- Lack of prescription drug coverage for people with Medicare
- Denial of payment for emergency room visits
- Denial of coverage for ambulance services

It is important for nurses to research and discuss the implications of proposed legislation as the effects of such legislation are far reaching. For example, legislation has affected the type of information that must be given to patients. To ensure that patients have been informed of their rights, multiple forms have been developed. The nurse is just one of the many health care providers who must ensure that patients understand their rights as presented in these forms. While seemingly innocuous, these changes result in operational issues for nurses regarding how the forms are administered and where health care providers will find the money needed to implement the new standards required by law.

Managed Care

Managed care was developed in an attempt to control health care costs. The roots of managed care go back to the 1920s when Henry Kaiser organized the first managed care plan (now known as Kaiser Permanente). In the 1980s and 1990s, enrollment in managed care grew rapidly as alarming increases in medical care costs caused employers and federal and state governments to seek lower cost alternatives. Although doctors and nurses have criticized managed care companies for interference in care decisions, shortened lengths of stay for patients, denial of reimbursement coverage, and rigid requirements for documentation, they also recognize the posi-

tive aspects of managed care. The increased emphasis on prevention services, the use of clinical practice guidelines, and disease management protocols are just a few of the positive outcomes related to managed care. Essentially managed care implies better control and requires better decision-making (McCullough, 2001).

Managed care, as defined earlier in this chapter, refers to a variety of strategies, systems, and mechanisms for monitoring and controlling the utilization of health services while maintaining satisfactory levels of quality health care. The goal of managed care is to match the patient's needs with the appropriate treatment while monitoring delivery of care and outcome of services in a cost-efficient manner. Torrens and Williams (2002) suggest that "managed care is an organized effort by health insurance plans and providers to use financial incentives and organizational arrangement to alter provider and patient behavior so that health care services are delivered and utilized in a more efficient and lower-cost manner" (p. 125).

Boland (1991) defined managed care as any system that manages the delivery of health care in such a way that cost is controlled either directly or indirectly. He proposed that managed care includes financial incentives and management controls which direct patients to efficient providers who provide appropriate medical care in cost-effective settings.

Managed care organizations (MCOs) define managed care as (a) the utilization of review mechanisms to contain costs and (b) case management interventions to facilitate quality of care through a credentialed network of providers across a continuum of care. Depending on the context in which it is used, managed care may refer to (a) a system of health care financing and delivery, (b) various techniques to manage the financing and delivery of health care, or (c) different types of organizations that practice managed care techniques.

TECHNIQUES OF MANAGED CARE

It is important to distinguish between the techniques of managed care and the organizations that provide managed care (McCullough, 2001). Managed care techniques include:

- Developing and maintaining a credentialed network of providers and facilities
- Providing prevention initiatives to the provider and patient
- Offering utilization management through monitoring access to services
- Continuing treatment review to establish authorization for continued care based on evidence-based medical necessity criteria

Other important tools in the managed care arsenal include an information system, quality and outcome measures, provider plan to control utilization, and capitation/risk sharing. Additionally, managed care requires that the insured individual is educated about the benefit plan. This education should include an understanding of the difference between managed care insurance and traditional fee-for-service type insurance (Torrens & Williams, 2002). Nurses can play a vital role in educating and advocating for patients involved with managed care health care programs.

HEALTH MAINTENANCE ORGANIZATIONS AND PREFERRED PROVIDER ORGANIZATIONS

In the 1980s and 1990s, managed care was provided predominantly by **health maintenance organizations** (HMOs). Today, most major insurance companies use managed care techniques in their **preferred provider organization** (PPO) and **point-of-service** (POS) products. A PPO is a health care plan that contracts with a group of providers on a fee-for-service basis to provide comprehensive services to individuals covered by the insurance plan. A POS plan allows the individual a choice at the time of service as to whether to use a member provider who has been contracted to provide services at a reduced rate or a nonmember provider who will offer services at a higher rate. The individual seeking health care pays for the higher fee out of pocket.

Techniques used by the HMO and PPO/POS to control health care costs in a managed care environment vary. The PPO and POS products will frequently require preauthorization for all inpatient and expensive services, but ultimately leave access up to the member with incentives to access network providers. The HMO product requires preauthorization for all services and treatment with access limited only to in-network providers and facilities. Furthermore, with these plans, an insurance plan member who goes to an in-network provider will receive 80% to 100% reimbursement, with the patient responsible for 0% to 20% of the provider's charge at the allowed rate. On the other hand, if the insurance plan member goes to an out-of-network provider, insurance will usually reimburse up to 70%, with the patient responsible for 30% or more of the provider's charge. Both of these plans differ significantly from the traditional indemnity health insurance plan that allows access and use of health care services with little or no management/control by the insurance company.

CRITICISM OF MANAGED CARE

Some who believe it is really managed cost in lieu of quality and freedom of choice or access criticize managed care. Physicians and hospitals contend that managed care alters decision-making by interjecting a complex system of financial incentives, penalties, and administrative procedures into the doctor–patient relationship. Other opponents to managed care point out that there is a growing consensus that managed care is not achieving intended objectives to reduce overall health care costs and stabilize health care premiums. Physicians believe managed care is a direct intrusion on professional judgment and autonomy in an effort to regulate and control health care costs (Sharfstein, 1990). Other critics believe inpatient care savings are offset by increased outpatient care costs and administrative costs of the utilization management. These costs include increased time spent (a) communicating with managed care case managers, (b) copying records, and (c) justifying the need for admissions and continued care.

Balancing Quality of Care with Financial Limits

The Joint Commission on Accreditation of Healthcare Organizations (JCAHO) (1992) views quality as the degree to which patient care services increase the probability of desired patient outcomes and reduce the probability of undesired outcomes given the current state of knowledge. In this stringent economic environment, using a universally accepted definition of quality as a guideline for measuring this concept becomes a mandate for health care providers. Balancing quality and maintaining a healthy balance sheet requires management skills unprecedented before the advent of managed care. The health care provider should therefore strive to provide optimal quality of care within the framework of reasonable costs.

Standards of Care and Budgets

The development of an institution's budget must be consistent with its mission statement and with the institution's annual goals and objectives. A **mission statement** reflects the reason an organization exists. It clearly states the overall purpose for the existence of the entity. For example, the mission statement of Saint Blaise Hospital, which is located in a rural community, is broadly stated within the context of available services. On the contrary, the mission statement for Saint Mary's Hospital, which is in a large city, is more restrictive because of the multiplicity of competitive services available in a metropolitan area. The **budget** reflects the expected revenue and expenses and serves as a guide to the financial administration of the organization. Revenue, costs, and quality are interrelated factors that must be understood if the resources of the organization are to be committed to the work necessitated by the mission.

The boundaries of professional practice within an institution are enhanced or limited by the mission and financial status or constraints of the organization. Therefore, it is not sufficient to be concerned solely about the delivery of care in the most ethical and prudent manner. It is also essential to have an awareness that the care is provided in a cost-effective manner. In other words, nurses must explore all alternatives to achieve desirable outcomes in a less costly manner.

Standards of care are written statements either of the care patients should expect to receive (process standards) or of the results of care already received (outcome standards) (Grohar & DiCroce, 2002). Standards of Practice for nurses are written and published by various nursing organizations. However, nurses are most often guided by the standards developed by the American Nurses Association (ANA). The ANA began preparing standards in the 1970s and has continued to update and add new specialty standards. Along with each state's Nurse Practice Acts, these ANA standards guide nursing practice in any setting. Knowledge of clinical practice guidelines along with adherence to the standards of practice within the framework of each state's Nurse Practice Act is essential to keep abreast of the latest clinical practices and evidence-based practice.

In theory, awareness of practice standards, practice guidelines, ethical guidelines, and efficiency should result in optimal care for patients. The relationship between the mission and the work of a health care provider can be depicted in a straight line, with the budget and ethics influencing the work determined by the mission.

Cost-Effective Use of Personnel

From 1985 to 1999, nursing departments experienced the frustration of cost containment strategies. Both hospital administrators and hospital finances were caught in a period of uncertainty and instability. Two economic principles that drove cost containment of that period were (a) supply and demand and (b) substitution.

As prospective payment (DRGs) spread as a form of reimbursement, hospital occupancy fell and revenues plummeted. A likely result would seem to be a decreasing need for nurses in these facilities. Implied in the economic theory of supply and demand is the notion that as demand decreases supply, prices will decrease. Administrators responded accordingly and the need for nurses decreased, thus creating a perceived oversupply. Even the Pew Health Professions Commission projected an oversupply and indicated that a number of schools of nursing should close. The Pew Commission advocated that the number of nursing programs should be reduced 10–20%; however, these closings should come with the closure of associate and diploma programs. (Pew Health Professions Commission, 1995).

The principle of substitution was used to control costs. As money was scarce, administrators substituted one worker (the nurse) with a worker (unlicensed personnel) who can do the work at a lower cost. Patient care technicians or assistants were trained and highly utilized as replacements for nurses in many circumstances. Unfortunately, what administrators could not foresee, measure, or predict was the impact the economically sound theoretical application of substitution would have on patient outcomes. Although assistive personnel can do much of the physical work of nursing, they cannot replace the professional nurse's critical thinking and judgment skills. These skills are acquired through education and strengthened through experience.

Since patients who remain hospitalized during these times are more acutely ill and frequently in unstable states, clinical decision-making by professional providers is crucial to their well-being. Sadly, there was and still is insufficient scientific evidence of the impact of a professional nurse's clinical judgment, decision-making, and interventions on patient outcomes. However, a number of investigators have studied the effects of decision-making, staffing mix, education, and experience on clinical judgment and quality of patient care. Akin, Smith, and Lake (1994) found lower mortality with higher skill mix (greater percentage of professional nurses to unlicensed assistive personnel). Benner's seminal work on nurses' decision-making is classic in that expert nurses (i.e., nurses with experience) made better decisions with fewer cues than did less experienced nurses with fewer experiences (Benner, 1984). Blegen, Goode, and Reed (1998) studied the relationships among total hours of nursing care, RN skill mix, and adverse patient occurrences. These adverse patient occurrences included unit rates of medication errors, patient falls, skin breakdown, patient and family complaints, infections, and deaths. Controlling for patient acuity, these researchers showed the higher the RN skill mix, the lower the incidence of adverse occurrences on inpatient care units. The economic question is "in addition to the insult to the patient who wants quality care, what does the adverse event cost the agency?" What if the infection caused four additional hospital days and the hospital is reimbursed at the DRG rate? What might be the costs of a Medicare patient's falling and breaking a femur while in the hospital?

Kovner and Gergen (1998) carried out a comprehensive study on nurse staffing and adverse events following surgery in U.S. hospitals while Kovner was a fellow at the Agency for Health Care Policy and Research (AHCPR), now known as the Agency for Healthcare Quality and Research (AHQR). This study showed that higher levels of staffing were related to lower levels of venous thrombosis, urinary tract infection, and pneumonia.

Similarly, in a major research study that included 799 hospitals in 11 states covering 5,075,969 discharges of medical patients and 1,104,659 discharges of surgical patients, Needleman, Buerhaus, Mattke, Stewart, and Zelevinsky (2002) found that a higher proportion of hours of care provided by registered nurses resulted in significantly shorter length of stay, lower rates of urinary tract infections, lower upper gastrointestinal bleeding, lower rates of pneumonia, and lower incidence of shock and cardiac arrest. In another major study on the effects of staffing and nurse–patient ratios, Aiken, Clarke, Sloane, Sochalski, and Silber (2002) found hospitals with high patient-to-nurse ratios had higher risk-adjusted 30-day mortality and failure-to-rescue rates, and nurses were more likely to experience job dissatisfaction and burnout. These studies are powerful indicators to the importance of registered nurses and adequate staffing levels in saving lives by surveillance, early detection, timely interventions, and the rescue of patients from life-threatening conditions. The same quality and economic questions as described earlier could be asked here. The evidence strongly suggests that if hospitals invest in adequate registered nurse staffing, preventable mortality can be averted and nurse retention can be increased.

Cyber Care

Electronic technology is revolutionizing health care. This technology includes (a) the electronic medical record, (b) transmitting diagnostic images to offsite locations for reading and viewing, (c) use of bar coding for charging patient-chargeable supplies in the hospital or controlling inventory in the hospital, (d) utilizing handheld computers to record patient vital signs and nursing documentation, (e) referring patients to the Internet for clinical information, and (f) electronic consultation for patients. Moreover, a survey by Harris Interactive (2001) found that 47% of all adults use the Internet to look for health care information.

The computerized patient record (CPR) has been around since the early 1990s, but recent changes have removed barriers that have impeded the development and use of the CPR during the last 10 years. For example, attitudes of health care providers toward the CPR have improved. Additionally, the existence of several economic factors will drive the rapid advancement in computerized patient record software. These include: (a) the need for more efficient documentation within managed care organizations; (b) the potential cost of HIPAA violations; and (c) the cost of malpractice insurance and the need for improved documentation of care and instructions provided to patients (Kadas, 2002).

Another exciting technology trend is the collaborative health record. This type of record focuses on the individual patient and can link health care providers at every encounter to collect details of conditions, assessments, and therapeutic interventions. This includes consumer-owned, physician-accessible online record storage and management systems. For example, My-Family MD, a Web-based consumer portal, enables members to chronicle health goals and progress, track medications, and contact physicians by secure means (Marietti, 2002). An additional trend is the integrated computing system or computerized physician order entry (CPOE). This system allows the physician to electronically input orders for medication, lab, and diagnostic interventions. The integrative system incorporates decision support to flag dosing errors, drug interactions, and drug allergies. California has actually passed legislation to require all urban hospitals to adopt a formal plan by 2005 that includes the use of a technology such as CPOE to minimize medication errors (May, 2002). "Improved organization, communication and time expenditures are just a few of the benefits of CPOE . . ." (May, 2002, p. 32). Still another enhancement in interactive patient services is the use of e-technology such as Patient Site, which lets patients view parts of their medical record and send messages to providers and staff, and enables physicians to direct patients to appropriate health information.

The ANA recognized the influence that the electronic media would have on its professionals and in 1999 published two monographs, *Competencies for Telehealth in Nursing* and *Core Principles on Telehealth* (ANA, 1999a, 1999b). These documents provide guidelines for nurses in this expanding telehealth market.

As anticipated, telehealth has been introduced into the market as a means of providing consultation for patients with an affixed cost. The first health plan to offer reimbursement to physicians for electronic consultation was established in 2000, noting that frequent office visits often prevent hospitalization and that the physician could achieve the same result through the use of electronic consultation with the patients (Maguire, 2000). Physicians are reimbursed the same amount, $25 per consultation, for preventive care visits. These decisions were made after research showed that 25% of the patients who use the Internet for health informa-

Research Application

You have been asked to investigate the benefits of establishing telehealth in the primary care practice where you have been working since graduation from a baccalaureate program in nursing. Although this assignment seems daunting, you know that you can carry out this assignment as you have a wealth of knowledge in health care and you had lectures in finance and economics in your nursing leadership course. You also had an introductory course in research in nursing.

- How would you plan this assignment?
- What search words would you use in surfing the Web for related studies?
- What search engines might be most helpful?
- What journals would be most helpful?

You remember reading a study in the Archives of Internal Medicine on telephone calls to discharged patients who had heart failure. Readmission rates were 36% lower for the patients who received telephone calls as follow up care. Would this be related to your assignment?

- What evidence of success would you look for?
- What comparisons might you use?
- What information do you need from your patients?

A number of private companies offer insurance plans specifically designed for international students. Quality varies, so request advice from the on-campus International Student Office and other international students—especially students who have had experience with insurance claims.

Important questions to consider include:

- Does the health insurance plan cover both accidents and sicknesses?
- Does the plan cover costs incurred outside of a hospital setting?
- Which doctors or hospitals does the plan recognize?
- What exactly are the exclusions and limitations?

Here are some basic insurance terms that will get you started in learning more about health care in the United States:

- *Premium*: The amount that you pay to purchase the insurance coverage.
- *Deductible*: The amount that the insured person must pay before the insurance company starts paying.
- *Co-insurance*: The percentage that the insured person pays after the deductible is paid; for example, if co-insurance equals 20%, then the insured person pays 20% and the insurance company pays 80%.
- *Expenses*: Costs for services such as surgery, hospitalization, x-rays, prescription drugs, and/or laboratory tests; expenses are defined in the individual insurance contracts (Miller, 2000).

tion would use it for physician encounters. As with all encounters of a private nature, the security of this information must be protected by secure passwords. Security rules have been written and are available from the Government Printing Office. The cost–benefit analysis and impact on patient outcomes of these electronic encounters will need to be determined before expansion of this model of care occurs with other providers.

With the increasing costs in health care it is prudent for health care decision makers to do a cost–benefit analysis before implementing new modalities, procedures, or programs. Nurses particularly must be mindful of the cost implications of their care in addition to the clinical implications. A cost–benefit analysis places a dollar value on what goes into the project and a dollar value on the outcome (Chang, 2001). Using the example of the physicians' online consultation, nurses need to answer these questions regarding nursing and consultation:

- Does online consultation require more time or less time than regular office visits on-site?
- Does online consultation require additional online follow-up?
- Are concerns/problems resolved sooner with online consulation?
- Are the outcomes the same?
- How many of the consultations could best be addressed by nurses? At what reduction in cost?

The nurse must also be aware of search engines that are available to access clinical information not only to enhance one's own knowledge, but also in the nurse's education role with patients. Most health care institutions are providing their clinical professional staff with online capability at the work site to access clinical information and the latest clinical research to enhance the quality of their work performance.

As the consumer becomes more computer literate, it is advantageous for nurses to recommend clinical information sites to aid in educating the patient and/or family, or be able to access appropriate information to give to the patient. Medline, a search engine that does not charge a fee gives access to more than 4,000 health care journals.

The fiscal impact of electronic technology on health care is expected to exceed $25 billion primarily due to implementation of HIPAA, the Health Insurance Portability and Accountability Act of 1996. This legislation created:

- Protection to assist Americans in keeping their health insurance when they change jobs
- Protocols for protecting the privacy and security of health care information
- Rules that standardize how health care information is electronically stored and transmitted
- An increased need for technology and security systems, software changes, and interfaces, as well as additional personnel, training costs, and possibly construction costs

Marketing and Development Strategies for External Funding

Health care has become a competitive business with all of the furnishings and equipment thus entailed. Just as with any other competitive business, health care providers are beginning to recognize the value of marketing. **Marketing** is a managerial process using promotion skills that reach out to consumers and inform them about the positive aspects of a product. Health care organizations market so as to draw consumer attention to a service.

In order to be effective, the marketing strategy must be aligned with the organization's strategic plan and goals as well as customers perceptions and preferences (Byers, 2001). Input into the marketing plans should be obtained from all stakeholders including nurses. This provides an opportunity for nursing to play a role in designing and implementing specific health care services. The involvement of the clinical staff ensures that the organization can deliver on the services promised, as it is the clinicians who provide the services. Marketing can occur via newsletters, newspaper, radio, television, billboards, intra- and Internet Web

---

Critical Thinking and Reflection

To ensure compliance with the new HIPAA regulations, what measures for patient privacy and security of patient information have been implemented in your clinical agency? Are they effective?

pages, and speakers' bureau. The quality of care provided and the patient's feelings regarding that care go a long way in marketing an institution. Patient word of mouth can be an invaluable marketing tool.

Professional Nurses' Role in a Managed Care Environment

Nursing professionals are currently in the middle of a struggle between payers and providers while trying to preserve quality of nursing care. Nurses tend to react to managed care in two ways, **reactionary** or **proactive.** An example of a reactionary response to managed care is perhaps seen in Weingart's (1991) articles lamenting about the "trouble with managed care" and with firms implementing strict utilization review mechanisms. The author advises readers to encourage patients to seek legal counsel should care be denied. The alternative nursing response to managed care is a proactive response to payer and employer demands for cost containment that is evidenced by the development of nursing case management by such nursing professionals such as Zander (1988) and Ethridge (1989, 1991). These programs are designed to proactively thwart any problems that the visionary nursing case manager might detect for either the patient or health care agency.

Why should nurses be concerned with preserving quality of care within the present health care environment? If nurses remain silent and apathetic, they will find themselves in a passive role waiting for external forces to define nursing within the new health care system. It is critical that nurses have a proactive role with managed care, thereby taking advantage of this excellent opportunity to define their own role in managed care, and positively impact health care.

Case Management

Case management has become quite popular in nursing within the last 10 years. Desimone (1988) defines case management as an informative technique appropriate to (a) identifying high-risk, high-cost patient care, (b) assessing opportunities to coordinate care, (c) assessing and choosing treatment option, (d) developing treatment plans to improve quality and efficacy, (e) controlling costs, and (f) managing a patient's total care to ensure optimum outcome. She further identified the following elements of care management: assessment, risk coordination, appraisal, treatment planning, services referral and treatment procurement, monitoring, tracking and assessments of progress, elevation, availability of continuity, and long-term accountability. Desimone (1988) also identified seven models of case management: social, primary care, medical/social, HMO, independent, insurance, and hospital in-house.

Guiliano and Poirier (1991) propose that nursing case management mobilizes, monitors, and rationalizes the resources that a patient uses over the course of an illness. In doing so, case management achieves a controlled balance between quality and cost. According to these authors, two tools are used in case management. The first tool is the case management plan, which is similar to the treatment plan currently used in most psychiatric settings to articulate problems and identify goals and interventions expected to resolve these problems. The second tool is the critical path, which articulates crucial incidents together with proper interventions that should take place on a given day of hospitalization to achieve standard outcomes within the allotted length of stay. The case manager's record documents deviations from the critical path, explores their causes within patient categories, and arranges for specific actions to be taken in response to the variances. Accumulation and analysis of variance data is then conducted to discover trends and directions for altering the practice environment and patterns of providers of care. The goal is always the improvement of the quality of outcomes and the costs of that quality. The critical pathway also helps to sequence interventions predictably and to avoid last minute complexities and oversights, which compromise effective discharge planning.

As with many goods and services, the relationship between quality and costs is not a direct one. That is, paying more for health care does not necessarily assure higher quality. If unnecessary care is provided, it may diminish quality. But even if the care provided is necessary, an efficient delivery system will deliver the same level of quality at a lower cost than will a less efficient one. The problem for the purchaser today is that there is little available information on the quality of individual systems. Without information it is impossible to know whether lower-cost providers are more efficient or whether they keep their costs down by withholding care or providing lower-quality care.

Medical Self-Care

Most efforts to contain health care costs have centered on controlling the provider, the supply side of the health care equation. HMOs and other managed care strategies, for example, achieve their savings by placing financial incentives on providers to avoid unnecessary procedures. While this strategy has worked well to reduce hospitalizations and some elective surgeries, it has failed to alter the upward spiral of health care cost increases that employers face at every insurance renewal.

One innovative system proposed to improve quality while decreasing health care costs is medical self-care (Kemper, 1993). Medical self-care is what the individual does for himself to recognize, prevent, and treat specific health problems. About 80% of all health problems are cared for at home without any help from a health professional (Kemper, 1993). Because of its breadth of impact, self-care is arguably the most important part of our health care system, and yet it is generally overlooked as a strategy for health care improvement. The primary goal of self-care programs is to improve quality of health care. Self-care programs are inexpensive, easily implemented, and well received by most patients and health care providers.

Medical consumerism is the term applied to an individual's role in medical decision-making. It is what the individual does to determine costs, risks, and benefits of treatment and provider options before agreeing to a particular treatment plan. It helps people improve the quality of care they receive without incurring unnecessary costs. Traditionally, medical consumerism has been stymied by a lack of access to information. Now that an increasing amount of information is reaching the public, more active roles for consumers are evolving. Ten action steps to reduce costs through medical consumerism include:

- Become an active medical consumer yourself.
- Build self-care concepts into all health promotion efforts.
- Increase access to medical information.
- Provide self-care training resources to employees.
- Eliminate consumer-squashing language.
- Support care counseling systems.
- Identify consumer-friendly providers.
- Reward people who use consumer skills.
- Track changes in the consumer models.
- Promote self-responsibility in health care reform (Kemper, 1993, pp. 445–446).

Trends in Health Care Reform

All health care systems face the same challenges: improving health, controlling costs, prioritizing allocation of resources, enhancing the quality of care, and distributing services fairly (Bodenheimer & Grumbach, 1998). The U.S. government has sanctioned improvement of health as a primary goal for all Americans. The explicit goals are outlined and discussed in *Healthy People 2000* and *Healthy People 2010* (DHHS, 1999). The economics for reaching this goal must be considered by all health care providers including nurses.

Controlling costs will remain a concern for the next several decades as the spiraling of health care costs is expected to reach new heights by the year 2020 (Feldstein, 1999). The allocation of resources will need to be addressed openly and forcefully as costs continue to escalate and resources are limited. Americans must face the issue of high costs of long-term care and prolonging life may be financially prohibitive. In the future, death with dignity will need to be addressed by health care professionals. Quality of care has been and will continue to be a focus of health care discussions as the measurement of quality remains elusive and individualized. Equal access to care or distributing services fairly will continue to be addressed. Affordability of insurance remains the greatest concern and will require a great deal of thought by health care providers, the public, and policy makers.

Now and in the future it is essential that health care and managing costs be viewed as one entity rather than two separate concepts. Both are required to meet the unique needs of the patient and the country as health care reform is implemented. Health care reform is likely to force physicians to move from solo to large group practices that will focus more resources on cost-effective treatment and management and care. In order to survive hospitals and health care providers will also need to focus on quality indicators, outcome measures, and practice standards. In the future, payments will be linked to these outcome measures and practice standards (Graham, 1995). Furthermore, health care reform is expected to:

- Assure access to care
- Provide preventative services
- Promote consumer input and evaluation
- Encourage research to validate utilization criteria and develop outcome monitors

Health care reform will require hospitals and other health provider agencies to focus on case management and multidisciplinary team care. While acuity of hospitalized patients remains high, revenues will need to be generated to not only meet inpatient needs, but also increase demands for outpatient services that focus on health promotion. Health care reform will force a movement from diagnosis and treatment to prediction and management (Graham, 1995). In addition, health care reform will need to address the following issues and concerns:

- Uninsured and underinsured individuals (e.g., children and the unemployed)
- Nursing shortage
- Patient rights
- Evidence-based practice
- Reductions in employer–provider health insurance
- Regulations for managed care
- Rationed care
- Alternative health care providers

There will most assuredly continue to be a debate concerning health care as right or privilege. In a free open market, a portion of the population would be denied health care if they were unable to pay. As health care costs escalate, this particular debate becomes even more important as a moral and political question for which answers will have to be found.

Demographics, technology, financing, and human resources drive the health care delivery industry. The age and composition of the U.S. population will be a principal influence on health care and health care reform in the twenty-first century. The elderly consume a higher rate of health care services, and the number of elderly are increasing at a rapid rate. In addition, the elderly represent a formidable political force, with very effective lobbying and a much higher rate of participation in local, state, and national elections than the general population. The aging population will also shift services from OB and mental health to services associated within more chronic and complex health threats such as cancer, heart disease, Alzheimer's disease, and cerebrovascular disease.

Job Availability for Nurses

The impact of recent changes discussed in this chapter will certainly influence the types of positions available to nurses in the next decade as well as the skills necessary to effectively practice. Important trends in regard to positions and skills include:

- Designers, managers and coordinators of care.
- Planners for implementing and evaluating nursing care based on the achievment of patient outcomes.
- Integrater of resources for private and public patients.
- Case managers integrating clinical and financial goals.
- Providers in a multidisciplinary environment for high-risk patients.
- Innovators to develop disease management programs.
- Marketers of Nurse Advice phone and Internet service.

Positions for nurses will continue to include the traditional inpatient and outpatient settings, but will also include increasing opportunities for nurses to design and implement new positions in insurance companies, disease management organizations, and other businesses. These opportunities offer an exciting time for both nurses as individuals and nursing as a profession. Now is the time to create meaningful roles for nurses in untraditional settings that improve care and control costs.

TRANSITION INTO PRACTICE

As a primary provider of health care services, the nurse must be knowledgeable of the economic aspects of health care. Nurses are in the best position to bring together quality care, patient advocacy, and sound economic practices (American Hospital Association, 2000). The novice nurse can transition into practice more successfully by understanding the effects of health care economics on staffing practices, care delivery models, and health care purchasing decisions. The nurse will need to recognize how these economic variables affect the patient's recovery and health care outcome.

Staffing practices represent one such economic variable that can be affected by health care economics as reimbursement for health care services must be divided between all the contributing sellers of service, including physicians, pharmacy, hospital operations, and other ancillary providers. If any one entity such as pharmacy begins consuming more of the health care dollar pie, the monies available for the remaining providers will shrink. This reality will drive decisions to staff nursing with less personnel or with less expensive resources. Without understanding health care economics, these staffing decisions may appear illogical to the nurse since the quality of service the nurse can offer is then jeopardized. The nurse who can understand the reality and reasons behind these uncomfortable staffing decisions can shift energy into offering creative solutions that instead contribute to improved staffing efficiencies and outcomes. This positive approach and realistic attitude may also assist the nurse with dealing with job burnout.

Another economic factor that has recently affected nursing is implementation of managed care programs. Managed care models require that the nurse develop excellent documentation and communication skills that effectively communicate the daily acuity and intensity of service required for the patient to meet medical necessity criteria for the level of service provided—otherwise reimbursement for treatment is denied. These same economic factors have created a greater number of nursing career options in nontraditional settings such as home health, ambulatory care, and other lower cost treatment services. In addition, positions as case managers will continue to increase as population-based care delivery models become more prevalent.

KEY POINTS

1. Health care funding is shared equally between public sources and private sources.
2. The goals of managed care are to increase financial risk sharing and decrease health care costs while maintaining quality of care.
3. Nationally, hospital care is the largest health care expenditure of the total expenditures on health care.
4. Investor-owned health care agencies (for profit) provide a monetary profit for their shareholders and pay local, state, and federal taxes.
5. The boundaries of professional practice within an institution are enhanced or limited by the mission and financial status of the organization.

6. The Health Insurance Portability and Accountability Act (HIPAA) of 1996 will demand vast investments in information technology to ensure compliance.
7. Three economic principles (supply and demand, substitution, cost–benefit analysis) influence decision-making in health care.
8. All health care systems face the same challenges: improving health, controlling costs, prioritizing allocation of resources, enhancing the quality of care, and distributing services fairly.
9. Drivers behind increasing health care costs and insurance premiums include: drugs, rising provider expenses, general inflation, increased demand, government mandates and regulation, impact of litigation, and fraud/abuse.

EXPLORE 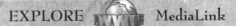 MediaLink

Critical thinking questions, essay questions, key terms, web links, activities, NCLEX review questions, and more interactive resources can be found on the Companion Website at www.prenhall.com/haynes. Click on Chapter 15 to select activities for this chapter.

REFERENCES

Abramowitz, K. S. (1991). Changing trends in health care delivery. In P. Boland (Ed.), *Making managed health care work* (pp. 48–50). New York: McGraw-Hill.

Aiken, L. H., Clarke, S. P., Sloane, D. M., Sochalski, J., & Silber, J. (2002). Hospital nurse staffing and patient mortality, nurse burnout, and job dissatisfaction. *Journal of the American Medical Association, 288,* 1987–1993.

Akin, L., Smith, H., & Lake, E. T. (1994). Lower Medicare mortality among a set of hospitals known for good nursing care. *Medical Care, 32*(8), 771–787.

American Hospital Association. (2000). *Reality check III*. Chicago: American Hospital Association.

American Nurses Association. (1999a). *Competencies for tele-health technologies in nursing*. Washington, DC: American Nurses Publishing.

American Nurses Association. (1999b). *Core principles on telehealth*. Washington, DC: American Nurses Publishing.

Benner, P. (1984). *From novice to expert: Power and excellence in nursing practice*. Menlo Park, CA: Addison-Wesley.

Blegen, M. A., Goode, C. J., & Reed, L. (1998). Nurse staffing and patient outcomes. *Nursing Research, 47*(1), 43–50.

Bodenheimer, T., & Grumbach, K. (1998). *Understanding health policy*. Stamford, CT: Appleton & Lange.

Boland, P. (1991). *Making managed health care work*. New York: McGraw-Hill.

Byers, J. E. (2001). Marketing: A nursing leadership imperative. *Nursing Economics, 19*(3), 94–99.

Chang, C. F. (2001). *Economics and nursing*. Philadelphia, PA: F. A. Davis.

Congressional Record. (1998, September 29). 144:H9183. Daily Edition.

Desimone, P. (1988, July). Professional nursing case management. *Continuing Care*, 22–23.

Duffy, J. (1993). *Economics*. Lincoln, NE: Cliffs Notes, Inc.

Ethridge, P. (1989). Professional nursing case management improves quality, access, and costs. *Nursing Management, 20*(3), 30–35.

Ethridge, P. (1991). A nursing HMO: Carondelet St. Mary's experience. *Nursing Management, 22*(7), 22–27.

Feldstein, P. J. (1988). *The politics of health legislation*. Ann Arbor, MI: Health Administration Press.

Feldstein, P. J. (1999). *Health care economics* (5th ed.). New York: Delmar Publishers.

Graham, N. O. (1995). Quality trends in health care. In N. O. Graham (Ed.), *Quality in health care: Theory, application, and evolution* (pp. 1–14). Gaithersburg, MD: Aspen Publishers.

Grohar, M. E., & DiCroce, H. (2002). *Leadership and management in nursing* (3rd ed.). Upper Saddle River, NJ: Prentice Hall.

Guiliano, K. K., & Poirier, C. E. (1991). Nursing case management: Critical pathways to desirable outcomes. *Nursing Management, 22*(3), 52–55.

Harris Interactive. (April 23, 2001). eHealth traffic critically dependent on search engines and portals. *Harris Interactive Health Care News, 1*(13), 1–3.

Joint Commission on Accreditation of Healthcare Organizations (JCAHO). (1992). *JCAHO accreditation manual for hospitals*. Chicago, IL: Author.

Kadas, R. M. (2002). The computer based patient record is on its way: HMOs, the economy, and HIPAA will drive adoption. *Health Care Informatics, 19*(2), 57–58.

Kemper, D. W. (1993). Controlling costs through medical consumerism. In *Driving down health care costs: Strategies & solutions* (pp. 440–449). New York: Panel Publishers.

Kovner, C., & Gergen, P. (1998). Nurse staffing levels and adverse events following surgery in U.S. hospitals. *Image: Journal of Nursing Scholarship, 30*(4), 315–320.

Maguire, P. (2000). How one health plan pays physicians for cybercare. *Observer, 20*(8).

Marietti, C. (2002). Collaborative health records: Power in partnerships. *Health Care Informatics, 19*(2), 29–30.

May, S. (2002). Computerized physician order entry: Patient safety drives refinement of systems. *Health Care Informatics, 19*(2), 32–33.

McCullough, C. S. (2001). Trends in healthcare change. In C. S. McCullough (Ed.), *Creating responsive solutions to healthcare change*. Indianapolis, IN: Center Nursing Press.

Miller, M. (2000). Health care: A bolt of civic hope. *The Atlantic Monthly, 286*(4), 77–87.

Minsky, H. P. (1996). Uncertainty in the institutional structure of capitalist economics. *Journal of Economic Issues, 30*(2), 357–368.

Mitsunaga, B. K. (1999). Transformation of the U.S. health care delivery system and it's consequences for the health professions. *Yonago Acta Medica, 42*, 141–145.

National Center for Health Statistics. (2001). *Health, United States, 2001 with urban and rural health chartbook*. Hyattsville, MD: Author.

Needleman, J., Buerhaus, P., Mattke, S., Stewart, M., & Zelevinsky, K. (2002). Nurse-staffing levels and the quality of care in hospitals. *New England Journal of Medicine, 346*, 1715–1765.

Pew Health Professions Commission. (1995). *Critical challenges: Revitalizing the health professions fort he twenty-first century*. The Third Report of the Pew Health Professions Commission. San Francisco, CA: The Center for Health Professions.

Sharfstein, S. S. (1990). Utilization management: Managed or mangled psychiatric care? *American Journal of Psychiatry, 147*(8), 965–966.

Sultz, H. (1991). Health policy: If you don't know where you're going, any road will take you. *American Journal of Public Health, 81*(4), 418–420.

Torrens, P. R. (2002). Historical evolution and overview of health services in the U.S. In S. J. Williams & P. R. Torrens (Eds.), *Introduction to health services* (6th ed.) (pp. 2–17). Albany, NY: Delmar Thompson Learning.

Torrens, P. R., & Williams, S. J. (2002). Managed care: Restructuring the system in the U.S. In S. J. Williams & P. R. Torrens (Eds.), *Introduction to health services* (6th ed.) (pp. 124–139). Albany, NY: Delmar Thompson Learning.

United States Bureau of the Census. (1998). *Statistical abstract of the United States: 1998*. Washington, DC: U.S. Government Printing Office.

United States Department of Health and Human Services. (1999). *Healthy people 2010*. Washington, DC: U.S. Government Printing Office.

Weingart, M. (1991). Commercially managed health care: An experience. *Nursing Management, 22*(1), 40–41.

Wilson, C. K., & Porter-O'Grady, T. (1999). *Leading the revolution of health care*. Gaithersburg, MD: Aspen Publishers.

Winegar, N. (1996). *The clinician's guide to managed behavioral healthcare* (2nd ed.). Binghamton, NY: The Haworth Press, Inc.

Zander, K. (1988). Nursing case management: Strategic management of cost and quality outcomes. *Journal of Nursing Administration, 18*(5), 23–30.

SUGGESTED READINGS

Blumenthal, D. (2001). Controlling health care expenditures. *New England Journal of Medicine, 344*(10), 766–769.

Burner, S. T., & Waldo, D. R. (1995). National health expenditure projections 1994–2005. *Health Care Finance Review, 17*(4), 221–242.

Carruth, A., Carruth, P., & Noto, E. (2000). Financial management: Nurse managers flex their budgetary might. *Nursing Management, 31*(2), 16–17.

Chang, C. F., Price, S. A., & Pfoutz, S. K. (2001). *Economics and nursing: Critical professional issues*. Philadelphia, PA: F. A. Davis.

Finkler, S., & Kover, C. (2000). *Financial management for nurse managers and executives* (2nd ed.). Philadelphia, PA: W. B. Saunders.

Goode, C., Tanaka, D., Krugman, M., O'Connor, P., Bailey, C., Dutchman, M., & Stolpman, N. M. (2000). Outcomes from use of an evidence-based practice guideline. *Nursing Economics, 18*(4), 202–207.

Gormley, K., & Verdejo, T. (2000). A systems approach— Budgeting for the 21st century: Turning challenges into triumphs. *Nursing Administration Quarterly, 24*(4), 51–50.

Ward, W. (1998). *An introduction to healthcare financial management*. Ownings, MD: National Health Publishing.

16

Policy, Politics, and Health Care Delivery
A Voice for Nursing

ELIZABETH FARREN CORBIN

> *The personal is political. Each of us is just one personal injustice away from being involved in politics.*
>
> *Dodd, 2001*

LEARNING OBJECTIVES

AT THE COMPLETION OF THIS CHAPTER, THE READER WILL BE ABLE TO:

- ➤ Discuss the concepts of policy, politics, and professional advocacy.
- ➤ Explain the apparent values in selected policies.
- ➤ Identify the role of professional nursing in the design, implementation, and evaluation of policy affecting health care.

- ➤ Discuss the application of policy, politics, and advocacy to the development of professional nursing.
- ➤ Address an issue of concern to nursing in the context of policy development.

MediaLink   www.prenhall.com/haynes

Additional online resources including NCLEX review questions, critical thinking questions, and real-world activities for this chapter can be found on the Companion Website at www.prenhall.com/haynes.

Nursing's involvement with policy and politics is concerned with advocacy and the need for nurses to control their own practice environment. Any basic writing on nursing explores the rich diversity of roles that make up this dynamic profession. That nurses are caregivers is fundamental. Caregiving is the primary focus, and for the novice, the ultimate goal to master.

In the evolution of professional development, nurses have extended care to an ever-widening circle. Once that focus embraces more than the individual patient, the nurse must develop additional skills and supplement singular interventions with collegial efforts. To control the professional practice environment, to influence the allocation of resources, and to advocate for more than one patient, the nurse must enter into and be a force in the development of policy, law, and regulation.

Health care in our country is governed, guided, and directed by policy. Government statutes (e.g., state nurse practice acts and professional rules and regulations) regulate providers and their practices. Accrediting bodies regulate health care agencies (e.g., hospitals, clinics, etc.). Organizations that reimburse health care costs (e.g., insurance companies) are governed by public law and their own organizational rules. Medical devices and pharmaceutical products are approved, regulated, and controlled by government rules. Health agency employees are governed by policies and procedures of the organization. All of this oversight and control, whether by law, ordinance, rule, or procedure manual, arises from policy.

Policy

Policy, whether public or private, gives voice to an individual's, a family's, or a group's intentions, values, and priorities. Policy impacts life at every turn (e.g., the life of the citizen, an employee, or a practicing professional). Policy is a formalized statement of committed direction. Every free country and every established organization is governed by policies that describe the response that entity will respond in a given situation. Many basic questions are answered by policy. For example, policy provides guidance as to how a citizen from another country enters the United States. Policy also addresses how a nurse licensed in one state can ultimately practice in another. Policy regulates care in health care organizations. Policy also regulates and guides a nurse to help or to criticize a struggling colleague.

Types of Policy

Policy exists on the most formal and lofty levels and on the most personal and intimate levels. Several categories of policy exist. **Public policy** refers to policies and laws formed by the government. These policies are applicable to all citizens and to all individuals of other countries visiting or residing in the United States. **Social policy** pertains to directives that promote the general welfare of the public. **Health policy** includes directives for specifically promoting or protecting the health of citizens and treatment of those ill or injured. It broadly includes designation of provider credentials, establishment of health care agencies, and identification of individuals or institutions responsible and financially accountable for health care. **Institutional policy** governs the workplace and directs institutional goals. It broadly includes how the institution will treat its employees and how its employees may work. **Organizational policy** is derived from an organization's goals and reflects its statement of philosophy or purpose. It guides the positions taken on issues of organizational relevance. **Personal policy** includes policy held by an individual. These individual policies are more commonly termed scruples, moral codes, or personal ethics. Examples of personal policy include: (a) being

---

Critical Thinking and Reflection

What are some of the policies at your school of nursing that most affect you? There would, no doubt, be a dress policy, a policy for missed exams, a policy for attendance. Do you find these policies supportive of your progress to your goals? Should some of these policies be improved? Strengthened? Eliminated? How would you go about changing policy there at your school?

helpful or critical; (b) striving for excellence or simply meeting the standard; (c) staying abreast; and (d) acting to influence the future.

Purpose of Policy

Policy drives but is not limited by laws, regulations, and rules. Once a policy is established, it may inspire or direct many laws, rules, and regulations, and may do so for many years. For example, the framers of the United States Constitution adopted a policy of protection of individual freedoms. From this policy generations of laws, beginning with the Bill of Rights have been established. This policy has been amended over time in the form of civil rights legislation, property rights, and many other protections for individual rights (U.S. Constitution, Article IV., sec. 2; Amendments 1 thru 10, 13, 14 sec. 1, 15, 19, 24, and 26).

A health care organization may have a policy to support research or teaching. Such a policy would dictate (a) the inclusion of research and teaching positions in the organization and (b) the budget or resources to accomplish education and research goals. A school of nursing may have a policy for admission of students that requires certain testing and prerequisite courses. Such a policy would direct admission of applicants based on policy regardless of the power or influence of any single individual. Both examples of policy illustrate the power a policy has to affect outcome.

Values: Apparent and Inherent in Policy

Policy also represents a statement of values. Clearly, the framers of the constitution valued individual rights and freedom. In the above examples, the health care agency valued teaching and research, and the school of nursing valued knowledge and preparation. Nursing as a profession has been very clear about values. The Code of Ethics for Nurses (American Nurses Association [ANA], 2001) is a policy statement of values (e.g., professional relationships, commitment to the patient, advocacy, responsibility and accountability, personal integrity, safety, competence, and professional growth). Some specialty nursing organizations also have codes of ethics that express their values (American Association of Occupational Health Nurses, 1991; American Holistic Nurses' Association, 1992). The Standards for Nursing Practice which, approved by the American Nurses Association express the value nurses assign to research, application of theory, and all aspects of caring for and managing patients.

To formulate a policy statement, many different values and opinions compete as the final position statement is formulated. Positions or actions that make up policy must be consistent with the expressed values of nursing as a whole. The sorting through of conflicting values and opinions and the forging of a single voice is a task accomplished using political strategies.

The Nature of Politics

Politics is a process of influence. It is a method of persuasion, negotiation, debate, and bargaining with the goal to adopt a particular viewpoint or path of action. Politics in a free society allows the expression of divergent points of view or conflicting values to ultimately be expressed as one policy, one voice. **Politics** can be defined as the process of putting the moral consensus of the community into practice (Bellah, 1987). In democratic politics, persons or groups with opposing views discuss their positions and work toward persuading opponents to their point of view. In the best of all possible worlds, this process can serve to increase information for decision-making and compel those involved to separate wants from needs.

Conflict develops as self-interest in positions grows. With feelings added to opinions, differences take on significant meanings and compromises or alternatives can seem like losses. How conflict is handled can determine the view many may have of politics. If the political process is open and fair, information and persuasive arguments from all sides of an issue can be heard. If the process is secretive or even punitive it can dissolve into a power struggle. In reality, the political process itself is innocent of harm, and can serve to forge true communal decisions; the guilty are those who engage in manipulative political practices. The distaste that is associated with politics has more to do with the behaviors of those handling conflict, than with the political process.

Mobilizing Forces for Change

The process of politics includes a wide variety of ways in which influence is brought to bear. In its best form, the process begins with information specific to an issue at hand. The force of information and sound critical debate can be powerful tools in negotiation. This is a natural process for nurses who are skilled at bringing all relevant information to bear on a problem. Nurses predicate their professional caregiving based on research and knowledge. These same diligent efforts in gaining knowledge and doing appropriate research on matters of policy can provide the nurse with a powerful influence for affecting a political outcome.

Commitment to a cause or an outcome is another powerful influence. The person or group who demonstrates an enduring effort to achieve an outcome can be a powerful political force. So many problems in society have been dealt with and even resolved by committed persons who work for better solutions. Witness Candy Lightener who, through tireless efforts, founded Mothers Against Drunk Driving (MADD). A grieving mother who lost a child to a drunk driver, Ms. Lightener worked to raise the consciousness of society regarding the plague of drunk driving. Through her efforts, and those of her supporters, policy and laws relating to alcohol, in general, and drunk driving in particular, were forever changed, with innumerable lives saved.

Witness also the late Princess Diana of England, who committed herself publicly and courageously to having international law changed regarding the use of land mines. She joined established organizations to draw attention to the innocent lives lost or maimed by land mines left behind after war. She made innumerable public appearances in mined fields using her public persona to raise consciousness of the problem; she committed her personal safety in an unprecedented way. Even today, years after her death, the image of the lovely youthful princess wearing a frag mask and walking through a mine field is a powerful motivation for change (Donnelly, 1997; Fried & Fried, 1997).

Action is another necessary ingredient in the political process. Hoping things will change and arguing

Research Application

Moskowitz, Griffith, DiScala, and Sege (2001, August) provide a perfect example of the use of research to discover knowledge that can be used to influence public policy. Researchers from New England Medical Center studied the incidence of assault injury to adolescents. They analyzed data from pediatric trauma centers in 45 states and national homicide data from 1989 to 1999 to determine if there were differences in victim characteristics, injury severity, and injury mechanisms among adolescent boys and girls.

The researchers found that adolescent girls were nearly twice as likely as adolescent boys to have preexisting cognitive or psychosocial impairments, which appear to have made them particularly vulnerable to attack. These factors have also been associated with risk of alcohol and other drug abuse linked to date rape. Adolescent boys were 1.75 times more likely to be injured in a public place and 2.27 times more likely to be injured in school than were girls. However, adolescent girls were more than twice as likely to be injured in their home or at another residence than a public place. This could indicate that girls are likely to be intentionally injured by a friend, an acquaintance, or an intimate partner.

Additional findings show that girls are more likely to be stabbed than shot, while the opposite is true for boys. Gunshot and stabbing injuries in the 10-year research period declined 28% for boys but only 7% for girls.

These findings suggest to the researchers the inadequacy of public health messages that focus mainly on violent risks to adolescent boys. They also plead the need to refine messages targeted to adolescent girls with forceful warnings and advice on how to prevent attacks at home or in the home of a friend.

With this very factually based research, one has a true and realistic knowledge of the problem of violence to adolescent girls. In addition, the research provides a strong rationale to seek support for additional efforts to prevent the violence uncovered by this longitudinal study of significant numbers of youth.

This study was supported in part by the Agency for Healthcare Research and Quality (National Research Service Award, training grant T32 HS00060).

that they should are only beginning steps. Without action these behaviors won't effect change. Eventually action is required. When research is complete and a commitment is made, action can be taken. There are many forums and avenues for action available to the informed and committed nurse. While a single voice, like a single candle does shed noticeable light, many voices are more illuminating. Whether an issue is public or private, local or national, widespread support is needed to affect any change in policy.

Mobilizing Support and Resources

The setting for proposed policy does not change the basic approach to the process. In the workplace, other interested and supportive persons must be enlisted to give stronger voice to the desire for change. Nurses may work through unit or agency committees, interest groups, or task forces. The resources of a group are most effective and available to the nurse when he or she has been a member of the group. One's voice carries more weight when one has been an integral member of a group, in service to achieve the group's goals. Working through the organizational chart is mandatory when enlisting aid and cooperation. The object always is to gain support for change, and that is best done by protecting existing interests as much as possible. Courtesy and respect for opposing positions and vested interests should always be a part of any negotiation. With careful and respectful work, the opposition will be limited to persons who truly oppose a policy change and will not include persons who have been ignored, offended, or insulted in some way by the tactics taken.

Affecting change in governmental policy is not much different from making changes in the workplace. Action must be preceded with the same research of the issue and a sorting through of possible remedies. The nurse must enlist like-minded supporters, and work through the governmental process. Support from like-minded nurses may, hopefully, be found in professional nursing organizations such as the American Nurses Association or various specialty-based organizations. These resources exist today because of the vision and sacrifices of their founding members.

History of Nursing in Policy and Politics

Nursing has a proud history of caring about and effecting policies of the government, health care agencies,

and its own professional organizations. From its modern beginnings, nursing has recognized the need to control not only nursing practice, but also the environment in which practice takes place.

Florence Nightingale

Florence Nightingale's inceptive work almost immediately extended to the arena of policy. Her work in the Crimea earned her the distinction of being regarded as the founder of modern nursing and a pioneer in the use of biostatistics (Coden, 1984). Much of her efforts were passionately directed at changing policy. She knew what the major killer of soldiers was, and she knew that all the compassionate nursing in the world could not fight rampant infection and contamination. She painstakingly compiled research data identifying infectious disease and malnutrition as etiologic agents. What was needed was a policy for sanitation and nutrition standards.

As history records, Nightingale heroically committed herself to years of writing to and pleading with military officials and then civil servants, to effect the needed sanitary conditions to protect the health of soldiers, the poor, and those in hospitals of all kinds. She fought for policy and standards so that the correct conditions could be maintained beyond her personal influence (Dossey, 2000). Further, she extended her concerns and teachings beyond her English shores in advice to nurses in the United States. In a letter written in 1872 to the founders of the nurse-training school, Bellevue Hospital in New York City, Nightingale differentiated between nursing and medicine. She spoke to the importance of having standards based on rationale understood by the practitioner, and cautioned new practitioners to maintain control of nursing by nurses (Nightingale, 1911).

While it seems clear that such issues as sanitation and standards of practice must be addressed by policy, it may seem strange that they were also political issues. It must be remembered that, at the time, there was no general knowledge of sanitation among the common citizens. Nor was it an accepted (or comfortable!) precept that women should work outside the home, have authority over serious endeavors, or control their own work. Thus, there remained not only the work of policy development, but also that of convincing the government and populace that these changes were needed, and were within the capability of professional nurses. For this work, organization and unity of the profession was needed.

"It did strike me odd, sometimes, that we should pray to be delivered from plague, pestilence, and famine, when all the common sewers ran into the Thames and fevers haunted undrained land and the districts which cholera visited could be pointed out. I thought that cholera came that we might remove these causes, not pray that God would remove the cholera" (Nightingale, 1859, p. 126).

Ms. Nightingale points out that sewers drain into the primary source for drinking water and that cholera visits specific geographic regions. What might she mean when she says that she thought "cholera came so that we might remove the causes?" Why would a nurse have an interest in sewer drainage? How would a nurse, in any time, go about having an effect on sewer drainage? What nursing roles would be employed?

The Woman's Movement

In the United States, nursing's notable step into the arena of policy and politics took place on behalf of the Woman's Movement and suffrage in particular. To have a voice, women would, at the very least, need to have an equal vote in the political processes in their own country. Nursing's most historical and enduring organizations in the United States all sprang from the desire to (a) establish nursing as a true profession based on a body of knowledge and (b) improve the care of the individual patient and the community at large. To accomplish these tasks, nurses recognized they would have to effect important social policy changes. To do this, at the very least, women would need the right to vote. Professional nursing organizations began to form in the late 1800s and early 1900s. While their initial intent was to define the profession, inform the public, and train recruits, nurses soon included social and health policies as critical to the mission of these new organizations. There were four major organizations formed in this time. Each had a special focus of concern, but as they matured and grew they found common ground in their concern for the health of patients and the social policies of the time effect health care and women.

Professional Organizations

The American Society of Superintendents was founded in 1893, renamed the National League of Nursing Education in 1912 and, finally, the National League for Nursing (NLN) in 1952. This organization of nursing instructors (superintendents), hospital chief administrators, and staff worked toward establishing standards of nursing care and uniformity of nursing curriculum (Lewenson, 1998). Since that time, the NLN has been a major force for standards of excellence and uniformity in nursing education and agency standards. It has been highly effective in setting policy for standards in nursing.

The Nurses' Associated Alumnae of the United States and Canada was founded in 1896 and renamed the American Nurses Association (ANA) in 1911. From its earliest beginning, the ANA advocated united action through political activity to accomplish its goals. The first editor of the organization's journal urged that state societies would form for the "definite and separate purpose of promoting legislation for state registration of nurses" (Palmer, 1909). Over the years, the ANA has had and continues to have a vital role and major impact on legislation affecting nurses, health, and health care. The ANA moved its national headquarters to Washington, D.C., in 1992 for the primary purpose of being close to the source of major policy decisions.

The National Association of Colored Graduate Nurses was formed in 1908, specifically to address and overcome racial hostility and to address professional nursing issues. Because of discriminatory practices in many professional nursing organizations, black nurses were banned from state training schools and from joining professional nursing organizations. This organization is a testament to the spirit and professionalism of African-American nurses, who were sadly limited from integration in society in general and even in nursing organizations until well after Word War II (Lewenson, 1998). By forming their own organization, these nurses triumphed to have a unique voice.

The National Organization for Public Health Nursing (NOPHN) was founded in 1912 by nurses who witnessed the threats to health of the growing urbanization of the United States in the throes of the industrial revolution. This organization was formed, as were the other nursing organizations, in order to ensure standards of nursing. This organization sought to specifically address the needs of the nation for clean water, decent housing, adequate sanitation, access to health care, and identification of and response to potential epidemics. From the beginning, NOPHN recognized the value in forming coalitions with interdisciplinary groups interested in common goals (Lewenson, 1998). Such broadly pervasive problems could only be addressed from a political policy perspective, with public will and public money.

Through these official organizations nurses debated and fought for the right to have a voice and to make a difference. They wanted control of their profession and their practice environment. They wanted nurses seated on boards of public and private health agencies. They realized that all of their goals would be more readily achieved if they, as a predominately female profession, had an equal vote; they turned their attention to the women's suffrage movement giving affirmative organizational support to the woman's right to vote documented in organizational resolutions in 1912, 1915, 1918, and 1919 (Bullough, Bullough, & Stanton, 1990).

Nursing recognized early on the need to be a full participant in the powers that would impact not only their practice, but also the health and resources of their patients. For contemporary nurses to fully implement their many roles as professional caregivers, they must, at every level, care about and take responsibility for policy. They must care about the social and health policies that affect their lives and the lives of their patients. They must care about the policies of their work environment and they must take responsibility for the policies of their own professional organizations. Policy is indeed a voice, and it must very clearly, and at every level, include the voice of professional nursing.

The rich tradition of policy development and advocacy for the profession and the people it serves continues today. Nurses are involved on every level, from the policy and procedure book on their unit to the standards and goals of their professional organizations, to social and health care legislation from the local, state, and federal governments. Much of this is accomplished through the political action committees of official nursing organizations and their astute coalitions with provider and consumer groups of all kinds.

Impacting Policy

For many nurses, policy closest to home is policy found in school, the state practice act, and on the job. Next in line would be actual social and health policies, national and local, that affect all citizens. Regardless of the level of policy, the process for influence is the same. What follows below is a discussion of the process with examples for practice. A brief summary of the process is provided in Table 16–1.

Policy Analysis

To impact policy, the nurse must have thorough knowledge of the policy. This is the requisite foundation for any action or reaction. One needs to understand the needs the existing policy meets. The nurse must also understand the needs that the existing or developing policy may not address by asking:

- What does the policy actually say?
- What is it intended to do?
- Is it doing that?
- If not, why not?

Policies, even legislative acts, are generally written in clear and understandable English, quite unlike a car insurance policy, for example. There may be ambiguity and vague statements that give rise to court challenges, but it is readable on its face. Read the actual policy carefully. It is not unusual, especially with long-standing policies, for people to relate to what they have been told a policy says. But what does it actually say? What specifics are mentioned? What issues are alluded to or implied? How much room for interpretation exists in the language? The *Americans with Disabilities Act*

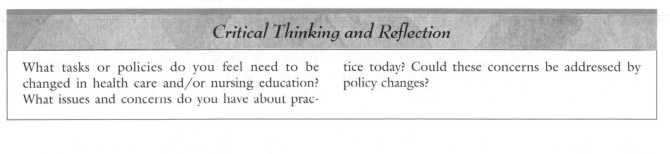

Critical Thinking and Reflection

What tasks or policies do you feel need to be changed in health care and/or nursing education? What issues and concerns do you have about practice today? Could these concerns be addressed by policy changes?

Table 16–1 Process for Policy Analysis or Development

Knowledge	Thorough understanding of the policy under analysis.
	Thorough understanding of the problem to be solved by proposed policy.
Intent	What is the intent of the policy under analysis?
	What is the intent of the proposed policy?
Outcomes	What outcomes are expected?
	How will outcomes be measured in proposed policy?
	What outcomes are demonstrated?
Values	What values are expressed in this policy?
	What values must be respected for this proposed policy to be accepted?
Economics	What costs are associated with this policy?
	What costs will be incurred or saved by this proposed policy?
Legality	Will this proposed policy be legal?
	Is there a legal contest associated with this policy?
	Would it require changes to other laws?
Politics	Who is advantaged and who is disadvantaged by this policy?
	Who would be for and who against the proposed policy?
	What coalitions of support might be possible?
	Are there favors to be called in?

(ADA, 1990), for example, specifically addresses the rights of the disabled. The definition of the word disabled, however, has occupied many legal minds in many instances of litigation in reference to the Act over the years. What was the climate in which the policy was first developed? What was the pressing need of that moment?

The intent of the policy is usually discoverable by a careful study of the policy itself and, perhaps, an interview of its authors or administrators. After thorough study of the policy as written, a clarifying discussion with administrators of the policy may be needed to ensure that an understanding of the policy is accurate. Perhaps, for example, nurses on a given agency unit are concerned about infections arising on their unit. They know there is an Infection Control Policy and so a study of this policy becomes essential. If some of the authors of that policy are available they might be able to share insight as to how and why the policy was developed and what some of the prominent considerations were at the time it was written. The policy may have been intended simply to spell out a procedural method for infection control. Or it may have been more broadly aimed at protecting patients and staff from the spread of infections and to comply with accrediting regulations.

The values inherent in the policy must be identified. These will be cultural values, that is, values generally accepted by the predominant culture that devised and accepted the policy. Understanding the why of the policy is important before any changes can be considered. For instance, does the policy address cost control measures as a primary consideration in planning infection control measures? The valuing of cost related to care must be considered in any analysis. It may not be the predominant value, but it is nevertheless important in understanding the climate from which the policy arose.

The next consideration is outcome of the policy. Is the policy accomplishing its intended goals? The answer to this critical question should include and may require a more formal process. Box 16–1 gives a list of various research techniques that may be employed in policy analysis.

Box 16–1 Research Strategies Applicable to Policy Analysis and Design

Nursing research is the backbone of nursing practice. It is the systematic process used to develop new knowledge, test the validity of accepted norms, and predict outcomes. Finding or doing research for policy work is a powerful tool for persuasion. Following are selected standard designs for research which lend themselves particularly well to the research needed to analyze a policy or to prepare a policy for proposal consideration.

Experimental Research

Experimental design processes include three qualities: manipulation of a variable, control over the experimental situation, and randomization. Manipulation of a variable means that the treatment would be intentional for testing. This is a design that could be used to test the success of a particular treatment, or *policy for treatment*. The nurse interested in giving evidence to policymakers that a specific treatment is successful and thus worth making into a recommended treatment, could cite or conduct experimental research to provide evidence of its effectiveness.

Quasi-experimental Research

This research is similar to experimental but does not have randomization. It is a very useful tool, though not as strong as experimental. It is often more practical for policy study because it can use treatments that are already established and ongoing. The experimental part happens when two or more treatment outcomes are compared. This method could be used to evaluate two similar groups of patients, for example, one of which was receiving a certain treatment, while the other group was not. Perhaps one group would be covered by a health care protocol that mandated certain health screening procedures while the other group did not receive this benefit. Comparing morbidity and mortality statistics of the two groups over time could provide good data for adoption or abolition of the screening policies.

Ex Post Facto Research

In this strategy, subjects in an experiment are selected on the basis of an existing variable that cannot or should not be manipulated. In considering a policy for counseling patients after a severe trauma, for example, one might gather data on the psychological well-being of persons who suffered a severe trauma and had professional counseling compared to similarly affected patients who did not have counseling. Finding a higher level of psychological well-being in the counseled group could be helpful in convincing policy makers to provide funds for a counseling program and to establish a policy of providing such counseling.

Epidemiological Research

An epidemiological approach is very helpful with a little studied problem. This strategy is very data intensive, looking at person, place, and time involvement with a problem (or solution). In design or analysis of a policy it is crucial to know who may benefit from a policy or treatment in terms of defining its need and also in terms of forming political alliances for policy support or defeat. This method would provide the nurse with knowledge of who might benefit from a policy and consequently who might be a good political alliance in getting a policy established.

Outcomes Research

Outcomes research is a natural for policy analysis. Nothing is quite as effective as being able to point to data that indicates that a certain goal was or was not obtained based on the policy in place. For example, did the infection rate on the postsurgical unit drop after the implementation of the new infection control policy?

Adapted from Polit, D. F., Beck, C. T., & Hungler, B. P. (2001). *Essentials of nursing research methods, appraisal and utilization* (5th ed.). Philadelphia, PA: Lippincott.

An epidemiological research approach could be used, for example, to determine the rate of infection for a given unit or service. If this were done using data before the establishment of the Infection Control Policy, and then done using data since the Infection Control Policy was applied, any difference in rates of infection would indicate the degree of success or failure of the policy to accomplish its goals. Knowing this, the only question remaining relative to existing policy is whether the policy is being applied faithfully and correctly.

Application of the Research Process

Observation or interview of staff or, perhaps, chart audit may bring to light either of the following possibilities as to application of the policy:

- Staff believes they are following policy; observation or chart audits will confirm or refute their adherence to the policy.
- Staff knows they are not following policy but have compelling reasons for not doing so (e.g., lack of knowledge, lack of supplies or equipment, shortage of staff, conflict of values).

With correct knowledge of the policy, data about its application, and epidemiological data indicating outcomes, the nurse could say with some assurance that a policy was or was not effective.

Evaluating a policy is a process that is important when considering existing policy, and is equally important in the consideration of proposed policy. Perhaps, instead of evaluating a policy, the nurses wish to establish a new policy relative to developing needs on their unit, in their community of service, or even on a regional or national level. The nurse must still begin with the process of evaluation, which means being fully prepared in knowledge, intent, values identification, and expected outcomes. The creation and development of policy also requires persuasion, and therein enters the value of knowledge regarding the political process.

Development of Policy

Policy is designed to provide guidelines and direction. Almost invariably its stimulus is to address a problem that is expected to arise again and again. The job of a policy is to provide a uniform set of directions for avoiding or solving an ongoing problem. The critical foundation to a policy is an accurate understanding of the problem to be solved and a reasonable assurance that the proposed policy is the best solution to that problem.

- Is the problem thoroughly understood? Has adequate research been done to understand the problem in its entirety, have all factors been considered?
- Is the policy as a proposed solution scientifically sound? Is it a rational solution?
- Is the policy realistic and workable? Is it workable in the existing structure for governance or reimbursement? What changes might be needed in order to implement this policy?
- How will outcomes be apparent? What data will indicate success or failure? Is it possible to capture this data?

Most solutions represent one of some, if not many possibilities. It is important to have the conviction that a proposed policy is not only a good and realistic solution to a problem, but also the very best solution possible. Thorough knowledge of the problem and the proposed policy would include knowing such things as if there are personnel who can carry out the policy and knowing if structural or legal changes would be required to implement the policy. It is of crucial importance from the beginning that one know which policy outcomes would indicate either success or failure. The current climate in health care is very much outcome focused (Aiken, Sloane, & Sochalski, 2001). How will the expected outcomes be measured? Are short- and long-term outcomes obtainable? These questions will eventually be asked by anyone who will need to vote for or approve the policy. Proponents of the policy must be prepared to address these issues convincingly to any person or group from whom they seek approval or support.

Consideration of Values and Ethics

For a policy to be acceptable to those who must vote for it, or approve it in some way, it must reflect the values of the predominant culture. Depending on the level of policy, that culture may be that of a nursing unit, a professional organization, or all of society. Some questions to consider when evaluating the values of a policy include:

- Is the policy under consideration compatible with contemporary values? With professional values and ethics?

- Does the policy contribute to equity, that is, would it be applied equally to all persons? Would some persons be granted exceptions from its limitations? Would some persons be excluded from its benefits?
- Is the policy just? Is it fair in its demands? Does it establish a prohibition or a benefit that is unjust in its outcome?
- Who would benefit from the policy? Is this benefit desirable to all?
- Who would be disadvantaged by this policy? Might this be acceptable to those who would be disadvantaged?
- Is the policy likely to generate other social problems?

These considerations are not necessarily deal breakers, but will always figure prominently. The ongoing conflict about abortion as a treatment in this country, for example, is about the conflict of values in our society as to the definition of life. Abortion legislation will always be in question while there remains a close division in social values. That is, one side seeking freedom of choice for the mother, and the other side seeking protection of the unborn. Either side would cite injustice as a cause for action.

Generally in America, we think in terms of equal application of the law. This is about the equitable application of the law to rich and poor, young and old, and to all individuals regardless of race, religion, or gender. In some instances, however, the values of a society will not only permit but may even dictate variations in equity or benefit. Some social legislation is designed to be unequally beneficial to certain subgroups of a society such as the young, the old, the infirmed, or the poor. The United States Tax Code, for example, has a minimum income cutoff at which point a citizen is exempt from paying income taxes based on membership in a financial category. Children have very few rights as compared to adults. Persons with certain clearly defined religious beliefs are exempted from select aspects of military service. In other words, some policies are designed to exclude some persons, and in so doing the policy supports society's contemporary values. A policy that defies society's values has very little chance of passage or acceptance.

Policies are almost always disadvantageous to some and more advantageous to others. Many public health policies weigh in this manner. Infectious disease laws, for example, are advantageous to those who are protected by the quarantine of those disadvantaged persons who are restricted in their movements due to their contagious disease.

Generating additional social problems is never the intent of any policy, and yet, over time, we have learned that it may very well be a consequence. The Hill Burton Act of 1946, just one example, increased the size and number of health care facilities in order to improve access to health care. Its continued implementation, however, is one reason the United States has focused provider activity on acute care, ultimately driving up the cost of health care to unbearable levels by the late 1970s (Sultz & Young, 2001). Efforts now at cost control risk the danger of reversing access, and so a policy, which was designed to increase access, has created a cost overhead structure that threatens to reduce access for a large segment of society (Harrington & Pellow, 2001).

Economic Considerations

Any decisions in the real world require that the cost of action taken or not taken be considered in the decision-making process. No policy is cost free, but some may be cost saving in either the long or short term. This will always be a pivotal decision point and must be addressed.

- Is the policy economical feasible? Would it be nice to have, or possible to have?
- Is the policy economically superior to other alternatives? That is, would this policy be more cost effective than existing policies aimed at the same problem?
- Is the policy workable, or might it require such massive structural changes or supports as to make it prohibitive?

Economics is now as much studied and researched in health care as is health care (Bodenheimer & Grunbach, 1995). Issues simply cannot be addressed without attention being paid to the economic repercussions of the change. The actual cost of the interventions mandated by a policy must be considered. Tangential implementation costs such as the need for additional providers, training to providers, and needs for additional equipment or facilities must also be considered. Third-party reimbursers and various consumer groups carefully watch proposed legislation for cost aspects. They are potent lobbyists in congressional work and influential with accrediting bodies. Costs of health care have become so burdensome that many times reimbursers freely oppose legislation due to cost. Policy proponents and adversaries must be knowledgeable of economic aspects of their ideas and must be prepared to justify costs.

Considerations of Legality

In all matters of policy, the question of legality must be addressed. No policy, public or private, may be enacted that is contrary to existing law. In matters of agency or organizational policy, it is important that a policy support the agency or organizational mission and goals. In considering proposed policy, ask:

- Is it legal?
- Is it congruent with existing law and the organizational mission?
- Would it require changes to existing law or policy?
- Are such changes feasible, acceptable, and realistic?

For nurses, a major consideration of legality will always be the Nurse Practice Act. No matter how desirable an innovation may be, actions by the nurse must be permitted under the applicable practice act. This is not to suggest that laws cannot be changed to permit innovation in policy. When new roles for nursing are developed, it is often the case that law must be changed to support the new role. The role of advanced practice nursing, for example, required new legislation in most states. Some states amended their practice act, some added new and separate advanced practice statutes, but in every instance the law was addressed.

Political Considerations

Policy is never a private matter. Once convinced that a proposed policy is worth commitment, the nurse must be prepared to involve supporters and be ready for opponents.

- To whom would the policy be politically acceptable?
- To whom would the policy be unacceptable?
- Who would have a stake in outcomes?
- Who might gain money, status, power, or influence under this policy?
- Who might lose money, status, power, or influence under this policy?

When dealing with matters of health, it is natural to think of other nurses who would likely be supportive. If the policy has real merit, however, it is likely that other providers, such as physicians, therapists, or pharmacists would be supportive. Who can be enlisted in the effort?

If the policy has patient benefits, patient groups or organizations might build coalition for support.

If the policy threatens the power or income of a constituency, opposition will likely be forth coming. Policies that define an activity as the sole province of one profession may be destined for opposition from other professions. When nursing, for example, expands its practice base with advanced skills, physician groups may oppose these changes, fearing the loss of prestige and even financial gain. When ancillary providers such as emergency medical technicians (EMTs) define their practice, nursing watches carefully to make certain policy language does not exclude nurses (as non-EMTs) from rights they previously held. Knowing the political repercussions of a policy is essential to building a base of support and anticipating opposition realistically.

Process and Power Applied to Changing Policy

Fully implementing the preparatory process thus far outlined will place the nurse in the best possible position for beginning the work of promoting or opposing proposed policy. Armed with thorough preparation the nurse can now turn attention to the political process of influence and persuasion.

Process and Power Applied to Organizational Policy

Impacting an organization requires understanding of its mission, goals, and political structure. An organization has a mission statement that reflects its goals and values. This mission statement will be key to indicating what changes would be acceptable to that particular organization. Most organizations have a corporate structure and a governance structure. The corporate structure will be identified in the organizational chart as line functions and the committee or governance structure will be identified as staff or advisory functions. The successful route for policy change in most instances will follow both structures; respecting existing policies and including interested parties on every level. The nurse who is interested in affecting organizational policy will first be an integral member of the organization. If this is a provider organization, the nurse must expect to speak for the providers or for the patients, or both. If this is a professional organization, the nurse must absolutely be a dues-paying, meeting-attending member of that organization. Giving service within an organization is an excellent way to learn and to demonstrate one's capabilities and genuine interest.

Committee membership will be important as a source of information and power in any organization. If one is concerned with practice policy, one should be serving on the practice committee. If one is concerned with the membership policies of an organization, one should become an effective member of that committee, gain knowledge, offer service, and build a cohesive group for action. Knowledge of an organization can best be gained from study of and participation in that organization, for while certain basic characteristics may be applicable across various organizations, organizations, like individuals, have their own intricacies. Serving as an officer, a member of the board, or a committee chair is a demonstration of higher commitment and generates more intimate knowledge of an organization. Such positions also carry intrinsic power that can be used in persuasion and debate. Isn't it more influential to hear ideas for action from persons truly immersed in the work at hand? Persons engaged in the work are more likely to know the playing field, where support might lie, where opposition might surface, and how best to answer concerns about proposed change.

Process and Power Applied to Political Process

Success in the process of change is more likely given when the political process allows for divergent opinions, shows respect for positions and preferences, and avoids creating winners and losers. Challenges to existing policies or suggestions for new ones are all about change, which can be difficult for the best practitioner. Alma Dixon reminds us that organizational conflict can be expected quite naturally in a work or organizational setting (Dixon, 1998). In the application of the process of policy development, one can expect intrapersonal, interpersonal, and intergroup conflict.

Intrapersonal conflict arises from competing values within the person for mutually exclusive goals. For example, a nurse might wish to see a firm absence policy to control understaffing, at the same time being sympathetic to working moms who are vulnerable to their children's sudden illnesses. **Interpersonal** and **intergroup conflicts** arise from persons and groups with competing interests. In order to preserve working harmony in an organization and still effect needed change, conflict management techniques should be applied. For example, conflict often arises between nursing work units with the flow of patient care.

Postanesthesia recovery may need to move patients to the unit to maintain safe staff to patient ratios. Unit nurses may resent the seemingly precipitous arrival of patients at times inopportune for their own workload. Conflict management processes can be employed to assist both groups to focus on patient care outcomes while supporting the needs of both work units to maintain patient safety.

As nurses work for policy changes, every effort should be made to preserve common goals and to incorporate as many preferences into a new policy as can be done and still preserve the intent and effectiveness of the policy. Such techniques as win–win solutions and principled negotiation should be employed so that as a new policy is created, working relationships are not destroyed. Both these techniques are designed to assist opposing groups to set aside personal agendas and work toward a common goal. Both techniques demand utmost respect of persons and positions during the process (Dixon, 1998).

Process and Power Applied to Government and Legislation

In all levels of government, policy exists from the constitution to laws, regulations, and ordinances. Indeed, the United States Constitution begins with the acclamation "We the people of the United States of America in order to form a more perfect union, to ensure domestic tranquility and to provide for the common defense, do ordain and establish this constitution . . ." (U.S.C.A., Constitution of the United States, Preamble). The signers, of that constitution and each person who accepts citizenship under that constitution, attest that this document gives voice to their philosophy of government, indicates their priorities, and describes their intentions. All laws in the United States must first be congruent with the constitution and then, through legislative process, be shown to reflect the desires of the citizens they will govern.

Laws in the United States come in several forms and all flow from the United States Constitution and the constitutions of the 50 states. **Statutory law** is devised in the legislative branch of our government. It may arise as a result of the need of the people or be identified by elected officials as necessary to the common good. Examples of such law would include the Americans with Disabilities Act (ADA, 1990) which describes American's policies for situations involving persons with disabilities and the various state Nurse Practice Acts, which describe the responsibilities of registered nurses to society. **Case law** is the result of a decision in the judicial branch of our government, which has considered an action already taken by individuals or organizations and deemed that action to be within the protection of existing law or in violation of it. The recent focus on the right to die issue which includes consideration of assisted suicide was the subject of a decision by the U.S. Supreme Court which ruled that there is no constitutional right to assisted suicide. (*Vacco v. Quill*, 1997; *Washington v. Glucksburg*, 1997).

State and federal regulations, once enacted, have the same weight as laws. Regulations come about through a process by which an official agency is allowed to spell out provisions for the accomplishment of its goals and the regulation of its work in conformity with legislative direction. This is usually in deference to the fact that the agency in question has very specific expertise that is not shared by the legislature, such as medical knowledge or engineering knowledge. The intent of the law is made clear to the agency or board by the legislature, and the board is left to draft regulations that best reflect the intent. These provisions then are reviewed by the legislative body, published in the federal or state register, and presented at legislative hearings for critique by the public. Once approved, they carry the same weight as statutes. Examples of such regulations would include the regulations stipulating the requirements for reimbursement of caregivers through Medicare and Medicaid, or the rules of nursing practice set forth by state boards of nursing. Regulatory law is a branch of law known as Administrative Law.

The Legislative Process

The legislative process for the state and the federal government is quite similar. It is complicated by many rules and procedures, but it is a learnable, workable process and should not be a barrier to a concerned citizen. Ideas for laws and policies can and should come from any interested party, and then be brought to the attention of legislators. Only a member of a legislative body, however, may introduce a bill for consideration as a law, though any citizen or group may petition a legislator to consider a suggested law. Bills may be introduced into either the House of Representatives or the Senate, or both concurrently. All appropriation bills must originate in the House of Representatives. Bills enter into consideration through various legislative committees, such as the committees on health, education, commerce, and so

on. Committee members must decide which of the many ideas introduced to their consideration are worthy of bill status. In these committees, wording of the desired bill is constructed in such a way that desired ends are identified and interested or antagonistic factions may be satisfied. Hearings are held by the committees to educate committee members and the public on the issue at hand and to provide a forum for supporters and opponents to speak. The bill very often will be amended through this process in some way. When the bill finally leaves the committee, it is accompanied by a report describing the intent of the bill and possibly the manner in which an agency is expected to interpret the law through regulations. The bill then is put on the calendar for consideration by the full legislative bodies of the House and Senate. Debate occurs among legislators and again, there may be revisions or amendments. Identical versions of the bill must pass in each house.

If different versions emerge, conference action must be taken. Leaders of each house, usually members of the committees who first proposed the bill, are appointed to reach a consensus. Again debate and compromise ensue until a single version of the proposed law can be offered back to both house and senate where it must once again be passed in its rewritten form. After passing both houses, a bill then goes to the chief executive officer.

Either the President of the United States or the Governor of one of those states has the power to sign the bill into law. Alternatively, he or she may veto the bill by returning it to the legislature *unsigned* and accompanied by a report addressing concerns or objections. Under the United States Constitution and in many states, the House and Senate may override a presidential or gubernatorial veto with an affirmative vote of two-thirds of its members. One additional possibility exists in this process. A bill may become law without a presidential signature if it is not signed within 10 congressional session days of being sent to the president. A president who wishes to make a statement of personal disapproval but does not wish to veto a bill may allow a bill to become law in this way. If Congress adjourns within those 10 days however, the bill dies and this is referred to as a pocket veto.

A final test of this "idea become law" may occur if the constitutionality of the law is ever questioned. This test would take place in the Supreme Court, in the form of a challenge in the application to a real-life case. Judicial decisions at this level may support existing law, nullify existing law, or become a new form of law called case law. Examples of case law include *Roe v. Wade*

(1973), the judicial decision that declared a Texas statute prohibiting the act of abortion of a living fetus to be vague and in violation of the ninth and fourteenth amendments.

Nursing's Role in Political Action

The most effective strategy for influence on policy is to come to the party early and to stay late. This means early involvement in the political process. The interpersonal process with legislators is key. While only a legislator may introduce a bill, bills can certainly be proposed to members of the legislature either by private citizens or special interest groups, such as nursing organizations. Know the legislators interested in the issues of concern to nursing. Know them by frequent contact and by working in their campaigns if they are worthy of support. Know the committees in the state or federal legislative bodies that deal with the business of those concerns. For example, know which legislators serve on the health committee and the education committee, as these are the committees most closely involved with issues of professional interest to nurses. A nurse, of course, will have interest in a variety of issues that come before the legislator. Issues of education, religious freedom, business practices, personal and public safety and recreation, and many other aspects of a full life all come before congress at some point.

If possible, work in the campaigns of legislators that have been helpful to nursing and the ones that will be involved in the work nurses wish to influence. Certainly, be a constituent. There is an old saying that one should "dance with the one who brought you." Legislators are most likely to respond to those who helped them gain their legislative position. This is good etiquette for formal dances and just as valid for political activity. Be part of what brings a congressman to elective office and expect to have greater influence.

Present concerns and ideas in a well-researched and knowledgeable format and seek the support of a legislator that is willing to carry the issue to the legislative body. Nurses can offer to help write legislation with legislative aids, thus increasing influence over the language of the bill and the bill itself.

When a bill is in committee, there will be public hearings and much negotiation between members. Nurses can be expert witnesses in hearings and serve as consultants to legislators on matters of health and health care. Continue advisory presence during the "mark-up" phase in which a bill may be strengthened or weakened. When a bill is about to reach the floor for vote, contact with legislators is crucial. This is the time to gather all possible support, to enlist all supportive parties to contact their own and other congressmen and women to encourage the desired action. Call, write, send a fax, or visit legislators in person.

If and when the final bill passes and moves for executive signature, be sure to contact the executive office, be it the President or Governor. Express support or dismay and give knowledgeable rationale for your position. Everyone responds to a report card. Thank yous and expressions of support are crucial in maintaining a sound presence.

Policies and Laws That Most Impact Nursing

Nursing serves at the pleasure of the public. As a servant of the public, it is subject to a certain amount of obligation and control. Obligation exists as the legal and ethical commitment nursing makes to its patients and as the legal empowerment and restraint it accepts. While the nature of nursing practice springs from the creative powers of its members and the needs of its consumers, the professional actions of its practitioners are very much directed by various policies and regulations

Critical Thinking and Reflection

How much does language matter? Currently, there is rising sentiment among physicians in regard to the word *provider* showing up in legislative language. Provider is an inclusive term. It permits an undefined description of who may carry out a health care service: physician, nurse practitioner, physician's assistant, licensed therapist. How much does this matter to you as a nurse? As a consumer of health care?

that have been developed over time. Awareness of such policies and regulations is an essential step to full professional practice. Control of those policies and regulations is the ultimate development of professional expression.

In the largest sense, most civil laws and agency policies impact nursing, the other professionals involved in giving health care, and nursing's intended patients. Laws affecting health care financing, for example, influence not only the size and nature of the patient population that may use nursing services, but can influence how ill a patient may allow himself to get before seeking health care. Laws allowing or outlawing smoking, addictive substances, and speed limits on highways all directly affect the public's health and consequently the need for care. Certain select laws and policies, however, very directly affect the practice of nursing. Primary among these are the state practice acts of the various 50 states, and the nurses' responsibilities to protect and ensure confidentiality, privacy, and consent.

State Practice Acts

State Practice Acts differ in every state but do share some basic similarities. These acts are designed to protect the public by setting forth obligations of a licensed professional nurse and to identify restraints to nursing practice that are deemed desirable by the people of that state. Most practice acts:

- Establish a State Board of Nursing that oversees licensure, evaluation, and discipline of licensed professional nurses.
- Define eligibility for licensure as a professional and retention of that license.
- Define nursing as it will be implemented in that state.
- Describe in very general terms the responsibilities of nurses in giving care.
- Establish and publish specific rules and regulations for the practice of nursing promulgated on the statutory directive (Guido, 1997).

It is always the nurse's responsibility to be aware of all rules and regulations of the state in which that nurse practices. This includes any changes that may occur over time, which could include additional responsibilities and loss of certain privileges or invoke new requirements for retention of license. Such issues as continuing education requirements for the nurse, support or punishment of the impaired nurse, and the relationship of the nurse to other health care providers may be addressed in the practice act. It is always incumbent on the nurse to voice concern over provisions that may unnecessarily or unfairly limit nursing practice and to work effectively for needed changes employing the full process for policy analysis and change.

Confidentiality and Privacy

Confidentiality is a duty owed the patient by the nurse. It is the protection of information shared by the patient with the nurse directly or through other providers in the medical record. The patient is protected from fear that his information will be shared with anyone other than those involved in his care. Few nurses would intentionally directly breach patient confidentiality. However, giving information that could be reasonably traced back to an individual patient might breach confidentiality. Confidentiality requirements arise from the concept of tort, or civil wrong. To breach confidentiality is to seriously wrong or injure another (Guido, 1997).

Privacy is the individual's right to be free from unreasonable intrusions into his or her private affairs. This also includes the person's right to have peace of mind, to be left alone without unwarranted publicity. It is the right of privacy that prohibits the taking of a patient's picture without expressed permission in the form of legal waiver. Privacy further protects the patient from being cast in a false light. For example, showing a picture of a patient leaving an abortion clinic, when that person was not actually a patient in that clinic is prohibited (Brent, 1997). It is the nurse's legal and ethical obligation to protect the patient's privacy and the confidentiality of any patient information.

Critical Thinking and Reflection

What do you know about the state nurse practice act in your state? What is its definition of nursing? Does it include the term nursing diagnosis? Does it make the nurse responsible for continual assessment of the patient? Do you think it gives a freeing or limiting definition of nursing?

Widely, both state and federal laws address the aspects of privacy and confidentiality. Remedies for breach of confidentiality and/or privacy are available through court action in the form of damages awarded to the wronged party. While few nurses question the wisdom of protecting a patient's privacy, some might question which patient aspects might be covered by this tort. Should a patient's HIV status, for example, be protected regardless of a needle-stick exposure to a caregiver? Should a provider be bound to silence regarding a patient's diagnosed sexually transmitted disease (STD), when there is a known sexual partner who is at risk of contracting a disease? These are issues that can and should be addressed by the nurse to improve practice and to appropriately protect both patient and nurse.

Laws of Consent

Laws of consent and informed consent are of great importance to the nurse. **Consent** is the authorization, implied or expressed, by the patient for the rendering of care. This legal concept is based in case law, *Schloendorff v. Society of New York Hospitals* (1914), and is about the patient giving permission for care that is offered. **Informed consent** is a separate concept that requires that the patient be given all necessary information for comprehension of the expected outcomes and possible risks that may accompany an aspect of his care, prior to being asked for his consent. This legal concept was not defined by law until 1957, again in case law, *Salgo v. Leland Stanford, Jr., University Board of Trustees* (1957). Proper execution of both of these responsibilities requires the nurse to actively seek the consent of the patient and to properly assess the patient's knowledge of expected and possible outcomes before accepting that consent. **Informed refusal** is a further obligation. It is about assuring that a patient who plans to refuse care fully understands the expected result of his refusal. For example, does the woman who refuses a Pap test at her well-woman exam clearly understand that she is refusing a procedure that could potentially discover a life-threatening cancer (Brent, 1997; Guido, 1997)?

Family Code Law

All states have civil laws defining and affecting aspects of family life. These include such concerns as definitions of marriage (who is legally married?), definitions of parents (who is a parent? who is a custodial parent?), legal majority (who is a minor and who can consent to medical care?). These laws are often grouped together and called family codes. These laws are very important to nurses as they deal with issues of consent. Who may authorize the treatment of a child, for example, or who may legally be given information about a patient without violation of confidentiality is defined in family law. These codes are critical in the protection of patients who may have few rights and should be evaluated by the nurse as to their ability to give appropriate protections where needed.

While the laws mentioned here have rather direct impact on nursing activities, there are many issues of health and safety that should be addressed for the protection of the nurse and/or the patient. Through thoughtful practice and political action, additional protections may be devised by caring and politically effective nurses.

Contemporary Political Issues for Nursing Practice

Today, health care exists in a climate of scarce resources and provider competition. Over the years, resource allocation has become a desperate problem. Most health care issues today are conflicted by the debate over the expenditure of resources, either human or material. The vast majority of health care dollars are spent in acute care settings during a patient's last 90 days of life. And yet, it is a widely known and accepted fact that the reason for the increased life span of modern man is due to public health advances and not to medical treatment (Sultz & Young, 2001). Nurses have the knowledge to design successful programs for health protection, health promotion, and health maintenance; they also have the knowledge to work effectively for needed funding for these interventions.

In the aftermath of the September 11, 2001, attack on the World Trade Center and Pentagon, there is renewed interest in public health protections. This is an opportunity for nurses to raise the knowledge level of society as it plans to shift emphasis from personal care to care of the public's health.

Many policy conflicts arise from issues of individual freedoms versus community rights. Especially in matters of mental health and communicable disease, it is vital that professionals with scientific knowledge join their voices to debates on policies that may unfairly disadvantage ill persons or fail to protect society.

Many of us would like to consider health care a basic right in the United States at the same time we struggle to plan for cost control. Nurses have specialized knowledge that is critical to this conundrum and should be involved on every level helping through research and advocacy to design the best possible system of health care. Box 16–2 offers some examples of specific problems that should be addressed by policy. This list offers only a small representation of problems that could be addressed by the policy process and very effectively addressed by nurses in concert with each other, their professional organization, and the many professional, political, and consumer groups working today for a better health care system and better health. Nurses need to have the confidence in our skill and power that others have in us. Nurses are perceived as having the knowledge and the concern to make a far-reaching difference. Witness the words of U.S. Senator Geraldine Ferraro:

> At no other time in our nation's history has our country so needed the expertise of nurses in the development of health policy. As our nation struggles to reverse the tide of rising numbers of uninsured children and adults, to increase consumer involvement in health

choices, and to care for our expanding aging population, we must turn to the expertise of nurses. These are complex issues that do not lead to simple answers.

You are the profession that can put a face to health. Your touch expertise is essential as we struggle to create caring health systems, redefine the role of government in providing care, and help consumers become knowledgeable about maintaining and improving their own health. Your voice is needed to move policy out of the realm of theory and into the everyday lives of real people with real health needs. You are closest to the patients and consumers of health care, and you have devoted your lives to empowering your patients. Now you must empower yourselves to help this country by taking an active role in the political and policy process.

I don't know one politician who would not welcome your support and your knowledge about health care. Policymakers need you, politicians need you, and the American public needs you to help us create affordable access to health care for every American. (Mason & Leavitt, 1998)

Box 16–2 Contemporary Issues for Policy Consideration

Homelessness

What are the health problems of the homeless population? What health threats might the homeless population pose to the general population? What services should be provided to this population at what share of the health care dollar?

Substance Abuse

Is substance abuse a crime or an illness? Should it be addressed by health care interventions or criminal prosecution? What are the substances of greatest concern?

Motorized Sporting Vehicles

In the United States, one needs to meet a criteria of knowledge and competence and obtain a license to drive a car or a motorcycle. However, there a few to no requirements in many states for the operation of powered vehicles for sport such as ski boats, ski-dos, and snowmobiles. Many injuries result yearly to both operators of these vehicles and to innocent bystanders. What is the physical danger and what is the cost to society for this permissive state of affairs?

Safety in Prisons

While health care of varying degrees of competence is offered incarcerated persons, the issue of safety remains a serious problem. Incarceration deprives a person of their resources to self-protect. In justice, prisoners are owed at least the basics of protection from theft, assault, and even murder. Contemporary stories from prisons indicate that these basic rights are not protected, and injuries and deaths do occur.

Provider of Care

Recently, the term provider has found its way into legislative language. The term is nonspecific enough to leave room for interpretation as to who the provider might be—a physician, a nurse practitioner, a physician's assistant. This seems dangerous on one level to the consumer who worries about who may be providing care; attractive to the consumer who wants a choice in what type of provider he may choose to select. This is currently very unattractive to physicians who, for many years, have perceived themselves to be the only providers. Is this a step up or a step down?

Student nurses are well versed in policy. Attendance policy, uniform policy, grading policies, and test-taking policies are an integral part of life. To be fully functioning, one must not only be aware of policies that impact student life, but must really understand them. In many schools of nursing, policy-forming committees like curriculum, admissions, and recruitment have student members to allow for adequate two-way communication between the school and the student. This is perfect training for the transition to practice, where many of the same concerns must be addressed. Volunteer to serve on one of these committees available to you.

In professional practice, policies will still impact dress and attendance. More importantly, policies will control practice in the form of the state practice act and policy and procedure manuals on the job. Evaluation of the nurse by peers and managers and even promotion eligibility will be governed by policy. The nurse must first endeavor to be fully informed of all policies, understanding intent of the law or policy as well as its actual stipulations.

Once knowledgeable of policies, volunteer to sit on committees that review or restructure policy in the workplace. Employ the process of knowledge, understanding intent and values, economic considerations, and legal impact of existing or proposed policies. Offer to participate in research to evaluate existing policy or to test proposals for new policy. Be a full participant in the work of the professional nurse who controls practice for nursing.

While establishing a base in practice, join the professional organization that will most enhance your practice, provide role models, and offer an opportunity for participation in the future of nursing. This may be the American Nurses Association and/or one of the many excellent specialty nursing organizations such as Association of Operating Room Nurses, American Association of Occupational Health Nurses, American Assembly for Men in Nursing, and many more. All of these organizations have political action committees. First and foremost, be a dues-paying and active member. Next, serve on one of the committees focused on policy formation. This may be in regard to the organizational policies themselves, proposed policies that will enhance practice opportunities or recommendations for social or health policies that will affect patients. Who better to influence social and health policies than the nurses who care for society's health?

Don't overlook the many consumer and political organizations that aspire to influence public policy. Parent groups, persons suffering from specific diseases, and families of mentally ill or challenged individuals often form voluntary organizations with vested interest in contributing to new policy or changing old ones. Examples include the American Cancer Society, Mother's Against Drunk Driving, the League of American Bicyclists, and the League of Women Voters, as well as the established political parties of our country: the Republican, Democratic, and other newer parties such as the Green Party. These groups are already committed to causes and make excellent forums for nurses with political agendas or aspirations. Yes, aspirations. What better public servant than a nurse dedicated to the health and well-being of others?

KEY POINTS

1. Policy is voice. It signals our intentions, our values, and our priorities. Policy impacts life at every turn: the life of the citizen, the employee, and the practicing professional. Policy is a formalized statement of committee direction.

2. Policy exists as public policy, social policy, health policy, institutional policy, organizational policy, and personal policy.

3. Policy drives laws, regulations, and rules, and it is larger than any of these things. Once a policy is established, it may inspire or direct many laws, rules, and regulations and may do so for many years.

4. Policy is a statement of values—what is held dear or supreme. Policy is the basis for the Code of Ethics for Nurses and the Standards of Nursing Practice.

5. Politics is a process of influence. It is a method of persuasion, negotiation, debate, and bargaining with the goal of seeing a particular viewpoint or path of action be adopted. Politics in a free society

allows the competition of divergent points of view or conflicting values. It is an essential exercise in a free society where many views and needs must ultimately be expressed as one policy, one voice.

6. Political action requires information, research and knowledge, commitment, and action.

7. From its modern beginnings, nursing has recognized the need to control not only nursing practice, but also the environment in which practice takes place.

8. Developing policy requires consideration of available information, values and ethics, economics, legal issues, and political influences.

9. The nurse who is interested in affecting organizational policy must first be an integral member of the organization.

10. To effectively influence policy requires early political and interpersonal involvement with decision makers.

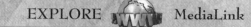

EXPLORE MediaLink

Critical thinking questions, essay questions, key terms, web links, activities, NCLEX review questions, and more interactive resources can be found on the Companion Website at www.prenhall.com/haynes. Click on Chapter 16 to select activities for this chapter.

REFERENCES

Aiken, L., Sloane, D. M., & Sochalski, J. (2001). Hospital organization and outcome. In C. Harrington & C. L. Estes (Eds.), *Health care policy: Crisis and reform in the U.S. health care delivery system* (3rd ed.) (pp. 163–169). Sudbury, MA: Jones and Bartlett.

American Association of Occupational Health Nurses. (1991). Code of ethics and interpretive statement. *American Association of Occupational Health Nursing Journal, 39*(10), 470 A–D.

American Holistic Nurses' Association. (1992). Code of ethics for holistic nursing: Developed by the American Holistic Nurses' Association. *Journal of Holistic Nursing, 10*(3), 275–276.

American Nurses Association. (2001). *Code of ethics for nurses with interpretive statements.* Washington, DC: American Nurses Publication.

Americans with Disabilities Act, 42 U.S.C.s 12101 et seq., Public Law 101-336, 140 Stat. 327, 1990.

Bellah, R. N. (1987). The quest for self. In P. Rubinow & W. M. Sullivan (Eds.), *Interpretive social science.* Berkeley, CA: University of California Press.

Bodenheimer, T., & Grunbach, K. (1995). *Understanding health policy: A clinical approach.* Norwalk, CT: Appleton & Lange.

Brent, N. (1997). *Nurses and the law.* Philadelphia, PA: W. B. Saunders.

Bullough, V., Bullough, B., & Stanton, M. P. (1990). *Florence Nightingale and her era: A collection of new scholarship.* New York: Garland Publications.

Coden, I. B. (1984). Florence Nightingale. *Scientific American, 250*(3), 128–133, 136–137.

Dixon, A. (1998). Conflict management. In D. Mason & J. Leavitt (Eds.), *Policy and politics in nursing and health care* (3rd ed.). Philadelphia, PA: W. B. Saunders.

Dodd, C. J. (2001). Can meaningful health policy be developed in a political system? In C. Harrington & C. L. Estes (Eds.), *Health policy: Crisis and reform in the United States health care delivery system* (3rd ed.) (pp. 373–382). Sudbury, MA: Jones and Bartlett.

Donnelly, P. (1997). *Diana: Tribute to a princess.* Philadelphia, PA: Courage Books.

Dossey, B. (2000). *Florence Nightingale: Mystic, visionary, healer.* Springhouse, PA: Springhouse Corp.

Fried, K., & Fried, N. (Eds.). (1997). *The people's princess: A memorial.* New York: Stewart, Tabori, & Chang, Inc.

Guido, G. (1997). *Legal issues in nursing.* Norwalk, CT: Appleton & Lange.

Harrington, C., & Pellow, D. (2001). The uninsured and their health. In C. Harrington & C. L. Estes (Eds.), *Health care policy: Crisis and reform in the U.S. health care delivery system* (3rd ed.). Sudbury, MA: Jones and Bartlett.

Lewenson, S. B. (1998). Historical overview: Policy, politics, and nursing. In D. Mason & J. Leavitt (Eds.), *Policy and politics in nursing and health care* (3rd ed.) (pp. 47–48). Philadelphia, PA: W. B. Saunders.

Mason, D. J., & Leavitt, J. K. (1998). Forward. In D. Mason & J. Leavitt (Eds.), *Policy and politics in nursing and health care* (3rd ed.) (p. xix). Philadelphia, PA: W. B. Saunders.

Moskowitz, H., Griffith, J. L., DiScala, C., & Sege, R. D. (2001). Serious injuries and deaths of adolescent girls resulting from interpersonal violence. *Archives of Pediatric and Adolescent Medicine, 155,* 903–908.

Nightingale, F. (1859). *Notes on nursing.* London: Harrison and Sons.

Nightingale, F. (1911). Florence Nightingale's letter of advocator to Bellevue. *American Journal of Nursing, 11*(5), 361–364.

Palmer, S. (1909). State societies: Their organization and place in nursing education. *American Journal of Nursing, 9*(12), 956–957.

Polit, D. F., Beck, C. T., & Hungler, B. P. (2001). *Essentials of nursing research methods, appraisal and utilization* (5th ed.). Philadelphia, PA: Lippincott.

Roe v. Wade, 410 U.S. 113, 1973.

Salgo v. Leland Stanford, Jr., University Board of Trustees, 317 P.2d 170 (Cal. Dis. Ct. App., 1957).

Schloendorff v. Society of New York Hospitals, 211 N.Y. 125, 105 N.E. 92, 1914.

Sultz, H. A., & Young, K. M. (2001). *Health care USA: Understanding its organization and delivery.* Gaithersburg, MD: Aspen Publishers.

Vacco v. Quill. (1997). U.S. Supreme Court, No 95-1958 (117 S. Ct. 2293, 65 U.S.L.W. 4695 [June 26, 1997]).

Washington v. Glucksberg. (1997). U.S. Supreme Court, No 96-110 (177 S. Ct. 2258, 65 U.S.L.W. 4669 [June 26, 1997]).

SUGGESTED READINGS

American Nurses Association. (1995). *Nursing's social policy statement.* Washington, DC: Author.

Ballau, K. A. (2000). A historical–philosophical analysis of the professional nurse obligations to participate in sociopolitical activities. *Policy, Politics, and Nursing Practice, 1*(3), 172–184.

Ennen, K. A. (2001). Shaping the future of practice through political activity: How nurses can influence health care policy. *AAOHN Journal, 49*(12), 557–571.

Gebbie, K. M., Wakefield, M., & Kerfoot, K. (2000). Nursing and health policy. *Journal of Nursing Scholarship, 32*(3), 307–315.

Jennings, C. P. (2002). Looking for a few good nurses: Be all that you can be! Become a nurse specialist in health and public policy. *Policy, Politics, and Nursing Practice, 3*(3), 207.

Mason, D. J. (2002). The politics of patient care: You have a duty to recognize the political nature of your work. *American Journal of Nursing, 102*(4), 7.

Milstead, J. (1999). *Health policy and politics: A nurse guide.* Gaithersburg, MD: Aspen Publishers, Inc.

Peters, R. M. (2002). Nurse administrators' role in health policy: Teaching the elephant to dance. *Nursing Administration Quarterly, 26*(4), 1–8.

Phillips, S., Dillard, C., & Burstin, H. (2002). The Agency for Healthcare Research and Quality (AHRQ) responds to emerging threats of bioterrorism. *Policy, Politics, and Nursing Practice, 3*(3), 212–216.

Pruitt, R. H., Wetsel, M. A., Smith, K. J., & Spitler, H. (2002). How do we pass NP autonomy legislation? *Nurse Practitioner: American Journal of Primary Health Care, 27*(3), 56, 61–65.

Vessey, J. A., Andres, S., Fountain, M., & Wheeler, A. (2002). Rx for the nursing crisis? The economic impact of mandatory RN staffing to patient ratios. *Policy, Politics, and Nursing Practice, 3*(3), 220–227.

17

Legal Concepts in Nursing Practice

GINNY WACKER GUIDO

"Standard of care means a nurse must have and use the knowledge and skill ordinarily possessed and used by nurses actively practicing in the nurse's specialty area."

King v. State of Louisiana, *1999*

LEARNING OBJECTIVES

AT THE COMPLETION OF THIS CHAPTER, THE READER WILL BE ABLE TO:

- ➤ Discuss and apply legal concepts to the practice of professional nursing.
- ➤ Enumerate the six phases of the litigation process.
- ➤ Analyze common sources of liability in professional nursing practice.

- ➤ Recognize and reduce liability exposure through intelligent nursing in clinical practice.
- ➤ Analyze workplace issues that place nurses at risk for liability.
- ➤ Analyze appropriate means to recognize errors and protect oneself legally.

MediaLink   www.prenhall.com/haynes

Additional online resources including NCLEX review questions, critical thinking questions, and real-world activities for this chapter can be found on the Companion Website at www.prenhall.com/haynes.

The quotation opening this chapter quickly reminds nurses of the vital impact that legal issues, most notably standards of care, have in the delivery of health care today. Nurses must have legal knowledge regarding aspects that apply to their area of practice. They must also be able to appropriately apply those concepts. Nurses today are legally responsible for their personal decisions and actions, which result from those decisions. This chapter assists nurses to acquire basic knowledge about selected legal issues in nursing.

▩ The Legal Process

Sources of Law

Laws are derived from constitutional, statutory, administrative, and judicial sources. The most basic source of law is **constitutional law**, which is a system of fundamental laws or principles for the governance of a nation, society, or other aggregate of individuals. For example, what is commonly known as the Bill of Rights (e.g., freedom of speech, freedom of religion, freedom of the press, etc.) offers the first ten amendments to The Constitution of the United States. These amendments are examples of fundamental rights and constitutional law. **Statutory laws** are those laws enacted by the legislative branch of the government. Nurses are more familiar with this source of law since the nurse practice act is an example of statutory law. This is an example of a law enacted by a state legislature. The United States Congress enacts federal laws or statutes.

Administrative laws are enacted by means of decisions and rules of administrative (or governmental) agencies, which are specific governing bodies charged with implementing selected legislation. When statutory laws are enacted, administrative agencies are given the authority to implement the specific intentions of those statutes by creating rules and regulations that enforce that statutory law. Boards of nursing are governmental agencies created under the authority of a state statute, the nurse practice act. The boards of nursing under the authority vested by the nurse practice act create rules and regulations (e.g., fees for licensure, continuing education requirement, etc.). These rules and regulations are examples of administrative law. Finally, **judicial (or case) laws** are created by the decisions of courts of law, interpreting legal issues that are in dispute. A variety of case laws will be discussed throughout the text of this chapter.

All laws, regardless of origin, are subject to change. Constitutional laws may be amended; statutory laws may be amended, repealed, or expanded; administrative agencies may be dissolved, expanded, or redefined (and their rules changed as well); and judicial laws may be modified or completely altered by subsequent court decisions.

An example of statutory and administrative law is a state's nurse practice act. The state nurse practice act is the single most important piece of legislation for nursing because it affects all aspects of nursing practice. The act defines a nurse's scope of practice, those actions and duties allowed and required by the profession, and establishes standards for nurses in a given state. Requirements for licensure and entry into practice, empowerment of a board of nursing to oversee practice, and the means for disciplinary action are all part of the nurse practice act. That act is the law which guides nursing within the state or territory. State boards of nursing cannot grant exceptions, waive the act's provisions, or expand practice outside the act's specific provisions.

Nurse practice acts typically define three categories of nurses: licensed practical or vocational nurses; licensed registered nurses; and advanced practice nurses. The acts, in concert with court-decided common law, set educational and examination requirements, provide for licensing by individuals who have met these requirements, and define the functions of each category of nurse. Some states have separate acts for licensed practical or vocational nurses, and some states do not have advanced practice roles defined.

Each state practice act establishes a board of nursing whose purposes are to (a) ensure enforcement of the nurse practice act, (b) regulate those who come under its provisions and prevent those not addressed by the act from practicing nursing, and (c) protect the public. Qualifications for board members, terms of office, and specific duties of board members are defined in the individual state's practice act.

Though the nurse practice act is a statutory law, judicial (or common) law may become involved in its application. In selected court decisions, the interpretation of the nurse practice act assists nurses to understand the full application of the law. For example, landmark court cases in 1983 upheld the right of nurses to practice as advanced nurse practitioners (*Sermchief v. Gonzales*, 1983) and in 1985 allowed a board of nursing to set educational standards for advanced nurse practitioners (*Bellegie v. Board of Nurse Examiners*, 1985). Nurses are cautioned that when courts or legislatures expand the nurse's role, the legal accountability owed by nurses also increases.

Types or Divisions of Law

Laws may also be classified into types or divisions. **Common law**, which originated in England, is defined as being derived from principles rather than rules and regulations. Common law is based on justice, reason, fairness, and common sense. **Civil law**, which originated in France, is based on rules and regulations. The terms common and civil law are often used interchangeably to describe law that affects individuals (rather than state entities), and is divided into a variety of legal specializations, including tort law, contract law, international law, and labor law.

Criminal law, sometimes referred to as public law, refers to laws which affect the state in its political capacity and that affects society as a whole. Criminal law may be divided into misdemeanors, or lesser crimes, and felonies, or more serious crimes that involve fines of greater than $1,000 and are punishable by prison terms of greater than one year or death. Table 17–1 gives examples of sources and types of law.

Common Sources of Civil and Criminal Litigation for Nurses

Nurses may become involved with the criminal justice system. The most common means of violating a state's criminal laws is by failing to renew one's nursing license in a timely manner. Once the nursing license expires, the nurse is then practicing nursing without a license, which is a direct violation of the nurse practice act. Other crimes committed by nurses frequently involve substance abuse, particularly if the nurse illegally acquires medications from clinical settings, as seen when patients are given placebos while narcotics are diverted to support a nurse's addiction. Less frequently, nurses have been charged with either intentionally or unintentionally causing the death of a patient.

Nurses are more likely to become involved in civil litigation (or commonly, lawsuits). Such litigation usually results from violation of **tort law,** defined as a wrongful act committed against another person or that person's property. Lawsuits involving tort law usually are termed nonintentional, intentional, or quasi-intentional wrongs.

Negligence and malpractice are the common terms for nonintentional wrongs. **Negligence** is either (a) the commission of an act that a reasonable and prudent person would not do in a given situation or (b) failure to act when a reasonable and prudent person would do so. It denotes conduct that is lacking in care and is usually seen as carelessness on the part of the care provider. **Malpractice**, sometimes referred to as professional negligence, elevates the standards of a reasonable and prudent person to the status of a professional person. Consequently, the question becomes what a reasonable and prudent nurse, having the same degree of education and expertise, would do in a similar situation.

Six elements are required to show malpractice (see Table 17–2). Note that if any element is missing, the nurse will not be found to have liability.

Some of the more common areas of malpractice for nurses include patient falls, medication errors, failure to assess the patient in a timely manner, failure to inform the primary health care provider of a change in patient status, and failure to provide adequate patient education. Compliance with nursing standards of care and following principles of basic nursing practice can help nurses prevent professional liability.

Nurses may also be found liable for **intentional torts**, a "tort" being generally defined as an action that violates another person's rights. In such actions, the nurse's actions must intend to interfere with the patient or their property, the nurse must intend to bring about the consequences of the act, and the act must be a substantial factor in causing the consequences or out-

Table 17–1 Sources and Types of Laws

Constitutional Law	Statutory Law		Administrative Law	Judicial Law
	Civil (Common)	**Criminal**		
Bill of Rights	Tort law	Penal codes	Boards of Nursing	Courts of law
Amendments to	Contract law	Misdemeanors	Regulatory boards	Trial level
the Constitutions	Patent law	Felonies		Appellate level
	International law	City ordinances		Supreme Court level
	Labor law			

Table 17-2   Elements of Malpractice

Elements	Examples of Nursing Actions
Duty owed the patient	Failing to monitor a patient for postoperative bleeding
Breach of the duty owed the patient	Failing to report a change in patient status
	Restraining a patient improperly and causing harm
Foreseeability	Failing to provide for the patient's safety
Causation	Failing to question an inappropriate medical order
Injury	Failing to provide patient education and discharge planning
Damages	Giving the patient incorrect advice

comes. Unlike malpractice, no actual harm is necessary for this tort—it is the violation of another person's rights that is the harm. The more commonly seen intentional torts in health care settings are assault, battery, and false imprisonment.

By definition, **assault** occurs when a patient fears, expects, or is apprehensive about being touched in an offensive, insulting, or physically injurious manner (e.g., one threatens the patient with an injection or the placement of a nasogastric tube). **Battery** goes further than the fear of being touched and is the actual contact with another person or the person's body or their property. Examples include forcing patients to ambulate against their wishes or restraining a patient so that a procedure can be implemented. For assault and/or battery to occur, there must be an absence of consent on the part of the patient.

False imprisonment is the unjustified detention of a person without the legal right to confine that person. The most obvious examples would be when a patient is physically prevented from leaving against medical advice or when nurses restrain a person in a confined space. Use of medications that alter a patient's ability to leave the health care setting (e.g., being heavily sedated) might also create this tort. As with assault and battery, consent is a vital element in this tort—mentally compromised patients who are restrained to prevent harm to themselves are not falsely imprisoned.

Tort law also recognizes a quasi-intentional tort. Unlike a true intentional tort, with a **quasi-intentional tort** there is no actual intent to injure or cause distress to another person. There is, however, an intentional act that causes injury or distress. Two quasi-intentional torts recognized in health care settings are defamation of character and invasion of privacy.

Defamation of character, also commonly known as libel and slander, is harming another's reputation by diminishing the esteem, respect, goodwill, or level of confidence that others have for that person. Individuals have the right to their good name. Defamation often occurs in medical record documentation. Nurses should use caution when deciding what and how to record patient data and descriptions in the medical record. A good rule for nurses to follow is to write in the medical record as though the patient and their family will be reading the record.

Invasion of privacy is a violation of a person's right to protection against unreasonable and unwarranted interference with his or her personal life. For a patient to show that their privacy has been invaded, the patient will need to show that (a) the nurse intruded on their privacy, (b) the type of intrusion would be objectionable to a prudent and reasonable person, (c) the intrusion concerns private or unpublished facts or pictures of a private nature, and (d) there was public disclosure of the individual's private facts. Examples of invasion of privacy include the taking of a patient's photograph without their permission, disclosure of medical facts to persons not entitled to those facts, and publishing information that misrepresents the patient's condition. For example, an employer might want or request medical information on an employee, the patient, but might not be entitled or authorized to know the information.

Breach of confidentiality, a form of invasion of privacy, concerns facts that are presented in the medical record. The majority of the cases concerning breach of confidentiality concern privileged conversations that are documented in the patient's medical record and the faxing or electronic conveyance of medical records. Health care professionals are cautioned to have procedures in place that permit the authorized disclosure of confidential data; the patient's written authorization to reveal selected information prevents a later complaint or lawsuit that privacy was invaded and there was a breach of confidentiality.

Standards of Care

Essential to showing that a nurse has breached the duty owed the patient is the concept of standards of care. What was the standard at which the nurse should have performed? **Standards of care** represent the minimal requirements that define acceptable nursing practice. Standards of care are written and established to assist nurses in knowing the acceptable levels of nursing care that must be maintained. Standards of care are based on what a reasonable and prudent nurse, in similar circumstances and with comparable education and experience, would do in any given circumstance. Nurses can exceed standards of care, but may not fall below the acceptable standard of practice.

Standards of care are not static, but rather are dynamic and changing and are established in a variety of ways. Usually, standards are divided into internal and external standards. **Internal standards** are those specific to a health care facility or the individual nurse. **External standards** reflect expectations of all nurses in multiple clinical settings. Most commonly, internal standards are established by the health care institution's policy and procedure manual. Other means of establishing internal standards of care are established by the requirements set out in the individual's job description and criteria for education and experience necessary for a particular job position. External standards are established through professional journals and textbooks, published standards of professional organizations, previous court decisions, and standing orders or protocols. Many specialty organizations, including the American Nurses Association, publish standards for practice.

In court, standards of care are established through testimony of expert witnesses. The purpose of an expert witness is to assist the judge and jury in understanding complex and technical concepts that the ordinary layperson would not know. Expert witnesses are allowed to use their experience and expertise, in conjunction with published standards and the health care institution's policy and procedure manual, in voicing their opinion about what constitutes the acceptable level of practice.

Typically, in a lawsuit, there are at least two (opposing) expert witnesses who will testify to the acceptable level of nursing practice. The expert witness for the injured party will often testify that a higher level of acceptable care is required than that level of care expressed by the expert witness for the defendant nurse and institution. A recent case illustrates this distinction. In *Sabol v. Richmond Heights General Hospital* (1996), a patient was admitted to a general acute care hospital for treatment after attempting a drug overdose suicide. While in this facility, the patient became increasingly paranoid and delusional. A nurse sat with the patient and tried to calm him. Restraints were not applied because the staff feared that restraints would compound the situation by raising his level of paranoia and agitation. Without restraints, the patient was able to get out of bed, fight his way past two nurses in the hallway, and jump from a third-story window, fracturing his arm and sustaining relatively minor injuries.

At trial, expert witnesses for the injured patient presented testimony supporting standards of care pertinent to psychiatric patients, specifically those hospitalized in acute care facilities with separate psychiatric units. The expert witnesses for the nurses introduced standards of care for patients hospitalized in nonpsychiatric centers or in institutions where there were no separate psychiatric units. The court ruled that the nurses in this general acute care facility were not professionally negligent in this patient's care. The court stated that the nurses' actions were consistent with basic professional standards of practice for medical–surgical nurses in an acute care hospital. They did not have, nor were they expected to have, specialized psychiatric nursing training and would not be judged as if they did.

Critical Thinking and Reflection

Reflect on one aspect of care you implemented for a patient recently encountered. What were the standards of care for that patient? What references or resources would you use to verify that standard of care for the patient? If asked to serve as an expert witness, how would you show the appropriate level of standards of care for that patient?

The Litigation Process

The American litigation process is complicated and essentially consists of six phases (Table 17–3). The **first phase** involves the initiation of a lawsuit. This phase commences when the complaining party (known as the plaintiff) seeks assistance of an attorney to begin the process of actually filing a case against the defendant(s), the answering party or parties. The plaintiff's attorney files a complaint with a court of competent jurisdiction to hear the case and has the defendant served with notice, a copy of the lawsuit, notifying the defendant that there is a lawsuit pending and that the nurse is a named party in the suit.

Nurses who have personal professional liability insurance, sometimes called malpractice insurance, should promptly notify their insurance carrier of the pending suit. Nurses should also notify the institution's administrative staff of the impending lawsuit. Notifying the institution allows the health care institution to better represent both the facility and the nurses' best interests. Nurses should not discuss the pending case with anyone other than their own attorney and the institution's attorney. The less said, the less likely it is that the nurse will be misquoted and the less likely it is that any comments made to others will be introduced into evidence at a trial.

Some states mandate that a process known as alternative dispute resolution be conducted at this early phase. **Alternative dispute resolution** refers to any means of settling disputes outside of the courtroom setting, including mediation, arbitration, early neutral evaluation, and conciliation. Some states use prelitigation panels as a part of this phase. Both alternative dispute resolution and prelitigation panels serve to ensure that there is a valid dispute prior to the actual court case.

The **second phase** of litigation involves pleadings and pretrial motions. A motion is basically a request by a party for the court to take some preliminary action needed for the case. In this phase, (a) attempts are made to ensure that the claim is fully understood by both parties to the lawsuit, (b) any evidence that would alter the lawsuit as filed is presented, and (c) any additional circumstances/facts specific to this case are heard. For example, motions about (a) the need for a speedy trial in the event that either the plaintiff or an essential witness is elderly or (b) the need for additional time to develop the case more accurately could be heard and ruled on before the trial commences.

Table 17–3   Phases in the Litigation Process

Phase One: Initiation of a Lawsuit

The complaint is filed by the plaintiff, an answer is filed by the defendant, and prelitigation panels, if mandated by state law, are held.

Phase Two: Pleadings and Pretrial Motions

Initial pleadings and answers to the pleadings are filed by both parties to the lawsuit, motions to dismiss (as applicable) are filed, and amended and/or supplemental pleadings are filed.

Phase Three: Discovery of Evidence

Interrogatories are served to both parties to the suit, depositions are taken, requests to produce evidence or additional examinations are made, and subpoenas of witnesses are issued. A pretrial settlement may be accepted during this phase of litigation.

Phase Four: Trial Process

The jury is selected, opening arguments are made, witnesses testify for both sides to the lawsuit, the case is given to the jury for its deliberation, and a verdict is submitted.

Phase Five: Appeals

The verdict is appealed to a higher court, if appropriate.

Phase Six: Execution of Judgment

Damages, if assessed, are paid to the plaintiff and/or the process of specific performance is initiated.

The **third phase** concerns pretrial discovery of evidence. Questioning of witnesses by opposing counsel prior to trial, the uncovering of relevant written documents, and possible additional medical examinations of the injured plaintiff prior to trial are all likely to occur during this phase of litigation. Pretrial questioning of witnesses may take two different forms: interrogatories and depositions. Interrogatories are written questionnaires mailed to opposing parties that ask specific questions concerning the facts of the case, which are to be answered in writing, under oath. Usually, the number of questions is limited, and only two or three sets of interrogatories may be sent to the same witness. Unlike interrogatories, wherein a witness has the written questions in advance, depositions are more spontaneous and require a witness to appear and respond to whatever questions are posed by the attorney. Depositions are witnesses' sworn statements, taken outside of court, that are admissible as evidence in court. Depositions are taken of witnesses who have vital information about the case, either directly because they were part of the event triggering the lawsuit or as expert witnesses. The primary purpose of the deposition is to assist opposing counsel in preparing for the court case by revealing potential testimony from witnesses before the actual trial. Depositions also record the testimony of witnesses who might not be available at the actual court hearing, such as elderly or very ill witnesses.

A court recognizes two types of witnesses at trial. **Lay witnesses** establish facts at trial, and state for the judge and jury exactly what happened, how it happened, and who was involved in the actual incident. Lay witnesses are allowed to testify only to their personal knowledge of the facts and may not draw conclusions or form opinions. **Expert witnesses,** those who explain highly specialized technology or skilled nursing care to the jurors, may draw conclusions and offer opinions. In a lawsuit involving care provided by a nurse, the primary purpose of the expert witness is to assist the jury and judge in understanding nursing care and outcomes.

During this phase, a variety of written documents are secured. Medical records (including nurses' notes), business records, x-ray films, or original laboratory reports may be obtained (such as the extent of a plaintiff's alleged injury). The court may also require a physical or mental examination of a party if the information to be obtained is pertinent to the upcoming court hearing. Generally, the scope of discovery is large and parties are allowed to discover all relevant materials that would be admissible in the subsequent trial.

The final aspect of the pretrial discovery process involves the pretrial conference, sometimes called a pretrial hearing. This is an informal session during which the judge and attorneys meet, agree on the legal and factual issues to be decided, and also settle final procedural matters. A settlement may also be reached at the pretrial conference, waiving the necessity for the trial itself.

The **fourth phase** of litigation is the actual trial of the case. A panel of jurors is selected, evidence is presented (primarily through the questioning of witnesses) facts are determined by the jury, principles of law are applied to the facts by the judge, and a verdict is formally reached. The order in which these events take place (such as questioning of witnesses and closing arguments) is prescribed by the state court system. Once closing arguments are made, the jury is given specific instructions and, hopefully, reaches a verdict. For example, the jury might be given an instruction defining negligence and be asked to decide whether or not a nurse was negligent in their care of the patient.

The **fifth phase** of litigation concerns potential appeals. For an appeal to occur there must be some error that occurred at trial that justifies the need for an appeal. Typically, these issues generally involve (a) procedural issues (e.g., improper evidence or testimony) or (b) monetary damages (e.g., damages assessed against the defendant deemed excessive by the defendant).

The **final phase** of the litigation process is the execution of judgment. Most lawsuits against nurses result in one of two possible conclusions—the award of money damages against the nurse–defendant or the dismissal of the case against the nurse–defendant.

Sources of Liability in Nursing Practice

The Nurse–Patient Relationship

One of the most fundamental aspects of malpractice law is the existence of a nurse–patient relationship. For a duty to be owed to the patient a nurse–patient relationship must exist. This may be accomplished by showing that a reliance relationship exists—one person depending on another person for competent, quality nursing care.

Lunsford v. Board of Nurse Examiners (1983) first established the concept of reliance in establishing the nurse–patient relationship. In that case, a patient experiencing severe chest pain sought assistance at a small, rural hospital in Texas. There was no emergency department at the hospital, but a nurse in the admitting office saw the patient. The nurse asked the patient some basic questions about his symptoms, did no physical examination of the patient, and sent the patient, via private car, to a major medical center after the nurse was instructed by an attending physician not to admit the patient. The patient died en route to the medical center. At trial, the defendant (the hospital) argued that no actual nurse–patient relationship had been established, therefore no duty was owed the patient. The court disagreed, determining that the patient was a person in need of health care assistance and that the patient had relied on the nurse for quality, competent care. The patient's reliance on the nurse established the nurse–patient relationship.

The core of any reliance relationship is trust and communication. Establishing rapport with a patient, informing patients honestly and openly of all aspects of their care, and allowing patients to make decisions for themselves provide nurses with a means of preventing potential liability. Nursing is a caring profession; part of caring is maintaining communications and ensuring that trust is established and continues throughout the interactions between the nurse and patient.

Informed Consent

While the doctrine of informed consent dates to the mid-1950s in America, the concept of consent has long been recognized under the law. Consent is an all-or-nothing proposition—a person will either allow a procedure to be done or refuse the procedure. Without consent, patients may not understand or may only vaguely understand what they are allowing.

The doctrine of informed consent requires that the primary health care provider disclose to the patient those needed material facts, in terms that the patient can reasonably understand so that an informed choice can be made. To allow a patient to make informed consent, descriptions of alternative procedures or therapies should be included as well as the risks and dangers involved with each alternative procedure or therapy. For informed consent, patients must receive, in terms they can understand and comprehend, the following information:

- A brief, but complete explanation of the proposed procedure or treatment.
- The name and qualifications of the person(s) performing the procedure or treatment.
- An explanation of any serious harm that could occur during the procedure or treatment. Pain and discomforting side effects both during and following the procedure or treatment should be included in the discussion.
- An explanation of alternative therapies to the procedure or treatment, including the risk of doing nothing at all.
- An explanation that the patient can refuse the procedure or treatment without having alternative care or support discontinued or that the patient can still refuse the procedure, even after the procedure or treatment has begun.

Consent may be obtained in a variety of ways. Nurses, and other health care providers, frequently rely on oral or expressed consent. The patient merely replies "Yes" when asked about beginning a given procedure or treatment. Health care providers may also obtain implied consent. Implied consent is obtained in response to the patient's conduct or is legally presumed in emergency situations. For example, the patient may merely extend an arm when asked about a specific injection or the patient may merely nod his or her head. In emergency situations, wherein a delay in providing care would result in loss of limb or life, the law presumes consent. Box 17–1 portrays the four elements of valid emergency consent.

Box 17–1 Elements of Emergency Consent

1. Delay in providing care will result in loss of either limb or life.
2. The care to be provided would be acceptable to a reasonable and prudent person.
3. The patient is not able to either consent or deny consent for the procedure or treatment.
4. There is no reason to believe that the person would not consent if the person were capable of giving consent.

There are a limited number of situations when informed consent is not required. One exception is the emergency situation described in the preceding paragraph. A second exception is patient waiver, seen in the instance in which the patient desires no further information. Prior patient knowledge is the third exception. Typically seen in situations in which the patient is undergoing a series of treatments, prior patient knowledge assumes that once the risks and benefits were fully explained the first time, the patient consents to the same risks and benefits in subsequent procedures or treatments.

The fourth exception, therapeutic privilege, is rarely used today. This exception allows health care providers to withhold information about the procedure or treatment if they feel that such knowledge would be detrimental to the patient; that is, full knowledge would hinder or complicate necessary treatment, cause severe psychological harm, or is so upsetting as to render a rational decision by the patient impossible (Rozovsky, 1990).

Patients have the right to what is now called informed refusal. Often, patients initially refuse invasive therapies or treatments, not understanding the full context of what could happen if such therapies or treatments are refused. The law has evolved to ensure that patients know the risks and potential complications of refusing recommended care, and it is the responsibility of the primary health care provider to explain what might happen if no course of therapy is initiated.

The physician or primary health care provider has the responsibility for ensuring that valid informed consent is obtained prior to initiation of a treatment or procedure. Nurses obtain informed consent prior to initiating nursing procedures. Nurses are continuously communicating with patients, explaining procedures, and obtaining the patient's permission. Nurses also accept the patient's refusal to allow a certain treatment or procedure. The responsibility of nurses when patients refuse consent is to ensure that the primary health care provider is notified of such refusal, in the event they may want to order additional therapy or alter already ordered treatments or medications in light of the patient's refusal. For example, intravenous antibiotics ordered for a patient with a severe infection cannot be given if the patient refuses the initiation of an intravenous line.

An important aspect of informed consent is assuring that consent has been secured from the appropriate person. An adult patient, 18 years of age in most states, and who is able to understand the consequences of their actions, is the appropriate person from whom to secure informed consent. Not always, though, will that adult be capable or competent to give or deny consent. In the case of the incompetent adult, one who either temporarily or permanently is unable to give consent, most states recognize a family consent doctrine. If the patient is unable to give valid consent, then the law, on behalf of the patient, recognizes family members in the following order: the patient's spouse; adult children or grandchildren; parents; grandparents; adult siblings; or adult aunts, uncles, nieces, and nephews. Consent by only one person is necessary; it is not necessary to have all the patient's adult brothers and sisters agree on a given procedure or course of treatment.

One of the problematic areas in informed consent involves working with persons who may have only intermittent periods of competency. Some elderly patients and certain psychiatric patients fall in this group. Courts generally have held that there is a presumption of continued competency. Assessment of competency should be done at the time that informed consent is requested and may be said to exist if (a) the person is of legal age in the state, and (b) the person is generally able to understand the consequences of his or her actions. It is not necessary that mental health practitioners assess the patient for continued competency; nurses are capable of determining if the patient is able to comprehend what is being asked of him or her.

Critical Thinking and Reflection

Think of an instance where a patient refused recommended care. How did you ensure that his or her refusal was informed? How did you document the care of the patient? Were the primary health care provider and/or immediate nursing supervisor notified of the refusal of care?

Sugarman, McCrory, and Hubal (1998) presented a structured literature review of published research articles concerning informed consent and older adults. The purposes of this study were to make recommendations for improving the informed consent process with this given population and to highlight areas requiring further research. Studies were included if they were reports of primary research data about informed consent and if older subjects were included in the study sample.

A total of 99 articles were included in the final analysis. Diminished understanding of informed consent information was associated with older age and fewer years of formal education. Older age was also associated with decreased participation in research, which may suggest that older adults are less likely to seek additional treatment or begin new therapies for themselves. Strategies to improve the understanding of these adults included: use of simplified, more storybook or video type presentations; quizzing of the adult more frequently and after major concepts are presented; multiple disclosure sessions rather than a single session; and use of health educators to present the information. Use of these strategies should be considered when approaching adult patients in any health care setting as informed consent relies on patient comprehension.

A limited number of states do not recognize a family doctrine in securing informed consent for adults who are unable to consent for themselves. The court, for the purpose of giving informed consent, may appoint a legal guardian or representative. Alternately, the patient may have a valid Durable Power of Attorney for Health Care, allowing another person, selected by the patient while still competent, to give consent regarding health care decisions for the patient if he or she becomes incompetent.

Minors, like incompetent adults, usually require that an adult either give or deny consent. However, the law recognizes exceptions to that rule when (a) the emergency doctrine applies, (b) the minor is an emancipated or mature minor, (c) there is a valid court order to proceed with the therapy, or (d) the law recognizes the minor as having the capacity to consent. Emancipated minors are those minors, while still under the legal age for majority within the state, who are no longer under their parents control and regulation and are managing their own financial affairs. Examples of emancipated minors include married minors, underage parents, or minors in the armed service.

Mature minors are recognized in some states as having the capacity to consent to their health care needs. Usually, the mature minor is between the ages of 14 and 17 and is fully able to recognize the nature and consequences of the proposed therapy or treatment.

There are also selected therapies for which the minor is allowed to give valid consent in all states. These include the diagnosis and treatment of infectious, contagious, or communicable diseases, drug dependency, drug addiction, or any condition directly related to drug usage, obtaining birth control devices, and treatment during pregnancy (so long as the care concerns the pregnancy).

Patient Rights

Health care providers are increasingly becoming more aware and respectful of patients' rights. In 1959, the National League for Nursing wrote one of the earliest statements regarding patient rights. At that time, the prevailing attitude in health care assumed that health care providers knew best and patients were expected to follow the advice of these health care providers. In the early 1970s, the American Hospital Association published *A Patient's Bill of Rights*, enumerating 12 rights that were to be afforded all hospitalized patients. These rights primarily concerned the patient's right to considerate and respectful care, informed consent concepts (including making treatment decisions based on informed choice), considerations of privacy, the right to know who will provide care, and the right to information about advanced directives. That document was revised in 1992. In its revised form (Appendix G) it addresses more forcefully (a) the health care institution's responsibility for providing medically indicated treatment and service, (b) the collaborative nature of health maintenance, and (c) the patient's rights to confidentiality, informed consent, and considerate and respectful care. Individual organizations and health care institutions have also published various patient bills of rights.

Today, nurses are much more cognizant of the rights of patients, including those not enumerated on printed documents. For example, the patient has the right to a facility that ensures the safety of its patients and visitors. Patients also have the right to full disclosure of information prior to becoming a subject in research studies. Prevention of liability begins with respecting the rights of the patient and ensuring that peer health care providers likewise respect and preserve those rights.

Hazards in Communication

Clinical practice involves all types of communications—verbal, nonverbal, and written. As part of the communication process, the primary purposes of the medical record are to (a) assist in planning patient care; (b) continue the evaluation of the patient's condition and ongoing treatment; (c) document the course of the patient's medical evaluation, treatment, and change in condition; (d) document communication between the practitioner responsible for the patient and any other health professional who contributes to the patient's care; (e) assist in protecting the legal interests of the patient, institution, and practitioner; and (f) provide data for use in continuing education and research (Joint Commission on Accreditation of Healthcare Organizations [JCAHO], 1999).

Documentation must show continuity of care, interventions implemented, and patients' responses to implemented interventions. Implemented interventions include patient education and any evaluation of the effectiveness of that education. Notes made in the patient record should be concise, clear, timely, and complete. Patient assessments should be performed and recorded by the nurse caring for the patient. Even if there is no noticeable change in the patient's condition, the absence of change should be noted.

Through a variety of court decisions, the American legal system has taught nurses what must be recorded and how that recording should be completed. Entries are made in the record for every observation made and intervention implemented, including the patient's response to that intervention. Once recorded, the legal system accepts the documentation as a true reflection of what has transpired. If there is a gap in the record or no information is provided about an event, then the jury can infer that no observation was made or that no care was given.

Nurses also have a duty to ensure that follow-up measures are taken; merely recording changes in a patient's condition is not sufficient. The landmark case of *Darling v. Charleston Community Memorial Hospital* (1965) concluded that follow-up and evaluation of a patient's responses to treatment were equally important to the initial assessment of the patient. In the *Darling* case, an 18-year-old football player broke his leg during a high school game. A cast was placed on the leg in the emergency department of Charleston Community Memorial Hospital, and the patient was admitted to the hospital for observation. The nursing staff continued to assess the casted leg over the next several days, noting repeatedly in the patient record Darling's deteriorating condition, the foul odor emitted from the casted leg, and the patient's ever-increasing levels of pain and elevated temperature. The nurses shared their observations with the attending physician, and he ordered additional antipyretics and pain medications. The nurses charted these additional measures, but took no further action. Ultimately, the patient was transferred to a tertiary hospital in an attempt to save his leg, but it was later amputated.

The court instructed that proper documentation, no matter how accurate and timely, could never be a substitute for quality nursing care. Rather, said the court, the nurses involved should have reported their observations and lack of subsequent medical interventions to the nursing supervisor. It then became the nursing supervisor's responsibility to inform the medical chief of staff.

Conversely, complete medical records also protect staff members. A recent case illustrates this point. In *Shahine v. Louisiana State University Medical Center* (1996), a patient sued, claiming ulnar nerve injury occurred during surgery. At trial, the court concluded from the documentation that the patient had been positioned in such a way that no pressure-related injury could have occurred. The records did not contain unsubstantiated judgmental assertions that the patient was "positioned properly" or "positioned in such a manner as to avoid injury." The nurse's documentation was a detailed factual statement explaining exactly how the patient was positioned. See Box 17–2 for guidelines regarding documentation.

Box 17–2   Guidelines for Documentation

1. Read the previous nurses' notes prior to assuming care for a given patient, as it is then possible to determine whether there has been a change in the patient's condition.
2. Make an entry, even if it is a late entry, and always use clear and objective language when charting.
3. Present a realistic and factual picture of the patient, particularly patients who refuse to comply with therapeutic regimens or who are difficult to care for because of abusive and threatening language. These latter patients are more likely to bring a lawsuit if they have less than the desired outcome, and documentation that the patient prevented the nurse from giving more complete care or that the patient was noncompliant with the interventions may prevent the lawsuit from even being filed.
4. Chart all patient education, including evaluation of the education. If a patient refuses care, include in the charting any education about the possible consequences of refusing such care.
5. Correct any errors in a timely manner, leaving the incorrect entry legible so that there is no later inference that there was something to hide from the patient or the jury.
6. Use standardized flow sheets or checklists as provided by the health care agency and clearly identify the recorder after every entry.
7. Use all lines in sequence so that no additional entries can be made later.

Computerized charting has assisted in making documentation more complete and accurate. Newer software programs prompt nurses so that vital information is not forgotten or overlooked, the spell-check function has assisted in ensuring that words are correctly spelled, and issues such as messiness and illegibility have been eliminated. However, computerized records raise areas of concern. These issues primarily involve a patient's right to privacy and confidentiality. Institutions that provide computerized records should ensure that there are few points of access into the system, that each person's access be restricted to a limited scope of information, that information sought through individual access codes be monitored for appropriateness, that passwords be changed on a frequent basis, that access to the system is terminated when the employee leaves employment, and that confidentiality statements are signed by users, acknowledging their awareness of legal and institution requirements for usage.

Potential hazards of communication, though, are much greater than just the lack of written entries. Nurses also have a responsibility to communicate with peers, interdisciplinary health care members, and with patients. This is especially true when there are changes in the patient's condition. Multiple court cases speak to this need for communication among staff and interdisciplinary members of the health care team. These include *Seal v. Bogalusa Community Medical Center* (1995), in which failure to report significant laboratory findings to the physician resulted in a patient's death; *Wingo v. Rockford Memorial Hospital* (1997), in which

failure to report signs and symptoms unambiguously to the physician resulted in the premature birth of a severely damaged infant; and *Rampe v. Community General Hospital of Suffolk County* (1997), in which the court ruled that nurses must keep notifying the physician of late decelerations until the physician has physically arrived at the institution and taken care of the patient.

Similarly, court cases have determined that nurses must listen to what patients are attempting to communicate. For example, in *Parker v. Bullock County Hospital Authority* (1990), a patient fell while showering. The patient recently had surgery and had informed the nurse who helped her to the shower that she was feeling light-headed and dizzy. Despite these statements, the nurse left the patient to shower by herself.

Reducing Liability Exposure—Smart Nursing

Recognizing Predisposing Factors

One of the ways to reduce liability exposure is to recognize that there exists a type of patient who is more likely to sue health care providers in the event that something untoward happens. This patient, labeled the suit-prone patient, typically has a psychological makeup that breeds resentment and dissatisfaction with all aspects of his or her life. Should the result of medical and nursing care not be what the patient anticipated, this patient is apt to file a lawsuit, naming all health care providers as defendants.

Suit-prone patients are easily recognized by their tendency to have common character traits (e.g., immaturity; overdependency; hostility; or uncooperativeness). In addition, they often fail to follow a designated plan of care. These patients are unable to be self-critical and shift blame to others as a way of coping with their own inadequacies. They project their fear, insecurity, and anxiety to the health care providers, overreacting to any perceived slight in an exaggerated manner.

Recognizing such patients is the first step in avoiding potential lawsuits. The nurse should react on a personal basis, such as expressing satisfaction with the patient's cooperation, showing empathy and concern with their suffering and setbacks, and repeating needed information to keep the patient less fearful of unknown treatments and procedures. An atmosphere of attentiveness, caring, and patience coupled with competent, quality nursing care may help prevent the suit-prone patient from filing a subsequent lawsuit.

Similarly, there are nurses who are more likely to be named in multiple lawsuits or have legal action pending against them. Known as suit-prone nurses, they are the equivalent of suit-prone patients. Suit-prone nurses may have trouble establishing close relationships with others; tend to be insecure; readily and consistently shift blame to others; tend to be insensitive to patients' complaints or fail to take complaints seriously; have a tendency to be aloof and more concerned with the mechanics of nursing and less concerned with establishing meaningful human interactions with patients and their families; and inappropriately delegate their own responsibilities to peers to avoid personal contact with patients. Nursing is a caring profession, one based in science and humanity. Nurses who fit the description of the suit-prone nurse need counseling and education to change behaviors and develop more positive attitudes. Classes in interpersonal relationships and working effectively with people help recognize a nurse's need to treat others with respect and compassion. Changes in the nurse's behaviors toward patients and others may well lessen the possibility of a future lawsuit.

Evidence-Based Practice and Application of Standards of Care

Nursing, as a discipline, has been involved in scientifically defining its scope and standards of practice since the mid-1950s. Early research in nursing concerned the education needed in order to practice nursing. Later research focused on describing the characteristics of nurses. Today, the focus of much nursing research concerns patient outcomes. With this movement toward scientific approaches to patient care and the testing of interventions, nurses have become much better consumers of nursing research.

Courts are beginning to recognize this trend toward evidence-based practice; questions directed at expert witnesses inquire about the standard of care defined by research. Increasingly more health care agencies are including evidence-based standards of care in their policy and procedure manuals. These trends indicate that nurses must be well read in nursing research, incorporating evidence-based practice into all aspects of their patient care. No longer is it sufficient to give patient care as learned in nursing school. Nurses now have a responsibility to ensure that evidence-based standards of care are practiced in their health care setting long after they have completed nursing school.

Perhaps the most effective strategy for the nurse in preventing liability is to ensure that the nurse knows the applicable standard of care and meets that standard. Doing so involves not only being technically competent, but remaining current with applicable nursing research concerning nursing interventions and evidence-based practice, meeting institution and peer expectations, and participating as an accountable member of the health care delivery team.

Critical Thinking and Reflection

Have you ever encountered a patient whom you thought could be suit-prone? Describe what behaviors and actions caused you to believe that this was a suit-prone patient. Describe the care you gave the patient after determining that the patient could be a suit-prone patient. What was your advice to other nurses who cared for this patient?

Box 17-3   Functions of Risk Management

1. Define situations that place the entity at some financial risk.
2. Determine the frequency of those situations that have occurred.
3. Intervene and investigate identified problems.
4. Identify potential risks that exist and opportunities to improve patient care.

Risk Management

Risk management is the process that identifies, analyzes, and treats potential hazards within a specific setting. The object of risk management is to identify potential hazards and to eliminate them before anyone is harmed. Risk management relies on data obtained from properly completed patient incidents and errors forms. Risk managers analyze and evaluate the data and then design ways to prevent or minimize losses in the future. The functions of risk management are included in Box 17-3.

All nurses participate in an organization's risk management program. Administration develops the philosophy that encourages safe, competent patient care. Administration also provides an atmosphere that encourages the prompt identification and control of risks within the health care setting. Staff nurses participate in their risk management programs through (a) attendance at continuing education programs, (b) adherence to institution policy and procedure manuals, (c) prompt reporting of identified risks and potential hazards in the environment and about patient equipment, and (d) in continually ensuring the competency of their patient care skills.

Risk management achieves these goals in a variety of ways. The first step is the identification of types of patient services to be performed in the setting. The next step is to determine who will need to be employed to ensure the competent care of potential patients; this involves calculating the number and mix of staff to be employed, given the number of patients anticipated to be served. Then, procedures are developed and put into place to be followed when patients experience unanticipated complications, such as when to transport patients out of the organization to a tertiary medical center. Finally, an evaluation process is designed, assuring that risks can be quickly identified and controlled.

Patient Advocacy and Nurturing Relationships

Nurses serve in the role of patient advocate, developing and implementing nursing diagnoses, and exercising competent patient judgment as they monitor the care given to patients by physicians as well as peers. The role of patient advocate is enumerated in state nurse practice acts.

Court decisions also emphasize this vital function of nursing. Courts have held that the nurse has a duty (a) to report medical care that jeopardizes the care of the patient (*Catron v. The Poor Sisters of St. Frances*, 1982); (b) to question incomplete or illegible orders, including those that deviate from the usual standards of practice (Fiesta, 1994); (c) to directly disobey a physician's orders if the order places a patient at risk for harm (*Cruzbinsky v. Doctors' Hospital*, 1983); and (d) to question a patient's early discharge from a hospital (*Koeniquer v. Eckrich*, 1988).

Closely connected to this duty to serve, as a patient advocate, is the nurse's duty to develop and nurture relationships in clinical settings. To be a true advocate, a nurse must empathize with how the patient thinks and what the patient would truly desire in a given situation. The nurturing relationship encourages the patient and family members to feel that they can trust the nurse and honestly, openly tell the health care provider their true desires and, thus, allow the nurse to be a better patient advocate. Remember, it is not what the nurse would want in a particular set of circumstances; rather, it is what the patient, with his or her own cultural biases, previous experiences, and perceptions of what is attainable, desires under the present circumstances.

Legal Rights and Responsibilities of the Employees and Employers

Legal rights that exist for nurses and responsibilities of employers are essentially the same. What is a right for one entity becomes a responsibility for another entity. Nurses are owed rights under the equal employment opportunity laws; these rights include (a) the right to a safe work environment, (b) the right to receive consideration as a person and be respected for individual worth, (c) the right to be free from intentional and quasi-intentional torts, and (d) the right to be compensated for any torts committed against them. They have a right to know expressed and implied contractual obligations of the employment, including scheduling of work time, work expectations, benefits, grievance policies, and promotion factors. They also have the right to negotiate for additional benefits.

Nurses responsibilities to the employer include (a) maintaining the standard of care as written in their state nurse practice act, (b) continuously upgrading their skills and education through mandatory or voluntary continuing education, (c) being a patient advocate as needed to assure quality care of all patients, and (d) knowing and applying legal concepts as they apply to all areas of patient care. They also have the obligation of maintaining appropriate licensure and credentials given their specific job description. Unless there is a contract to the contrary, nurses have an obligation to assist in staffing alternate units within their institution, ensuring that all patients have access to competent care.

Preventing Nursing Liability in Health Care Settings

There are several ways nurses can legally protect themselves when working in health care settings. Based on legal principles, the means to prevent potential liability are enumerated in Box 17–4.

Box 17–4   Preventing Potential Liability

1. Treat all others with respect, communicating in an open and honest manner.
2. Maintain standards of care at all times. Know the institution policies and procedures, remain current in nursing practice through continuing education, and ensure that your nursing care is reflective of standards of care.
3. Base your care on the nursing process. Using all steps of the process prevents overlooking any essential step, particularly the evaluation of implemented care.
4. Use your nursing knowledge to make appropriate nursing diagnoses and implement nursing interventions as appropriate. You have an affirmative duty to give competent care; the beginning of that care is correctly identifying appropriate diagnoses and acting on those diagnoses.
5. Document completely care given the patient, including his or her reactions to the implemented care. Chart entries as soon as possible, ensuring that facts and observations are not overlooked or forgotten.
6. Respect the patient's right to education about his or her diagnosis, ensuring that the patient and/or family is (are) taught about essential etiology, therapy, and possible complications.
7. Delegate patient care wisely, and know the scope of practice for yourself and those you supervise. Never accept or allow others to accept more responsibility than they are able to competently accept or than they are allowed by law to accept.
8. Maintain patient privacy and confidentiality and ensure that others in the health care setting do likewise. Know and enforce the patient's right to be free from assault, battery, and false imprisonment in the health care setting.
9. Treat all patients with the same competent, courteous care that you would demand for yourself or your family member.
10. Know and apply legal principles in all aspects of health care delivery.

As nurses begin their professional nursing practice, issues in the workplace sometimes seem overwhelming. The new nurse no longer has the same safeguards afforded the nursing student: He or she is expected to care for multiple patients rather than two or three selected patients; often the mentor, either the clinical instructor or agency preceptor, who seemed ever present when there was a question or concern is gone; and many more decisions seem to rest solely on the new nurse. Additionally, this new nurse is most often working in a clinical setting other than the setting in which he or she had clinical experiences while in school, thus policy and procedure is not as familiar as it once was. Finally, the new graduate may have chosen to work in a setting where there are not the numbers of support staff that once existed; gone may be the institution that had medical students and an active residency program as well as nursing students.

There are several measures that will assist this new graduate as he or she transitions into "real world" nursing. The first is to know and understand the job description. What are the expectations that this new graduate is expected to fulfill? Question any portion of the description that is unclear and insist that you are able to competently practice in the setting. If there are expectations for skills that you do not have, ensure that you are given the necessary education to perform the skills. Likewise, ensure that you understand the agency's policies and procedures fully, including any unwritten policies that might exist.

Recognize your own limitations and strengths. Too often, the new graduate sees only his or her limitations. Remember, you also have a variety of strengths, including your communication skills. Often, this is the new graduate's greatest asset—the ability to listen to what the patient or other health care provider is saying and asking the appropriate questions to further clarify the issue at hand. If a patient questions a treatment or medication, find out why he or she is questioning it and do the same. Perhaps the physician has told the patient that the treatment was being discontinued and that order had not yet been transferred to the patient care form or the previous nurse gave the medication early and merely neglected to chart it.

Learn to communicate effectively and appropriately. If you are sure of the correct action to take, then implement the action. If you are unsure of the significance of a new symptom or sign in a given patient, use clinical resources wisely. Question physicians if that is the appropriate action to take, regardless of the time of day or night. Too often, nurses hesitate to question physicians about subtle and pertinent patient changes during the night hours, especially if the institution is not a medical training facility. Communicating when appropriate ensures that patients receive the care that they require when it is required. It also assists in ensuring that your concerns will be taken seriously, for this is an instance in which you need assistance and could not have implemented correct action on your own.

KEY POINTS

1. The state nurse practice act is the single most important piece of legislation for nurses because the practice act affects all aspects of nursing, from the definition of professional nursing, to requirements for licensure, standards of nursing practice, and disciplinary actions.

2. Nurses may be involved in civil and criminal causes of action. The most frequent means of incurring criminal action is by failure to renew one's nursing license in a timely manner because, once the license has expired, the nurse is then practicing without a license.

3. Complying with standards of care as well as following principles of basic nursing practice assists in preventing liability for malpractice.

4. Two types of witnesses are recognized by the legal system: lay witnesses who establish facts at trial level and expert witnesses who explain highly technical and skilled nursing practice to jurors. Both types of witnesses are critical to the American legal system.

5. The doctrine of informed consent mandates that primary health care providers disclose needed material facts in terms that patients can reasonably

understand so that the patient can make an informed choice.

6. Documentation must show continuity of care, interventions implemented, and patients' responses to implemented interventions. This includes patient education and any evaluation of the effectiveness and level of understanding of the education.

7. Nurses have a responsibility to communicate with peers, interdisciplinary health care members, and with patients, particularly in respect to changes in patients' conditions.

8. Courts are recognizing the trend toward evidence-based practice; questions now raised concerning

patient care is centered on standards of care as defined by research data.

9. Nurses serve in the role of patient advocate, developing and implementing nursing diagnoses and exercising competent patient judgment as the nurses monitor the care given to patients by physicians as well as peers.

10. Discrimination in the workplace involves treating others differently based on stereotypes about groups of people; discrimination may involve sex, gender, racial, ethnic, age, or disability.

EXPLORE 🌐 MediaLink

Critical thinking questions, essay questions, key terms, web links, activities, NCLEX review questions, and more interactive resources can be found on the Companion Website at www.prenhall.com/haynes. Click on Chapter 17 to select activities for this chapter.

REFERENCES

Bellegie v. Board of Nurse Examiners, 685 S.W. 2nd 431 (Tex. Ct. App.-Austin, 1985).

Catron v. The Poor Sisters of St. Francis, 435 N.E. 2nd 305 (Indiana, 1982).

Cruzbinsky v. Doctors' Hospital, 188 Cal. Rptr. 685 (Cal. App., 1983).

Darling v. Charleston Community Memorial Hospital, 33 III. 2nd 326, 211 N.E. 2nd 253 (1965). cert. denied 383 U.S. 946 (1965).

Fiesta, J. (1994). Failing to act like a professional. *Nursing Management, 24*(7), 15–17.

Joint Commission on Accreditation of Healthcare Organizations. (1999). *Accreditation manual for hospitals*. Oakbrook Terrace, IL: Author.

King v. State of Louisiana, 728 S. 2nd 1027 (La. App., 1999).

Koeniquer v. Eckrich, 422 N.W. 2nd 600 (South Dakota, 1988).

Lunsford v. Board of Nurse Examiners, 648 S.W. 2nd 391 (Tex. App.-Austin, 1983).

Parker v. Bullock County Hospital Authority. (1990). A90A0 762 *Medical Malpractice: Verdicts, Settlements, and Experts, 6*(10), 28.

Rampe v. Community General Hospital of Suffolk County, 660 N.Y.S. 2nd 206 (N.Y. App., 1997).

Rozovsky, F. A. (1990). *Consent to treatment: A practical guide* (2nd ed.). Boston: Little, Brown and Company.

Sabol v. Richmond Heights General Hospital, 676 N.E. 2nd 958 (Ohio App., 1996).

Seal v. Bogalusa Community Medical Canter, 665 S.W. 2nd 42 (La. App., 1995).

Sermchief v. Gonzales, 660 S.W. 2nd 683 (Mo. en banc, 1983).

Shahine v. Louisiana State University Medical Center, 680 So. 2nd 1352 (La. App., 1996).

Sugarman, J., McCrory, D. C., & Hubal, R. C. (1998). Getting meaningful informed consent from older adults: A structured literature review of empirical research. *Journal of the American Geriatrics Society, 46*(4), 517–524.

Wingo v. Rockford Memorial Hospital, 686 N.E. 2nd 722 (III. App., 1997).

SUGGESTED READINGS

Bernzweig, E. P. (1996). *The nurse's liability for malpractice: A programmed text* (6th ed.). St. Louis, MO: Mosby.

Brent, N. J. (1997). *Nurses and the law*. Philadelphia, PA: W. B. Saunders.

Dempski, K. (2000). Serving as an expert witness. *RN, 63*(2), 65–70.

Eskreis, T. R. (1998). Seven common legal pitfalls in nursing. *American Journal of Nursing, 98*(4), 34–40.

Fiesta, J. (1999). Do no harm: When caregivers violate our golden rule, part 2. *Nursing Management, 30*(9), 10.

Fiesta, J. (1999). Nursing malpractice: Cause for consideration. *Nursing Management, 30*(2), 12–14.

Guido, G. W. (2001). *Legal and ethical issues in nursing* (3rd ed.). Upper Saddle River, NJ: Prentice Hall Health.

Hall, J. K. (1996). *Nursing ethics and law*. Philadelphia, PA: W. B. Saunders.

Steckler, S. L. (2000). Nursing case law update. *Journal of Nursing Law, 7*(1), 55–64.

Unit 5

Career Management and Professional Growth

18

Obtaining Professional Employment

LINDA C. HAYNES

> "A career is a life's work, success in one's chosen profession; a path and a journey. For many, career and life visions emerge with great clarity. For others, such career visions take shape gradually through identifying personal and professional passions, preferences, interests, and strengths."

The University of Iowa College of Nursing
Men in Nursing, 2002

LEARNING OBJECTIVES

AT THE COMPLETION OF THIS CHAPTER, THE READER WILL BE ABLE TO:

- Identify strategies important to a successful job search.
- Investigate employment opportunities.
- Complete a self-appraisal and develop a career trajectory.
- Identify responsibilities of interviewers and decision makers.

- Prepare a resume and cover letter.
- Analyze interview topics and formulate answers to interview questions.
- Discuss resignation and transfer.

MediaLink   www.prenhall.com/haynes

Additional online resources including NCLEX review questions, critical thinking questions, and real-world activities for this chapter can be found on the Companion Website at www.prenhall.com/haynes.

To graduates who are prepared, initial employment should represent more than a first job. It should be the initial step in a carefully thought out, well-developed career plan. This chapter should help the nursing student develop a career trajectory. The process for seeking employment, suggestions for investigating employment opportunities, and steps for a successful job search will be presented. Information to guide job selection is discussed. Strategies for future job searches and procedures for resignation and transfer are also included.

Employment Opportunities: Past, Present, and Future

The current nursing workforce shortage, unlike previous cyclic deficits, is of unprecedented severity and is expected to endure long into the future (Marshal, 2001). Presently, 126,000 nurses are needed to fill vacancies in the nation's hospitals (American Hospital Association, 2001); according to the Bureau of Labor Statistics, it is projected that more than 1 million new nurses will be needed by 2010 (Hecker, 2001). Of available employment opportunities in acute care facilities, 75% are for nurses. In March 2000, the average age of currently employed registered nurses was 43.3 years. It is expected that by 2010, 40% of all employed nurses will be over the age of 50 (Bureau of Health Professions Division of Nursing, 2001). While the total number of nurses has continued to increase, the rate of increase has slowed. Data from the Division of Nursing's *National Sample Survey of Registered Nurses March 2000: Preliminary Findings* indicate that of the total number of registered nurses, 58.4% work full time, 23.2% work part time, and 18.3% are not employed in nursing. The National Council of State Boards of Nursing (NCSBN) report that the number of first-time U.S. graduates to sit for the NCLEX-RN declined by 26% from 1995 to 2001.

Of employed nurses working in hospitals as many as 40% report being dissatisfied (Aiken et al., 2001). In the same study, up to one-third of nurses under the age of 30 reported that they plan to leave their current job within 1 year. Moreover, one in five report they intend to leave the patient care setting within 5 years for reasons other than retirement.

Relief from the nursing shortage is limited by a shortage of available nursing faculty. The average age of current doctorally prepared nursing faculty in the United States is 53.5 (American Association of Colleges and Nursing [AACN], 2003). There is expected to be a wave of retirements, which will peak in just 10 years (AACN, 1999). Schools of nursing already experience and anticipate increasing difficulty in recruiting new faculty (Brendtro & Hegge, 2000). Implications of the nursing faculty shortage for both education and clinical practice are serious. The shortage is likely to limit nursing school enrollment, which will (a) compound the current nursing shortage, (b) result in burnout of presently employed nurses and nursing faculty, and (c) lead to a decline in the quality of educational programs and, subsequently, health care across the country.

While the nursing shortage intensifies, there are demographic signals to suggest a need for increasing numbers of nurses to care for the aging population. It is expected that the ratio of available caregivers (nurses and other care providers) to those in need of care (growing numbers of elderly, ages 60 to 80) will decrease by 40% over the next 20 years (University of Illinois, Nursing Institute, 2001).

These daunting statistics clearly indicate new graduate nurses will have no difficulty finding employment. In most cases, new nurses can expect to find a job working in the specialty field they have chosen, on the shift they desire, and at a salary higher than that of their predecessors. New graduates can also expect greater availability of internships, better orientation programs, and competitive incentive packages.

Research Application

While the current nursing workforce shortage is not surprising, the public seems surprised that one out of every five nurses currently employed in nursing is considering leaving the profession within the next five years. A nationwide survey was conducted on behalf of the Federation of Nurses and Health Professions (2001). A sample of current direct-care (700) and former direct-care (207) nurses was surveyed to examine their perspective on nursing and the current shortage.

(continued)

Not surprising to nurses, the survey found that the present nursing shortage will be compounded as current nurses leave the profession for reasons other than retirement. Overall, these direct care nurses described working conditions as poor. They cited stress, irregular hours, low morale, and an inadequate supply of nurses as reasons for dissatisfaction. When asked how to improve recruitment and retention of nurses, these nurses suggested (a) better staffing ratios, (b) more patient time, (c) more input in decisions, (d) higher salaries, (e) performance bonus, (f) flexible schedules, (g) availability of part-time employment, (h) financial support for continuing education, and (i) better insurance coverage.

Nurses who were seriously considering leaving nursing stated they would stay with better pay, staffing, schedules, and more respect. Nurses who had left nursing cited the need for higher salaries and better staffing and schedules in order for their return to the profession.

The nursing student and new graduate should find the above information discouraging at best. At worst, one would expect these individuals to feel hopeless and helpless and thus seek other careers. However, this author would suggest an alternative—political activism and involvement in professional organizations to make a change for nurses and patients today and in the future. The theme and goal of many of the chapters of this textbook has been the need for nurses to band together to make change and to end intraprofession discord for the betterment of individuals, families, and communities.

Beginning the Job Search

A successful job search begins with a career plan that includes short- and long-term personal/professional goals. As already suggested, the job market is wide open for new nurses. But nursing is not simply a job, it is a career; the opportunities are abundant, and as with any career, new nurses should carefully consider what they might wish to do with their career and life before accepting that first professional position. Rather than striking out impulsively taking just any job, the nurse's first job should be selected as part of a very carefully outlined plan for career management.

Self-Appraisal

Prior to establishing career goals, the nurse should first take a thorough, critical inventory of personal and professional skills. Significant others (e.g., friends, family, colleagues, and former nursing faculty) can help the nursing student or new graduate with this self-appraisal. Most nursing students tend to focus on their psychomotor skill competence; however, it is important for the new nurse to consider all skills, not just those he or she may value. Other skills, including the ability to teach, counsel, problem solve, and function under stressful conditions, are equally important to job satisfaction. The nurse should also carefully consider strengths and needs for growth regarding interpersonal skills.

Personal values, interests, needs, and strengths/weaknesses should also influence job selection. Some nursing students have no difficulty identifying their strength and weaknesses; they may also have clearly defined values, interests, and needs. Others require guidance from other sources (e.g., peers, mentors, or family) to identify these important personal attributes that may influence job satisfaction.

VALUES

Values are the basis for thoughts, choices, feelings, and actions (Uustal, 1992). Each person has a set of values, and those values guide behavior. Few individuals put their values into conscious thought. Too often, individuals do not take time to seriously consider their value system. In order to avoid a conflict of values, the new nurse must make a conscious decision to understand what is valued and then should carefully compare these values with the values of a possible employing institution. The values of the institution will be reflected in the institutions mission and philosophy, the care provided patients, and the actions of employees. New nurses can gain insight as to what an employer values by reviewing the mission and philosophy of the organization and observing care provided and actions taken by employees. This information can then be compared with the nurse's own values. Table 18–1 provides the nurse with a venue for identifying most cherished values.

INTERESTS

Interests or activities/things the individual enjoys, values, appreciates, and/or finds challenging, should be considered when initiating a job search (Henderson & McGettigan, 1994). A wide range of interests suggests flexibility. The flexible nurse is more likely to adapt during times of challenge and change. The interests listed in Table 18–2 are not designed to determine nursing interest, but rather to reflect personal interest. These interests are divided into six categories: realistic, investigative, artistic, social, enterprising, and conventional interest. From these six categories, the nurse can recognize personal interests and apply these interests to available employment opportunities. Employment decisions should in part reflect an individual's interests.

Realistic interests reflect an awareness of things as they are. Individuals with realistic interests enjoy activities that involve mechanical or technical skills. A nurse with strong interests in mechanical or technical skills may not be satisfied in a position that focuses on psychosocial needs (e.g., mental health nursing). The

emergency department or intensive care setting may prove more satisfying. Nurses with **investigative interests** are likely to use mental strategies that involve logic and analysis of data. These individuals observe details and seek answers to questions (e.g., research-oriented nurses).

Artistic interests are present in individuals highly aware of art or beauty. There is a tendency to express feelings through such activities as art, acting, and creative writing. School nurses can use art and role playing to teach health promotion to young children. Further, nurses with creative writing interests may enjoy developing teaching tools for patient education. People who enjoy **social interest** tend to enjoy the company of others. They are especially skillful at listening, counseling, leading, mentoring, negotiating, or supervising. A nurse with social interest is likely to enjoy working in any environment that allows for people contact and interaction. This nurse would likely enjoy mentoring new nurses and spending time providing discharge teaching, and would be adept at providing supportive services for families and patients. **Enterprising interests** are found in nurses who initiate and are eager to face challenge. The nurse with enterprising interest is likely to enjoy an administrative position or supervisory role. This nurse might also consider a nontraditional position (e.g., self-employment or advanced practice). Finally, individuals who have strong **conventional**

Table 18–1   Most Cherished Values

Instructions: Rank the values listed below from 1 (most cherished value) to 20 (least cherished).

• Achievement		• Physical health	
• Adventure		• Meaningful work	
• Personal freedom		• Affection	
• Authenticity		• Pleasure	
• Expertness		• Wisdom	
• Emotional strength		• Family	
• Service		• Recognition	
• Leadership		• Security	
• Money		• Self-growth	
• Spirituality		• Intellect	

Adapted with permission from Henderson, F. C., & McGettigan, B. O. (1994). *Managing your career in nursing* (2nd ed.) (p. 86). New York: National League for Nursing.

Table 18–2   Interest Inventory

Instructions: For each category of interest 12 activities are listed. Score each activity as either: 0 (no interest), 1 (low interest), 2 (moderate interest), or 3 (high interest). Sum scores for each of the six categories of interest.

Activities	Score	Activities	Score	
Set A Realistic		**Set B Investigative**		
1. Biking		1. Assessing others		
2. Cooking		2. Using logic		
3. Dancing		3. Experimenting		
4. Designing objects		4. Observing		
5. Adjusting equipment		5. Clarifying problems		
6. Operating equipment		6. Researching		
7. Woodworking		7. Surveying		
8. Needleworking		8. Analyzing		
9. Sailing		9. Diagnosing problems		
10. Swimming		10. Testing ideas		
11. Running		11. Critiquing		
12. Skiing		12. Evaluating		
Set A (Realistic) Score		Set B (Investigative) Score		
Set C Artistic		**Set D Social**		
1. Applying theory		1. Caring for others		
2. Creating new ideas		2. Coaching		
3. Developing models		3. Counseling		
4. Designing visuals		4. Editing		
5. Creating works of art		5. Listening		
6. Directing productions		6. Designing educational materials		
7. Drawing		7. Leading groups		
8. Composing music		8. Negotiating		
9. Acting		9. Writing letters		
10. Predicting		10. Writing reports		
11. Taking pictures		11. Reading		
12. Writing poetry		12. Translating		
Set C (Artistic) Score		Set D (Social) Score		
Set E Enterprising		**Set F Conventional**		
1. Initiating ideas		1. Keeping deadlines		
2. Planning changes		2. Carrying things out in detail		
3. Taking risks		3. Making contracts		
4. Assigning tasks		4. Organizing records		
5. Setting standards		5. Classifying data		
6. Coordinating activities		6. Filing		
7. Implementing policies		7. Processing forms		
8. Managing conflict		8. Inventorying		
9. Speaking in public		9. Keeping financial records		
10. Competing in games		10. Managing budgets		
11. Telling stories		11. Allocating resources		
12. Using humor		12. Following through others' instructions		
Set E (Enterprising) Score		Set F (Conventional) Score		

Adapted with permission from Henderson, F. C., & McGettigan, B. O. (1994). *Managing your career in nursing* (2nd ed.) (pp. 87–90). New York: National League for Nursing.

Table 18-3   Needs Assessment

Instructions: Rank the needs listed below from 1 (most essential) to 22 (least essential).

• Independence			• Self-respect		
• Being well known			• Creativity		
• Beauty			• Money		
• Orderliness			• Belonging		
• Pleasure			• Insight		
• Intelligence			• Giving and receiving love		
• Intimacy			• Physical vitality		
• Altruism			• Being praised		
• Excitement			• Sense of accomplishment		
• Meaningful work			• Being good at something		
• Ability to handle inner feelings			• Security		

Adapted with permission from Henderson, F. C., & McGettigan, B. O. (1994). *Managing your career in nursing* (2nd ed.) (p. 92). New York: National League for Nursing.

interests are likely to enjoy the status quo or established standards. These individuals can be depended on to work within deadlines and attend to detail.

NEEDS

A human needs model suggest that all individuals have needs that are met in a hierarchical fashion (e.g., physical/safety needs, security, belonging, personal growth, and self-actualization). An individual's needs are determined by past experiences as well as availability of resources. Table 18–3 assists the nurse to identify and rank needs and Table 18–4 assists in creating values, interest, and needs profile for nurses.

Developing a Career Trajectory

Initiating a job search should be about creating a career. New graduates should have no difficulty finding a first job; however, the search should be for a job that suits or fits the needs, values, and interest of the new graduate. A career trajectory provides guidance for a professional career in nursing. The first job should be selected as part of a well-thought-out plan.

Table 18-4   Values, Interests, Needs Profile

Instructions: Write the three most cherished values, highest-ranked interest themes, and most essential needs identified using Tables 18–1 through 18–3 in the space provided below. Consider this information while making decisions regarding professional employment.

Values	Interests	Needs

Adapted with permission from Henderson, F. C., & McGettigan, B. O. (1994). *Managing your career in nursing* (2nd ed.) (p. 94). New York: National League for Nursing.

Once the nurse or nursing student has identified values, interests, and needs it is important to analyze the data. Table 18–4 allows the nurse to summarize information collected in Tables 18–1 through 18–3. This summary can guide the nurse to an accurate self-appraisal that will hopefully promote job satisfaction. Look at the three most cherished values, interests, and needs and consider how this information can be an integral part of the job search. When you look at the mission or philosophy of an institution, how does it compare to your own mission or philosophy of health care? Analyzing your interests, what type of job might be most satisfying? Consider your needs. Will your needs be met in the job area you find most interesting, or is this an area that requires more preparation?

Career Goals

The new nurse needs to identify what they intend to do with their career by narrowing the clinical focus, care setting, and functional category desired. Clinical focus refers to a special area (i.e., medical, surgical, women's health, pediatrics, or psychiatry). If the desired clinical focus is medical nursing, the new graduate would next need to determine if there is a specialty focus within the clinical focus. While a nurse may choose to obtain employment on a medical unit, there is also the option for selecting a specialty area such as neurology, renal, or cardiovascular, to name just a few.

The nurse must also decide which care setting is desirable. For example, nurses are employed in inpatient, outpatient, acute care, long-term care, and community-based care settings. Each of these settings also has specialty settings that offer further employment opportunities. Historically, nurses who worked in community-based care settings served as public health nurses. They were employed by health care agencies, provided home visits, and established limited outpatient clinic services. Today, community-based care may involve home care, but it could also involve care in other sites such as school health, occupational health, or specialty out patient clinics (e.g., dialysis and wound care centers).

The nurse can also use functional categories as a means for establishing career goals. Most new graduates will serve as direct care providers; however, nurses are also needed in leadership, supervisory, educational, service, and research roles. Table 18–5 offers the nursing student a mechanism for identifying the clinical focus, care setting, and functional category, which are most desirable.

Initiating the Job Search by Surveying the Marketplace

Today's nurse may begin a job search via the Internet; however, jobs can also be found through employment agencies; human resource departments; friends, family, and professional contacts; newspapers and professional journals; college and university career centers; and career/job fairs. While employment opportunities in the first decade of the twenty-first century are abundant, the nursing student should remember certain jobs, internships, and employment packages are very competitive; therefore, it is important that the new graduates prepare to "market themselves" as a viable, strong candidate for a desired position. It would not be prudent for a nurse or nursing student to assume the current shortage will guarantee employment in any position that is desired. Employers continue to look for the best available employees using enticing hiring bonuses and other incentives to attract new nurses. While the incentive may be enticing, the nurse must remember that the goal is to obtain employment consistent with his or her values, needs, and interests. The sign-on strategies used by some employing agencies are at times nothing more than deplorable practices designed to bribe the nurse into accepting employment.

Marketing Yourself

The cover letter and resume introduce applicants to prospective employers. A well-written introduction serves to excite an employer enough to call the applicant. It provides the reader with information that will stimulate that person's desire to read on and meet an employment candidate. The resume provides the

Table 18–5 Focusing Career Goals

Instructions: Fill in the following blanks: (a) under clinical focus rank the specialty areas according to interest 1 (most interested) to 5 (least interested); (b) for your highest-ranked clinical focus list 3 to 5 specialty areas to consider in order of most to least interested; (c) rank care settings and functional categories, if you have a preferred setting or category not listed fill it in; and (d) complete the sentences, which follow the ranking.

Clinical Focus					Care Setting	Functional Category
Medical	Surgical	Ob/Gyn	Pediatrics	Psychiatry	Acute care	Direct care provider
List subspecialties for the clinical focus selected					Long-term care	Supervisory
					Community-based	Educational
						Service
						Research
						Leadership
						Other

My desire is to work in an area with a clinical focus on _____

The nursing specialty within the clinical focus that I most desire is _____

Desired care setting _____

Desired specialty _____

Desired functional category _____

Desired specialty functional category _____

reader with a more detailed description of the prospective employees' attributes. Cover letters and resumes are generally sent to the human resource department of an employing institution. Some employers want initial communication to be via e-mail with attachments or via some other route on the Internet. The applicant should review the prospective employer's Web site to verify the employer preference regarding applications.

Most human resource specialists take less than 3 minutes to read and formulate an initial opinion of an applicant based on initial information received. Some will scan the material in as little as 40 seconds and place the documents aside to be reread later when time is available. The applicant writing these documents (e.g., cover letter, resume, electronic application) wants to provide the human resource specialist with a reason to thoroughly reread the materials so that a fact-to-face interview is offered.

Cover Letter

Always remember that the cover letter is the key to getting a resume read and is the first step to obtaining an interview. Consider the following when writing an effective, concise cover letter.

- All cover letters should be written on bond stationery, preferably white or ivory. They must provide an adequate heading with information as to how the prospective employer can reach the applicant. Cover letters are always typewritten. A professionally appearing cover letter might begin by providing the reader with the applicant's name, address, phone number, and e-mail address. While there is a standard format for writing a business letter, the applicant may wish to deviate from the standard format in favor of a more contemporary style. Computer processing today allows the appli-

Table 18–5 can help a nursing student focus goals. If you know some day you hope to return to school for graduate education to teach or engage in advanced practice you can use the table to help work out the steps needed to reach that long-term goal. For example, you may know you wish to be involved in medical–surgical nursing, you have a special interest in oncology, and desire to work as a direct care provider, but your ultimate goal is education. What steps do you need to take to develop clinical expertise, complete educational requirements, and ultimately serve in an educational role? Do you wish to teach undergraduates or graduates, patients, or nurses in clinical settings? What obstacles may need to be overcome to achieve these goals? Develop a plan and a timeline for dealing with these obstacles.

cant to creatively produce letterhead-type stationery. Consider the following:

Joan Smith
2536 Newton Street
Dalworth, Texas 75235
214.111.1111
joan_smith@easytoreach.com

- The cover letter must be addressed to an individual. Avoid "To whom it may concern." This phrase may cause the reader to scan your letter rather than read it thoroughly. When addressing the reader, include his or her title. An applicant can usually find this information either from an employment Web site, by calling the Human Resource Department, or through networking with other professionals currently employed by the institution. The applicant should avoid assumptions. Do not assume the human resources representative is a nurse. The following provides a guideline for the traditional salutation.

January 13, 2004

Joan Recruiter
Human Resource Specialist
Human Resource Department
Best Hospital
2222 Market Street
Dallas, Texas 75244

Dear Ms. Recruiter,

- In the first paragraph the applicant should provide an introduction and quickly inform the reader of the purpose for the letter. This introduction should include a statement as to how the applicant knows a position is available. For example: "While researching employment opportunities for gradu-

ate nurses in the Dallas health care marketplace on the Internet, I learned of openings at your facility. I would like to be considered for a position in the emergency department. My resume is enclosed."

- In the second paragraph the applicant provides a brief description of qualifications, a concise overview of educational and work history, and any skills the nurse possesses that may help him or her perform the job. The applicant also explains why he or she is qualified to work for the institution in the available position. This paragraph should not be a rehash of the resume; however, if the applicant has significant accomplishments or relevant experience this information should be included. The second paragraph might read: "In May 2004, I will obtain a Bachelor of Science in Nursing from Johnston University. The program at Johnston is intensive and has provided me with hands on experiences through clinical rotations. In these rotations, I have worked with a variety of clients on several units including medical–surgical, psychiatry, pediatrics, and obstetrics. In addition, I completed an elective clinical rotation in the Level 1 Emergency Department at Jones Hospital. In this elective I was fortunate enough to be involved in all aspects of emergency care, including initial triage, acute care, advanced life support, and discharge planning. This spring I will complete a six-week, 150-hour clinical internship under the supervision of a nurse preceptor in the surgical intensive care unit of the Mark Healthcare System."

- The third paragraph states the nurse's confidence in his or her ability to perform the tasks required by the job and the potential asset he or she expects to be to the organization. In this paragraph the applicant also provides the potential employer with information as to how the applicant can be reached. The applicant reaffirms interest in the opportunity provided by the prospective employer and asks for an interview. For example: "I am confident my skills and experience would prove beneficial to your organization. I would welcome the opportunity to discuss my qualification with you in person. I can be reached after 6 PM at area code/phone number or via e-mail at joan_smith@easytoreach.com."

- The cover letter should close with an expression of appreciation of the reader's consideration of the application and should be signed professionally (e.g., "Sincerely," or "Respectfully,"). As the resume is attached to the cover letter, a notice of enclosure follows the applicant's name. Applicants always take care in signing their name. *The cursive signature is always legible.* The cover letter might end: "Thank you for your attention and consideration."

Respectfully,

Joan Smith

Enclosure

A professionally written cover letter increases the likelihood of having a resume read. An example of a complete, professionally written cover letter is available in Box 18–1. Remember the goal of the cover letter is to stimulate the interest of the reader so that he or she will read the resume. The following is a list to carefully double check after a cover letter is written:

- The name of the institution and the name of the human resource department's representative are spelled correctly.
- The cover letter has the correct address of both the applicant and the prospective hiring institution.
- The letter is addressed to a person and the person's correct title has been used.
- Words are spelled correctly, there are no typographical errors, and grammar is correct.
- Bond stationery was used, and the letter was folded in a trifold manner, and inserted into a matching envelope.
- All enclosures, including the resume, that were referred to in the cover letter were enclosed.
- In the cover letter the applicant asked for an interview and provided times of availability.

Resume

Building a resume is not effortless. There are a number of Internet sites and resume-building programs; however, it is likely these resources are costly and time con-

suming when a school of nursing library and texts such as this offer the nurse an easy formula for successful resume writing. Not every resume is appropriate for every job. The applicant may wish to modify a resume to attract individual employers. The following is designed to help the nursing student, new graduate, or experienced nurse obtain professional employment. The principles for building a successful resume remain the same regardless of experience. Factors that contribute to a successful resume include:

- A focus on skills with the use of action words to describe job/education-related experiences.
- A resume that is easy to read and understand.
- A resume that is visually powerful, yet free of gimmicks.
- A resume that is brief, yet concise. Most entry-level nurses will require no more than one page for the resume, though two pages are acceptable; experienced nurses should build a resume that is no longer than two pages.
- A resume with proper grammar and spelling with consistent use of tenses is essential.
- A resume that is formal (e.g., no contractions or abbreviations).
- A resume that is computer generated.
- A resume that is printed on high-quality paper, preferably white or ivory; other colors may copy poorly (e.g., gray) or have a less than professional appearance (e.g., pink, blue).
- The sections of a resume are presented in chronological order with most recent work- or education-related experiences first.

ORGANIZING THE RESUME

The resume can be developed using either a chronological (Tables 18–6 and 18–7) or functional/skills style (Table 18–8). The chronological style is used for an individual who "has training and/or experience consistent with the career objective [or qualification summary], has relevant job titles, or is applying for a job in a highly traditional field. This style is the most effective for the majority of new college graduates" (Baylor University Career Services, 2001, p. 12). The functional style emphasizes skill areas and is most helpful for applicants who wish to emphasize their abilities for the job. Skills listed in this type of resume should be ranked in a manner that best supports the objective or qualification summary.

The resume must be "scanner friendly," as many employers are using scanning technology to file and access the document for future use. Scanning technol-

Box 18–1 Cover Letter

Name
Complete Address
City, State, Zip Code
Area Code/Phone Number
E-mail Address

Date

Name
Pediatric Intensive Care Coordinator
Agency Name
Address
City, State, Zip Code

Dear Ms. Name,

I became interested in City Hospital while researching employment opportunities for nurses in the Dallas/Fort Worth area. I recognize your facility as a world-renowned children's hospital with a special focus on education and research. I am currently working as a Nurse Technician in the pediatric intensive care unit at City Hospital. I am drawn to remain at City Hospital due to the teamwork, caring attitude, and commitment to excellence demonstrated by the staff. I would now like to be considered for a Graduate Nurse position in the Pediatric Intensive Care Unit.

In month of year, I will complete my Bachelor of Science degree in Nursing from State University. The clinical rotations in medical–surgical, obstetrics, psychology, pediatrics, and community health care have provided me with hands-on experience in a variety of clinical environments. My pediatric clinical experience gave me the opportunity to develop skills in pediatric assessment, medication administration, and collaborative health care. In addition, I completed an elective in emergency room nursing at University Medical Center. The high intensity and critical thinking required in that environment were challenging. In nursing school I have had the opportunity to work as a nurse technician at City Hospital, where I have been able to gain additional nursing and time management skills. This spring I will complete a four-week, 120-hour internship in Labor and Delivery at City Hospital.

I am confident my skills and experience would prove beneficial to your organization. I welcome the opportunity to discuss my qualifications with you in person. I can be reached during the day by e-mail at (e-mail address) or by phone at area code/phone number. If I am not available, you may leave a message and I will promptly return your call.

Thank you for your time and consideration. My resume is enclosed.

Respectfully,

First and Last Name

Enclosure (1)

Table 18–6 *Chronological Style Resume for a New Graduate*

Name

Present Address: Permanent Address:
Street   Street
City, State, Zip Code   City, State, Zip Code
Area Code and Phone Number   Area Code and Phone Number
E-mail Address   E-mail Address

OBJECTIVE   To obtain a graduate nurse position in a pediatric intensive care unit.

EDUCATION   **STATE UNIVERSITY**
                         City, State
                         Bachelor of Science in Nursing, to be awarded, Month Year
                         Cumulative Grade Point Average: 3.67/4.0

CLINICAL EDUCATION   **Community Health—Community Center**
                         Provided immigrant patient population with information needed to access health care
                         in the United States. Organized community resources for elderly patients.

                         Pediatric Clinical—City Hospital
                         Provided care to children of all stages of development on a general pediatrics unit.
                         Focused on developmental issues, medication administration, and provided support
                         and education to family and patient.

                         Psychiatric Clinical—Psychiatric Hospital
                         Participated in care of patients with a variety of mental health disorders.
                         Worked to improve therapeutic communication and mental health assessment skills.

                         Emergency Department Clinical Elective—University Medical Center
                         Enhanced clinical skills including triage, assessment techniques, medication administra-
                         tion, and cardiac monitoring. Performed a wide range of complex nursing skills includ-
                         ing intravenous therapy and management, wound care, and nasogastric tube mainte-
                         nance.

                         Obstetrics Clinical—City Hospital
                         Provided care for mothers and infants in high-risk antepartum, labor and delivery, post-
                         partum, and neonatal intensive care units. Monitored status and provided intrapartum
                         care to at-risk mothers and newborns; taught new mothers infant care.

                         Medical–Surgical Clinical—University Medical Center
                         Provided care to patients admitted to general medical–surgical units, focused on clinical
                         assessment, assisting with activities of daily living, cardiac monitoring, teaching, med-
                         ication administration, patient rehabilitation, and comfort measures.

EXPERIENCE   **City Hospital—Dates**
                         City, State
                         Pediatric Intensive Care Unit
                         Nurse Technician
                         Responsible for monitoring patient status prior to transport, assisted in stabilizing new
                         patients admitted to PICU, and gathered supplies and prepared patients for proce-
                         dures.

HONORS   Golden Key Honor Society
                         University Presidential Scholarship Recipient

Table 18–7   Chronological Resume for a New Graduate Using a Qualification Summary

Name
Address
Phone Number and E-mail Address

QUALIFICATION SUMMARY

In my experience at State University, I have focused on polishing my clinical skills, performing patient teaching, and caring for patients holistically, and am currently interested in pursuing a position in the NICU to fulfill my goals in nursing.

EDUCATION

STATE UNIVERSITY
City, State
Bachelor of Science in Nursing, to be awarded, Month Year
Cumulative Grade Point Average: 3.67/4.0

CLINICAL EDUCATION

State University—City, State
Level II Fieldwork (year to present)

City Hospital Neonatal Intensive Care Unit—City, State
Worked one-on-one with a nurse preceptor during a 4-week, 120-hour clinical internship caring for high-risk infants. Drew labs, fed infants by gavage and nipple, performed developmental care, assessed blood gas values, and consulted with physicians, respiratory therapists, families, and other health care staff to plan holistic care for patients.

City Hospital Emergency Department—City, State
Triaged emergency room patients, started IVs, inserted Foley catheters and nasogastric tubes, assisted staff during traumas, and conducted discharge teaching.

Children's City Hospital—City, State
Calculated pediatric medication dosages, administered medications via syringe pump, conducted play therapy sessions, and collaborated with pediatricians, nurses, and families to organize patient care.

Psychiatric Hospital—City, State
Communicated therapeutically with patients, assisted patients with recovery process, and conducted teaching sessions regarding medication regime.

Level I Fieldwork (year to year)
University Medical Center—City, State
Assisted patients with activities of daily living, administered oral and perenteral medications, and assisted patients with rehabilitation exercises.

University Medical Center—City, State
Interpreted electrocardiograms, assessed heart sounds, administered medications, prepared patients for cardiac procedures, and customized plan of care.

University Medical Center—City, State
Assessed high-risk antepartum patients, guided patients through the labor process, monitored fetal heart tones, and implemented pain relief and relaxation measures.

OTHER EXPERIENCE

City Hospital—Dates
City, State
Nurse Extern—Mother/Baby Unit (PRN, Month year to present)
Performed perineal care, assisted mothers with breastfeeding, monitored intake and output, and assessed, bathed, and fed newborn infants.

MEMBERSHIPS

University Student Nurse Association (year–year)

Table 18-8 Functional/Skills Resume for an Experienced Nurse

Megan D. Jones
2222 Smith Circle
Dallas, Texas 75246
214/222-2222

OBJECTIVE	Staff nurse position in a level one trauma emergency department.
SKILLS	**Psychomotor** Fully qualified to provide a wide range of skills including physical assessment across the age spectrum. Able to initiate and maintain cardiac monitoring and IV therapy, perform gastric lavage; experienced in safely administering and monitoring the effectiveness of a wide range of medications; and accurately follows protocols using central (PIC, port-a-cath, triple lumen, etc.) and peripheral lines. Able to function as any needed member of a CPR team. Familiar with current medication management in emergency services. Able to correctly administer a variety of volume expanders. **Interpersonal** Have worked effectively as a team member; able to recognize the emotional needs of patients, families, and peers. Experienced in conflict management. Sensitive to legal protocol and interpersonal needs of victims of violent crimes. **Critical Thinking and Judgment** Experienced in triaging a wide range of patients under demanding circumstances. Able to establish priorities based on clinical presentation of patients; recognize lethal arrhymias and initiate appropriate response; and accurately differentiate between urgent and emergent patient needs while reassuring and instilling confidence in patients and families regarding needed care.
EDUCATION	**Baylor University** Louise Herrington School of Nursing, Dallas, Texas Bachelor of Science in Nursing, May 1996 Minor: Spanish

EXPERIENCE	Hill Community Hospital, Waco, Texas Staff Nurse 4E Trauma Services	June 1996–May 2001
	Pinecrest Memorial Medical Center, Dallas, Texas Staff Nurse Medical Intensive Care Unit	June 2001–present
Additional Information	CPR Basic Life Support Certification CPR Instructor	May 1995–present August 2000–present
	American Heart Association Advanced Life Support Certification	July 2001–present
	Bilingual: Spanish	

ogy allows the employer to access the resume based on keywords or "buzzwords" that identify the resume, and thus the applicant as a potential employee. When a job description is posted, key words tell the applicant whether he or she is qualified for the job. These same words can be used in conjunction with scanner technol-

ogy to locate a qualified applicant who has submitted a resume. Keyword searches are usually based on skills, abilities, and competencies; experience; and accomplishments. For example, a human resource specialist may use scanner technology to search for all applicants whose resumes reflect the following:

- Current RN license or interim permit
- BSN
- Current CPR
- Hematology/oncology position

To ensure that a resume is scanner friendly, the font should be simple, with 11 or 12 point font. Italics, script, and underlined passages tend to be problematic, while bold print is generally acceptable, though capital letters can be a substitute. Horizontal and vertical lines should be used sparingly. Resumes printed on plain, white letter-quality paper using a laser printer are most easily scanned. The name of the applicant is best placed on each page of a resume with contact information appearing on the first page only. Resumes that have been faxed are also problematic. To decrease the likelihood of errors in a faxed resume, set the machine on "fine" rather than "standard" mode.

RESUME WRITING PITFALLS

The resume should be a concise statement of the nurse's background. Most new graduates are able to provide this information in one page. More experienced nurses may require two pages. No resume should exceed two pages. The resume must be without typographical, grammatical, or spelling errors. The quality of the resume is seen as a reflection of the professionalism of the applicant. Applicants should have at least two other people critically proofread the resume. The applicant should avoid having friends read the resume who are unwilling to provide constructive input.

Resumes should always be easy to read; therefore, it is imperative that they be typed and copied in a professional manner. The font should be no smaller than 11 point. The resume is a summary document; therefore, complete sentences are not required. The applicant should avoid being wordy or using phases that "sound good" but are so vague as to be meaningless (e.g., "able to provide holistic patient-centered care" sounds good, but what does it mean?). It is equally important to give enough information. Simply stating that past employment included a position as a nursing technician at a certain hospital does not tell the reader much. The applicant would want to include job duties, experiences obtained, or type of patients cared for.

Even a new graduate with no work experience will soon find that one page is very short when it comes to developing a resume; therefore, irrelevant information should not be included (e.g., social sororities, marital status, age, sex, children, height, weight, health, church membership, hobbies). Both the resume and cover letter should be customized to a specific job. One resume does not fit all positions. Generic resumes are passed over for the resume that clearly presents the candidate as qualified for a given position.

As a final consideration, it is important the resume is not too snazzy, boring, or modest. The applicant should portray a professional but accurate presentation of skills and abilities. Most health care facilities tend to be conservative, so pink, blue, or violet stationery may not reflect the image that is being sought. Similarly, black ink is professional and does not need to be offset by blue or red. To avoid boring the reader the applicant should use action verbs, outline what he or she has accomplished, and avoid starting every sentence or section with the same word. No matter how modest the nurse is the resume should reflect competence without misrepresenting ability.

Job Application Form

All prospective employers will expect applicants to complete a job application form. The resume is not a substitute for the application form. The applicant should never write on an application form "See Resume." Job applications can be obtained directly from an agency's human resource department; for convenience, many institutions have handy online application forms. If possible, the job application should be filled out completely prior to the interview. The applicant should take care in providing a legible, neatly writ-

---

Critical Thinking and Reflection

So it is time to get a job. Make sure your cover letter and resume don't scream "I need a job and any job will do." The fact is, any job won't do and if you present as an applicant for any job, then in all likelihood, given the current nurse shortage, you will get the job no one else wants. List three to five pieces of information about you that make you stand out as a candidate for a *specific job*. How can you include this information in your resume or cover letter?

ten or typed application. The applicant must avoid errors in grammar and spelling. Black ink is best suited for both copy purposes and professional appearance. The applicant should take care in signing the application by providing the reader with a legible signature. Remember, both legible and illegible handwriting will make an impression.

It is imperative that the application form be filled out completely and accurately. Since application forms always require dates of past employment, the applicant should maintain an employment file in which these dates and the name of relevant supervisors can be readily accessed. Any erroneous information provided on an application can be construed as fraudulent and provide the basis for later termination of employment.

DRESS FOR SUCCESS

Appearance, attitude, and behavior are important factors to consider when preparing for an interview. Regarding attitude and behavior, the nurse applicant must remember that these need to be displayed not only to the interviewer, but also to his or her representatives (e.g., secretaries and administrative assistants). Behavior is monitored in every contact with the prospective employer, from first contact through acceptance of the job. Even phone behavior is closely scrutinized. A written record of each contact with an employing institution is likely to be maintained to monitor prospective employees. The behavior of the nurse is under scrutiny by management as well as staff throughout the interview process. The interview is a time to display those qualities that attract employers; therefore, the applicant must demonstrate professional behavior. Employers recognize that how an interviewee treats a receptionist may reflect how that interviewee may treat a patient or other staff members when frustrated.

Both the potential employer and the applicant form first impressions. A good way to begin that first impression is with a firm handshake and a smile. Most individuals hope to obtain employment based on qualification, but the reality of today's world is that appearance often makes a significant difference. It is an unfortunate reality that individuals are judged, whether consciously or unconsciously, on appearance including clothing, makeup, hygiene, body size, gender, cultural symbols, and age. In most cases these impressions are not ethically, legally, or morally correct; however, the interviewee has no power to control judgments made by the interviewer and in most cases will be unaware of these judgments. At the time of the interview, the nurse has no control over body size, gender, or age. The interviewee does have the power to present him- or herself in the most favorable light possible for the interview. The applicant does control hygiene and dress, and should make conscious decisions regarding the impression being sought. In all cases the nurse must be clean, well groomed, and free of body odors including fragrance from perfume. Generally, clothing should be professional, though in some interview environments more casual clothing may be preferred (e.g., outpatient or walk-in clinics where business dress could cause discomfort for the clients). The key is to know the institution. Applicants should not purchase expensive suits, restrictive clothing, or short skirts for the interview. It is better for the applicant to err on the side of conservative than to be overdressed. The interviewee's appearance should not distract the interviewer (e.g., keep jewelry to a minimum).

The Interview

While dressing for success is extremely important, it is equally important for the new graduate to do his or her homework in preparing for the interview. To prepare for the interview the nurse should learn about the institution, its mission, purpose, and philosophy. This information is generally available via the Internet or can be obtained directly from the institution prior to the interview.

Remember that while the prospective employer is interviewing the prospective employee, the reverse should also be true. The interview should be a two-way conversation. Generally, interviewers go into an interview with a set of questions designed to determine the competency, interest, and suitability of an interviewee. Box 18–2 provides applicants with a list of commonly asked questions. Preparation for an interview includes planning responses to potential questions and practice with a peer or family member who is willing to serve as a human resource representative role model.

The American Association of Colleges of Nursing publishes a "tip sheet" detaining *What Every Nursing Student Graduate Should Consider When Seeking Employment* (1999). In that document, students are encouraged to ask, "Does your potential employer . . .

- Manifest a philosophy of clinical care emphasizing quality, safety, interdisciplinary collaboration, continuity of care, and professional accountability.
- Recognize the value of nurses' expertise on clinical care quality and patient outcomes.
- Promote executive level nursing leadership.
- Empower nurses' participation in clinical decision-making and organization of clinical care systems.

Demonstrate professional development support for nurses (1999)."

Interview behavior should be positive, polite, and professional. Most interviewers respect and look for enthusiasm and an energetic, positive attitude in potential employees. Giddy nervousness, immaturity, and hyperactivity are not the same as enthusiasm. While physical appearance should not distract the interviewer, neither should behavior. It is important for the applicant to monitor behavior throughout the interview. The applicant should avoid being overly casual/familiar while being professional and receptive. The applicant should make eye contact with the interviewer but also remember to blink and avoid staring at the interviewer or the ceiling. Formal titles should be used when addressing the interviewer (e.g., Mr., Mrs., or Ms.). Interviewers should not be addressed by their first name unless they have initiated this familiarity.

The interviewee should also prepare a set of questions designed to determine the suitability and compatibility of the hiring institution with the applicant's personal and professional values, interests, and needs. By preparing for the interview, the new graduate is more likely to obtain employment that will provide long-term professional satisfaction.

Job interviews tend to be somewhat stressful; therefore, the nurse may wish to write questions down prior to the interview. The nurse can be certain the interviewer will ask if the applicant has any questions. Several questions should be prepared beforehand to (a) ensure that the applicant has acquired all information needed for making an employment decision, (b) show interest in the prospective employer, and (c) avoid uncomfortable silences, which will come if the applicant is nervous. Box 18–3 offers a list of questions applicants may wish to ask employers. These questions are designed to help the applicant make final employment decisions. It is important that this data is collected from all prospective employers for comparative analysis of available employment opportunities.

The nurse is wise to bring a nice pen and notepad to the interview to take notes for later reference when evaluating employment alternatives. Note taking helps the applicant appear engaged in the interview. The interviewer will most likely take notes throughout the interview, though some interviewers defer note taking

---

Box 18–2   Common Interview Questions

Nursing Philosophy
- Tell me what you want from your first nursing position.
- What do you find rewarding about nursing?
- What do you like about nursing? What do you dislike?
- How would you describe your philosophy of nursing?
- What turns you on about nursing? What turns you off?

Personal Attributes
- What are your least and most favorite aspects of nursing?
- What motivates you to put forth your greatest effort?
- Tell me about yourself (your short-term goals/long-term goals).
- What is one strength that makes you a good candidate for this position? Tell me about your greatest professional weakness. How will this affect the way you approach a job as a staff nurse?
- How would you describe your personality?
- How would you describe yourself, a leader or a follower? Explain?

Personal Goals and Planning
- Is there any particular area you are interested in?
- Why did you select to interview at this institution?
- What do you plan to do for continuing education?
- Tell me something about your academic background (i.e., clinical and theory classes). Which one(s) did you like most? Why? Which one(s) did you like least? Why?
- Professionally, where do you want to be in 2 years? 5 years? 10 years?

(continued)

Box 18–2   (continued)

Ability

- What are your strengths and weaknesses?
- What do you feel you can offer our institution?
- How do you feel about working under pressure? Nursing shortage sometimes creates pressure situations due to staff shortages. How will you deal with this type of pressure?
- What qualifications do you have that make you feel that you will be a successful nurse in this position?
- What is your GPA? Overall? Nursing?
- What technical skills do you feel comfortable performing?
- What technical skills have you performed?

Work Setting

- How do you feel about working evening or overtime shifts?
- What influenced you to apply at this hospital/agency?
- What type of clinical experience do you hope to obtain by working with us?
- What type of position are you looking for?
- I see from your resume that you are interested in _____. Tell me why this is your first area of interest. Would you be willing to work in another area?
- Due to the current nurse staffing pattern, nurses are periodically pulled to other units. How do you feel about this?

Critical Thinking and Judgment

- Tell me about your most memorable client/patient. Why is this patient memorable? How did you influence the care of this individual?
- Tell me how you would respond to a patient that presented with
  - Hypoglycemia?
  - Malignant hypertension?
  - An angry family?
  - Drugs/alcohol abuse?
- Describe your most challenging patient situation.
- What lessons have you learned from your clinical experience?
- What types of patients do you have trouble working with?

and write down impressions immediately following the interview.

The applicant will wish to bring one or more copies of the resume and list of references. These may have been mailed to the institution, but the applicant should be prepared and have ready access to these documents during the interview. If the applicant is interviewed on several units within an institution, readily available resumes and references will be useful.

INTERVIEW TOPICS FOR DISCUSSION

The interview format can be formal, wherein the interviewer asks a set of prepared questions, or it may be more informal, wherein the recruiter allows the conversation to follow a more relaxed format. Most recruiters will initially try to "break the ice" with applicants by talking about a wide range of subjects, from the weather to current sport events. While this type of conversation may be pleasant and not appear to be part of the interview, informal conversations such as this allow the potential employer or employee to find out valuable information needed for hiring decisions (e.g., interpersonal skills, communication abilities). The applicant should pay as much attention to casual conversations during the interview as he or she does to the professional-focused interview and job-related questions. Care should be taken to avoid spending the entire interview discussing anything but the job. Table 18–9 offers the applicant a useful guide designed to present appropriate and inappropriate responses to interview questions.

Box 18–3   Questions to Ask Potential Employers

Please describe the duties of the job for me. What are the key responsibilities?
What kind of person are you looking for?
What kind of supervision, mentoring, and assignments might I expect the first six months of the job?
Does your agency encourage further education?
How often are performance reviews given?
Do you have plans for expansion?
Have you cut your professional staff in the last three years?
How do you feel about creativity and individuality?
Do you offer flex time?
In what ways is a career with your institution better than one with another agency?
What is the largest single problem facing your staff now?
What is the usual orientation time?
Has there been much turnover in this job area?
What qualities are you looking for in the candidate who fills this position?
What skills are especially important for someone in this position?
What opportunities for professional growth are available with this institution?
What is the next course of action? When should I expect to hear from you or should I contact you?

IMPROPER QUESTIONS

Early in the interview the recruiter will attempt to make the applicant feel comfortable. This can be achieved with carefully selected job-related questions. Recruiters generally avoid non-job-related questions; nurses should be aware that these questions may be intended to gain information about the applicant that is discriminatory and specifically not allowed by law. Legislative control of interview questions is designed to discourage discriminatory employment decisions. It is presently illegal to ask about an applicant's age, marital status, ethnic background, sexual orientation, national origin, social/religious/political preference, or arrest record. Questions regarding marital status and family plans are sometimes asked; however, these questions are illegal in many states.

Responses to particularly difficult or possibly illegal questions should be carefully worded. Rather than a direct response, which challenges the authority of the recruiter, the applicant may wish to take a more indirect response by asking how the information is needed for the particular position being sought. Most likely, the interviewer will provide an answer and move on to another line of questioning.

THE APPLICANT'S ROLE

Applicants can help guide the interview by actively taking a role in the process and avoiding monosyllabic answers. Discussions should be steered toward the career interest and qualifications of the applicant. The applicant should strive to (a) show they know about the hiring agency; (b) gain information needed to make an employment decision; (c) demonstrate interest, good interpersonal skills, and intelligence; and (d) allow the recruiter the opportunity to gather information. Initial topics the applicant may expect include:

- Clinical experience
- Positions available
- Career goals
- Long-term opportunities
- Corporate culture

Later in the interview the applicant can expect to discuss salary, benefits, retirement programs, holidays, and other benefits associated with the job. The informed applicant comes to an interview with knowledge regarding area and national salary norms and other benefits. If by the end of an interview the human resource representative has not discussed salary or benefits, it is acceptable for the applicant to ask questions regarding this information.

FOLLOW-UP

If the interviewer does not make a job offer, it is reasonable for the applicant to ask for information regarding the next step in the hiring process. At the completion of the interview, thank the interviewer, shake hands, and exit. A friendly smile, thank you, and good-bye should also be offered to others as the nurse

Table 18–9 Interview Questions

Questions	Answers	
	The Good, the Bad, and the Ugly	
What about this institution led you to apply for a position?	"I understand City Hospital is well known for its commitment to patient care excellence. As a teaching hospital I am also aware opportunities for my professional growth will be abundant."	"Well it's close to my home."
What are you looking for in your first job?	"The opportunity to provide total patient care with a combined emphasis on psychosocial, spiritual, and physiologic needs of patients. I am hoping to work in an institution that will provide me mentorship while I prepare to function autonomous."	"One with a lot of skills."
Tell me about your nursing school clinical experience.	"I had a wide variety of clinical experiences including rotations in medical–surgical nursing, obstetrics/gynecology, psychiatry, pediatrics, and community health. These rotations provided me with hands-on experience in a variety of clinical environments. In addition, I completed an elective in emergency room nursing at University Medical Center. The high intensity and critical thinking required in that environment were very exciting and challenging."	"It was great, I had the best instructors." Or "Well, I am sure you have heard my school of nursing isn't the best."
What clinical did you like best/least?	"I really enjoyed my pediatric clinical experience. This experience gave me the opportunity to develop skills in pediatric assessment, medication administration, and collaborative health care. Regarding my least liked clinical experience I would have to say that was my rotation on a psychiatric unit. Though I learned a lot about therapeutic communication and I use those skills daily in working with patients, I guess I just like hands-on patient care.	"All of them."
What nursing skills do you want to develop more fully in the next 12 months?	"I feel very comfortable providing basic patient care, but I continue to need support and supervision with more complex skills such as starting IVs, cardiac monitoring, and management of a cardiac emergency. The nursing program at State University placed strong emphasis on critical thinking, clinical assessment, and collaboration. I look forward to using these skills in my first job as an RN."	"All of them, I didn't have much experience in nursing school."
What rewards do you expect from your career?	"Providing care to patients is rewarding, but every once in a while there is that one patient that you feel you have really bonded with and had an influence in their life."	"Just the privilege of helping patients get well."

(continued)

Table 18–9 (continued)

Questions	Answers	
	The Good, the Bad, and the Ugly	
How would your clinical instructors describe you?	"Enthusiastic, motivated, and impulsive at times, but still able to recognize my limits."	"I have no idea."
What is your GPA?	"My overall GPA is a 2.5 and my current nursing GPA is a 2.8. As a student I supported myself through college. Working 20 hours a week did distract me as I am sure is reflected in my GPA. In my clinical rotations, my grades were predominantly Bs."	"2.5"
Tell me about a situation where you went above and beyond to help a co-worker or fellow student?	"During the winter of my senior year I participated in a medical missions trip to Mexico. This trip was offered to some as a clinical elective, but since I had already taken an elective I chose to take the trip to expand my knowledge of more diverse populations. I further enjoyed the opportunity to provide care for medically underserved patients."	"My nursing school was so full of busy work that I really didn't have time for much more."
Tell me about a situation where you made a mistake and how it was corrected?	"I once drew up the wrong medication. Fortunately, at State University we are well supervised by our clinical faculty. My instructor watched me draw up the wrong medication, walked with me down the hall, and then as I got ready to walk into the patient room, I checked the medication again and noted my error. My instructor smiled at me and said, 'I wondered when you were going to notice the mistake.' After I provided the patient with the right medication, my instructor and I reviewed my procedure and came up with ways for me to avoid mistakes such as this in the future. I think this experience may have made me a better nurse. I sure know I double check myself more."	"Where do I start? I gave medication to the wrong patient once but it didn't cause a problem."
How have you responded to other students or staff nurses when they have encouraged you to take short cuts that were not consistent with safe nursing practice?	"A nurse once told me not to worry about gowning and gloving as I wasn't going to really be doing much when I went in to my patient's room. This patient had VRE, was on contact precautions, and had multiple draining wounds, which were frequently not self-contained. I visited with my instructor regarding my concerns and we developed a plan. The plan included my role-modeling appropriate isolation technique during the time I cared for the client. My instructor visited with the unit supervisor regarding concerns. As a result, the unit had an in-service that I really think improved overall care and safety for all patients and staff on that floor."	"I listened and then did what I knew needed to be done."

If you are being interviewed and you are asked a question that is potentially illegal, how will you respond?

leaves. The applicant should not linger when the interview is complete.

Thank you letters should be sent to all individuals who help the applicant with the job search process. They serve to express appreciation, reemphasize qualification, restate interest, and provide supplemental information. Though not an essential feature of the job search process, the thank you letter is a courtesy overlooked by some and appreciated by many. A thank you letter should be sent promptly, within 24 hours of the interview or assistance. It should be sent to each person who interviewed the applicant. Additionally, thank you notes should be sent to those providing recommendation for the applicant. A sample thank you letter is found in Box 18–4.

The thank you letter may be handwritten on simple stationery or typed and formal using a business format. While this letter is a more personal form of professional correspondence, handwritten thank you letters that are not legible lose their value. If the applicant's handwriting is poor, it must be typed.

Selecting the Right Job

All job options should be carefully considered. Applicants should avoid making a quick decision that may later be regretted. In today's job market, the appli-

---

Box 18–4   Thank You Follow-up Letter

Name
Complete Address
City, State, Zip Code
Area Code/Phone Number
E-mail Address

Date

Name
Pediatric Intensive Care Coordinator
City Hospital
Address
City, State, Zip Code

Dear Ms. Name,

Thank you for spending the time with me during my interview for the graduate nurse position in the pediatric intensive care unit at City Hospital. I enjoyed our meeting and was able to gather valuable information about the unit, City Hospital, and the positions available for graduate nurses.

As a result of the interview, my desire to begin work with children in an intensive care setting has increased. I feel my education, clinical experiences, and skills fit with the job requirements.

I wish to reiterate my desire to become a member of your staff. Please call me at xxx/xxx-xxxx or contact me via e-mail at email.candidate if I can provide you with additional information. Again, thank you for the interview and for considering my application for employment as a graduate nurse in the pediatric intensive care unit at City Hospital.

Respectfully,

First and Last Name

Whether a nurse is offered a position in an interview or not, it is worthwhile to take time to evaluate the interview. Many factors contribute to the hiring of a nurse. It is good to review the interview experience in order to better prepare for future interviews. Ask yourself: (a) were you prepared, (b) did you convey your strengths and goals, (c) were your qualifications consistent with what the employer was seeking, and (d) did you look and behave your best?

---

cant may have several job offers. Selection decisions should be based on job requirements, the work climate, opportunities for career development, benefits, and availability of supervision/direction. Many applicants will face a dilemma regarding job selection when offered a job prior to completing the job search. When an offer is made, the applicant can choose to accept, decline, or ask for time to make a decision. Many new graduates ask if they should inform the prospective employer that they have not completed the job search. If the applicant is not ready to make a decision regarding a job, that applicant should simply ask for a specified period of time for making the decision. This implies that the applicant has not completed all interviews. During the time that a prospective employer waits for an applicant to make a decision, that employer is not obligated to "save" the position for the applicant if an equally or better qualified applicant seeks the position. Whenever deferring an employment decision, the applicant is taking a risk that another nurse may obtain the position. This is a risk a nurse should be willing to take when feeling undecided as to whether the job provides the right fit.

Consider the following when making an employment decision:

- Job content
  - Does the work appear satisfying?
  - Do you possess the appropriate skills?
  - Does the job offer a challenge?
  - Are there opportunities for professional growth?
- Development
  - Is the initial orientation/preceptorship/mentorship period sufficient and well organized?
  - Is continuing education offered by the agency?
  - What support (financial or work release time) is there for continuing education?
- Direction
  - What supervision is available?
  - What is the agency's philosophy of supervision?

- Work Climate
  - Is the work climate formal or informal, structured or unstructured, complex or simple?
  - Do the employees look professional and content?
  - Is the unit laid out in a comfortable manner that supports work efficiency?
- Compensation
  - What is the potential for an increase in salary?
  - How is work performance reviewed?
  - Is there a correlation between performance and increases in salary?

Negotiating What You Want

Negotiating can involve salary, work hours, and other forms of compensation. While many things about a first job may be nonnegotiable, the new graduate should not assume a position of powerlessness. Nurses in general, and more specifically women, are taught to be polite. Assertiveness has not traditionally been a cultivated personality trait. When assertiveness is employed individuals generally have increased self-confidence and find the results rewarding. Assertiveness may result in better compensation.

In one new graduate's job search, she was offered a set salary for a position in an emergency department. The hospital had not previously accepted new graduates, yet this senior nursing student conveyed confidence and experience through nursing school rotations that made her a viable candidate for the position. The graduate was also offered a sign-on bonus, which was very attractive. Recognizing that accepting the position required she relocate, the student asked about relocation benefits. The student later admitted she was simply doing what she had been told to do in her nursing class related to obtaining professional employment and really did not expect to receive an allowance for relocation. The graduate was told no allowances were offered for relocation.

When offered a job, this student had genuinely not completed the interview process and asked for two weeks to make final employment decisions. Two days after the interview, the human resource representative called the graduate to confirm the offer of employment, outline the sign-on bonus, and add a relocation incentive. This example is not intended to encourage the applicant to be manipulative in order to obtain better employment packages, but rather to outline how assertive behavior can possibly (a) result in employment in a position that had not previously been designed for graduate nurses and (b) improve the benefits package.

Preemployment and Postemployment Screening

Preemployment screening may be part of the selection process for new employees or it may be used after a nurse has accepted a position. According to Strader and Decker (1995), preemployment screening may include:

- Drug screening tests
- Verification of nursing license
- Two/three references of past employers or clinical instructors
- Educational transcripts
- Interviews with the nursing team
- Skills competency testing
- Criminal record verification

After an employee is hired, the employing agency may wish to obtain further information as a condition of employment. Employment may be conditional, based on information gathered during the screening process. For example, the applicant may be hired conditionally while verification of licensure is being sought. Further screenings that may be required include a physical examination with selected blood analysis or personality testing with standardized inventories. Most health care institutions will require intermittent/annual skill competency testing. Some may require occasional drug screening and criminal background checks.

TRANSITION INTO PRACTICE

This chapter has focused on obtaining professional employment, but what happens if it turns out the job selected is the wrong job? Generally, new graduates should remain in their first position for at least one year. While frustrating, it may take up to a year for a new nurse to sufficiently adjust to a position. Nurses who change positions frequently soon develop a reputation that makes employers reluctant to offer them positions.

If a nurse finds there is a need to change positions it is important to not only consider his or her needs, but also the needs of the staff, patients, and employer. It is always advisable to leave a position under amicable circumstances. Certain steps taken by the nurse will foster the likelihood of just such a change. The following should be considered when leaving a position. First, depending on the reason for the change, many encourage the nurse to notify an employer prior to making a final decision or accepting a new position. This may seem counterintuitive to quitting a job; however, in light of the nursing shortage, an employing agency may wish to work with the nurse to prevent that nurse from leaving the institution. The employer may have a more desirable position that the nurse would consider rather than terminating the relationship with the agency. In contrast, some will recommend that a notice of termination should not be issued until a final decision has been made to leave and another job obtained. Regardless of the decision the nurse makes regarding notification of an employer, the nurse should never "bluff" in order to manipulate a current employer to improve the employee's agency status.

When resigning a position, a nurse should provide a 2- to 4-week written notice. Care should be taken to avoid sharing the intent to resign with peers prior to the official notice to the employer. The nurse should remember that a reference may be required from the employer and should therefore resign in a courteous and private fashion. Resignation letters should simply and professionally state the (a) intent to resign, (b) effective date of the resignation, and (c) reason for the resignation. The letter should be unemotional, with no hint of vindictive animosity and in fact express a genuine appreciation of the experiences gained while employed. Finally, the letter should close in a gracious manner. A sample resignation letter is offered in Box 18–5.

If the nurse has signed an internship or work agreement, the commitment must be fulfilled in order to avoid possible financial penalties. Many employing institutions will work with the nurse to help him or her fulfill the obligation, if not on the assigned unit, then possibly at another site within the institutions.

Most institutions will have a formal termination process that may include a terminal interview, return of hospital property (including keys, badges, etc.), a mechanism for reaching the nurse for final paychecks, and a method for dispensation of any employee benefits (e.g., health insurance or unused vacation or leave time).

In today's mobile society it is doubtful any nurse will work for one employer throughout his or her career. It is more likely that several institutions will employ the nurse over a career. It is important that as the nurse moves on to new employment opportunities, current or old employers are treated respectfully and with courtesy. Professional behavior always increases the likelihood of a positive recommendation and the possibility of a return to the agency in the future.

Box 18–5   Resignation Letter

Name
Complete Address
City, State, Zip Code
Area Code/Phone Number

Date

Name, Title
Human Resources
City Hospital
Address
City, State, Zip Code

Dear Ms. Name,

I regret to inform you that following my marriage on June 1, 2004, I will be relocating to Reno, Nevada. Consequently, I am tendering my resignation May 15, 2004.

I have enjoyed my time at City Hospital. My tenure on 4N-ICU has been very satisfying. The staff are competent and supportive, the experiences challenging yet fulfilling, and the environment a one of respect and value of the professional staff. The mentorship and support of the staff on 4N-ICU have allowed me to develop professions with regard to my technical, interpersonal, and problem solving skills. I am proud to have been a member of the staff on such a competent and caring unit.

Thank you for the privilege of working at City Hospital. If I can be of assistance in preparing for my departure please feel free to contact me.

Respectfully,

First and Last Name
CC Joan Clark, RN
Coordinator 4N-ICU

KEY POINTS

1. The current nursing workforce shortage is of unprecedented severity and is expected to endure long into the future.
2. A search for a first job begins with a career plan that includes personal/professional goals based on a critical inventory of personal and professional skills.
3. A career trajectory provides guidance for a professional career in nursing. The first job should be selected as part of a well-thought-out plan.
4. It is important to be prepared to market yourself as a viable, strong candidate for a desired position.
5. The behavior of the nurse throughout the interview process is under scrutiny. The interview is a time to display professional behavior and those qualities that attract employers.
6. The applicant may have several job offers. Selection decisions should be based on job requirements, opportunities for career development, work climate, compensation, and availability of supervision/direction.
7. Consider job content, development, direction, work climate, and compensation when making an employment decision.
8. Preemployment screening may be part of the selection process for new employees. This screening generally can involve drug screening tests, verification of nursing license, references, educational transcripts, interviews, skills competency testing, and criminal record verification.

EXPLORE MediaLink

Critical thinking questions, essay questions, key terms, web links, activities, NCLEX review questions, and more interactive resources can be found on the Companion Website at www.prenhall.com/haynes. Click on Chapter 18 to select activities for this chapter.

REFERENCES

Aiken, L. H., Clarke, S. P., Sloane, D. M., Sochalski, J. A., Busse, R., Clarke, H., et al. (2001). Nurses' reports on hospital care in five countries: The ways in which nurses' work is structured have left nurses among the least satisfied workers, and the problem is getting worse. *Health Affairs, 20*(3), 43–53.

American Association of Colleges of Nursing. (1999). *Hallmarks of the professional nursing practice setting: What every nursing school graduate should consider when seeking employment.* Washington, DC: Author.

American Association of Colleges of Nursing. (May 2003). *AACN White Paper: Faculty Shortages in Baccalaureate and Graduate Nursing Programs: Scope of the Problem and Strategies for Expanding the Supply.* Washington, DC: Author.

American Hospital Association. (June 2001). The hospital workforce shortage: Immediate and future. *TrendWatch.* Dallas, TX: Author.

Baylor University Career Service. (2001). *The bear facts: A career development and job search guide.* Dallas, TX: Baylor University.

Brendtro, M., & Hegge, M. (2000). Nursing faculty: One generation away from extinction? *Journal of Professional Nursing, 16*(2), 97–103.

Bureau of Health Professions, Division of Nursing. (2001, February). *The national sample survey of registered nurses March 2000: Preliminary findings.* Washington, DC: Author.

Bureau of Labor Statistics. (November 1999). *Occupational employment projections to 2008.* Washington, DC: Author.

Hecker, D. E. (2001). Occupational employment projections to 2010. *Monthly Labor Review, 124*(11), Washington, DC: U.S. Department of labor, Bureau of labor Statistics.

Henderson, F. C., & McGettigan, B. O. (1994). *Managing your career in nursing* (2nd ed.). New York: National League for Nursing.

Marshal, E. E. (2001). Nursing workforce in practice and education: What can we learn from the current crisis? *Journal of Perinatal and Neonatal Nursing, 15*(1), 16–25.

Strader, M. K., & Decker, P. J. (1995). *Role transition to patient care management.* Norwalk, CT: Appleton & Lange.

The Nurse Shortage: Perspectives from Current Direct Care nurses and former direct care nurses. An opinion research study conducted by Peter D. Hart Research Associates on behalf of the Federation of Nurses and Health Professionals April 2001.

University of Illinois, Nursing Institute. (May 2001). *The future of health care labor force in a graying society.* Kaiser Family Foundation, Washington, DC: Author.

University of Iowa College of Nursing. (2002). *Men in nursing.* Iowa City, IA: The University of Iowa.

Uustal, D. B. (1992). The ultimate balance: Caring for yourself—Caring for others. *Orthopedic Nurses, 11*(3), 11–15.

SUGGESTED READINGS

Abrams, S. L. (2000). *The new success rules for woman.* Roseville, CA: Prima Publishing.

Allen, S. R., Thrasher, T., Wesolowski, C., Carroll, S., Schaffer, P., Eckstein, L., et al. (1998). Notes from the field. Peer interviewing: Sharing the selection process. *Nursing Management, 29*(3), 46.

Bernzweig, E. P. (1996). *The nurse's liability for malpractice: A programmed text* (6th ed.). St. Louis, MO: Mosby.

Bove, L. A. (2002). Tap Internet employment resources: Planning to you're your job search on line? Here's how. *Nursing Management, 33*(6), 51–52.

Crepeau, E. B., Thibodaus, L., & Parham, D. (1999). Academic juggling act: Beginning and sustaining an academic career. *American Journal of Occupational Therapy, 53*(1), 25–30.

Saver, C. (2000). Nursing in the new millennium. *Imprint, 46*(1), 35–36.

Serembus, J. F. (2000). Teaching the process of developing a professional portfolio. *Nurse Educator, 25*(6), 282–287.

Serumbus, J. F. (2000). Pocket full of miracles: A professional portfolio can be a powerful force in your career advancement. *American Journal of Nursing, 100*(11), 67.

Tanner, C. A. (1999). Developing the new professorate. *Journal of Nursing Education, 38*(2), 51–52.

19

Transition into Practice

Linda C. Haynes

> *Be the change you wish to make in the world.*
>
> *Mahatma Gandhi*

LEARNING OBJECTIVES

At the completion of this chapter, the reader will be able to:

- Explain the importance of successful role transition.
- Describe the process of professional socialization.
- Recognize the nurse's responsibility for ensuring successful transition into professional practice.
- Identify factors that influence successful bicultural socialization.

- Discuss essential skills for successful transition into professional practice.
- Apply selected models to professional socialization.
- Discuss reality shock.
- Explore the benefits of workplace orientation programs, preceptors, mentors, and internships.

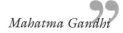 MediaLink www.prenhall.com/haynes

Additional online resources including NCLEX review questions, critical thinking questions, and real-world activities for this chapter can be found on the Companion Website at www.prenhall.com/haynes.

A positive, successful transition into professional practice is in the best interest of novice nurses, health care employers, the public, and the nursing profession. Transition is best embraced as a challenging opportunity. Novice nurses face exciting prospects for learning as newfound autonomy is explored. New graduate nurses have an extensive repertoire of skills for successful role transition from nursing student to professional nurse.

Preparing for the challenge of role transition can be compared to preparing to run a marathon. Successful achievement of this goal requires hard work and dedication. The marathon transition to professional practice requires hard work, dedication planning, and preparation. As with any other training program, preparation helps to avoid mishaps along the way. It is important for new nurses to recognize that the way they handle themselves during the transition is key to making the transition less painful. Successful transition requires that the new graduate:

- Gain greater self-awareness
- Handle that inner voice, which discourages, questions, warns, and leads to paralyzing feelings of helplessness
- Learn to make conscious choices by exploring beliefs and how they influence choices
- Take responsibility
- Gain awareness of inner strengths
- Explore vocabulary and speak to inner strength and authenticity
- Raise self-esteem
- Accept fear and discomfort as part of life and embrace it positively
- Analyze decisions made and the process used
- Dream
- Plan life
- Have a life

This chapter is intended to help the nursing student make the transition from student to professional nurse as successful as possible. The process of transition along with strategies for success and pitfalls to avoid will be discussed.

The Process of Transition

Transition is the process of moving from one state, stage, or place in life to another. Schumacher and Meleis (1994) classify four major types of transitions: (a) developmental, (b) health–illness, (c) organizational, and (d) situational. Examples of developmental transitions include puberty, becoming a parent, and retirement. Health–illness transitions are exemplified by adopting new health habits for a healthy lifestyle or for managing a chronic illness. Organizational transitions include changes in leadership, changes in staffing patterns, or even a change in the philosophy of an organization. Situational transitions include graduation, marriage, and beginning professional employment.

Whether developmental, health–illness, organizational, or situational, transition is synonymous with change. Change, as a threat to status quo, can be difficult. Nurses experience transition whenever moving from one role or setting to another. For nurses, one of the most significant and often most stressful transition occurs at graduation when the nursing student takes the title and assumes the responsibilities of the professional nurse (Godinez, Schweiger, Gruver, & Ryan, 1999). This transition may be simple requiring only minor adjustments or more complex marked by geographic, economic, social, and psychological upheaval.

Regardless of the complexity of the transition, the cumulative result is still change. David Welsh (2001) describes managing change as similar to navigating the white waters of a river. New nurses can apply Welsh's strategies for "navigating the white waters of change" to their transition to professional practice. In planning for this transition, Dr. Welsh advises that it is important to recognize the inevitability of change (e.g., graduation) and the predictable discomfort that accompanies growth (e.g., assuming responsibility for finances). New nurses who experience change are encouraged to remember previous successes (e.g., acceptance to nursing school and successful completion of course work), maintain a balance in life (e.g., good nutrition and exercise), and consider what life would be like without the change (e.g., care plans and exams). During change, it is especially important to recognize areas of relative constancy (e.g., faith, family, and friends). Finally, it is important to avoid feelings of victimization during change (e.g., redefine stress by labeling it as an opportunity or challenge). Table 19–1 summarizes Dr. Welsh's suggestions.

Professional Socialization: A Step in the Transition Process

Historical and societal factors combine with individual health care experiences mold an individual's percep-

Table 19–1   Navigating the "White Waters" of the Transition to Professional Practice

Strategy	Reality
Accept the reality of change.	The student has now graduated and can either return to school in a new student role, move into the workforce, or in some other way make a life change. No matter what else occurs in this student's life, the fact is the student has graduated and nothing will change that fact.
Recognize that pain accompanies growth.	Just as with any other growth experience in life, the transition from nursing school will be painful. How painful the experience will be and how much effort it will take to adjust to the pain is unknown, but the fact is growth is accompanied by pain.
Remember previous successes.	By remembering past success, the new graduate will have a frame of reference to draw from as he or she faces the challenges of transition to professional practice. Just as the nursing student was successful in that first visit with a patient, so can the new graduate be successful in role transition.
Explore the other side of change.	Students should remember that without graduation, they would still be writing care plans and studying for exams. While the thought of returning to the comfort and security of school may initially appear attractive to new graduates, the ultimate benefits of graduation will be realized with time.
Maintain balance in life.	Change associated with graduation will be difficult; the nursing student needs to have established a life outside school prior to graduation. When school is gone, as it will be at the time of graduation, the new graduate needs to have activities that will fill the void (e.g., reading, exercise, friendships).
Identify areas of relative constancy.	As a nursing student approaches the transition to professional practice, there must be recognition of something bigger than them as individuals. The new graduate should look around and find those constants that remain with them and help define who they will ultimately become within the professional group.
Refuse to be a victim.	Individuals who recognize that there is a finite time to life also recognize that there is not time to waste being a victim. Becoming a victim, just like becoming a victor, is to a great extent a choice. Choose to be a victor.
Redefine "success."	If success is earned, achieved, or acquired, then, with time and change, success can be taken away. To be successful in the transition into professional practice, the new graduate should make certain the definition of success is realistic.

tions of nursing. Critical early childhood health care experiences influence an individual's understanding of who nurses are and what they do. How a child interprets treatment during immunization experiences or routine physical exams clearly influences long-term expectations of nurses and other health care experiences. Books, television, and movies further influence an individual's perception of nursing. Students come to nursing with an image of nursing portrayed by nurses they have seen. A student's lay perception of nursing is transformed to a more professional understanding that is acquired in nursing school.

This process, called **professional socialization**, is the development and internalization of a professional identity. During the socialization process, values, behaviors, and attitudes necessary for assuming the role of nurse are learned along with knowledge and skills necessary to the role. As professional socialization to nursing progresses, each of these attributes become part of a nurse's personal and professional self-image and behavior.

Educational experiences play a vital role in socialization of nursing students as they observe and experience the culture of nursing (e.g., rites, rituals, and valued behaviors of the profession). Formal socialization occurs in both the classroom and clinical setting, where nursing students learn to assess needs; analyze data; and plan, implement, and evaluate effective care. Informal socialization occurs through lessons learned by observing or interacting with other health care providers.

Time spent in the clinical setting is a less structured educational experience that can be more powerful and memorable than formal classroom instruction. In the classroom, procedural steps are taught and emphasis is placed on the importance of each step, using specific scientific principles. The contextual influences of the clinical setting cannot be duplicated. Students are quizzed, evaluated, and observed using these formal techniques and steps. When students move into a clinical setting, they provide care and observe care given by other professionals. The action of a single nurse performing a task using precision and expertise can be a more powerful form of instruction than any formal classroom instruction.

Professional socialization, like learning, is lifelong and is especially important in a dynamic profession like nursing, where new technology and evolving roles demand continuous adaptation. Although socialization to the profession may begin in and be most strongly influenced by nursing school experiences, each nurse is accountable for continued lifelong professional growth and continued socialization.

Models of Professional Socialization

It is useful to think about the process of professional socialization using theoretical models. While the process of socialization may at first appear simple, it is in fact one of the most complex and critical aspects of becoming a professional. Models help explain how socialization takes place. Becoming an active participant in socialization, and evaluating personal progress through transition, will allow a nursing student or nurse to take an active role, thus influencing outcomes. The following models serve as a guide to active participation in socialization.

BANDURA'S MODEL

Bandura (1977) developed a model to explain the acquisition of new knowledge and behavior by modeling the actions of others who typically demonstrate the desired behavioral outcome. Using this approach to socialization, a nurse actively observes and makes conscious efforts to model actions similar to behaviors demonstrated by selected role models. In order to effectively achieve professional socialization through modeling, the new nurse identifies, observes, and learns from one or more experienced nurses who typify the behaviors, values, and attitudes most desired. From the observed behavior the novice learns both the professional role and expected patterns of behavior within that role. Observation (e.g., of experienced nurses, mentors, or preceptors) is followed by (a) intentional simulation of behavior and (b) evaluation of the new nurse's behavior by an experienced nurse, mentor, or preceptor.

DAVIS'S MODEL

While Bandura's model serves as a guide for acquisition of any new knowledge or behavior, Davis (1975) developed a model to explain the initial socialization experiences of nurses. He identified a set of sequential phases that describe the socialization process. The model focuses on the transition of a student's nonprofessional imagery of nursing to the development of a professional perspective for practice. Davis offers six stages to describe the process of professional socialization.

In stage 1, initial innocence, students new to college have an altruistic, service-oriented image of nursing. This stage is quickly followed by stage 2, incongruity, when the student realizes that learning to care for ill patients involves much more than physical care and includes (a) health and illness prevention; (b) forming therapeutic relationships; (c) technical mastery supported with clinical judgment; and (d) accountability and responsibility. In stage 2, students are able to articulate the incongruencies they have noted between the public image of nursing and the professional demands of becoming a nurse. As the realities of education and clinical practice collide students experience dissonance (a lack of harmony, discord, and discomfort). Students may see prerequisite educational requirements as more of a nuisance, hindrance, or even a roadblock that delays their ultimate goal of becoming a registered nurse. Once in basic nursing courses, patient care plans, theoretical models, and other seemingly mundane educational activities seem to further delay the ultimate "mission," which is care of patients. While providing care, patients themselves may further disillusion students. Nursing students are ill-prepared to deal with intractable pain, patients who are angry, or even patients who fail to recover. At this stage of the socialization process, students begin to question their career choice and some opt to leave nursing. Others become angry, frustrated, and disheartened.

As socialization continues and the student begins to identify more with selected role models, some will experience guilt and a sense of insincerity with the role being emulated (stage 3—"psyching out"). These students may feel they are performing to placate the instructor rather than fulfilling the role of professional nurse. As students become more successful with the role imitation, they become more comfortable (stage 4—role simulation). For example, therapeutic communication, a technique that had felt awkward and insincere becomes more natural and second nature. Technical skills are being performed with greater ease.

In stage 5, provisional internalization, the student will continue to cling to some of their old images and ideals while continuing to move forward and incorporate new ideals. As socialization continues, the nursing student is exposed to both positive and negative role models. This exposure helps to further strengthen the bond the student is developing with the nursing profession as selected skills, values, beliefs, and behaviors are internalized. Stable internalization, stage 6, is achieved when the professional image of nursing is fully integrated. The student has moved beyond the media-based image of nursing, and has accepted and is comfortable with the realities of professional nursing practice. There is a balance between academic, professional, and personal expectations.

Reality Shock

There is great disparity between what is taught and what is possible to achieve within an 8- to 12-hour shift, 3 to 5 days a week. In her landmark study, Kramer (1974) described first work experiences of new graduate nurses as a "reality shock." **Reality shock** sets in when a student or new graduate applies idealistic expectations from nursing school to the workplace. When the graduate moves from the classroom to the work setting, priorities and pressures change. In nursing school, the dominant value taught is based on comprehensive, individualized patient care with family involvement. Judgment, autonomy, cognitive skills, and decision-making are strongly reinforced. In the work setting, organization, efficiency, cooperation, and responsibility are highly valued. As new graduates strive to balance the needs of the patient with the needs of the health care setting, conflict arises.

Individuals of many professions experience reality shock; it is not specific to nursing. As a group, however, new graduate nurses consistently experience intense levels of reality shock. The four phases of reality shock: honeymoon, shock or rejection, recovery, and resolution are summarized in Table 19–2.

HONEYMOON

The honeymoon phase is short lived; it begins and may end in nursing school. During this phase there is a naïve excitement or fascination with the daily prospect of nursing. Initially, the novice cannot believe how wonderful everything is. Years are spent in preparing for and achieving the ultimate goal of becoming a nurse.

Internships and mentoring serve to support newfound freedoms and enthusiasms; however, they also serve to delay the reality shock associated with employment and autonomy. New graduates see their salary as an added bonus to the clinical work they had once performed for free as students. A regular paycheck means bills can be paid and new clothes bought. In this phase, students and new graduates are concerned with two major activities: (a) mastery of skills and routine and (b) social integration.

SHOCK (REJECTION)

Once orientation is over reality begins to set in as the student or new graduate begins to care for patients. The reality of daily assignments and responsibility for patient care can be overwhelming. No longer does the new graduate have an instructor to rely on, short clinical days, and two-day workweeks. Performance of skills by observation or under supervision no longer cushions the new graduate's reality. Excitement is replaced with shock, fear, and confusion. When the new graduate tries to accomplish a goal and finds the path blocked by personal inadequacies or system realities, there is further shock and frustration.

These realities are complicated by the fatigue associated with long work hours. The shock phase is characterized by moral outrage, rejection, fatigue, and perceptual distortion. Rejection of school or the work scene can be expected. With rejection of school, the new nurse can project blame onto the quality of past instruction or the inadequacy of instructors. By rejecting the work scene, the novice nurse can project blame on the staff and may change positions or leave nursing. The new nurse experiences increasing levels of fatigue, which can lead to somatic discomfort. Perceptions become distorted and the new graduate is as negative as he or she had once been positive during the honeymoon phase. The graduate's views are negatively polarized; there is difficulty receiving information without negatively distorting it with preconceived opinions. This phase cannot go on forever, since anger, moral outrage, and frustration are exhausting.

RECOVERY AND RESOLUTION

For nurses who learn to work within the system to make change, recovery is the next predictable phase of

Table 19–2   Kramer's Stages of Reality Shock

Phase	Presentation	Duration	Defining Statement
Honeymoon	Excited, naïve, fascinated with the daily prospect of coming to work	Begins shortly after orientation and is usually short lived	The novice nurse can't believe how wonderful everything is; there are no complaints and as an added bonus the novice is now receiving a paycheck.
Shock and Rejection	Excessive fear and mistrust; increasing somatic complaints, decreased energy and fatigue; hypercritical; displays a sense of moral outrage; blames others and is unable to effect positive change	Duration varies; many nurses fail to resolve the sense of shock, rejection, and disappointment	The novice nurse may be heard to say, "I've never done this," "Who will supervise me?", "Let me watch one more time," or "That wasn't the way we did it in nursing school."
	To adapt to shock and resistance rejection the novice nurse may:		
	• Go native	• Seeks the path of least resistance	• "That is the way we do it here."
	• Become a "runaway"	• Chooses a different occupation or returns to school	• "By returning to school I can teach others what it means to be a nurse."
	• Develop protective "rutters"	• Nursing becomes a means to an end, a paycheck	•"I'll just do what it takes to get by."
	• Burn out	• Conflict is bottled up	• "It's just not worth the aggravation."
	• Become a loner	• Just does the job, keeps quiet, and stays to themselves	• "Working nights you just don't have to hassle with the bureaucracy."
	• Seek to remain the "new kid on the block"	• Changes jobs frequently	• "I'm new here, just tell me what to do."
	• Become an agent for change	• "Bicultural trouble makers" (Kramer, 1974) work within the system to make change	• Keeps the welfare of the patient at the forefront
Recovery	A return of humor	Varies with the individual; some nurses never recover from reality shock	The nurse begins to develop confidence and a belief that skills and care will improve and become more efficient.
Resolution	An adjustment to the new environment	Professional growth and lifelong learning continue throughout a professional career.	Work expectations are more easily met and the nurse is able to elicit change.

reality shock. Recovery is marked by the return of a sense of humor. The new nurse can begin to laugh at those things about nursing and the job that may have once caused shock, annoyance, or frustration. No longer does the graduate view everything as a challenge. During this phase the nurse begins to develop confidence and a belief that skills and patient care abilities will improve and become more efficient.

Successful recovery from reality shock leads to the final stage, resolution or adjustment to the new work environment. Once the nurse has reached resolution, there is greater ease in meeting work expectations. This nurse is able to influence change.

The Responsibility for Clinical Competence

Attrition from nursing is greatest among new nurses (Dearmun, 2000). The vast majority of new graduates choose to begin their careers in hospital settings. Though new graduates are clearly prepared for positions outside acute care settings, most generally chose familiar acute care settings because they feel the need to boost clinical skills (Kelly, 1996). At the time of graduation, a theory/practice gap exists between what a new graduate knows to be theoretically true and the amount of time this nurse has spent in clinical practice to develop clinical competence. This theory/practice gap creates a dynamic tension, which motivates actions needed for adaptation during transition (Rafferty, Allcock, & Lathlean, 1996). The ability to fill this gap and merge school values, knowledge, and beliefs with those found in the workplace is known as **biculturalism** (Kramer, 1974).

Experienced nurses play an important role in the bicultural socialization of new nurses who lack confidence in their technical skills, which may, in fact, be as good as those of many staff nurses. While experienced nurses can help new graduates appreciate their abilities and avoid devaluing themselves, the new graduate must take the responsibility to create a personal environment conducive to successful transition. Self-statements of inadequacy serve as self-fulfilling prophecies. It is important for new nurses to have a realistic sense of self and competency. In taking personal responsibility for successful transition the graduate nurse evaluate clinical skills against realistic rather than perfectionist standards. Mentors and preceptors have an invaluable role in helping nursing students and novice nurses avoid exposing themselves to undue self-criticism.

Most nurses desire to be the best nurse—not just an ordinary nurse but rather a "super nurse" (Davidhizar & Shearer, 1999). Most nursing students are oblivious to the fact that being a super nurse is not only unrealistic, but also in the long run impossible. When new graduates are unable to meet all the needs of both patients and the institution, they experience a sense of failure. This type of self-evaluation based on perfectionism can lead to frustration, anxiety, depression, dissatisfaction, and potentially a career change. Many individuals remain in nursing just long enough to prove to themselves that they can do the job. Once this need is satisfied, the new nurse may move on to a new position or even leave nursing for something more attractive. The loss of these new graduates is a loss to the institution, the patient, and the profession. For each new nurse who leaves nursing, the profession loses both a prospective leader and the caring potential of that individual. To better prepare new nurses for transition to the workplace and thus decrease attrition, faculty and experienced nurses are becoming increasingly more resourceful in assisting students to realistically evaluate their competency and the expectations they set for themselves.

Nursing students generally express concern about competency or the "possession of the skills, knowledge, and understandings needed to do the job of a nurse" (Schmalenberg & Kramer, 1979). Discussions involving competency usually refer to technical, interpersonal, and organizational competency. In these discussions, it is important to recognize that individuals and employers perceive competency differently. For the new nurse, the question of competence is not really one of knowledge, organization, or even technical ability. At this point, most new nurses are actually asking "Do I have it in me to do this job?" From the institutional perspective, the question is not "Can the new graduate do the job," but "How much supervision does the new nurse need to do the job safely?" Health care providers are very interested in knowing when a new nurse will be able to function independently.

For nurses today, there is more knowledge to gain and more technology to master. Furthermore, there is a renewed commitment, by the profession, for these nurses to understand and integrate the core values of professional practice. Because there is so much for the novice nurse to learn, institutional personnel recognize that teaching is not the sole responsibility of nursing faculty and that learning is not complete at the time of graduation. While both the new graduate and the employer are clearly concerned with competency, neither should be under the impression that the new graduate is a finished product who is ready to function independently without supervision. In order to gain the knowledge, skill, and understanding to be an effective nurse the employer and new graduate share the responsibility for continued professional development.

When evaluating your own competency, what do you perceive to be your strengths and weaknesses? What are the responsibilities of faculty, staff, and the employer for ensuring your competence for providing safe care to patients? What are your responsibilities for attaining, maintaining, and sustaining competence in light of ever-changing technology and patient demands? Does the responsibility for competence lie with the profession, the institution, or the individual?

Developing Emotional Competence

Nurses, along with the general public, are taught that success is dependent on intellectual ability, a strong work ethic, and personal motivation. In nursing school, students are taught that they must also be able to critically think and have technical expertise in order to be successful. Despite our beliefs regarding intellectual ability, critical thinking, and the ability to perform technical skills, not all bright, motivated, skilled nurses are successful. In fact, neither cognitive intelligence nor the ability to perform highly technical activities is a guarantee for success. Furthermore, nurses who believe that the road to professional autonomy and success is via high-tech activities that attract power, prestige, and a nod from the elite in the profession are ensuring nurses will remain assistants to the medical profession and an exploited workforce within the bureaucracy of the health care institutions (Stevens & Crouch, 1998).

While cognitive ability, motivation, critical thinking ability all influence achievement, Daniel Goleman (1994, 1998) suggests that emotional intelligence may be one of the best predictors of an individual's ability to be successful. **Emotional intelligence** is a measure of the:

- Capacity to recognize and manage one's own feelings
- Ability to identify feelings in others
- Power to motivate oneself
- Capacity to handle relationships
- Ability to manage emotions in oneself

Emotional competence is a learned capability based on emotional intelligence. The practical skills related to emotional competence are based on self-awareness, self-regulation, motivation, empathy, and social skills. Table 19–3 summarizes these skills.

Self-awareness is characterized by the ability of a nurse to recognize his or her own feelings. This awareness also involves the ability to use this understanding to guide decision-making. Nurses with emotional awareness are alert to how they may respond emotionally and how their feelings can affect thinking and performance. Self-awareness is based on realistic self-assessment abilities. Nurses who are capable of realistic self-assessment (a) are able to reflect on past performance and learn from experience, (b) are open to feedback and the perspective of others, (c) seek continuous learning and self-development, and (d) maintain a sense of humor and perspective about themselves and their situation. Some of the specific "blind spots" to an accurate self-appraisal include ambition, unrealistic goals, relentless striving, power hunger, insatiable need for recognition, preoccupation with appearances, and the need to be perceived as (if not be) perfect (Goleman 1994, 1998).

Self-regulation, the ability to manage internal emotional states, impulses, and resources, is the second personal competency necessary for the development of emotional competence—it is characterized as handling emotions in a manner that facilitates rather than interferes with task completion. Self-regulation involves the ability to be conscientious and delay gratification when working toward a goal. With self-regulation, a new graduate can recover from emotional stress versus "getting even" or holding a grudge. Self-regulation involves self-control, the capability to manage emotional responses and impulses, to be composed and positive, and to think clearly so as to be able to focus under pressure. Self-regulation involves the ability to take responsibility for personal performance. The self-regulated nurse is innovative and comfortable with novel ideas, approaches, and information. The innovation may be a willingness to participate in an innovative fashion or a willingness to develop innovative evidence-based strategies for

Table 19–3 Emotional Competence

Skill	Definition	Characteristics of the Nurse with Emotional Competence
Self-aware	The ability to recognize one's own feelings	• In touch with his or her own feelings and values • Has an accurate sense of personal strengths and weaknesses • Sense of self-confidence • Recognizes feelings are important and provide valid information about stressful situations
Self-regulated	The ability to manage personal feelings/emotions	• Able to handle emotions while allowing passions to emerge • Able to control distressing emotions such as anger, sadness, and anxiety • Accepts responsibility for emotional responses • Defines situations as challenging rather than stressful
Self-motivated	The drive for achievement, commitment, initiative, and optimism	• Recognizes emotions affect performance • Manages setbacks effectively • Asks "What can I fix?" rather than "What is wrong with me?" • Knows what can be changed and what he or she is powerless to change • Able to focus attention
Empathy	The ability to recognize and respond to the emotions of others	• By expressing empathy, this nurse can create empathy in others • Recognizes that emotions affect measurable goals and productivity • Knows that problem solving may include a recognition and validation of feelings
Social skills	A culmination of all of the other skills that make up emotional competence and lead to collaborative interpersonal relationships	• Able to influence and persuade others to a higher level of collaboration • Builds consensus and supports team goals • Motivates and inspires

patient care. Certainly innovation requires accurate knowledge.

This nurse can stay committed, feel in control, and be challenged rather than threatened by stressful conditions. Handling multiple demands and adjusting one's daily or ongoing priorities with appropriate personal responses and tactics are examples of the adaptability found in self-regulated nurses.

Self-regulation requires trustworthiness and conscientiousness. These capabilities allow the nurse to act ethically and above reproach, to build and sustain trust through reliability and authenticity, owning personal mistakes and confronting others for unethical actions even if the cause is unpopular. Keeping promises, showing up, being accountable and responsible, and being both organized and meticulous in job performance are examples of the actions of the conscientious nurse (Goleman 1994, 1998).

Motivation is the third personal competency. Motivated individuals love what they do and expect excellent performance from themselves. The motivational component of emotional competence includes the drive for achievement, commitment, initiative, and optimism. Achievement involves being results oriented, having drive to complete challenging goals with calculated risk, and seeking new knowledge and skills to meet goals and improve performance. Commitment involves aligning with the goals of a work group or organization and may involve:

• Offering self-sacrifice for larger goals
• Having a sense of purpose congruent with the larger mission
• Taking on the group's core values
• Seeking opportunities to contribute to the group's mission

Using a motivational framework, initiative is almost synonymous with being proactive and optimistic while being persistent. Nurses who demonstrate initiative seize opportunities, go beyond basic expectations, mobilize others, and "bend the rules" or cut the red tape to get the job done and accomplish the goals of the group. The optimistic nurse is persistent, with a "hope for success," and recognition that setbacks are not personal flaws but opportunities that are manageable (Goleman 1994, 1998).

Empathy, the fourth personal competency, involves the ability to recognize the feelings, interests, needs, and reactions of others. This is a skill that all new graduates have been taught, if empathy can be taught. Empathy goes beyond an understanding of others. It also involves helping others to develop by assisting them to determine their need and the nurse acts to bolster the individual. Finally, empathy involves political awareness. This awareness allows the nurse to recognize emotional currents and the power structure of the patient, family, unit, or organization (Goleman 1994, 1998).

Social skills, the fifth competency contributing to emotional competence, is broadly representative of the interaction patterns of successful practitioners. Social skills require that the new graduate is able to influence, communicate, manage conflict, lead, initiate and manage change, build bonds, collaborate and cooperate, and effectively work with the health care team in pursuit of the collective goal. This capability has to do with "handling" another person's emotional responses and inducing desirable responses in others. Emotion is "contagious." Pessimism can permeate a group if not recognized and dealt with. As pessimism permeates a group, productivity is reduced and satisfaction is diminished. Conversely, enthusiasm and satisfaction are also contagious and can lead to productivity and job satisfaction.

When a new graduate is able to use social skills to influence others change is possible. New nurses need to be able to recognize the need for change, champion for change, and model the expected change for others. Good social skills require communication that includes active listening and clearly stated convincing messages to deal with even difficult issues and situations. Along with communication skills, the new graduate also needs (a) skills for dealing with conflict and (b) beginning leadership skills (Goleman 1994, 1998). Table 19–4 offers a do-it-yourself guide a new nurse can use to assess readiness for role transition.

Easing the Transition

Hospital nursing is stressful. The new graduate often faces unrealistic expectations by the staff, role conflict, role ambiguity, value conflicts, and lack of support. New graduates fear failure, fear total responsibility, and fear mistakes. Generally, new nurses perceive themselves as powerless to make change. They feel power overwhelmingly resides with the system and the past generation of nurses. They expect their values to come in conflict with hospital practice. Despite these expectations they are rarely prepared for the degree of conflict they experience or how to deal with the conflict experienced.

Conversely, new graduates are motivated to learn and make a difference. They value the right of the patient to be treated with respect and to know what is happening to them. New graduates value having a voice in their own fate. They value the little things about nursing, which include combing the patient's hair, cleaning their dentures, going for a walk around the halls, and simply sitting with a patient in a time of need. New graduates also value fitting in and going along with the system while retaining their own ideas and values (Kelly, 1996).

Originally, nurses entered the profession as apprentices who were trained using a task-based model of patient care. As the education of nurses has moved into college and university settings, there has been a movement to concept-based education. Simultaneously, the number of hours spent at the patient bedside has dropped dramatically. Novice nurses may be comfortable with the concepts and theory of patient care; they may be able to synthesize, analyze, and evaluate data in

---

Critical Thinking and Reflection

Are you ready to accept responsibility for your socialization to professional nursing? How can you apply each of the behaviors listed in Table 19–4 that are designed to help you adjust to your role as a professional nurse?

Table 19–4   A Do-It-Yourself Assessment of Readiness for Role Transition

Listed are pairs of behaviors (role accepting or role resisting). The transition to professional practice will require adaptation to workplace challenges. For each pair of behaviors, place a check next to the behaviors that most commonly describe you. An honest appraisal of past behaviors may be useful in preparing for role transition.

Role-Accepting Behavior	✔	Role-Resisting Behavior	✔
1. Involved with classmates; readily and quickly forms/joins groups		1. Physically isolated from peers both in class and clinical	
2. Initiates discussions with others; contributes equally with group members		2. Does not initiate interactions with others; does not contribute equally with other group members	
3. Asks for clarification		3. Responds only if called upon	
4. Meets deadlines; negotiates for extensions when needed		4. Forgets or suppresses assignment dates	
5. Accepts and welcomes evaluation by others		5. Self-conscious about being evaluated by others	
6. Effective in time management		6. Has difficulty setting priorities; waits for others to initiate priority setting	
7. Takes initiative in resolving conflict situations		7. Lacks initiative to deal with conflicts	
8. Aware of and uses available resources		8. Unaware of available resources	
9. Able to reward self		9. Elicits performance rewards and feedback from others	
10. Eager to try out new skills; takes risks; volunteers to demonstrate new behaviors		10. Last to volunteer to demonstrate new behaviors	
11. Searches for continuity and structure but can adapt to unstructured clinical settings		11. Needs a structured clinical setting to further develop	
12. Generally on time, interested, and open to learning opportunities		12. Demonstrates disengaging behaviors (late, uninterested, resistive to learning opportunities)	
13. Identifies role models in clinical setting; articulates need for change and professional growth		13. Sees past experiences as ideal and denies need for change; resists using newly developed skills, more comfortable with previous level of performance	
14. Realistic about own achievements and progress in educational system		14. Too ideological or overly critical of others	
15. Appears to enjoy learning and performing in clinical settings		15. Frustrated with nursing as a career choice	
16. Participates in professional organizations; values symbols of profession (using assessment tools, RN name tags)		16. Does not participate in professional organizations	
17. Demonstrates pride in new role behaviors and shares with others in work settings		17. Feels no increased esteem in performing new role behaviors; avoids giving feedback to agency personnel	
18. Seeks out instructor for additional learning, information, and professional growth opportunities		18. Meets minimal requirements and sees instructor only in evaluative role	
19. Takes calculated risks (questions level of care, seeks multiple learning opportunities, shares level of expertise, elects to test out required/elective courses)		19. Selects patients with common familiar clinical disorders	
20. Able to realistically appraise strengths and weaknesses		20. Has difficulty with realistic appraisal of abilities (either overly critical or overly confident)	

Scoring: Use this checklist as a means to identify role-accepting and role rejecting behaviors you have used in the past. Examine each of your role-resisting behaviors and think about how you can change that behavior to facilitate a successful transition to professional practice. If the majority of your behaviors are role accepting, congratulations. See if you can begin using some of the remaining behaviors to have a positive influence on future role transition.

Adapted from Throwe, A. N., & Fought, S. G. (1987). Landmarks in the socialization process from RN to BSN. *Nurse Educator*, 12(6), 15–18.

The current nurse shortage is evident across all specialties. Recruiting and retaining perioperative nurses is particularly problematic given the challenging, stressful environment. A collaborative program was developed between the School of Nursing at Oakland University and St. Joseph's, a 250-bed tertiary hospital. The purpose of the program was recruitment and retention of nurses for employment in perioperative environments. With no guarantee of employment following successful completion of the program, a perioperatiave fellowship program was offered to nursing students following graduation. The program included 196 hours of didactic contact and approximately 250 hours of clinical experience. Development and implementation of the course content was provided by a visiting professor from the university. The primary goal of the program was to orient nurses to perioperative competencies based on the Association of Operating Room Nurses' (AORN) standards in a protective and nurturing environment.

As the students involved in the fellowship program were not guaranteed employment or committed to employment at the hospital, it was the challenge of both the students and the staff members to develop relationships with one another. The overall result of the program was that the staff nurses wanted all students hired. Of the 11 students completing the program, 10 assumed positions in perioperative settings. One year following the program all but one student remained in perioperative nursing.

Though the sample was small, data support the need for a structured, protected, and nurturing environment for new nurses. Studies (Coeling, 1990; Hamilton, Murray, Lindholm, & Myers, 1989; Mathews & Nunley, 1992) of new graduates have suggested that 30% to 60% change their place of employment within the first year. The unique and innovative approach of this program was that it placed equal emphasis on (a) adaptation to the stressful environment and (b) learning course content and gaining clinical expertise.

the classroom. However, they may be entering the work environment with significantly less clinical experiences than the nurses that preceded them.

Novice nurses are acutely aware of their inexperience and are eager and motivated to learn. Just as their education differs from that of their predecessors so does their style of learning. Today's learners approach learning in much the same way as they approach their ATM machines (Anderson, 2000). They expect convenient and efficient access to knowledge.

Facilitating Transition of Nursing Students Through Preceptorship

Recognizing the learning needs and style of new graduates, many schools of nursing have begun offering preceptorships near the end of the nursing student's educational program. These programs combine didactic learning with the opportunity for a concentrated clinical experience. Often, students are able to select a specialty area for focused study. Preceptorships are generated through a cooperative arrangement between a health care agency and the educational institution. The health care agency provides **preceptors**—experienced nurses

working in the clinical setting who are willing to model the professional role desired, affirm progress of the future graduate, and supervise care provided. The school of nursing provides instructors who arrange preceptor relationships, provide didactic instruction, and collaborate with preceptors in the evaluation of student learning.

New Employee Programs to Ease Orientation of New Nurses

While preceptor programs prior to graduation may influence successful transition into professional practice, many new graduates continue to feel inadequately prepared to meet the demands of professional employment. Employer expectations of competency combined with increasing patient complexity has lead to more innovative approaches to orienting new graduate nurses. Included in the 1999 Practice Analysis of Newly Licensed Registered Nursing in the United States completed through the National Council of State Boards of Nursing (Hertz, Yocom, & Gawel, 2000) were questions related to type and length of orientation programs offered to new graduates.

These data indicate that most employers offer one or

more orientation formats to ensure successful transition of new graduates. The most frequently reported length of orientation programs reported was four or more weeks. The most common (81%) type of orientation to the work setting tended to be through preceptorship with an experienced nurse. In addition, many new graduate orientation programs to work included formal classroom instruction (57%), evaluation with reference to a checklist (57%), and competency-based orientation/competency testing (42%). Of survey respondents 5.4% reported formal orientation programs, internships. Of the new graduates responding, 12.7% reported no orientation at all (Hertz, Yocom, & Gawel, 1999). Of new graduates responding to the 2001 RN Practice Analysis Update, only 5% had no orientation; most (57.4%) respondents reported an orientation of greater than 4 weeks (Smith & Crawford, 2002).

Orientation programs serve to assimilate a new employee into the workforce and assure the safety and competency of the employee prior to assuming sole responsibility for care of patients. While orientation programs generally follow a structured format determined by the employer, it is best that the individual needs of the new graduate be considered. Orientation is intended to provide a bridge for the theory practice gap that exists at the time of graduation.

Many new graduates do not find traditional orientation programs adequate to meet their transition needs. To further ease the transition process many health care employers are offering **internships** and other prolonged, structured orientation programs. Internships vary in length and degree of structure. Internships are often used to attract graduates of baccalaureate programs. These programs usually provide the novice nurse with an intern advisor(s) who functions to guide new nurses. While the framework for the internship program may vary, the intern advisor usually meets regularly with interns to guide, evaluate progress, and problem solve. Internship programs may also involve didactic, classroom instruction. In some programs the intern may elect to rotate the clinical experience between two or more units. Generally, operating room and critical care rotations are reserved for longer and more structured internship experiences.

Internship programs provide not only clinical experience and orientation but also emotional support for novice nurses. By increasing the self-confidence and clinical reasoning of novice nurses through skill development and improved time management, it is the goal of many internship programs to decrease staff turnover.

Internship programs tend to thrive during times when health care agencies are seeking to attract new nurses. In times of adequate nurse availability, the short-term expense of internship programs has overshadowed the long-term benefit of staff stability.

Employment preceptor programs, much like preceptorship programs offered by some educational institution, are also used to assist new graduates through transition to professional practice. These programs provide an employer the chance to recognize experienced nurses. The opportunity to precept a new graduate offers experienced nurses an extraordinary opportunity to be involved in the professional development of a new nurse. Nurses, who precept new graduates, work with novice nurses to assist them to gradually take on assignments consistent with unit expectations.

Most new graduates find preceptorships and internships very helpful; however, there are potential hazards associated with internship and preceptor programs (e.g., role confusion, apathy, delayed socialization). Marquis and Husted (2000) indicate that the potential hazards of internships and preceptorships may be avoided with:

- Careful selection of preceptors
- Selection of preceptors with a strong desire to be a positive role model
- Preparation of preceptors for their role by providing formal instruction
- Monitoring of preceptors and new graduates by experienced staff development personnel and supervisory staff

Selecting a Mentor to Facilitate Transition

Mentors are individuals who are willing to take a special interest in a nursing student or new graduate. A mentor inspires, encourages, and assists with career development. A strong relationship between a new graduate and a mentor serves to further successful transition to clinical practice (Vance, 1999).

The mentor–protégé relationship has traditionally been a relationship established between a new nurse and an older more experienced nurse who is admired. Today's mentors can differ greatly from the traditional model. As compared with the preceptor relationship, the mentor relationship is informal and can be either short or long term. Mentor–protégé connections can be diverse in terms of age, experience, education, and culture. Mentors provide novice nurses with (a) career guidance, (b) role modeling, (c) intellectual stimulation, (d) inspiration and expectations, (e) advising and coaching, and (f) emotional support (Vance, 1990).

Mentorship benefits the protégé, the mentor, the workplace, and the profession. Novice nurses can sur-

Imagine you are a new graduate in the third week of your first job. You have just received an order to infuse two units of packed red blood cells. Imagine you turn to your preceptor for advice on how to initiate the order. The preceptor responds in one of two ways:

- "Go look in the policy and procedure book. After you have read the policy get the slips that go to the blood bank, and we will go from there."

- "Let's go look the procedure up in the policy and procedure manual then we can go from there."

Anxiety is a powerful emotion that blocks learning. Facilitated learning does not mean furnishing all information needed to make a clinical decision. Reflect on how the preceptor in each situation helped or hindered learning for the new nurse. What is the new nurse's responsibility for learning unfamiliar information?

vive without a mentor, but the transition to professional practice can be made less difficult with the support of a caring, active mentor. Mentor relationships are common throughout a nurse's professional career. These relationships serve to:

- Strengthen the profession
- Enhance the self-esteem of the individual
- Boost personal and professional satisfaction
- Promote leadership preparedness
- Support career success and advancement

Either the mentor or protégé can initiate the mentor–protégé relationship. The new nurse's behavior often has the strongest impact on the development of this relationship. Successful relationships are most often established when the new nurse:

- Takes the initiate to seek advice or information from another nurse
- Is serious about his or her career
- Is a self-starter in initiating the relationship
- Maintains his or her own identity (Vance, 1999)

Both the mentor and the preceptor have powerful roles in facilitating professional and personal development by means of role modeling and counseling (Atkins & Williams, 1995). These role models help to provide learning that extends beyond clinical practice issues into socialization issues related to what it means to be a nurse. The greatest contribution of the preceptor and mentor comes from their willingness to demonstrate appropriate clinical skills, attitudes, and behaviors in a reality-based clinical setting.

TRANSITION INTO PRACTICE

Throwe and Fought (1987) sought to explain socialization of registered nurses who return to school seeking baccalaureate education. When registered nurses return to school as nurse learners they are inculcated with the knowledge, values, beliefs, and role expectations of the professional registered nurse. The RN is not socialized to nursing but rather *resocialized* to a new role. According to Marquis and Husted (2000), "resocialization occurs when (a) new graduates leave the socialization of nursing school and enter the work world; (b) the experienced nurse changes work settings, either within the same organization or in a new organization; and (c) the nurse undertakes new roles" (e.g., RN learner) (p. 238).

Resocialization, for these nurses, can be fraught with tension producing conflicted emotions. Throwe and Fought developed a framework to explain the process of professional resocialization of RN learners based on the eight stages of development identified by Erickson (1950). These eight stages represent those tasks adults master as they grow from infancy into adulthood. These stages were used as a framework to design an assessment tool that registered nurses (RN learners), enrolled in BSN programs, can use to measure their progress in the resocialization process. Role-resisting and role-accepting behaviors characteristic of the resocialization process listed in the tool offer receptive individuals a guide for role development. The tool is also useful for faculty and others who wish to help guide not only the RN learner through the resocialization process but any nurse undergoing role change.

1. Successful role transition is in the best interest of the individual novice nurse, health care employers, the public, and the nursing profession.

2. Failed role transition is personally and professionally devastating and financially costly to the employer.

3. Professional socialization involves the development and internalization of a professional identity, which includes the values, behaviors, and attitudes necessary for assuming the role.

4. Models help to explain the process of socialization.

5. Reality shock sets in when a student or new graduate applies idealistic expectations taught in nursing school to the workplace.

6. Most new graduates clearly prepared for positions outside acute care settings most generally chose these familiar settings because they feel the need to boost clinical skills.

7. It is important for new nurses to have a realistic sense of self and competency.

8. Mentors and preceptors have an invaluable role in helping novice nurses avoid exposing themselves to undue self-criticism.

9. Discussions involving competency usually refer to technical, interpersonal, and organizational competency.

10. Individuals and employers perceive competency differently. Employers are generally interested in patient safety and realistic estimates for when a new nurse can function independently.

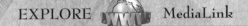

EXPLORE MediaLink

Critical thinking questions, essay questions, key terms, web links, activities, NCLEX review questions, and more interactive resources can be found on the Companion Website at www.prenhall.com/haynes. Click on Chapter 19 to select activities for this chapter.

REFERENCES

Anderson, C. A. (2000). Our obligation to the next generation. *Nursing Outlook, 48*(4), 149–150.

Atkins, S., & Williams, A. (1995). Registered nurses' experiences of mentoring undergraduate nursing students. *Journal of Advanced Nursing, 21*(5), 1006–1015.

Bandura, A. (1977). *Social learning theory.* Englewood Cliffs, NJ: Prentice Hall.

Coeling, H. V. E. (1990). Organizational culture: Helping new graduates adjust. *Nurse Educator, 15*(2), 26–30.

Davidhizar, R., & Shearer, R. (1999). The "super nurse" syndrome. *Seminars for Nurse Managers, 7*(2), 59–62.

Davis, F. (1975). Professional socialization as subjective experience: The process of doctrinal conversion among student nurses. In C. Cox & A. Mead (Eds.), *A sociology of medical practice* (pp. 116–131). London: Collier Macmillan.

Dearmun, A. K. (2000). Supporting newly qualified staff nurse: The lecturer practitioner contribution. *Journal of Nursing Management, 8*(3), 159–165.

Erickson, E. (1950). *Childhood and society.* New York, NY: W. W. Norton.

Godinez, G., Schweiger, J., Gruver, J., & Ryan, P. (1999). Role transition from graduate to staff nurse: A qualitative analysis. *Journal for Nurses in Staff Development, 15*(3) 97–110.

Goleman, D. (1994). *Emotional intelligence: Why it can matter more than IQ.* New York: Bantam Books.

Goleman, D. (1998) *Working with emotional intelligence.* New York: Bantam Books.

Hamilton, E. M., Murray, M. K., Lindholm, L. H., & Myers, R. E. (1989). Effects of mentoring on job satisfaction, leadership behaviors, and job retention of new graduate nurses. *Journal of Nursing Staff Development, 5*(4), 159–165.

Hertz, J. E., Yocom, C. J., & Gawel, S. H. (2000). *1999 practice analysis of newly licensed registered nurses.* Chicago, IL: National Council of State Boards of Nursing.

Kelly, B. (1996). Hospital nursing: "It's a battle!" A follow-up study of English graduate nurses. *Journal of Advanced Nursing, 24*(5), 1063–1069.

Kramer, M. (1974). *Reality shock: Why nurses leave nursing.* St. Louis, MO: Mosby.

Marquis, B. L., & Husted, C. J. (2000). *Leadership roles and management functions in nursing: Theory and application* (3rd ed.). Philadelphia, PA: Lippincott.

Mathews, J. J., & Nunley, C. (1992). Rejuvenating orientation to increase nurse satisfaction and retention. *Journal of Nursing Staff Development, 8*(4), 159–164.

Rafferty, A. M., Allcock, N., & Lathlean, J. (1996). The theory/practice "gap": Taking issue with the issue. *Journal of Advanced Nursing, 23*(4), 685–691.

Schmalenberg, C., & Kramer, M. (1979). *Coping with reality shock: The voices of experience.* Wakefield, MA: Nursing Resources, Inc.

Schumacher, K. L., & Meleis, A. I. (1994). Transitions: A central concept in nursing. *Image, 26*(2), 119–127.

Smith, J., & Crawford, L. (2002). *NCSBN research brief: Report of findings from the 2001 RN practice analysis update.* Chicago, IL: National Council of Sate Boards of Nursing.

Stevens, J., & Crouch, M. (1998). Frankenstein's nurse: What are schools of nursing creating? *Collegian, 5*(1), 10–15.

Throwe, A. N., & Fought, S. G. (1987). Landmarks in the socialization process from RN to BSN. *Nurse Educator, 12*(6), 15–18.

Vance, C. (1990). Is there a mentor in your career future? *Imprint, 36*(5), 41–42.

Vance, C. (1999). Mentoring—The nursing leader and mentor's perspective. In C. A. Snderson (Ed.), *Nursing student to leader: The critical path to leadership development* (pp. 200–211). Albany, NY: Delmar Publishers.

Welsh, D. (2001). *Navigating the with water of change,* June 29, 2001, Fourth National Conference on Nursing Skills Laboratories, San Antonio, Texas.

SUGGESTED READINGS

Boyle, D. K., Popkess-Vawter, S., & Taunton, R. L. (1996). Socialization of new graduate nurses in critical care. *Heart and Lung: The Journal of Acute and Critical Care, 25*(2), 141–154.

Brown, H. (2000). Lifeskills training. You've read the book . . . Now it's time to apply it to life! *British Journal of Perioperative Nursing, 10*(1), 30–33.

Coudret, N. A., Fuchs, P. L., Roberts, C. S., Suhrheinrich, J. A., & White, A. H. (1994). Role socialization of graduating student nurses: Impact of a nursing practicum on professional role conception. *Journal of Professional Nursing, 10*(6), 342–349.

Fredey, M. (2000). What every new nurse needs to know. *On Call, 3*(6), 12–15.

Jonson, K. (1998). Learning the ropes through mentoring. *The Canadian Nurse, 94*(2), 27–30.

20

Licensure

FRANCES EASON

"Knowledge is power and what you don't know, can hurt you!"

Unknown

LEARNING OBJECTIVES

AT THE COMPLETION OF THIS CHAPTER, THE READER WILL BE ABLE TO:

➤ Discuss the purpose of licensure.

➤ Explain the process for regulation of nursing practice.

➤ State the purpose, characteristics, and format of the NCLEX.

➤ Identify requirements for maintaining licensure.

➤ Describe the concept of multistate licensure and interstate compact.

➤ Identify future trends including the process of differentiated licensure.

MediaLink www.prenhall.com/haynes

Additional online resources including NCLEX review questions, critical thinking questions, and real-world activities for this chapter can be found on the Companion Website at www.prenhall.com/haynes.

*N*urses have not always been required by law to have a license. Prior to 1903, no state had any requirements for an individual to be called "nurse." In fact, most nurses had little or no education in the field of nursing except through life experiences and on-the-job training. Nurses simply cared for an individual or group of individuals who were unable to care for themselves. Early nurses went to the home of the ill individual. The nurse not only provided care, but also served as a maid to the family, cooking meals, providing child care, and cleaning house. There were no standards for nurses to follow; they either did what others had done before them or they followed the physician's orders. This chapter reviews the historical march toward licensure for nurses. A plan for NCLEX preparation is presented along with other current trends and issues related to the licensure process.

Historical Perspectives and the Board of Nurse Examiners

The Civil War marked the beginning of an organized concentration of women called to public service. This "call" for women to volunteer as nurses in the hospitals was the beginning of organized health care (Wyche, 1938).

As medications became available, nurses had a new responsibility; they dispensed medications such as quinine sulfate and morphia. Many substitutes for these essential drugs were also available, such as dogwood berries to replace quinine, and blackberry roots and persimmons combined to form a cordial to treat dysentery, while castor beans yielded oil for constipation, and the poppy plant yielded opium for treatment of pain (Wyche, 1938).

Despite added responsibilities, standards did not exist in any state to regulate the practice of nursing. The public had no method by which to assure that a "nurse" providing care had the competence that was required for that care. Little to no training was available or required for employment. The few nursing programs in existence varied from 6 weeks to 3 years in length, and there were no outcome measures to indicate the competence of a person who completed the program.

As early as 1867, Dr. Henry W. Acland suggested licensure for nurses in England. In 1892 the American Society of Superintendents of Training Schools for Nurses organized and supported licensure in the United States. In 1896, the Nurses' Associated

Alumnae of the United States and Canada was created; one goal was to establish legal licensure for nurses. It was not until 1901 that the first nursing licensure in the world was established in New Zealand (Ellis & Hartley, 2001).

On December 5, 1902, the North Carolina State Nurses Association was incorporated and on March 3, 1903, the North Carolina Legislature passed into law the first Nurse Practice Act. This first Act created a Board of Nurse Examiners (BNE) to be composed of two physicians, elected by the North Carolina Medical Society, and three registered nurses from the North Carolina State Nurses Association. The election of the nurse members to the BNE took place in June 1903. In 1903, three other states, New Jersey, New York, and Virginia, passed laws to create a Board of Nurse Examiners. The first nurse practice acts allowed for optional licensure, it was not until 1938 that New York passed the first mandatory practice act that required licensure of nurses (Kalisch & Kalisch, 1995).

The first Boards of Nurse Examiners (a) designed and administered an examination and (b) issued a license to those who passed the examination. The examination was intended to assure the public that a nurse with a license had met a minimum standard for safe patient care. The first examination was given in North Carolina on May 24, 1904, and certificates (now licenses) were issued to six graduates of nursing schools in North Carolina. The members of the Board of Nurse Examiners wrote the examination, with each board member writing items (Wyche, 1938).

Activities of Boards of Nurse Examiners proved to be an important step in the educational advancement of nursing. These boards influenced nursing curricula and determined the length of time a student was to be engaged in theory and clinical experiences in order for a diploma to be issued at the time of graduation (Wyche, 1938).

Later, Boards of Nurse Examiners (BNE) broadened their responsibilities to encompass more than licensure examinations. As responsibilities changed, so did the names for established BNE. For example, in February 1917, the North Carolina Board of Nurse Examiners changed the name to Board of Examiners of Trained Nurses in North Carolina, and again in 1931 the name was changed to the North Carolina Board of Nurse Examiners (Wyche, 1938). From those early names most boards became known as "The State Board of Nursing"; even today, most are known by the appropriate state name with the words "Board of Nursing" to follow.

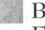

Board of Nurse Examiners Today

Today, the Governor or a branch of the Legislature appoints the member of most Boards of Nursing. In some states, health-related groups nominate board members with the final approval left to the Governor. In 1981, North Carolina became the first state to have a nurse practice act that allowed licensed nurses the privilege of electing the 13 nurse members, while the Governor continued to appoint the two public members. Today, North Carolina is the only state that offers nurses the opportunity to have input into the regulation of nursing by electing board members. In some states, qualifications for board membership are determined by the nurse's background (e.g., clinician, educator, etc.). This encourages boards to have a variety of nurse representation and not just nurses from one type of practice arena. Since nurse members to the board represent a practice area and not individual nurses nor specialized groups of nurses, a variety of practice sites are represented. The trend today is to have a larger number of public members serving on Boards of Nursing, with most states having at least two public members.

Currently, over 60 Boards of Nursing exist in the United States; some states have two boards, one for the practice of registered nursing and one for the practice of licensed practical (vocational) nursing. The majority of states have one combination board that regulates both registered and practical nursing. The legal mandate for Boards of Nursing is that mandatory licensure of all who engage in the practice of nursing is necessary to ensure minimum standards of competency and to assure nurses meet minimum standards to provide safe nursing care to the public (North Carolina Board of Nursing [NCBON], 2001).

Supervision of Education

In the 1800s as hospitals were being established, it became clear that there must be nurses to provide care to the patients. Nurses were employed who had no education or varying levels of education. No standards existed for nursing practice except the prescriptions for care as written by physicians. In the mid-1800s, most nursing education was under the auspice of the Catholic sisterhoods. In the latter 1800s, the American Medical Association established a committee to study the shortage of trained nurses and recommendations were made that every large hospital establish a school of nursing. Hospitals began to establish schools of nursing primarily based on an apprentice type of education. Many of these schools were designed to support on the job training; doctors and practicing nurses taught classes. The main objective was not the education of students, but rather to provide a source of free or inexpensive labor to increase the workforce of hospitals. Students were assigned patient responsibility without a great deal of supervision. Often, they were the only caretakers on a hospital unit with only a single registered nurse hospital supervisor. The assignment was often beyond the educational level of the student; however, this type of student role prepared graduates for the real world of nursing at that time. Graduates were in great demand as they completed educational requirements. Many of the graduates remained at the hospital where they were trained after completing their education since many hospitals offered them benefits to remain, for example, uniforms, free laundry, low-cost housing, and free or low-cost meals (Wyche, 1938).

In the 1900s, the Boards of Nurse Examiners began to implement rules dictating the specific number of hours of classroom and clinical experiences. As standards were adopted, the hospital schools of nursing were required to meet these standards. The hospital diploma schools were very popular as few vocational opportunities were afforded women other than teaching (Wyche, 1938). Today, many states have diploma schools that stand alone or are affiliated with community colleges or baccalaureate programs offering students some college credit. The diploma school met a great need and provided young women with an education at no cost or a low cost. Even as late as 1962, a student could complete a nursing program for as little as $300 for the 36 month training period. This exceptional deal included textbooks, room and board, the education, and uniforms.

Supervision of the Scope of Nursing Practice

Boards of Nursing are typically empowered to supervise nursing through licensure, discipline, education, and practice. Today's Board of Nurse Examiners (Boards of Nursing) not only influences education, but also defines the scope of practice for nursing. Generally, Boards define and describe activities that require licensure and provide legal protection for the title of "registered nurse" or "licensed practical nurse." Further, the Board may describe what activities do not require the professional judgment of a licensed nurse; these then become common tasks or procedures that may be delegated to unlicensed persons.

The scope of nursing is often defined in broad terms to allow agencies to have input into the role of their employees. However, some Boards prescribe, either in the law or in rules, specific activities that are permissible for nurses to perform. In this case, the employer does not have the privilege to prevent the nurse from practicing nursing within the scope of practice as required by the nursing practice act. On the other hand, the employer does not have the liberty to allow or demand a nurse to perform activities that the Board has indicated are not within the scope of nursing practice. The Board supports safe, effective practice by not allowing nurses to be assigned activities that may cause the nurse to exceed the scope of practice.

Many practice acts are written using a nursing process format that has a companion document available from the Board to further explain the act. This companion document may then become part of the rules that the Board is empowered to enact without legislative approval. In many practice acts, the first section of the act includes a listing of definitions including the legal definition of nursing. The act then spells out the scope of practice (Ellis & Hartley, 2001). In nursing, the scope of practice for nursing is continually evolving as more and more nurses receive advanced education and become certified as advanced practice nurses (APN).

Advanced practice nurses have functioned in the United States for more than a century (American Association of Nurse Anesthetists [AANA], 1997). From a historical perspective, the first APRN were the certified registered nurse anesthetists (CRNA). Many CRNA graduated from diploma schools and later attended a program of anesthesia. Today, schools of anesthesia usually require a master's degree in nursing, which most often require a baccalaureate degree in nursing for admittance (Kelly & Joel, 1999).

LICENSURE OF FOREIGN NURSE GRADUATES

The Board of Nurse Examiners regulates licensure in relation to the requirements for initial licensure, renewal, and for the process of endorsement. In addition, the Board regulates the process by which foreign nurse graduates seek licensure in the United States through examination. That regulation requires that the nurse educated outside of the United States pass a test administered by the Commission on Graduates of Foreign Nursing Schools (CGFNS). This examination consists of three sections to (a) validate the nurse's cre-

dentials as compared to those of a registered nurse educated in the United States, (b) test the nurse's knowledge base, and (c) test English language proficiency. The CGFNS has been deemed to be an accurate predictor of success on the state licensing examination. This role of the BNE was established in the 1970s when a shortage of nurses forced hospitals to recruit foreign nurses to increase the pool of available nurses (Mitchell & Grippando, 1993). Again in the 1980s and early 1990s, recruitment of foreign nurses increased, as the United States faced a continued shortage of nurses or at least a problem with the distribution of nurses.

The contemporary nurse shortage is also expected to lead to recruitment of foreign nurses. If the nurse's credentials are varified, the knowledge base confirmed, and English language proficiency determined, the public must ask the moral/ethical question about the effect of this type of recruitment on the nation loosing the nurses during the world-wide shortage.

DISCIPLINARY ACTION

The Board of Nursing regulates discipline of nurses. The Board has the responsibility to investigate any and all complaints that are presented in relation to potential violations of the nursing practice act. After an investigation, the Board can initiate charges against the nurse if the evidence indicates a violation of the nursing practice act. Depending on the severity of the charges and if this is the first time that the nurse has been a subject of investigation, the Board may allow the licensee to voluntarily surrender the license, meet in a settlement conference (if the Board has such a procedure), or go before the Board for a hearing. At either the settlement conference or hearing, the Board can issue a reprimand, which is generally the least sanction that the Board implements. In addition, the Board can require that the licensee take remedial courses such as an ethics course, a pharmacology/drug course, or any other course that the Board deems necessary. The licensee has a limited time to complete the requirement and if the requirement is not met, the licensee may receive a restricted license. A restricted license allows the licensee to keep a license to practice, but with limitations in relation to the time (hours of the day) that the licensee can work or in which sites that the licensee can be employed. Other limitations may include a restriction from administering narcotics or even from administrating any medication in general. Finally, the licensee may be required to have their charge nurse or manager submit written evaluations of their performance with special emphasis on the reason that the license was restricted. In addition to time, site, medication administration, or performance evaluations, the Board may place any other restrictions that are deemed necessary, and may enforce the restrictions indefinitely or for a prescribed period of time (NCBON, 2001). For more serious violations, the license may be suspended. During the time of suspension, some Boards of Nursing allow the nurse to function as a certified nurse assistant (CNA) while other Boards do not have this provision.

Generally, the nurse must petition to have the license reinstated after a suspension. Most Boards will issue a restricted license initially for a period of time to allow the licensee to readjust to nursing while still receiving Board supervision. Likewise, the nurse may be required to petition the Board to have restriction(s) removed after they have been in place the specified time period. In the case of a restriction or a suspension, the Board has the authority to require the licensee to be assessed by a qualified psychiatrist or psychologist to determine their propensity toward certain behaviors. These may include the use of alcohol, drugs, or theft. The Board may also require the licensee to participate in all treatments as prescribed by the clinician completing the assessment. All of the contingencies must be met before the Board of Nursing will return the license that was in abeyance (NCBON, 2001).

The primary role of the Board is to protect the public. The disciplinary process is a necessary requirement to assure safe practice. Every nurse also has a role to assure public safety. In one sense nurses watch over and supervise one another to prevent unsafe behaviors while on duty. Nurses share the responsibility to protect the public by reporting unsafe nurses (NCBON, 2001).

All licensed nurses are required to know their scope of practice and to practice at that level. It is within the nurse's legal right and obligation to decline to perform any activity for which the nurse is not prepared or for which the nurse understands is not within their legally approved scope of practice (Deloughery, 1998).

EDUCATION

In relation to education, the Board of Nursing has been empowered to write standards for education programs and to survey the education programs to determine compliance with established standards. The Board may routinely visit schools of nursing to determine compliance or to determine if they may accept without any additional steps the reports from an accreditation agency, such as the American Association of Colleges of Nursing (AACN) or National League for Nursing Accrediting Commission (NLNAC) as the Board's approval process. Allowing accrediting agencies to perform this duty is a trend that is cost effective for both the Board and schools of nursing.

PRACTICE

The last area that the Board is empowered to regulate is the area of practice. The Board makes decisions as to what is basic nursing practice and what is considered to be practice beyond the basic level. Generally, basic nursing is taught in the college and four year nursing programs; nursing activities that are beyond the basic school of nursing education are considered advanced practice.

Within their scope of practice nurses delegate health care activities to other providers. Since the early 1990s the role and training of unlicensed assistive personnel (UAP) has been an issue of concern for many Boards of Nursing and to that end, the Boards have written interpretive statements to describe the registered nurse's role in delegation (Eason, 2000).

When delegating care, the nurse is accountable for all acts performed by the UAP or other licensed personnel. Registered nurses must provide the appropriate level of supervision to all personnel when patient care tasks are delegated. The registered nurse must be knowledgeable of not only the scope of practice for licensed personnel, but also for the action of the UAP. The entire gamut of delegation including accountability, tasks which can be delegated, teaching of UAPs, and the relationships among levels of care providers continues to be a focus for Boards of Nursing (Eason, 2000).

In addition to the roles of UAP, Boards of Nursing also regulate nursing practice by focusing on clinical issues and/or questions related to roles, technology,

Critical Thinking and Reflection

Review the nurse practice act in your state. What tasks can the registered nurse delegate to UAP? Are there any laws in your state that empower UAPs beyond the scope of practice as is outlined in the nurse practice act?

and other new directions in nursing. The Board often issues interpretive statements in response to concerns of nurses, health care administrators, and the public. Issues such as management of pain, professional boundary issues, and accountability of practitioners for care will continue to be in the forefront of review by Boards of Nursing.

The Board is the regulatory body for professional practice of nurses today and students in nursing programs who will be established practitioners in the future. Today, this would include all advanced practice areas (e.g., nurse midwifery, nurse anesthetists, nurse practitioners for all ages and specialties, and clinical nurse specialists) (Eason, 1999).

NCLEX

From the early days of the Boards of Nurse Examiners, examinations have been part of the licensing process and the license has been a measure of knowledge and competency. In the early years the examination was generally written by individual board members and may have contained both a written and a skill performance section. Later, when the National League for Nursing (NLN) was contracted to prepare and grade the examination, it was made up of five sections: medical, surgical, pediatrics, obstetrics, and psychiatry. A failure on any one section required that section to be retaken. In 1978, the National Council of State Boards of Nursing (NCSBN) was formed and presently serves as an umbrella organization with delegates from each state that forms a decision-making group, the Delegate Assembly. The NCSBN contracts with testing agencies for the administration, scoring, and compiling of statistics for the licensure examination. In 1981, the National Council administered the first National Council Licensure Examination (NCLEX). In 1987, the NCSBN designed the NCLEX based on a study of knowledge deemed necessary for entry into nursing practice. At that time an overall passing score was established; any new graduate with a score below the numerical passing level was required to retake the entire examination. In 1989, the NCLEX was first reported as Pass/Fail rather than as a numerical score. A failure on the examination required that the graduate repeat the entire examination. Currently, job analysis studies continue to be administered and the test plan redesigned to reflect contemporary nursing practice. The Delegate Assembly of the NCSBN approves changes to the test plan and the composition of the examination is changed to reflect the new plan (National Council of State Board of Nursing, 2000).

The test plan is basically designed to reflect patient needs including a safe, effective care environment; physiologic integrity; psychosocial integrity; and health promotion and health maintenance (Silvestri, 2002). Since April 1, 1994, the test has been administered using a Computer Adaptive Testing (CAT) format. The four areas of patient needs have remained the same after computer utilization except the percentages have been modified to provide a structure for defining nursing actions and competencies across all settings for all patients. This test is not subdivided into five content areas, as was the previous plan. The new test plan, based on four patient need categories, is further divided into subcategories (NCSBN, 2000). This test plan is more descriptive than previous plans and has percentages assigned for each of the subcategories rather than the major categories. In addition, the test plan has six additional concepts and processes integrated throughout the examination including caring, communication and documentation, cultural awareness, nursing process, self-care, and teaching/learning. When preparing to write the NCLEX, the candidate should obtain information regarding the current test plan since the plan is subject to change based on the most recent job analysis.

In 1999 at its annual meeting, the NCSBN presented a plan to add test items to the NCLEX using innovative formats. The NCSBN developed and researched these items as part of a continuous quality improvement system and as of April 1, 2003, these items were included on the NCLEX examinations.

These items use technology, which allows formats other than the usual four-option, multiple-choice question. Innovative test formats vary. For example, some allow for more than one response to a traditional four or more option question, some require the test taker to fill in a blank by typing in an answer, while still other test items may direct a candidate to answer a question by identifying an area on a picture or a graph. Any of the innovative test items on the examination may also include charts, tables, or graphic images. Regarding calculations, historically, test takers have been required to calculate answers and then select from four possible answers. An innovative test item may require the candidate to perform a calculation without the opportunity to select a response. The candidate would simply type in the calculated answer.

The current test plan and test length remain unchanged. The innovative items are not expected to replace a significant number of traditional test items. Presently, there is no established number of innovative test items that a candidate can expect on the examination. Just as with traditional NCLEX test items, these new items will be scored, as either right or wrong and no partial credit will be given.

While the new format may initially cause candidates to experience a variety of emotions related to this change in format, the candidate should remember that these items (a) make up only a very small portion of the overall exam and (b) should not require any additional time.

The same system of item design including development, validation, pretesting, and evaluation was utilized to develop the innovative test items. As with all other test items these items will allow the candidate to demonstrate entry-level competence. It is expected that this different format may assess content and competencies more readily and authentically, and thus improve assessment of entry-level nursing practice. Candidates will receive information about innovative items in the *NCSBN Examination Candidate Bulletin*. Additionally, update information is included on the NCSBN Web site.

Since NCSBN implemented computerized adaptive testing (CAT), candidates have the opportunity to take the NCLEX in locations in any state, and receive a license from another state. The CAT has many advantages, but the one that often appeals to the candidates is the fact that the results are available within a short time frame (as early as 2 to 3 weeks) after the examination is completed (National Council State Boards of Nursing, Inc., 2001).

The role of the Board of Nursing in licensure examinations continues to be multifaceted; the board authorizes the candidate to take the examination, provides the candidate with notification of the NCLEX score, and serves as the source of information for the candidate. In addition, the board determines the location of test centers and approves procedures for testing in the state (National Council State Boards of Nursing, Inc., 2001).

In some states candidates are required to pay an additional fee for a criminal background check, which accompanies the application for licensure. This requirement is in keeping with legislative mandate to protect the public (NCBON, 2002).

The NCLEX for the practical nurse has a similar format of patient needs but is based on the job analysis focus directed at long-term care settings and patients over 65 years of age. The percentage of items in each category is slightly different from those on the NCLEX-RN examination. The testing procedure and the scoring procedure are similar to the NCLEX-RN and are reported as a "pass" or "fail" (Silvestri, 2002).

Purpose

Many ask the purpose of an examination after graduation. After all, every school administers tests at the conclusion of every course. The NCLEX is intended to measure the minimum competence for entry-level practice. Passing the NCLEX provides notice to the prospective employer and to the public that the registered nurse has demonstrated entry-level competence.

Characteristics

Since 1950, when the Bureau of State Boards of Nurse Examiners was formed, each state administered an identical examination. That test was referred to as a State Board Test Pool Exam. Each state established its own passing score so that automatic endorsement from state to state was not possible. Eventually, all states adopted a uniform passing score which facilitated endorsement on the national level (Kalisch & Kalisch, 1995).

Today the NCLEX is administered in all states and territories of the United States and is prepared under the oversight of the NCSBN. The National Council of State Boards of Nursing contracts with a testing company to design and administer the test written according to the approved test plan.

In order to take the NCLEX, a candidate must complete two applications. These applications may be combined or they may be separate. One application registers the candidate with the testing organization while the other is an application for licensure in a particular state. Each individual state has its own application and requirements for licensure; cost may vary. For example, one state may require the application to be notarized, another may require an actual transcript from the nursing school, while another may only request verification of graduation from the program director or registrar. Most boards have a Web site that provides directions regarding obtaining an application. Candidates must submit the appropriate fee in the form of a money order, certified check, or cashier's check to both the testing organization and the appropriate Board of Nursing (National Council State Boards of Nursing, 2001). Appendix B offers contact information for each State Board of Nursing.

Once eligibility to take the examination is established, the candidate is notified and can obtain an appointment for the examination. The examination is administered in every state and territory. One of the benefits of having a computerized national examination is that candidates are not required to take the examination in the state to which they have applied for licensure (National Council State Boards of Nursing, 2001).

Computer Adaptive Testing (CAT) Format

Since 1994, testing has been via a computer adaptive testing (CAT) format which allows for adaptation to the individual candidates' ability. The CAT consists of a bank of examination items that have been proven to be reliable and valid. On every candidate's examination there will also be test items labeled "try outs," integrated throughout the examination which are being reviewed for reliability and validity. The test items are not included in the overall calculation of the candidates score. (National Council State Boards of Nursing, 2001).

For the RN exam, the candidate can complete testing with a minimum of 75 items or a maximum of 265 items. On the PN exam the minimum is 85 items and the maximum is 262. Every candidate will receive at least the minimum number of items and may receive any number over the minimum. The difficulty level of the items that the candidate can answer successfully determines the actual number of items on an exam. Every candidate's test is adapted to the examinee as the exam progresses. Based on the testing format, it is almost statistically impossible for any two candidates to experience the same test. It would not be a wise use of time to attempt to determine every item that a classmate or friend answered on the NCLEX, as no two candidates are likely to receive one or more of the same items. The test bank is updated often to keep the items current so even the candidate who wrote the exam 91 days prior will not have the same items repeated on the second examination. This is one of the reasons that a candidate may not rewrite the examination before 91 days following a failed examination (National Council State Boards of Nursing, 2001).

During the actual testing the computer is scoring the test. Based on the computation as the applicant progresses, additional items are presented to clearly determine whether the applicant meets the standard for passing the NCLEX based on the four areas of patient needs. Basically, as an applicant answers an item successfully, the next item is at a higher difficulty level. If the answer is incorrect, the difficulty level of the next item is less difficult. If a candidate can successfully answer 75 items at a consistently high difficulty level, then the computer will automatically end the test as the candidate has demonstrated the minimum knowledge required for entry-level nursing practice. Likewise, if an applicant is unable to answer a sufficient number of items with a higher difficulty level, they also may have only 75 items. This applicant will have demonstrated that they do not have the knowledge to practice entry-level nursing and the computer will end the test. If there are only 75 items, 15 are "try outs" and the remaining 60 are real items that are the basis for the score of pass or fail. The number of "try outs" is always 15 regardless of the total number of items (National Council of State Boards of Nursing, 2001).

Preparing for NCLEX

Every candidate must determine their own best method to prepare for the NCLEX examination. As was the case in school, candidates have individual styles of learning that should be considered when it is time to prepare for the NCLEX. Graduates can prepare for the

---

Research Application

Beeman and Waterhouse (2001) analyzed data from 289 individuals who graduated from a baccalaureate nursing program between 1995 and 1998 to determine if there were variables that would predict success on the Computerized Adaptive Testing (CAT) currently in use with the NCLEX-RN. Using discriminate analysis, 21 variables were identified. Interestingly, the researchers report that for their sample population, the data to predict NCLEX-RN was available by the first semester of the students' senior year; therefore, at-risk students identified as early as five months prior to graduation could take advantage of this information in preparing for the exam. Further, these authors report that these predictors provide for earlier identification than is possible using either the HESI or other assessment exams such as Mosby's.

In their study, the authors found they could, with 92% accuracy for failing and 94% accuracy for passing, predict NCLEX-RN results. Within the limits of their sample population the authors found that grades in selected nursing courses (including pathophysiology) were predictors of success on the NCLEX-RN. These authors did not study the predictive ability of the HESI, NLN test scores, and Mosby Assess Test. However, SAT and GPA results were analyzed and found to have no significant predictability for the CAT NCLEX-RN as opposed to previous paper and pencil formats of licensure examinations.

When evaluating study results the researchers indicate that data were collected on graduates from a single baccalaureate school of nursing. Since nursing curricula vary widely; therefore, application of these results is limited. Nursing students may wish to ask faculty about predictors and predictions for NCLEX-RN success at their own school. This knowledge can provide future graduates with information helpful to preparing for their individual readiness for the exam.

exam in a variety of ways. They can (a) review course notes and class textbooks; (b) purchase NCLEX textbook and/or accompanying compact disc; and (c) complete, NCLEX review courses. In addition, there are online courses available and face-to-face review courses that may be offered in locations accessible to most candidates. Each candidate must take studying for the NCLEX very seriously and map out a plan for success.

If test anxiety is a concern, there are programs available that will assist the candidate and courses that are designed to improve study habits. These programs may assist a student with test taking prior to graduation as well as with the NCLEX. As a graduating senior, using an NCLEX review book may be a good review for course work and will serve to familiarize the candidate with the type of items included on the NCLEX.

One suggestion for preparation is to answer as many test items as possible and to time oneself so at least one item is answered each minute. This is the average time it takes to answer a four-option multiple-choice item. Candidates should spend as little time as possible when they find that they cannot even make an educated guess. Time should not be wasted. The best choice is to answer those items that one is not sure of an answer as quickly as possible since that is the only way to get to the next item that may offer an easily identified correct option. In preparing for the NCLEX, this manner of test taking is useful.

Since buying several review books may be costly, rather than buying several books, answer the items on a separate paper and do not write in the test book. By utilizing this method, it is possible to exchange review books with another candidate and each have the opportunity to answer the items, and the candidate can answer the same items more than once. In other words, recycle the test book. Generally, it is difficult to sell or share a test book that has all of the test items already answered.

Another suggestion for NCLEX study is to use a variety of methods in preparation for the exam, as this will assist the candidate in maintaining interest in the study process. For example, use a test item book and review items in a particular chapter. It may be wise to answer only a limited number and then determine the correct answers. For each item, answered either correctly or incorrectly, review rationale as presented in the NCLEX review book. Then answer 20 to 25 more items and repeat the process. During that same study time, review a video on particular content. This method is more effective than sitting for long periods to answer test items from a test book. Preparation time should be a rewarding time, as candidates are generally surprised to find that they know more than they had anticipated and it is gratifying to be making progress.

Finally, one may study with another person or group if he or she finds that this is an effective, satisfactory method for study. The important thing is to go to the group study session prepared. Assigning each group member a section to present to the total group is helpful. If a group member attends without having completed the assignment, then that member should be asked to not continue with the group. Teaching content or explaining to someone forces the teaching partner to be prepared. This method can be successful but also can be a poor utilization of time if the group members use the time as a social event rather than a time to study.

The old adage that "practice does make perfect" is true in relation to answering items, as it programs the candidate to become familiar with responding to four-option multiple-choice items. It is also very helpful for the candidate to review NCLEX programs on a computer whether it is CAT formatted or not. Since the use of the CAT, every item on the NCLEX stands alone. There is never a situation in which multiple questions relate to the same situation. The test on the computer offers an integrated format. Many graduates have never taken a test in which one item relates to newborns and the next item may relate to an elderly patient. The integrated approach is difficult for some new graduates who are seeing an integrated test for the first time; a practice test can help reduce this fear.

In consideration of the time involved in taking the NCLEX, many students are accustomed to having a 50-minute test and a 10-minute break every hour, so it is hard for them to concentrate for more that 50 minutes without a break. On the NCLEX exam, the first break is scheduled after 2 hours. Some candidates report that they did not realize how tired they would be, as they had never taken a test for 2 hours without a break. The candidates may prepare themselves by sitting at a computer responding to items for a longer period of time to get the feel of the NCLEX procedure.

Picking the Best NCLEX Review Course

Many review courses are available. All courses have "good points" and points that some individuals would say are not so good. As with every problem or question encountered in the nursing profession, step one should be to complete an assessment of the review course. The first thing that most students ask is "How much does it cost?" After that question is asked, then find out the number of hours required to complete the entire course. Then calculate the cost per hour. In 2002, an informal survey regarding the cost of five courses revealed the cost ranged from $5.66 per hour to $8.62 per hour. Cost per hour may be more important than the total course cost. Courses generally vary from 30 to 40 hours in length (American Nursing Review, 2000).

Another factor to consider is whether or not there is a guarantee related to NCLEX success. A money-back guarantee means that money will be returned if the candidate does not successfully pass the NCLEX. On the other hand, if a course offers a guarantee, this means that the course can be taken again or audiotapes may be sent to review in preparation for the next attempt. Many candidates prefer the money-back guarantee and use the money for another type of course or to purchase materials to use for home study. It is important to understand what guarantee is offered before making a deposit and registering for a review course.

In selecting a review course it is also important to know if there are a minimum number of participants that must take the course to ensure the course will be held. If the answer is yes, ask if a company representative will call within a time frame that allows for registration in another course. If at all possible, get the facts regarding a second course and keep the phone number in mind in the event that the class is canceled.

When considering a review course ask whether a review book is included in the cost of the course. If it is not, the candidate may consider making the purchase prior to the course to begin utilizing it in advance. If a

Critical Thinking and Reflection

Preparation for NCLEX-RN informally begins the day a student enters nursing school. Formal preparation for NCLEX-RN begins later. Some students voice the intent to take the exam once, without study or preparation, in order to get the practice. This is a *very* bad idea. Failure to pass the exam the first time has serious consequences. When do you plan to begin preparation for the exam? How do you plan to prepare? Do you need a formal classroom review, an online review course, or are you ready now to take the exam?

review book is included, the candidate should find out the title so that the same book is not purchased prior to the course. Many companies will not discount the course cost if the candidate does not need the book that is included with the course. In relation to the review book, consider the two types of books. One type contains test items only, while the second type is a combination of content and test items. If the candidate has access to nursing school texts, then a book containing content may not be needed, though review books with question rationale offer valuable insights.

When considering a review course ask if there is a free computer disc offered with the course, and, if so, whether it is CAT formatted or just a test on a computer. Some NCLEX review courses charge extra for the computer disc and for other study aids that are available during the week of the review. Another feature of some review courses is that a diagnostic test may be included to assist in determining what content should be reviewed. Know in advance exactly what has been purchased when signing up for a review course. If the materials that were paid for are not available, ask for information regarding when the material will be received.

When registering, ask about the format of the class. If students are allowed to ask questions during the class time, the content may not be covered entirely. Some courses have a policy that no verbal questions are allowed but the instructor will consider written questions, which may be answered aloud for all of the participants.

Since the late 1990s there have been classes offered online to prepare for the examination. Included in both online and traditional courses may be content on how to study, how to reduce fear, and how to use memory clues or relaxation techniques to assist the candidate to concentrate during the examination. Be aware, however, that some courses review very little content, but rather offer memory games to help one memorize. Generally, a few memory games may be beneficial, but if the entire review course is based on cartoons or gimmicks to assist with memorization, then this course may not be as much of a review as it is a form of entertainment.

Generally, the value of a review course can be determined by discussing the merits of the course with other persons who have taken the course and were successful on the examination. Remember when purchasing a product know as much as possible about that product before making payment. Let the buyer beware! Ask questions. There is not one best course. The candidate must decide what course is best for his or her situation, learning style, and resources.

Licensure

Once a nurse has successfully passed NCLEX the applicant should be qualified for licensure. State practice acts usually include the basic requirements for initial licensure. The requirements include being a graduate or having earned the equivalent of a high school diploma, and having graduated from an approved nursing program. Approved nursing program refers to a school of nursing approved by the Board of Nursing, which is different from being accredited by a national nursing organization, such as the AACN or NLNAC.

Some examples of requirements for licensure that differ from state to state may include a specific short-term course on a particular clinical issue, such as "the care of patients with AIDS" or a course on "caring for the elderly." The schools of nursing usually meet these requirements in that state, but graduates outside of the state must meet them before they can be issued a license even if they are successful on the NCLEX. Other Boards of Nursing may have requirements for a specific number of continuing education hours on an annual basis (or renewal period basis), whereas some states have no education requirements beyond the basic nursing school education. In 1976, California was the first state to implement a policy that continuing education was a requirement for licensure. Since 1976, several other states have also required a specific number of approved hours in continuing education as mandatory for renewal of licensure. The important thing to know is that states may have similar but different requirements for obtaining an initial license in addition to passing the NCLEX, and there may or may not be continuing education contingent for license renewal.

Today, some boards require first time applicants to pay an extra fee, which has been added to the cost of the license, for a criminal background check. If an applicant has a criminal record or convictions, this may not absolutely prevent licensure. The Board of Nursing may allow the new graduate to write the NCLEX and, if successful, they may call for a hearing before the Board to consider the application. Convictions will be reviewed on an individual basis, and a decision may be dependent on how long it has been since the last conviction and the nature of the conviction. After the hearing, the Board may then issue the license, place restrictions on the license, or deny the application until certain requirements are fulfilled. Students in nursing programs need to know that "what they don't know about the process of licensure can hurt them" when they apply for licensure. This is especially true if they were not aware that the Board has the responsibility to protect the public by monitoring those that receive a license or maintain a license. Even a conviction for driving while intoxicated or for selling alcohol to a minor while working in a food store may have implications for licensure. If this is a one-time conviction, and it was many years prior to the application, there may be no action by the Board except to review the situation and grant the license if the applicant meets all other requirements. The most important advice for candidates is to be truthful, to not withhold information, and report all convictions to the Board.

Eligibility for Renewal

In addition to the procedure described above, the nurse must also consider some of the factors that will prevent a license renewal. Each state may have differing requirements that will prevent or cause delay in the license renewal process. The best sources for a listing of requirements would be the practice act, the Web site for the Board, or by direct contact with the Board of Nursing via telephone or e-mail. Most of the practice acts indicate that selected misdemeanors or felony convictions must be reported to the Board of Nursing on the application for renewal. When a nurse requests a renewed license, no action may be taken because of a misdemeanor or felony conviction, but the Board of Nursing may require a remediation course or require that an applicant obtain an assessment from a Board-approved psychiatrist or psychologist and follow all treatment plans after the assessment. In addition, if a nurse is involved in a crime, during the case presentation in criminal court, the judge may require that the clerk of the court send the nurse's license to the Board of Nursing, either for a specified time period, or allow the Board of Nursing to determine the time period that the license is suspended. This is not a second trial for the same offense, but rather a hearing for being convicted of a crime that may undermine the public trust. This action usually results from convictions related to drug theft, the selling of drugs, or other crimes that may undermine the public trust and safety. This

action is referred to as a court-ordered surrender, and the Board must hold the license in abeyance for the time period as ordered by the court before the license can be returned (NCBON, 2001).

An overall authority of Boards of Nursing includes regulation of those that practice nursing. To this end, the nursing practice acts usually allows for sanctions to be placed on nurses' licenses until specified requirements are met. These sanctions may include completing certain educational courses such as an ethics course or a pharmacology/drug administration course or even courses related to behavior control (e.g., anger control). In addition to education, the Board of Nursing may issue a reprimand. The licensee can then petition the Board of Nursing to remove the reprimand through a process called absolution. The time period is dependent on the type of practice act violation in which the nurse was found guilty (NCBON, 2001).

For more serious violations, the nurse may receive a restricted license that allows him or her to keep the license, but restrictions are added. The restrictions may include working only during a specific time frame of the day (such as days only), or a specific type of work site, such as not being allowed to work with the aged or a pediatric population. A license may also have restrictions that do not allow the nurse to administer any narcotics or have access to any drugs. The nurse may also be required to notify the Board of Nursing if drugs are prescribed for him or her. When a license is restricted, the licensee may be required to have the charge nurse or nurse manager complete quarterly reports, which are sent to the Board of Nursing regarding the nurses performance. These reports must speak clearly to the reason that the license was restricted. If an unsatisfactory report is received, the licensee may automatically lose the license or be summoned to the Board for a hearing.

The Board may remove the restrictions or reinstate a license when there is evidence that the reasons for the restrictions or suspension are no longer in existence and the Board finds that the nurse can reasonably be expected to safely and properly practice nursing (NCBON, 2001). Generally, prior to reinstatement of a license, the nurse must petition the Board and a hearing may be conducted to determine if restrictions will be placed on the reinstated license. The Board of Nursing is empowered to implement these restrictions and suspensions as part of its role in protecting the public (Deloughery, 1998).

In 1986, Congress passed the Health Care Quality Improvement Act (HCQIA) in response to a rise in the number of malpractice cases in the United States. This act provided for the establishment of the National Practitioner Data Bank as an information and reporting system. This group maintains information about (a) payments made by medical malpractice insurers; (b) disciplinary actions taken by any state licensing board; (c) disciplinary actions taken by a state licensing board or agency against other health care providers; (d) disciplinary actions about incompetence or unprofessional conducts by hospitals, group medical practices, and health maintenance organizations (HMOs) that adversely affect clinical privileges of physicians and dentists; and (e) actions by a professional society for incompetence or unprofessional conduct that affects membership in that society. This reporting system collects data on nurses and is available to hospitals and other agencies that employ nurses. Nurses should be aware that any reports and guilty verdicts by a licensing board will be listed in this national data bank and is available to potential employers (Brent, 2001).

Licensure Renewal

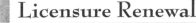

Renewal forms are directed to practicing nurses and serve as the request for licensure for future years. Boards of Nursing generally require license renewal every 2 years on the nurse's birthday, the last day of the birth month, or on December 31 every 2 years. Renewal notices are sent to the nurse prior to the expiration date. It is the responsibility of the nurse to keep the Board of Nursing informed of a current address to ensure timely receipt of forms. Many nurses have a false belief that the post office will forward mail for an indefinite period of time. Generally, that period may be limited to as few as 30 to 45 days.

After that period, the mail is returned to the sender (Board of Nursing), in which case the nurse may never receive the renewal form. Whether a renewal notice is received or not, the nurse may not practice nursing without a current license. In the future many states may require or offer nurses the opportunity to renew their license on-line.

Nurses and not their employers are accountable for maintaining current licensure. This responsibility cannot be delegated to an employer. However, the chief nurse responsible for employment of a nurse may also be subject to disciplinary action if a nurse is employed without a current license. Though both the nurse and the employer may share the responsibility for this illegal practice of nursing, the ultimate accountability rests with the nurse (NCBON, 2001).

Multistate Licensure

Multistate licensure (nurse licensure compact) was considered by the National Council of State Boards of Nursing (NCSBN) as early as 1996 and was finally approved in 1998. The first four states that implemented the registered nurse (RN) and licensed practical nurse (LPN)/licensed vocational nurse (LVN) compact were Maryland, Texas, Utah, and Wisconsin. These four states enacted the law for the compact on January 1, 2000 (NCSBN, 2001).

The **Nurse Licensure Compact** is a mutual recognition model of nurse licensure that allows a nurse to have one license (in his or her state of residency) and to practice in other states subject to each state's practice laws and regulations. In order to achieve mutual recognition, each state must enact legislation authorizing the Nurse Licensure Compact. As of 2001, the multistate licensure applies only to registered nurses and licensed

Critical Thinking and Reflection

Take a few minutes to look up requirements for renewal of licensure in your state. Consider any costs involved in licensure renewal. If continuing education is mandated for renewal, consider the costs of continuing education not only in terms of costs for the course, but also cost to you for time off from work. When interviewing for a job, it is important to ask prospective employers about provisions for continuing education. Are courses available at the employing institution? Will the employer provide paid time off for the nurse to pursue continuing education hours?

practical nurses. Consideration by the National Council of State Boards of Nursing is being given to the possibility of advance practice nurses (APN) also being included in a compact. The rationale for the APN being included in the mutual recognition model at a different timeline is that a base of comparable licensure requirements does not currently exist for APN (NCBON, 2002).

Overall, the mutual recognition model allows the nurse to use one license to practice in multiple states. To this end, multiple licensure privilege grants the authority to practice not only in the primary state of residency, but also in remote states within the interstate compact. Multistate licensure is not an additional license that one has to apply for or pay an additional fee. If fact, part of the interstate compact mandates that an individual hold only one license (multistate license) and not multiple state licenses. The interstate compact supersedes state laws and may be amended by all party states agreeing to change individual state laws (NCBON, 2002).

Multistate licensure requires the nurse to meet the requirements of the Board of Nursing in their primary state of residence. The primary state of residence refers to the nurse's fixed, permanent, and principal home (NCBON, 2002). If a nurse with an unencumbered license has a license in a state that is part of the interstate compact, they will be issued a "**multistate privilege to practice**" in any of the other compact states. The state of their permanent residence address is called the primary state and the second, third, and other states in the compact are called remote states. The home (primary residence) state as well as the remote states may take disciplinary action and can address the out-of-state nurse's behavior. The compact authorizes the nurse licensing board of any compact state to investigate allegations of unsafe practice by any nurse practicing in that state. Based on findings of the investigation, the remote state may deny the nurse's multistate privilege to practice in that state. The compact does not diminish the current authority of the home state to discipline, but allows for ready exchange of investigatory information among the states. In addition to the actions that may be taken by the home state, the remote state has the authority to issue cease-and-desist orders on the licenses. Reports will be sent to the home state where actions to the multistate license can be taken (NCBON, 2002).

If the nurse changes primary residence to another state, there is usually a 30-day period of time in which they can practice before they must have a license for the state in which they have primary residence. Any licensed nurse that is changing residency from one state to another should contact the new state prior to relocating to obtain specific information regarding licensure in the second state. Currently there are only 13 states in the interstate compact so it cannot be assumed that the second state belongs to the compact. Lastly, the Nurse Practice Act in a state belonging to the Compact usually contains information about the Compact. The National Council State Boards of Nursing (NCSBN) Web site contains a listing of the states in the Compact and information on the mutual recognition model.

Differentiated Practice

According to Dorothy Jones as published in *Nursing Issues in the 1990s* (Strickland & Fishman, 1994), there are at least three purposes for the differentiated practice including (a) the explosion of knowledge within health care, (b) the expanding knowledge base within the various health care disciplines, and (c) the need for more cost-effective health care. These factors have led health care providers to assess carefully the unique contributions each health care discipline offers in providing patient care. Harkness, Miller, and Hill (1992) define **differentiated practice** as "practice expectations that are consistent with expected competencies of graduates from different kinds of education programs" (p. 26).

Historically, differentiated practice was first recognized following World War II when a nursing shortage existed; licensed practical nurses and nursing assistants were introduced to relieve that shortage. A great need then existed to define the roles in order to make clear where the accountability and responsibility for patient care outcomes resided. At that time differentiated practice was established by the role the care provider held as either case manager or care associate (Primm, 1987). Differentiated practice has also been used to describe one's work contingent on philosophy and educational preparation.

An educational-based model differentiated practice based on educational preparation has been proposed (Jones, 1994). The premise for this discussion was that the BSN graduates functions in the professional role and the ADN graduates function in a technical role. This model existed in theory until North Dakota, in 1987, required nurses to have a baccalaureate degree for licensure as a professional nurse. Since then, graduates from associate degree programs are licensed as technical nurses, while baccalaureate graduates are licensed as registered nurses. Interestingly, in the almost 15 years since North Dakota instituted this requirement no other states have followed suit.

After the 1987 North Dakota decision, an all-professional model emerged in many employing institutions, which encouraged all nurses be prepared at the baccalaureate level. It was soon learned that there were not enough available nurses prepared at the baccalaureate level to implement the model in its purest form. Today, some employing institutions have implemented the all-professional model in selected clinical areas such as intensive care and emergency departments.

In 1995, the Pew Commission submitted a report advising that nursing distinguish between the different levels of nursing. The report suggested that associate degree preparation focus on knowledge and skills for entry level hospital setting and nursing home practice, and that baccalaureate preparation be directed toward hospital-based case management and community-based practice. The report advised that the master's degree be reserved for the specialty prac-

tice in the hospital and for independent practice as a primary care provider. The Pew Commission's advice supports the definition of Harkness, Miller, and Hill (1992) in relation to differentiated practice; however, even with this recommendation, states have failed to amend nurse practice acts.

Differentiated practice may be the future of nursing, however, there is again a shortage of nurses particularly in acute care settings. Some believe that educating more individuals to be nurses is the answer; others believe the answer may be differentiated practice and educating nurses based on public health care needs. Still others believe that nurses graduating from Baccalaureate programs be licensed at a higher level of practice than nurses graduating from Associate Degree programs. Currently, there is a trend for more nurses to practice at advanced levels as primary care providers; nurses are working in areas not previously available. Even with the requirement of an advanced degree, advanced practice has drained from the pool of already practicing nurses. A shortage will always exist when the entering number remains constant while the practice site opportunities are increasing.

TRANSITION INTO PRACTICE

Fifteen percent of new graduates who take the NCLEX are not successful on their first attempt (National Council of State Boards of Nursing, 1999). As a result, these nurses will experience several adverse consequences. Most will experience a financial loss due to the resultant change in job status or loss of employment. Many will lose highly coveted internships. Nurses who fail the NCLEX often experience pain associated with the stigma that accompanies failure. Furthermore, failure to pass NCLEX can lead to a fear that the exam will never be passed and, thus, an inability to prepare adequately to take the exam a second time (Dennis et al., 1990; Zuzelo, 1999).

While the literature is replete with articles that provide students and new nurses with guidance for preparing for the NCLEX, there are relatively few articles geared to helping the graduate who has experienced failure. Poorman and Webb (2000) undertook a qualitative study designed to increase understanding of noncognitive variables that influence NCLEX success. In their study, they found three themes present in the

thoughts of a sample of new graduates who had failed the NCLEX. The first theme common to the thoughts of these nurses was one of failure. The nurses felt they had lost their identity as "nurse" and thus were at a loss as to what direction to take next; they doubted their abilities (e.g., engaged in negative self-appraisal, questioned their knowledge) and experienced frequent somatic complaints. The second theme associated with thoughts of these graduates was one of "wanting" (e.g., wanting more from their lives and wanting support). The final theme that permeated the thoughts of theses graduates involved feelings of hope and determination. While these researchers offered a structured supportive program for the graduates, several retook the exam more than once and one had failed to pass the exam by the end of the study.

With regard to the literature it is clear that no single forecaster exists to predict failure on the NCLEX. It is also clear new graduates are not afforded the same opportunities and support from faculty and schools of nursing that they had experienced prior to failing the exam. If a new nurse is faced with the requirement to retake the exam, the individual graduate should assess his or her strengths, weaknesses, and needs. It is important the graduate develop a positive attitude, seek support of a tutor or review course, use review textbooks, develop test-taking skills, and continue to gain clinical experience within a health care setting. Clinical experience is often helpful in developing priority setting and clinical judgment skills. Furthermore, unit managers and other nursing personnel can offer the graduate support and encouragement as he or she prepares to take the next exam. Some individuals faced with repeating the NCLEX will also need to seek counseling for test anxiety (Todd & Gruber-May, 1993; Vance & Davidhizer, 1997). Such courses offer the graduate the ability to deal with feelings of anxiety and help him or her place the test in a realistic perspective. Finally, the graduate must take personal responsibility and control for learning and thus success on the NCLEX.

KEY POINTS

1. Boards of Nursing mandate licensure to ensure minimum standards of competency and to provide the public safe nursing care.

2. Boards of Nursing are typically empowered to perform functions related to the licensure, discipline, education, and scope of practice of nurses. Further Boards of Nursing often describe what activities do not require the professional judgment of a licensed nurse and these become common tasks or procedures that may be delegated to unlicensed persons.

3. In the area of licensure the Board regulates licensure in relation to the requirements for initial licensure, renewals, and for the process of endorsement of nurses educated in both the United States and its territories and of foreign nurses seeking licensure by examination.

4. The Board serves to protect the public. In order to fulfill this mission the Board may suspend, restrict, or revoke a nurse's license.

5. In relation to education, the Board of Nursing is empowered to write standards for education programs and to survey the education programs to determine compliance with the standards.

6. The Board makes decisions as to what is basic practice and what is considered to be practice beyond the basic level. Generally, basic nursing is that which is taught in the nursing program while nursing activities that are beyond the basic school of nursing education is considered advanced practice. These are different from the scope of practice taught in the curriculum of the advanced practice nurse at the master's level.

7. Nurses may delegate tasks to UAP; however, as the nurse remains accountable for the tasks delegated he or she must (a) know what can be legally delegated, (b) understand the skill level of the UAP, and (c) maintain open communication with the UAP regarding patient response to care provided.

8. The NCLEX measures minimum competence for entry-level practice; successfully passing the test indicates that the registered nurse has the competence to practice at the entry level.

9. The NCLEX test plan is (a) based on a job analysis survey, (b) reflects patient needs including safe effective care environment, physiologic integrity, psychosocial integrity, and health promotion and health maintenance, and (c) has six concepts/processes integrated throughout (caring, communication and documentation, cultural awareness, nursing process, self-care, and teaching/learning).

10. For the RN exam, there is a minimum of 75 items and a maximum of 265 items. Every candidate will receive at least the minimum number of items and may receive any number over the minimum. The actual number of items on an exam is determined by the difficulty level of the items that the candidate can answer successfully.

11. Every candidate must determine the best method for him or her to prepare for the NCLEX.

12. Boards of Nursing generally require license renewal every 2 years. Renewal notices are sent to the nurse. It is the responsibility of the nurse to keep the Board of Nursing informed of a current address. It is the responsibility of the nurse not to practice without a current license.

13. The Nurse Licensure Compact is a mutual recognition model of nurse licensure that allows a nurse to have one license (in his or her state of residency) and to practice in other states subject to each state's practice laws and regulations.

EXPLORE MediaLink

Critical thinking questions, essay questions, key terms, web links, activities, NCLEX review questions, and more interactive resources can be found on the Companion Website at www.prenhall.com/haynes. Click on Chapter 20 to select activities for this chapter.

REFERENCES

American Association of Nurse Anesthetists. (1997). *Providing anesthesia into the next century: Executive summary.* Park Ridge, IL: Author.

American Nursing Review. (2000). *An analysis of NCLEX-RN review courses* [Brochure]. Washington, DC: Author.

Beeman, P. B., & Waterhouse, J. K. (2001). NCLEX-RN performance: Predicting success on the computerized examination. *Journal of Professional Nursing, 17*(4), 158–165.

Brent, N. J. (2001). *Nurses and the law: A guide to principles and applications* (2nd ed.). Charlotte, NC: W. B. Saunders.

Deloughery, G. (1998). *Issues and trends in nursing* (3rd ed.). St. Louis, MO: Mosby.

Dennis, E. K., Edwards, S., Grau, W. H., Henning, E. D., Lee, B. T., & Moses, D. L. (1990). Enhancing the success of NCLEX-RN retesters. *Nursing Connections, 3*(3), 43–50.

Eason, F. R. (1999). Riding the tides of change in the NP and RN markets. *Advance for Nurses, 1*(1), 6.

Eason, F. R. (2000). The four A's of delegation: A primer. *Advance for Nurses, 2*(22), 11–12, 30.

Ellis, J. R., & Hartley, C. L. (2001). *Nursing in today's world.* Philadelphia, PA: Lippincott, Williams & Wilkins.

Harkness, G. A., Miller, J., & Hill, N. (1992). Differentiated practice: A three-dimensional model. *Nursing Management, 23*(12), 26–27, 30.

Jones, D. A. (1994). Advanced practice. In O. L. Strickland & D. J. Fishman (Eds.), *Nursing issues in the 1990s* (pp. 133–165). New York: Delmar Publishers.

Kalisch, P. A., & Kalisch, B. J. (1995). *The advance of American nursing* (3rd ed.). Philadelphia: J. B. Lippincott.

Kelly, L. Y., & Joel, L. A. (1999). *Dimension of professional nursing* (8th ed.). New York: McGraw-Hill.

Mitchell, P. R., & Grippando, G. M. (1993). *Nursing perspectives and issues* (5th ed.). New York: Delmar Publishers.

National Council of State Boards of Nursing. (2001). *About NCSBN events, news, views, & nursing regulations* Washington, DC: Author.

National Council of State Boards of Nursing, Inc. (2001). *NCLEX examination candidate bulletin* [Brochure]. Chicago, IL: Author.

National Council of State Boards of Nursing. (2000). *Test plan for the National Council of Licensure Examination for registered nurses.* Chicago, IL: Author.

National Council of State Boards of Nursing. (1999). *Report summary of NCLEX results.* Chicago, IL: Author.

North Carolina Board of Nursing. (2001). *Nursing practice act, State of North Carolina.* Raleigh, NC: Author.

Pew Health Professions Commission. (1995). *Critical challenges: Revitalizing the health profession for the 21st century.* San Francisco: UCSF Center for Health Professions.

Poorman, S. G., & Webb, C. A. (July/August 2000). Preparing to retake the NCLEX-RN. *Nurse Educator, 25*(4), 175–180.

Primm, P. L. (1987). Differential practice for ADN and BSN prepared nurses. *Journal of Professional Nursing, 3,* 218–225.

Silvestri, L. A. (2002). *Q & A review for NCLEX-RN.* Philadelphia, PA: W. B. Saunders.

Strickland, O. L., & Fishman, D. J. (1994). *Nursing issues in the 1990s.* New York, NY: Delmar Publishers.

Todd, C. M., & Gruber-May, J. (1993). Surviving NCLEX-RN reexamination. *MEDSURG Nursing, 2*(4), 304–306.

Vance, A., & Davidhizer, R. (1997). Strategies to assist students to be successful the next time around on the NCLEX-RN. *Journal of Nursing Education, 36*(4), 190–192.

Wyche, M. L. (1938). *The history of nursing in North Carolina.* Chapel Hill, NC: University of North Carolina Press.

Zuzelo, P. R. (1999). Professional practice and the NCLEX examination: A bottom-line approach. *Nurse Educator, 24*(3), 11–12.

SUGGESTED READINGS

American Association of Colleges of Nursing. (2002). Public policy update: Nurse licensure compact. *AACN News, 19*(6), 17.

Accord, L. G. (1999). Education: The case for differentiated practice. *Journal of Professional Nursing, 15*(5), 264.

Barkley, T. W., Rhodes, R. S., & Dufour, C. A. (1998). Nursing and health care perspectives. *Predictors of success* on NCLEX-RN among baccalaureate nursing students, *19*(3), 132–137.

Davis, C. R., & Nichols, B. L. (2002). Foreign-educated nurses and the changing U.S. nursing workforce. *Nursing Administration Quarterly, 26*(2), 43–51.

Eddy, L. L., & Epeneter, B. J. (2002). Journal of nursing education. *The NCLEX-RN experience: Qualitative interviews with graduates of a baccalaureate nursing program, 41*(6), 273–278.

Hall, B. (2002). Imprint. *Tips on Taking the NCLEX Exam, 49*(1), 43, 45.

Joel, L. A. (2002). Education for entry into nursing practice: Revisited for the 21st century. *Online Journal of Issues in Nursing, 7*(2), 8P.

Nibert, A. T., & Young, A. (2001). Computers in nursing. *A Third Study on Predicting NCLEX Success with the HESI Exit Exam, 19*(4), 172–178.

Prothero, M. M., Marshall, E. S., & Fosbinder, D. M. (1999). Implementing differentiated practice: Personal values and work satisfaction among hospital staff nurses. *Journal for Nurses in Staff Development, 15*(5), 185–192, 223.

21

The Stress of Life and Professional Survival

ELIZABETH FARREN CORBIN
LINDA C. HAYNES

Life is difficult.

Peck, 1978

LEARNING OBJECTIVES

AT THE COMPLETION OF THIS CHAPTER, THE READER WILL BE ABLE TO:

- Discuss the dynamics of stress.
- Recognize unique sources of stress for nurses.
- List techniques that promote health and increase stress hardiness.
- Distinguish between effective and ineffective strategies for coping with stress.
- Explain the relationship between stress and such pathologic states as burnout, compassion, fatigue, depression, and addiction.
- Develop effective personal and professional self-care strategies.

MediaLink   www.prenhall.com/haynes

Additional online resources including NCLEX review questions, critical thinking questions, and real-world activities for this chapter can be found on the Companion Website at www.prenhall.com/haynes.

In today's fast-paced world individuals experience a wide range of stress-related symptoms and/or diseases including headaches, backaches, indigestion, hypertension, fatigue, and insomnia. Health promotion strategies, home remedies, prescribed medications, alternative therapies, over-the-counter drugs, and in some cases illicit/illegal drugs are being used to treat or reduce symptoms of stress. Nurses experience stress caused by the physical, mental, and spiritual strain of everyday life as well as the responsibilities of a professional nursing career. Today's nurse is expected to do more for more people, care for patients who are sicker, and maintain up-to-date knowledge and skills in a rapidly changing health care industry that is plagued by a workforce shortage, declining budgets, and intense scrutiny by public and health care regulators. Despite professional demands and the challenges of everyday life and family, nurses continue to provide for others while often neglecting to care for themselves with the same level of compassion they provide others. This personal disregard for their own physical, mental, and/or spiritual health makes nurses prime candidates for developing adverse stress-related disorders.

Occupational stress can result in high levels of absenteeism and attrition from the profession. Some studies have suggested that stress in nurses is also associated with higher error rates (Charnley, 1999). To combat stress individuals employ a number of coping strategies. Some of these strategies are effective and lead to increased job satisfaction and work productivity, while others result in poor work performance, impaired interpersonal relationships, addictive behavior, and chemical dependency.

This chapter focuses on the nature of stress and addresses the unique vulnerability nurses have to the consequences of stress. The dynamics, causes, and manifestations of stress are reviewed. Practical techniques for effectively managing self and coping with stress are discussed.

Dynamics of Stress

Stress is defined as "a physical, mental, psychological, or spiritual response to a stressor" (Narasi, 1994, p. 73). A **stressor** is any experience an individual evaluates to be burdensome and threatening to his or her well-being (Huber, 2000). Individuals respond to stress in uniquely personal, emotional, and physical ways.

While the term stress is often associated with negative events, joyous celebrations (e.g., graduation, wed-

dings, childbirth, etc.) as well as unpleasant experiences (care plans, clinical evaluations, NCLEX preparation, etc.) cause stress. The terms eustress and distress are helpful in drawing a distinction. **Eustress** is stress that is sufficient to motivate and engage one's attention and energy, but not sufficient to overwhelm or discourage the individual. Eustress is a positive form of stress. **Distress** is a painful and toxic level of stress. The amount of stress necessary to cause distress varies with individuals and varies for the individual at different times in life. For one person, a certain amount of stress may seem challenging or invigorating. At another time or for another individual the same stress may seem overwhelming and punishing. There is a fine line between stress that leads individuals to be productive and stress that works against personal comfort. Stress is positive when it stimulates performance, and destructive when it inhibits growth, stifles creativity, drains energy, and lowers achievement. The effect stress has on individuals depends on their ability to successfully deal with the stress provoking stimuli.

The benchmark work of Cannon (1932) characterized the essential response to stress in physiological and metaphorical terms as a "flight-or-fight" response. Selye's (1956) general stress adaptation theory helped further the human understanding of stress. Selye proposed that stress was a nonspecific state or syndrome, which can lead to acute and chronic health problems. As a physiological response (a) the sympathetic nervous system is activated, (b) the adrenal medulla is innervated, and (c) catecholamines, especially epinephrine and norepinephrine, are released. The behavioral response to stress is dependent on the nature of the stressor, the individual's perception of the stress, the availability of support systems, and the individual's overall state of health.

Long-term or chronic exposure to stress can lead to depression, a weakened immune system, cardiovascular disease, infertility, miscarriage, and premature birth (Nies & McEwen, 2001). Similarly, short-term stress can impact health and well-being in the form of irritability, tension, headaches, and muscle pain. When feeling stressed, individuals may eat too much or too little and may find bowel function altered, concentration diminished, and sleep disturbed. Given the degree of discomfort stress can cause, it is not surprising interpersonal relationships can also be adversely affected.

There is a significant body of evidence to support the stress response as outlined by Selye. However, the preponderance of supportive data was gathered from studies of males, more specifically, male rats. Until

Taylor et al. (2000) explored the female stress response, which, like all human stress-mediated behavior, had been characterized as a "flight-or-fight" response. The preponderance of evidence supporting the human stress response has been conducted on males. These researchers hypothesized that females "create, maintain, and utilize social groups" (p. 411) to manage stress. The attachment-giving system was proposed based on neuroendocrine evidence that oxytocin, other female endocrine hormones, and endogenous opioid peptides may be at the core of the female response to stressful stimuli.

"Tend and befriend" represents another behavioral hypothesis to explain the female stress response.

This theory suggest "that woman's responses to stress are characterized by patterns that involve caring for offspring under stressful circumstances, joining social groups to reduce vulnerability, and contributing to the development of social groupings" (p. 422). The authors readily admit the "tend and befriend" model represents a "relatively primitive neuroendocrine model," which merits additional empirical study.

They argue that the present "flight-or-fight" model has merit and health care implications (e.g., early development of cardiovascular disease especially in men). However, they propose that the stress adaptation model as currently taught may be much more complex than originally believed in both males and females.

1995, women constituted only 17% of participants in laboratory studies. Although the flight-or-fight response is the primary physiological response to stress, some researchers have found neuroendocrine evidence that links oxytocin, some specifically female hormones, and endogenous opioid peptides to a uniquely female stress response (Taylor et al., 2000). These researchers suggest that the female stress response is modulated by a tendency to "tend and befriend." They hypothesize that females create, maintain, and utilize social groups to manage stress. They tend to care for others under stressful circumstances and join social groups to reduce vulnerability.

Preparation for Stress and Health Promotion

Hans Selye (1956) described stress as universal. "The soldier in battle, . . . the beggar who suffers from hunger and the glutton who overeats, . . . the house wife who tries to keep her children out of trouble, the child who scalds himself with coffee and especially, the particular cells of the skin over which he spilled the boiling coffee, they too are under stress" (p. 4). Few would argue that the actress competing for an Academy Award, the athlete in competition, and the entrepre

neur at the creation of a venture are all also under stress. Stress cannot be avoided. Individuals, however, can and should prepare for and learn to manage stress.

If stress is seen in both the coveted academy award and the dreaded wounds of battle, it would seem reasonable to suggest that preparation for stress is simply preparation for a rich and hopefully rewarding life. In its most basic form, preparation for stress involves health promotion via protective behaviors. "**Health promotion** is behavior motivated by the desire to increase well-being and to actualize human health potential. **Health protection** is behavior motivated by a desire to actively avoid illness, detect it early, or maintain functioning within the constraints of illness" (Pender, Murdaugh, & Parsons, 2002, p. 7).

Most individuals enter the nursing profession with an avowed dedication to care for the ill, prevent disease, and promote health. They simply do not apply this same dedication to their own health. Nurses depend on scientific and intuitive knowledge to devise appropriate plans of care for their patients. The same skill and preparation can and should be applied to the self-care necessary to create and sustain a joyful and energetic life for themselves both personally and professionally. A true advocate of self-care, Dr. Selye (1956) dedicated his book "to those who are not afraid to enjoy the stress of a full life, nor too naïve to think that they can do so without intellectual effort."

Nutrition

Nutrition is foundational to health, and even members of the health professions don't get to break the rules. While no one would send an athlete into competition on an empty stomach, many nurses begin their shift on an empty stomach or, worse, with their circulation coursing with caffeine. A nurse would never needlessly deprive a patient of lunch; however, many nurses deprive themselves every day. Everyone knows that fuel is required if a car is to operate; fuel is neither an indulgence nor an extravagance. Just as fuel is necessary for a car, good nutrition is necessary for every human being, including nurses. Adequate nutrition provides energy, satisfies hunger, and promotes a physical sense of well-being. Poor nutrition may be present in nurses who experience fatigue, cravings, hunger, and feelings of being bloated.

To ensure a proper diet, food selection should be based on sound nutrition science. Cravings, especially for refined and processed foods, often result from serious lack of essential nutrients or long-term habits of poor choice. Nurses have a professional advantage in knowing what constitutes good nutrition; however, adhering to proper nutrition can be difficult and requires planning. There are many insightful and instructive works on practical nutrition. One example is from Deepak Chopra, noted physician and author who, in his brief work *Boundless Energy*, speaks from the perspective of Ayurveda, a holistic Indian approach to health.

Chopra (1995) emphasized the importance of nutrition, writing "Everything you do and accomplish, every day—from the beating of your heart, to the millions of microscopic processes happening in every one of our cells, to walking and thinking and working—everything requires energy, and it is derived from the food you eat" (p. 31). The following basic nutritional principles, identified by the U.S. government in 1977, offer guidelines that remain valid today:

- Meet basic requirements for all nutrients on a regular basis.
- Eat approximately the amount of calories that will be expended on any given day.
- Increase consumption of fresh fruits, vegetables, and whole grains to 48% of daily intake.
- Keep fat consumption to below 30% of daily intake, saturated fat to 10%.
- Keep cholesterol consumption to 300 grams per day.
- Limit intake of salt to 5 grams per day.

Proper nutrition and healthy dietary habits require planning to ensure availability of the right foods. Many nurses eat poorly because they allow work to conflict with nutrition. They do not set priorities or allow time for meals, snacks, and breaks. Despite the busy work schedule of most nurses, it is possible to plan for healthy nutrition. Fresh fruits, vegetables, and whole-grain breads are transportable, require little preparation, and can easily be brought to work. When refrigeration is available, yogurt or a healthy sandwich from home offer nutritious alternatives. By making nutrition a priority, the nurse is building a foundation for lifelong health.

Sleep and Rest

Rest and sleep are two additional physiologic needs that individuals often overlook or take for granted. While people often complain about fatigue, they rarely plan for rest and relaxation. Only when individuals find themselves burdened by fatigue do they consider sleep a priority and allow themselves the opportunity to rest, relax, or sleep. Often, busy people see sleep time as flextime, during which they can finish more chores, watch TV, or catch up on personal errands. These activities may insidiously erode targeted bedtimes and result in loss of sleep and rest.

One should expect to feel rested and refreshed by sleep. Concentration and focus should come easily. Drowsiness and actual fatigue can be remedied only by

---

Critical Thinking and Reflection

List the signs and symptoms of mild to moderate intoxication. In a separate place, list the signs and symptoms of hypoglycemia. What are the similarities? Would you attempt to give nursing care after a few alcoholic drinks? Should you attempt to give nursing care without an appropriate meal when you are potentially hypoglycemic?

adequate sleep and rest and should never be addressed with caffeine or other stimulants. Table 21–1 is designed to assist the nurse in assessing current sleep habits.

Factors that prevent the nurse from meeting minimum requirement for sleep should be addressed aggressively. Physiologic signs of sleep deprivation include slowed reflexes, loss of equilibrium, nystagmus, ptosis, decreased respirations, and cardiac arrhythmias. Common psychological signs include irritability, sluggishness, decreased mental agility, memory failure, limited attention, and bizarre behavior. None of these outcomes is pleasant or compatible with feelings of well-being. Serious sleep problems may require the attention of a professional, but most individuals can significantly improve sleep habits by:

- Having a stable bedtime and bedtime routine
- Preparing for sleep with restful activities such as pleasant reading or conversation
- Avoiding stimulation or stress just before bed

- Avoiding alcohol or beverages with caffeine prior to sleep time

Each individual has unique sleep patterns, which follow a 20-hour circadian rhythm. Consistent with these unique patterns, there really are night people and morning people. Individuals who recognize their peak and trough energy times are more likely to meet critical energy needs through sleep and rest. By lovingly structuring and prioritizing responsibilities around energy needs individuals can expect better health and enhanced work capability.

Rest is not interchangeable with sleep. The human body needs both. Rest, like sleep, is individual and cyclical and is expressed on an ultradian rhythm. In most adults this rhythm includes 90 to 120 minutes of activity followed by 20 minutes of rest. Individuals who are able to maintain this psychobiologic rhythm are able to replenish energy more naturally (Rossi, 1991). The cyclic ultradian rhythms alert individuals to hunger, creative tension, and the need for solitude

Table 21–1   Sleep Questionnaire

Directions: Answer the following questions. Use your answers to evaluate your sleep habits and quality of sleep. An affirmative answer to three or more of the questions could indicate a possible sleep disorder and support referral to a sleep specialist for further evaluation.

1. Do you have trouble falling asleep?
2. Do you have trouble staying asleep?
3. Do you feel that your sleep is not refreshing or restful?
4. Has anyone ever told you that you snore?
5. Has anyone ever told you that you are restless when sleeping?
6. Have you ever been told that your legs jerk, twitch, or kick while you are asleep?
7. Has anyone ever told you that you stop breathing while you sleep?
8. Do you experience frequent headaches upon awakening from sleep?
9. Do you frequently have to get up at night to go to the bathroom?
10. Do you experience symptoms of gastric reflux that awaken you from sleep?
11. Do you frequently feel sleepy in the daytime?
12. Have you ever fallen asleep while at work or while driving a car?
13. Do you feel suddenly unable to move your limbs or speak when falling asleep or awakening?
14. Do you sometimes feel unusual sensations like "pins and needles" or a crawling feeling in your legs while at rest?
15. Do you have periods of the day when you have trouble paying attention, remembering things, or staying awake?
16. Do you have high blood pressure?
17. Have you ever experienced a sudden loss of muscle strength when laughing, angry, or excited?
18. Have you recently experienced decreased sexual drive or impotence?
19. Do you walk in your sleep?
20. Do you take daytime naps on a regular basis?

Source: Mary Ann Yantis, Louise Herrington School of Nursing, Baylor University. Printed with permission from Mary Ann Yantis.

or social contact. Prolonged overactivity results in physiological distress secondary to the release of neurochemicals. Honoring the cycle allows the body to replenish and sustain productive levels of activity (Dossey, 1995).

Many equate rest with taking a nap; however, any activity of a different pace or different orientation may result in feeling rested and/or refreshed. For example, rest may be experienced when switching from an intellectual activity to a physical activity or from a solitary activity to a social activity. To achieve rest the nurse should balance 90 to 120 minutes of physical activity, such as direct patient care with 20 minutes of intellectual activity, such as charting. Ninety to 120 minutes of study might be balanced with 20 minutes of physical activity such as cleaning the bathroom, playing with a pet, or going for a brief walk. When possible, true rest in a quiet, comfortable, and pleasant environment is a sound investment in future energy.

Exercise

Human beings are very much physical beings. The joy of using one's full potential as a physical being is, in contemporary society, often overshadowed by the "should" of well-intentioned experts. Exercise has become a prescriptive "should." Feeling guilty, many individuals feel they "should" be exercising. In gym class one "should" do a minimum number of push-ups or a prescribed distance of running. The simple fun and feeling of well-being in movement has somehow gotten lost.

Sadly, after a day at work many nurses feel they have had plenty of exercise. Unfortunately, what the nurse experiences on the job is repetitive and fatiguing activity, but not real heart-, lung-, or muscle-stimulating exercise. Exercise has been shown to have great impact on physiologic stability and emotional functioning. It is effective in the promotion of health and the prevention of disease (Pender, 1996). Furthermore, activity can be a vehicle for physical and mental stress relief, socialization, and above all, a connection to the whole self.

Assessment of one's own kinesthetic state is very important. The President's Council on Physical Fitness and Sports reveals that 60% of adults and 49% of youths (ages 12 to 21) are not regularly active (U.S. Department of Health and Human Services, 1996). Physical stamina, muscle strength, and adequate range of motion are essential to supporting the activities of every person and most especially, the professional nurse.

Structured exercise can be planned to achieve many objectives, including body sculpture, strength training for injury protection, weight reduction, and skill development. Many women have poor upper body strength. Strength training can help prevent cervical strain and back injuries, which are common among nurses. As with all other health promotion activities, implementation of an exercise regime requires planning. Exercise is doable even for busy, overworked nurses. There are a variety of exercise programs available. It is important that the nurse consider time limitations, financial constraints, and personal interest when selecting lifelong activity programs.

Physical fitness has no universal definition at this time, despite recent increased attention. A useful definition is the ability to perform activities of daily living without undue fatigue or spontaneous injury. Health-related fitness is seen to have five components: body composition, aerobic capacity, muscular strength and endurance, flexibility, and balance. All can be measured and all can be addressed in an individual program of fitness.

For some time the standard recommendation for minimal physical activity has been vigorous activity (60% or more of maximum heart rate) for 20 minutes, three times weekly (Pender, 1996). More recently, recommendations focus on improvement of baseline fitness in all the component areas. Fitness programs should be individually tailored, building on strengths and remediating deficits (Elder, 2002).

Exercise and activities should be selected with at least as much thought as is given career selection. A life's work is selected on the basis of capabilities, strengths, and preferences. Exercise plans should be approached in the same manner. If a person is socially oriented, a team sport like volleyball, soccer, or softball might be attractive. For nurses who spend their days intensely involved with others, a solitary pursuit like running, walking, swimming, or biking might be a pleasant diversion. For the athletic nurse or the nurse who is an overachiever, a competitive sport might prove invigorating. Just as no single career is appropriate for everyone, no single plan for exercise is congruent with the nature of every person. Though the goal of vigorous and regular exercise is beneficial to all persons, the method of meeting that goal can vary widely and still be effective.

Exercise includes any movement that calls for additional effort and results in an elevated respiratory and heart rate. Dancing is excellent form of exercise whether pounding at a disco, floating in a ballroom, or simply swaying to the music. Painting walls, gardening, and yard care all call for more activity than most get in daily routines. Physical activity of moderate to vigorous intensity burns 3.5 to 7 kilocalories per minute. Biking, walking briskly, swimming, or dancing meet this definition for physical activity. Vigorous activity that burns more than 7 kilocalories per minute includes jogging, swimming continuous laps, or bicycling uphill (Pender et al., 2002, p. 171). A sustained heart rate over prescribed periods of time will increase fitness; however, any activity that is beyond the routine, especially if it is pleasant, is going to reduce stress. Bringing the fun of physical movement back into daily life can open up potentials for increased well-being and a healthy focus on personal needs.

Unfortunately, time constraints are often a deterrent to getting needed, even wanted, exercise. The nurse can find time for exercise by tucking it into existing activities. For example, breathing deeply and fully frequently during the day relieves tension and improves oxygenation. Walking from the farthest parking place, taking stairs instead of elevators, and striding the length of athletic fields while watching children's events can add exercise to an otherwise sedentary lifestyle. Substituting active pursuits for sedentary habits is a time-conservative option that brings activity to one's life. A walking or activity date, in lieu of a movie and fast food, is a healthy option that provides an even better opportunity for getting to know a companion. Listening to a novel on a walkman while walking is a good substitute for reading in a chair.

Mind/Spirit

Nourishing the body through optimal nutrition, rest/sleep, and physical activity support self-development. It is equally important to promote and enhance cognitive abilities and deepen communication with the spirit in order to control stress.

A nurse's educational experience focuses on the acquisition of knowledge related to the science of health care. Despite the rigor of education the nurse must not forget his or her lifelong personal journey. This journey includes continual exploration of personal interest and unique interpretation of life. Reading, discussion, art, and music all enrich the mind and are just as necessary to personal development as is the in-service that explains a new clinical procedure. Pressure to read about and learn professional material should never replace the freedom to grow and explore other intellectual or personal pursuits. Indeed, given the multifaceted nature of nursing, it is hard to think of an intellectual, spiritual, or social pursuit that wouldn't have some application to nursing.

A relationship with oneself requires time and attention just as time and attention are required for relationships with others. Time with oneself must be scheduled with the same sense of commitment as other appointments involving work and family obligations. Personal reflection, meditation, and prayer require undisturbed time and regular practice. The investment in self will be apparent in physical, mental, spiritual, and cognitive growth and well-being. Spending just moments a day in undisturbed quiet can result in a centered, steady flow of energy and the clarity of knowing one's true goals and truths.

While knowing oneself is important, so are sustained personal relationships, which tend to vex and intrigue most human beings. Establishing and maintaining healthy human relationships takes time, effort, and skill. Relationships with others bring forth emotions,

---

Critical Thinking and Reflection

Take a piece of paper and divide it into four sections. In each section, list things that give you pleasure. In the first section, list things you can do in 5 to 10 minutes; in the second section, things you can do in 30 minutes; in the third section, things you can do in a half day and in the fourth section, things that require more than a day. How many things do you have in each section? How many things do you have in section one and two?

- You need to have lots of things in the first two sections because it is more likely that you will have 5 to

30 minutes for pleasure activities most days. Those activities that take up a half or whole day may require planning in order to experience their pleasure.

- You need to have a list of things in mind that will relax and bring you pleasure. If you only have 5 free minutes, you don't want to spend most of them trying to think of what to do!
- If you had trouble thinking of anything to go into any of the sections, you might consider that your pleasure tank is running on empty.

which increase the range of the human experience. Recognizing one's own feelings for what they really are is a skill that allows one to bring another dimension of knowing to conscious awareness. Sharing feelings and confidences appropriately with trustworthy people can often help to clarify feelings and give insight to emotions and moods. Accepting positive and negative feelings as valid is a part of learning about oneself.

Students are vulnerable to priorities set by the rigors of the nursing curriculum and graduate nurses are vulnerable to their demands of the job setting. Despite these rigors and demands, it is always important to reflect on what gives life meaning and joy. Though choices may change over time, the nurse should always protect the ability to pursue and support personal choices. Time and other personal resources must be dedicated to ensuring access to those things that give life meaning. Time to engage in art, sports, learning about the world, worship, and camaraderie are all essential to protecting the spirit and wholeness of the individual. A music lesson, a religious service, a soccer game with friends, and personal moments of prayer are not indulgences; they are investments in the hardiness of the human spirit.

Stressors in the Nursing World

Stressors commonly identified by nurses have changed little over the course of time. Florence Nightingale (1860) wrote in *Notes on Nursing* of the obligation of nurses to ensure a healthful environment (e.g., cleanliness, noise, air, temperature, clutter) for the patient, to see to the condition of the patient, the care and feeding of the patient, the medications offered the patient, the conduct of visitors, the management of the house or institution, and the need for continual education of the nurse. Even in the 1800s, the job of nurses was overwhelming, never ending, and therefore stressful. Nightingale gave the following sound advice: "At all events, one may safely say that the nurse cannot be with the patient, open the door, eat her meals, take a message all at one and the same time. . . . Let whoever is in charge keep this simple question in her head (*not* how can I always do this right thing myself, but how can I provide for this right thing to always be done)" (Nightingale, 1860, pp. 37, 40–41).

For nurses, the number one stressor seems to be the truly large and complex amount of work. Clearly, the number of tasks and the complexity of tasks is chal-

lenging even to the most industrious and experienced of nurses. The new graduate or the nurse new to a specific clinical area may face an even greater challenge. It is likely Nightingale would advise these and other nurses to set priorities and delegate.

Delegation

Delegation is the act of assigning a task or a series of tasks to another, while retaining responsibility for the outcome. Delegation requires careful planning and carries with it legal implications that never relieves the delegator of ultimate responsibility. When used wisely, delegation (a) promotes comprehensive care, (b) is economically prudent, and (c) serves to develop skills and initiative in subordinate colleagues. Far from being a handoff of undesirable tasks, delegation can be a chance for others to employ existing skills or to learn new ones. The first step to effective delegation is to form a clear picture of the work to be accomplished. The more overwhelming a situation may seem, the more important it is to break it down into smaller tasks. Developing an inventory of tasks to be accomplished and professional responsibilities can put a day's workload into better perspective. Frequently, nurses spend much of their workday on non-nursing activities. Such tasks are best delegated to appropriate personnel.

In matters of patient care, the nurse should plan for appropriate delegation after asking which tasks really must be done by the nurse, and which can be legally and safely delegated. Care must always be taken to delegate tasks to those colleagues who have the necessary skills and credentials to perform them. Delegation requires mutual acceptance. The delegated task must not only be within the competence and experience of the person accepting the task, but must also be accepted by the individual who has been delegated the task. By delegating early in a shift, all personnel involved have a chance to plan their workload and can avoid the pitfall (and stress) of having to interrupt others to seek help. Many patient care interventions lend themselves well to delegation. It is most important that delegation always follow policy and procedure rules for a given work setting.

Delegation is a tool that should not be confined to the workplace. Nurses may also find opportunities for delegation in their private lives. Delegation can relieve stress, reduce work, and provide opportunities for growth not only for colleagues but also for friends and family members. Delegation of a task to a child, for example, can create an opportunity for learning and lead to increased confidence and self-esteem for that child. The rules for delegation are equally important in both the personal and professional settings. The same courtesy, mutuality, and opportunity for negotiation must prevail. Even in the case of parent and child, a mutual agreement about responsibility for accomplishing tasks should be achieved. The delegated task must be within the competence of the person taking on the responsibility and adequate support must be given to ensure success.

Mutual recognition of one person's need to lower his or her workload may be sufficient to reach an agreement about delegation of a task or a responsibility between two or more persons. Sometimes mutual agreement may involve a trade of duties to achieve balance. For example, one spouse cooks and washes the dishes while the other spouse takes on the shopping and the errands; one nurse works out staffing patterns for the unit, while the unit manager attends budget meetings. Through whatever method, delegation can serve as a useful tool for reducing stress.

Time Management

Contemporary discussions of time management always address the issue that time management is really self-management. No one is able to actually increase time itself, nor can time be managed. Management involves the ability to handle, wield, and control work (Friend & Guralnik, 1958). While time cannot be saved, increased, or managed, individuals have the ability to handle/manage themselves and thus control their expenditure of time. With thoughtful planning, time can work for, rather than against, desired ends. Some of the most common problems involving self-management involve the unplanned and unnoticed expenditure of time.

ESTABLISH GOALS AND SET PRIORITIES
Nurses know how to set both long- and short-term goals for patients. This is basic to the nursing process

and a fundamental aspect of nursing education and professional practice. Establishing goals is also essential if the nurse is to successfully conduct his or her personal and professional life. To address goals, the nurse must first identify them. Goal identification requires the nurse to assess and plan. Short-term goals may be accomplished in a matter of minutes, hours, or days. Long-term goals may require days, months, or even years. The achievement of long-term goals usually results when a succession of short-term goals are accomplished. Oddly enough, it is sometimes the focus on short-term goals that sabotages the accomplishment of the long-term project. For example, in an effort to create order in the work area, some nurses focus so exclusively on clerical minutia that patient needs are overlooked. Steven Covey (1989) offers some intriguing advice applicable to time management. He suggests classifying tasks as important/unimportant and urgent/nonurgent. Some tasks are very important, but not urgent. Some are urgent and important. Some are urgent but not very important. Thankfully, some are neither important nor urgent.

Evaluating daily tasks in this objective manner can help the nurse focus time and energies effectively. By analyzing the importance of each task or activity the nurse is forced to ask:

- "Is the task really important?"
- "Is the task urgent?"
- "If urgent but not important, does it really deserve time?"

People often feel compelled to do tasks that are not important. It is not unusual to be tempted to do an unimportant task if that task is both pleasant and guaranteed to be successful. Sometimes these tasks help individuals feel good about themselves. By completing tasks, individuals can raise their self-esteem, renew their confidence, and improve their outlook. Therefore, this type of task diversion is not necessarily bad, but can create problems if carried too far. Diverting valuable time

---

Critical Thinking and Reflection

Make a realistic list of duties that you face on a regular basis. Could any of these duties be delegated? Who would be the appropriate person? How do you think another person would feel about accepting these tasks? How would you feel about relinquishing those tasks? What would you do with the released time were someone else to do some of the tasks you usually do? Would you simply add more tasks?

to this type of task is of concern only when time to complete a task is limited and the use of time on such a task decreases the likelihood that more important or urgent tasks will be accomplished.

BE DECISIVE

It is not uncommon for people to redo or duplicate tasks. The way most individuals handle the mail, particularly bills, provides a good example of task duplication. Many people open and sort mail with the intent of establishing priorities for later disposition. While sorting and prioritizing may seem like an efficient thing to do, mail that is not dealt with usually requires rereading prior to decision-making and action. Many individuals find they handled mail several times before acting on, filing, or disposing of the mail. Similarly, a nurse who takes notes while caring for patients and later transfers those notes to the medical record may be attempting to be efficient. Note taking, however, can result in needless duplication if there is no reason to delay writing directly onto the record.

Needless duplication can also occur when communicating with staff, family members, or roommates. Difficult as finding meeting times can be, having a short meeting may prevent needless repetitive conversations that repeat even the briefest communication over and over. A convenient time for professional communication may be during shift report when groups of individuals are gathered. Similarly, a memo or note on a unit or family note board offers a convenient format for communication.

AVOID PROCRASTINATION AND PERFECTIONISM

Perfectionism is often associated with procrastination, and nurses are particularly vulnerable to both. **Perfectionism** is the desire to be perfect and to do things perfectly. Nurses at all levels of skill and experience are vulnerable to the "super nurse" syndrome (Davidhizar & Shearer, 1999). Most nurses wish to be the best nurse possible, a goal which is realistic and admirable. But when this desire denies the nurse the latitude to be anything less, no matter the circumstance, serious stress can result. When the nurse sets lofty and idealistic goals for herself or himself and/or for the patient, and these goals are not met, the nurse may have difficulty reconciling reality with the expected ideal. This difficulty can result in stress-related feelings of guilt and inadequacy.

Few nurses admit to thoughts of perfectionism, while many expect no less than perfection from themselves and sometimes from others. Instead of helping reach higher levels of performance, the need for perfection can lead to discouragement and dissatisfaction. These feelings serve to rob the nurse of initiative and enthusiasm. Striving for excellence is inspirational and admirable. Striving for perfection is unrealistic and stress producing. Seeking guidance from teachers, supervisors, or mentors to set realistic expectations at any level can help nurses avoid perfectionism and the internalized "super nurse" image. Soliciting another professional's opinions can help to maintain a more realistic view of success.

Whether a function of perfectionism or not, many nurses also procrastinate. To **procrastinate** is to unnecessarily "put off" an action that is needed. This is not about planning a better time for an activity. This is about waiting until the last minute or, indeed, never getting a task accomplished. Procrastination ultimately effects patient care. While medications are generally given on time and procedures performed in a timely manner, other tasks (e.g., getting a procedure book up to date or a policy manual reflective of current practice) are put off. The nurse may put off such tasks to when "there is more time." This type of procrastination is unfortunate, as it is the out-of-date procedure manual that may cause less-than-optimal technique or actual errors in patient care. It may also be a time waster if the experienced nurse has to demonstrate or correct the procedure of newer nurses because the manual is no longer a good reference.

There are many causes of procrastination. Fears of not meeting a perfect standard may cause the task to take on exaggerated importance. For example, a nurse can never ensure that revisions to a manual will be completely accurate, comprehensive, and up to date. This subconscious fear can result in endlessly putting off the work. Viewing a project as a work in progress can considerably reduce pressure and consequently open the door to a hopeful and timely beginning.

Skill may be another reason for procrastination. If a nurse has doubts about the outcome of an anticipated project because of a possible skill deficit, the nurse may delay taking on or completing the task. In such a case, the nurse may wish to delegate the task to a colleague who has this skill. The nurse could then consider some form of education to better equip him- or herself for similar activities in the future.

Procrastination can also be a symptom of chronic fatigue, overload, and even burnout. Care should be taken to evaluate habits in a loving, not punitive way so that appropriate remedies can be applied to improve performance.

FOCUS AND COMMIT

Ambivalence, conflicting priorities, and guilt can contaminate time by influencing an individual's focus and effort so that time is not used efficiently (McGee-Cooper, 1983). Successful use of time requires focus and commitment. Extraneous thoughts and activities like daydreaming or carrying on unnecessary conversations while ostensibly working can sabotage efforts. For example, the nurse may experience ambivalence, guilt, conflicting priorities, or resentment, which interfere with productivity in each of the following situations:

- Sitting at a desk daydreaming about being "off" because a spouse or children are at home
- Turning down a desirable invitation for a social activity because some work has to be finished, and then failing to do the work
- Attending a meeting at work, yet worrying constantly through the meeting about what patient care activities may not get completed on time
- Attending a social occasion and yet worrying throughout about the work that isn't being done

In each of the above examples time goes by, but neither work nor relaxation is accomplished. The time is essentially wasted. To avoid such waste, seek an alternative solution when possible. If, for example, it is important to be home on a family day off, try to arrange to have that day off. Avoid feeling guilty about the request and use the time to renew, rebuild, and reenergize. If it is not possible to have the requested day off, try to plan an alternate family event that is possible. Commit to work while knowing an alternate day off is "in the bank."

Objectivity is another useful tool. If a nurse knows his or her presence is more valuable in the work setting at a given time than at a scheduled meeting, every effort should be made to make that choice when possible. It is much better to miss one meeting to address pressing work than to worry through a meeting making little contribution to either work or the meeting.

When work time is consistently contaminated by intrusive thoughts, the nurse most likely needs rest and relaxation for either a brief or extended time. Seldom do people "snap out" of the need for rest or change, any more than they "snap out" of the need for food or water. Nurses accept the legitimacy of rest and relaxation for patients. They must also accept this need for themselves. Rest and fun provide an investment in future productivity.

ENSURE CLEAR COMMUNICATION

Clear communication goes a long way toward organization in work and home settings. It eliminates misunderstandings, gives everyone an equal footing regarding information, and promotes solid interpersonal relationships. Communication is a dual responsibility of the speaker/writer and the listener/reader. Personal and public communications should be clear and to the point. The receiver bears the responsibility to clarify anything that was not understood. If, for example, after reading a memo, the nurse is not sure how to respond or comply, it is his or her responsibility to seek clarification. In personal communications, it is especially important that conclusions drawn from a communication be "checked out" by the receiver.

Messages that have, or are perceived to have, an emotional component are especially sensitive. If criticism, for example, is inferred from a communication, it is most important to clarify. Saying "Do you mean that my work was inadequate or that a different method should be tried next time?" enables the speaker to clarify the intended meaning. Clarifying in this way increases the likelihood that the receiver receives the message that was intended. No more. No less.

ORGANIZING THE CHAOS

The necessarily rigid scheduling of nursing responsibilities can leave little room in a day for reflection and planning. Without planning, however, a demanding schedule can become chaotic and tyrannical as one races the clock to complete tasks and solve crises. It is necessary to plan in order to avoid being taken captive by competing demands. Having a planning session with oneself and ideally with one's co-workers is an important control measure. Making "to do" lists is useful on several levels. Working with colleagues and shared "to do" lists allows others to know what demands each member is trying to satisfy. Making a "to do" list also helps rank priorities. These lists can be especially helpful should new priorities arise. Tickler files, brief outlines of essential information, can also be of great assistance. A tickler file is a simple recipe for an activity or a process that is likely to be repetitive, but infrequent. Such a task is performed so infrequently that most people forget exactly how to do the task and spend and respend valuable time figuring it out again and again. The "tickler" may simply be the name and phone number of needed services that are used infrequently. It may be a few notes on how to access and use a computer program for a once-a-year report. Perhaps a task is done quarterly. It may be difficult to remember how something was done three months ago. Rather than beginning anew with trial and error, a "tickler file" could quickly remind how best to get this task done.

Scheduling blocks of time for direct care, documentation, and review of lab work or procedure schedules can prevent the nurse from feeling fragmented in a chaotic work environment. Activities that must be done at a stipulated time can form the skeleton of a schedule. Other tasks can be worked in around the edges of these non-negotiable deadlines. Filing systems can also prove useful by keeping needed information readily available. If the workplace has no mechanism for accessing important papers (e.g., teaching guides, patient information tools, in-service records), then the nurse can begin the process for getting such a system up and available to those who need it. Such things eliminate the stress of recreating things that can't be found easily when needed.

LEARN TO SAY "NO" AND SET LIMITS

Setting limits and saying "no" cannot only conserve energy, but can also help avoid the confusion of competing and unrelated tasks that seem to crop up in the natural flow of events. If an activity was not planned into the day, it is important to analyze its actual value. If it is both important and urgent, it must be accommodated. If perhaps it is important but not urgent, then it may be most appropriate to say no and plan for the activity at a later date. If it is neither urgent nor important, saying no is likely to be the best response.

Saying "no" requires assertiveness, determination, and good assessment and interpersonal skills. Saying "no" generally does not feel good at first, especially for nurses who became nurses to help "everyone." Dr. Ann McGee-Cooper describes a merciless master that lives in many of us. "You can recognize a Merciless Master in you when, no matter how hard you work, or how well you do, it is never enough. The Merciless Master always wants more" (McGee-Cooper, 1983, pp. 7.2–7.16). She is referring to self-talk. Too often, when a request is made of the nurse, the nurse thinks "I should be able to do that" rather than "Does that need doing?" or "Am I the one who should do this?" The Merciless Master, of course, thinks it's the nurse's job to do that and every other task to the highest possible standard. Quite practically, not every task is deserving of the highest standard of execution. There are times when anything more than adequate is a waste of time and energy. Certainly, patient care should always be done to the highest standard. Many times, however, ancillary tasks simply need to be done adequately. An organized office system, for example, is just as serviceable as a fanatically organized system.

Sadly, failing to set limits and taking on more than a reasonable amount of work usually results in chaos, confusion, and poor patient care. Nurses need to see limit setting as a mechanism for chaos control. Nurses can control unreasonable demands set by others and establish organization in the work setting. This same technique, taken home, can have the same impact. Setting limits and compromising while ensuring safety and quality is a necessary survival skill. Doing fewer things with grace and focus makes as much sense in the home as it does in the workplace and often leaves all involved feeling better in the long term. A simple sandwich and cup of soup, for example, may be more nourishing with a relaxed Mom, than a four-course meal with an exhausted homemaker.

CHECK REALITY

Stress is not unique to the nursing world. The stress and strain a nurse experiences is not greater or of a more serious magnitude than that experienced by individuals of other occupations. True, a mistake by a nurse could result in the loss of a life, but air traffic controllers, railway switchmen, and drug manufacturers can cost lives when a mistake is made. Financiers risk losing money, often the money of other people. The loss could mean life or death, success or failure to families or corporations. Nurses are under stringent time pressures in their jobs, as are broadcast persons, bus drivers, assembly line workers, and fast food employees. Nurses are expected to do multiple tasks simultaneously, as are all parents raising children, commercial chefs, and small business entrepreneurs. Nurses are constantly exposed to other people's tragedies, as are child protection workers, lawyers, and social workers. Perhaps one of the greatest stressors to nurses is the attitude that nursing is one of the most stressful jobs and that solutions must be found that are specific to nursing. In reality, each human being faces challenges of time, energy, precision, organization, and compassion. This is good news, because it means that lessons and solutions from across society can be brought to bear on difficulties faced by the nurse in seeking a happy and fulfilled life.

From Stress to Distress

Stress can sometimes overpower the best of intentions and strategies and result in serious distress in a variety of forms. It may be that stress prevention measures are not started soon enough or that the measures taken are not sufficient to tame the intensity of the stress experienced. It may be that stress sneaks up on the unsuspecting, and insight isn't gained in time for remedial actions to be taken. For whatever reason, sometimes stress, continued stress, or excessive exposure to stress in personal or professional life overwhelms the individual. Stress may then provoke unhealthy responses that contribute to, rather than work against, the ravages of job and personal pressures. Just as with any threat to health, it is at this time that early diagnosis and prompt treatment may be the best tool for return to optimal well-being. Signs of stress buildup include the following feelings and behaviors:

- Irritability more frequent or more profound than previously experienced
- Lack of interest in work
- Dreading going to work
- Feeling emotionally drained
- Bringing work-related problems home with you
- Losing one's temper over minor things
- Over- or undereating
- Indulgence in alcohol or recreational drugs for relief
- Feeling pessimistic about life and work
- Finding decision-making difficult on any matter
- Feeling out of control of one's life
- Engaging in addictive behaviors such as smoking, gambling, or inappropriate sexual encounters (Malakh-Pines & Aronson, 1988)

In addition, argumentative behavior and lack of intimacy in previously satisfactory relationships are serious signs of distress. Discovering these signs in oneself or having a colleague or family member identify these behaviors can enable the nurse to recognize a dangerous situation and take steps to obtain assistance in regaining perspective, energy, health, and joy. There is no quantitative answer as to how much stress is neces-

sary to move an individual from simple fatigue to burnout, from needing a day off to needing psychotherapy. Each individual has a limit for stress, and likely that limit varies over the course of a lifetime.

When the amount or duration of stress finally gets one's attention, effective coping is of the utmost importance to avoid serious personal consequences. Stress management requires an awareness of stress and its consequences. Stress management also involves a belief that change is possible, and an individual's commitment to take action. Individuals who manage stress find they are able to "let go" of stress-related emotions. While not as effortless as it may sound, "letting go" of stress may simply involve (a) resolving that the stressor is not all that important, or (b) electing not to dwell on the stressor. In dealing with stress it is important to acknowledge what control one does have and what factors are outside personal control. Nurses who are able to recognize what control they do have and what pieces of a situation cannot be controlled (e.g., the feelings of another person, the ultimate decision of a competent adult, or the thoughts of others) have a better chance of managing stress than do nurses who are rigid and controlling. It is also helpful for the nurse to realize that dealing with some stressful stimuli can be delayed. For example, it is best to avoid dealing with stressful stimuli when feeling anger or when fatigued. Furthermore, it is best to have all available information before attempting to deal with a stressor. It is important to fully diagnose a problem before attempting remedies. Dealing with only part of a problem can perpetuate the effects of a problem and add to stress. Seeking help from appropriate persons involved in the situation is important in terms of not only gaining assistance, but in sharing responsibility. Continued distress with any situation can ultimately lead to more serious problems. The critical aspect of self-care is the recognition of deepening threats to health and well-being before stress turns to distress.

Burnout

Occupational or job stress results from pressure related to the demands of a professional role or job. Job stress can lead to **burnout,** a syndrome comprised of emotional or physical exhaustion, depersonalization, and reduced job productivity. Nurses who experience burnout move from enthusiasm and dedication in their jobs to a feeling of disinterest, even distaste. They may actually find themselves unable to perform beyond that which is minimally required to maintain employment.

Burnout is an occupational risk for all nurses, indeed for any person who takes on sustained responsibility for critical work. Though burnout is not inevitable, nurses who work in chronically understaffed, highly intense, or toxic environments where their personal philosophy of care cannot be actualized are especially at risk.

Nurses generally enter the helping profession because of a desire to care for others. Changes in health care economics and managed care have resulted in capitation, cost containment, and shortened hospital stays that may not be compatible with the emphasis many nurses have for quality patient care and service.

Psychosocial hazards faced by nurses include the expectations, attitudes, and behavior patterns of patients, families, other health care providers, and nurses themselves. Nurses who work against overwhelming odds of heavy patient loads, short staffing, and increasing responsibility without relief are at high risk. Workplace issues such as challenging patients, violence (verbal and physical), and lack of human or material support in the workplace are all the components of a stressful job setting.

Burnout is further influenced by a nurse's problem-solving skills, health habits, relationships with support systems, and self management skills. Other factors influencing a nurse's response to stress and the potential for burnout include age, sex, pressures of private life, education, and past experiences with stress. Additionally, nurses whose interests and satisfactions are limited to work are more prone to the effects of job-related stress.

Nurses are also at risk for burnout due to occupational hazards they face daily—biological, chemical, physical, and psychosocial. Biological hazards faced by nurses include the possible contraction of communicable disease. Chemical hazards associated with health care include not only chemotoxins but also environmental toxins such as cleaning products, latex antigens, and other substances used on a daily basis in the health care setting. Physical hazards are associated with patient care as the nurse assists with the transfer, positioning, and mobility needs of patients.

Goliszek (1992) identified four stages of burnout, including (a) high expectations and idealism, (b) pessimism and early job dissatisfaction, (c) withdrawal and isolation, and (d) irreversible detachment and loss of interest. Early in their careers, nurses have high expectations and tend to be enthusiastic and idealistic. When high expectations and idealism collide with the reality of the workplace, the nurse begins to experience pessimism and job dissatisfaction. These feelings can be associated with physiological and psychological symptoms of stress. As feelings escalate and needs are unmet, the nurse characteristically experiences anger, hostility, and negativism. Both physical and psychological symptoms worsen.

Interventions aimed at developing more realistic goals, changing attitude, and altering behavior can reverse burnout. Without these interventions, the nurse becomes increasingly withdrawn and isolated. Ultimately, the nurses can experience an irreversible detachment and loss of interest as physical and psychological symptoms worsen and self-esteem declines. Behavior is marked by absenteeism, negativism, and cynicism (Tappen, Weiss, & Whitehead, 1998).

Compassion Fatigue

Akin to burnout but different in a number of ways is a condition recently described as compassion fatigue. Some classify compassion fatigue as a post-traumatic stress disorder, while others describe it as an acute form of burnout. Compassion fatigue is a state of physical distress, emotional pain, and spiritual exhaustion. Some describe compassion fatigue as a result of "caring too much." It is important to differentiate compassion fatigue from burnout and to recognize that neither is currently a disorder listed in the *Diagnostic and Statistical Manual of Mental Disorders*, Fourth Edition (Text Revision) (DSM-IV-TR). While burnout develops over time and nurses often have time to adapt, compassion fatigue develops in response to an acute incident. There is little time to adapt. Affected nurses continue to give of themselves fully while nurses who are burned out are not committed to nursing, their employer, or the patient. Compassion fatigue usually affects front-line workers such as firefighters, police, paramedics, nurses, counselors, and pastors. Of these, front-line workers, those less satisfied with their professional effort and those unable to disassociate from the patient or their work, are most likely to develop compassion fatigue.

Sadly, rescue workers in disasters such as those offering assistance following the September 11, 2001, terrorist attacks in New York City and Washington, D.C., are most at risk for developing symptoms. Those dedicated workers experienced extreme grief and frustration, as so few lives could be saved. In addition, the months involved in the massive recovery effort and the pressure to complete the process as quickly as possible further drained and exacted a toll on untold numbers across the nation. There was little time to disassociate from the effects of the disaster. Even counselors who provided emotional support had little time to separate themselves from the overwhelming needs of the workers, families of victims, and a nation in grief.

All front-line workers, including nurses, must recognize their vulnerability to compassion fatigue. Unfortunately, as nurses mature and gain professional experiences they become less sensitive to their own stress. They tend to ignore their own personal emotions as they seek to be not only good nurses, but also "super nurses." Individuals with compassion fatigue (a) relive aspects of the trauma they experienced, (b) avoid anything potentially related to the trauma, and (c) experience physical symptoms such as sleep disturbance. As with burnout, compassion fatigue over the long run ultimately takes its toll not only on the nurse, but also on the workplace in the form of increased absences, higher turnover, decreased productivity, and patient dissatisfaction. Workers may even choose to leave a profession as an attempt to avoid further trauma.

Prevention of compassion fatigue is essential. For a nurse to prevent experiencing compassion fatigue it is important to (a) remember it is normal for people who care very much to experience pain, (b) recognize when fatigue is present, and (c) to adopt a lifestyle with habits that replenish the soul. Nurses who experience compassion fatigue need to remain connected with friends and family. They must maintain daily habits that reenergize the body, mind, and spirit. They also need quiet time alone. More severe cases of compassion fatigue, which are associated with depression, anxiety, or other symptoms of post-traumatic stress disorder, may require professional intervention.

Abuse and Addiction

DRUG AND ALCOHOL USE IN NURSES

The First National Symposium on the Impaired Nurse was convened at Emory University School of Nursing in 1982. Some attention had been given the problem in the early 1970s, but no organized effort had been made to identify or assist nurses so afflicted. Since that first forum, most states have addressed chemical dependency in nurses and much has been written. The primary goals in addressing this problem are protection of the public and treatment and support of the nurse (Hack & Hughes, 1989).

Chemicals are used freely in our society to remedy a host of problems. Health care providers are grateful for the modern arsenal of chemicals available to relieve pain, decrease anxiety, and treat depression. Nurses spend a great deal of time and effort learning about the administration and skillful selection of medications to treat patients. Early sociological research into the genesis of drug and alcohol use suggested that dependence would be high in people with (a) access to dependence-producing substances, (b) freedom from negative proscriptions concerning their use, and (c) role strain (Winick, 1974). Recent work by Alison Trinkoff et al. (2000) supports the utility of this theory as applied to the study of chemical dependence among nurses. Nurses clearly have access to a wide variety of drugs, have specialized knowledge of drug use that would banish negative proscriptions, and often experience job strain or role stress.

Many nurses start using the substance they will ultimately become addicted to while in nursing school. Figures from the American Nurses Association (1987) indicate that 6% to 8% of nurses have a drug/alcohol-related problem. More recent estimates indicate that the use of drugs and alcohol is at about the same rate as found in the general population; however, nurses who work in certain stressful specialty areas may be more prone to substance abuse. Emergency and critical care nurses are three times more likely to use cocaine and marijuana, oncology and administration nurses are twice as likely to engage in alcohol abuse, and psychiatric nurses are more likely to smoke cigarettes (Trinkoff & Storr, 1998). The validity of these figures is difficult to determine based on the high rate of denial among effected nurses. Furthermore, most nurses perceive self-reporting as dangerous. Employer data are generally unreliable as they are often reluctant to make accusations that can be difficult to prove and thus their data may underestimate the use of drugs and alcohol of employees. Often, nurses suspected of drug involvement are simply allowed to resign and no records of a drug or alcohol problem are maintained.

Common behaviors indicative of chemical dependency have been identified in numerous studies. Table 21–2 offers a list of selected warning signs of abuse and/or addiction that can be used to identify nurses with problem behaviors. A nurse who exhibits some or many of these identified behaviors deserves the attention of co-workers and supervisors who are concerned for the well-being of the nurse as well as the patients under that nurse's care. Nurses who are indeed using

Table 21–2   The Chemically Dependent Nurse: A Comprehensive Profile

Important: The following is designed to provide a frame of reference. Look for patterns or changes. **Not all characteristics need be present to indicate that a problem exists.**

Alcoholic Nurse	Drug-Addicted Nurse
Physical and Behavioral Indicators	
• Irritability, mood swings	• Extreme and rapid mood swings
• May become isolated; wants to work nights, spends break-time alone, avoids staff get-togethers	• Pupillary changes, weight loss
• Elaborate excuses for behavior, such as being late for work	• Activity level changes (i.e., lethargy to hyperactivity)
• Unkempt appearance	• Diaphoresis, pallor
• Experiences blackouts (periods of temporary amnesia)	• Wears long sleeves all the time
• Impaired motor coordination, slurred speech, flushed face, red or bleary eyes	• Frequently absent from unit, frequent use of restroom
• Numerous injuries, burns, bruises with vague explanations	• Blackouts
	• Usually works evenings, nights
	• May request prescriptions from staff physician
	• Consistently signs out more controlled drugs than anyone else
	• Waits until alone to open narcotics cabinet
	• Disappears into bathroom directly after being in narcotics cabinet
	• Often medicates other nurses' patients
	• Patients complain that pain medication dispensed by this nurse is ineffective, or patient denies receiving medication charted
	• Always uses maximum PRN dosage
	• Initiates an order for or a change in PRN medication
	• Violates procedure for wastage of narcotics
	• Signs out larger dose than ordered and wastes excess amount, when required dose is available on unit
	• Consistently volunteers to be medication nurse
	• Entries on narcotic control record are out of chronological sequence
	• Discrepancies exist between time drug is signed out on control sheet and time documented on nurses notes or medication administration record or not charted in patient care record at all
Job Performance Changes	
• Job shrinkage, does minimum work necessary	• Frequent medication errors
• Difficulty meeting schedules and deadlines	• Illogical or sloppy charting
• Illogical or sloppy charting	• Errors in judgment
• Errors in judgment	• Treatment missed, IVs empty, and other indicators of declining job performance
• Slow to respond to emergency situations	

Table 21–2 *(continued)*

Time and Attendance Changes	
• Increasingly absent from duty without adequate explanation, long lunch hours • Calls in to request time off at beginning of shift • Frequent "no show" status	• Frequently absent from unit • Comes to work early and stays late for no apparent reason • Volunteers for overtime • May work two jobs • Appears on unit during off time • Never takes breaks

Nonspecific Indicators	
	• Incorrect narcotic counts • Narcotic records disappear • Fictitious names appear on narcotic control record • Vials/packaging appear altered • Empty vials/packaging found in bathroom • Unusual amount of syringes used on unit

substances, legally or illegally, should also use this list for self-analysis. Nurses can ask themselves if any of these behaviors are becoming part of their own behavior profile, and if so, seek help for impaired functioning.

THE PROCESS OF CHEMICAL DEPENDENCY

The process of dependency and addiction usually begins as the nurse seeks to relieve physical or psychological pain. The degree of unrelieved pain often parallels the rate of addiction. The first step in the addiction process, the **experience**, occurs with the introduction of the drug or alcohol. The first encounter with the drug or alcohol is called the **initiation.** The nurse may first encounter the substance in either a therapeutic (prescribed drug) or social context. When the nurse associates the drug or alcohol with relief of pain (physical or psychic) a connection is made. Once this connection is made the nurse may begin to experiment with drug or alcohol use to continue to meet the need for pain relief. During this experimentation the nurse is attempting to gain control, heal, and/or reintegrate.

The second step in the process of chemical dependency involves **commitment**. The nurse makes a commitment to the drug of choice and makes it a part of his or her lifestyle. Acquisition of the chemical is a problem

if the drug of choice is not alcohol. Initially, the nurse engages in self-dialog as a way to justify, deny, or bargain with him- or herself as the chemical use continues. During this step in the process of chemical dependency the nurse begins to disengage or withdraw from co-workers, friends, and family in an attempt to prevent interference. The nurse begins to withdraw from former values. Routine chemical use becomes part of the nurses life. The nurse's behavior begins to include conning, stealing, lying, or whatever other behavior is necessary to cover up the now physical dependence on the chemical. The nurse feels powerless to stop and overwhelmed by feelings of guilt and terror that others will uncover the secret.

In the final step, **compulsion**, all energy is focused on getting and taking the drug or alcohol. Cravings take over, the nurse drinks or uses the drug to live. The nurse surrenders to the chemical and engages in bizarre and dangerous behavior (e.g., car accidents, suicidal behavior, accidental overdoses). Rather than a means for pain relief, the chemical becomes the vehicle for destruction (e.g., malnutrition, abscesses, liver damage, septicemia, and cardiac problems). In this final stage, mental health is adversely affected and work and family problems result. The addicted nurse may feel that death is the only outlet. Depression is common among individuals who abuse drugs and alcohol.

FROM ADDICTION TO RECOVERY

When addiction is undetected and untreated, the nurse lives a lonely and tragic life. Addicted nurses pose a hazard to themselves, co-workers, employers, patients, and their family. These nurses tend to (a) be unproductive workers; (b) use more benefits, including sick time; (c) place other employees, their patients, and the employer at risk; (d) cause more errors and perform poor patient assessments; (e) are forgetful; (f) demonstrate sloppy charting; (g) work at half the level of efficiency; (h) use more supervisor time because of poor work performance; and (i) adversely impact morale because of the attempt by others to cover for the impaired nurse.

Treatment is best aimed at detecting the problem early and educating staff members so as to help the addicted nurse avoid the path to self-annihilation. While it is the legal and ethical obligation of all nurses to confront the impaired nurse as soon as possible so as to protect patients, most nurses have difficulty confronting one another. Nurses are taught to be nurturing and caring; their tendency to enable the impaired nurse comes naturally. Additionally, nurses fear litigation if they confront a suspected peer of drug or alcohol use. Fortunately, this type of lawsuit is generally not upheld as long as proper procedure is followed and confidentiality is maintained.

To report the impaired nurse should be perceived as neither cruel nor threatening to the nurse's livelihood. Reporting this nurse may be a way of saving a life. When a nurse is confronted either by an individual or via a formal intervention, the following are important to remember:

- Staff should not confront the nurse alone.
- Consult with a supervisor and know policy and procedure.
- Evidence should be gathered and documented regarding problem behaviors and staff and patient complaints.
- It is unethical, and in most cases illegal, to quietly sit back and allow a nurse to practice in an unsafe manner.
- Nurses who are "found out" are generally relieved.

Peer assistance programs for nurses will vary in availability from state to state. Many employers have peer assistance programs for employees with drug or alcohol addictions. Support and information from these programs offers useful guidelines for intervening with the addicted nurse. Intervention begins with careful documentation of behavior. Documentation is verified for accuracy and includes verbal testimony as well as written evidence (e.g., medication records and nurses' notes). The goal of an intervention is to help an individual recognize problematic behavior. The intervention team is generally made up of a trained interventionist, a representative from nursing administration, a concerned co-worker or friend, a peer assistance program representative, an immediate supervisor, and possibly the nurse's family. A preintervention meeting is held to discuss the purpose and goals of the meeting, define member roles, cover the documented facts, and reach a consensus as to the consequences the nurse will face should he or she refuse to follow a recommended treatment plan.

During the intervention, information is presented in a nonpunitive, caring manner with respect for the nurse's legal rights (e.g., maintaining confidentiality). The nurse is encouraged to listen quietly with as few interruptions as possible. After all evidence is presented, the nurse is provided the opportunity to respond. The nurse will be provided with choices, though theses choices are generally unacceptable to the nurse (e.g., treatment or termination and referral to the Board of Nurse Examiners). Because the choices are generally unacceptable to the nurse, there is an element of coercion in intervention. Treatment varies and may include inpatient or outpatient care. Regardless of the outcome of the intervention, the nurse must be escorted (e.g., by a friend, family member, or treatment representative) to his or her destination following the meeting.

In recovery, most nurses will be welcome to return to work. A return-to-work conference is held. The recovering nurse and involved co-workers receive education and support when the nurse returns to work. During the initial phases of recovery the nurse may be restricted as to (a) access to narcotics and other addictive drugs, (b) hours of employment (e.g., day hours versus night and evenings when there is less supervision), and (c) the type of employment allowed (full-time staff nursing versus floating or agency PRN work). It is also likely that the nurse will be required to (a) submit to drug or alcohol testing and (b) attend follow-up meetings (e.g., NA or AA). Recovery from addiction is a lifelong process. Relapse is a normal aspect of this disease that is not necessarily inevitable. Self-care is not selfish. It is true dedication of the profession when the nurse chooses to protect and nurture the health of all persons including him- or herself.

NURTURING MIND, BODY, AND SPIRIT

Health promotion and the prevention of illness have become major objectives for the world community. In

June 2000, the Fifth Global Conference on Health Promotion was held in Mexico City, Mexico. Here was a conference attesting to the commitment of a world of cultures and nations to the improvement of the health of their people (Pender et al., 2002, p. ix). Surely, the welfare of the nurse is included in that commitment.

The distinguished nursing leader Jean Watson tells us that "all nursing must be more holistic, regardless of practice setting or patient population. We now see more clearly . . . that nursing becomes transpersonal and even metaphysical" (Dossey, 1995, p xxii). Dr. Watson is telling us that not only does the mind, body, and spirit of the patient deserve caring and healing, but that the mind, body, and spirit of the nurse enters into the equation as well.

In *Holistic Nursing: A Handbook for Practice*, nurse authors Dossey, Keegan, Gazzetta, and Kolkmeier challenge nurses to "explore the inward journey towards self-transformation and to identify their growing capacity for change and healing" (Dossey, 1995, p.

xxvii). Their entire book places a dual focus on the nurse and the patient because they realize that nursing is a transactual process. While all patients are deserving of care, healing, and growth, there is no patient more inherently deserving than the nurse. What better to offer the patient than care in which the nurse has confidence gained from self-care?

Care of the nurse is care of a precious resource. It is the responsibility of those who believe in the value of human beings and in the value of the caregiver and healer. Care of the nurse must begin with the nurse him- or herself. This chapter has provided a holistic approach to care of the mind, body, spirit, and career of the nurse. There are reminders for health promotion, suggestions for specific prevention of problems, and interventions for real problems. It remains for nurses to dedicate themselves to preservation of their own mind, body, and spirit in the belief that their knowledge of health and healing is more than a job, more than a career—it is a path to peace and fulfillment.

TRANSITION INTO PRACTICE

The sole purpose of this chapter has been to help the new graduate make a smooth and healthy transition into practice and to maintain the joy and achieve the fulfillment that motivated his or her desire to be a nurse. Unfortunately, not all individuals receive the hoped-for rewards, either esoteric or material, that were sought as they began their careers. A nurse who apparently suffered disappointment and disillusionment in her career wrote the article that follows. Eventually, as she describes, she left the profession. Read through this sad chronicle and then reflect on the questions that follow.

In writing her article "One Nurse's Response to the Profession," Barnet (2001) cited reasons she chose to retire from nursing, a job that she described as the "most stressful job in the world." She compares the media stereotype of nursing with the vastly different reality most nurses face as they care for sicker patients in an economic environment that has resulted in staff reduction when there is already a shortage of nurses. Ms. Barnet states that "nurses today are expected to do much more with less, so they have little time to spend with patients. High-tech breakthroughs, combined with the 'quick fix' cures seen on ER, have created unrealistic expectations in the public's mind" (Barnet, 2001, p. 27A).

She further describes nursing as a profession in which care providers are constantly "putting out fires," are caring for eight or more patients, and frequently do without bathroom breaks and meals in order to ensure positive outcomes for their patients. She very eloquently writes that while visitors to health care facilities see nurses actively providing care they are truly unaware of the responsibilities, high stress, and burnout experienced by many nurses that may include juggling calls, checking equipment, reviewing orders, inputting data, and comforting patients while also dealing with verbally and occasionally physically abusive patients.

Ms. Barnet addresses the trend in hospitals is to refer to patients as "customers." Many nurses take exception to this term. As she points out, nurses are not salespeople, maids, or waiters. Rather, nurses are professionals who care for patients with health care needs while being paid less than some trash collectors.

Stating she was overworked, underpaid, and unappreciated, Ms. Barnet chose to walk away from nursing. In her article she reported a feeling of relief but added "With fewer people choosing to enter nursing as they become aware of its declining status, low salaries, and impossible demands, who will care for me?" (Barnet, 2001, p. 27A).

After reading the Transition into Practice feature of this chapter and the nurse's chronicle of her career as a nurse, the authors of this chapter ask you to reflect for a few moments and consider some questions. As you answer these questions realize that you can only hypothesize, and should certainly not judge or second-guess the decision of any nurse to leave nursing. Remembering this, do you believe that many nurses have a realistic picture of nursing when they enter the profession? Do you believe you have a realistic picture of nursing as a profession? What was the first "stress report" that you identify in this nurse's writing? What aspects of self-care may have been overlooked? When you read this chapter, were you convinced that good nutrition and physical self-care were important, or did you see this chapter as simply one of many stress management discussions you have had while in nursing school? Do you have any new insights as to how self-care neglect can affect a career if not a life.

As you read this nurses report of duties, were you excited or dismayed? Do you see these incidents as part of a normal day or as assaults on the nurse's peace of mind? Which of the self-care activities discussed in this chapter do you think might have made a difference for this nurse? Which ones do you think will make a difference for you? How committed will you be to making sure that while you are working at your career, your career is also working for you?

Realistically, self-care may not be all that is required of nurses in order to keep nurses in nursing. Nurses must also develop and express a collective voice for change. As you enter the profession, consider how your voice can be heard so that while you are working to maintain your own physical, psychological, and spiritual health you are also advocating for a healthy work environment.

The authors of this chapter have a combined 68 years in nursing. We are alive, well, working in nursing, and happily enjoying our careers and are able to make time for our families and communities. We also see ourselves as voices for change and advocates for a healthy work environment. And we most heartily are hoping you enjoy the same success in your professional and personal life!

KEY POINTS

1. Nurses experience stress caused by the physical, mental, and spiritual strain of everyday life as well as the responsibilities of a professional nursing career. Today's nurse is expected to do more for more people, care for patients who are sicker, and maintain up-to-date knowledge and skills in a rapidly changing health care industry that is plagued by a workforce shortage, declining budgets, and intense scrutiny by public and health care regulators.

2. Some nurses disregard their own physical, mental, and/or spiritual health; this disregard makes them prime candidates for developing stress-related disorders.

3. Nurses should apply their skill and knowledge to the self-care necessary to create and sustain a joyful and energetic life.

4. Nutrition, exercise, and rest/sleep are fundamental to health and even members of the health professions don't get to break the rules.

5. One of the greatest stressors a nurse faces is the truly large and complex amount of work. To effectively manage stress the nurse must learn to delegate and manage self.

6. Self-management requires the nurse to establish goals and set priorities, be decisive, avoid procrastination, focus and commit, be organized, learn to say "no" and set limits, and perform routine reality checks.

7. Stress can lead to distress in the form of burnout, compassion fatigue, and dependency/addiction.

8. Health promotion and the prevention of illness have become major objectives for the world community; nurses should strive to ensure their own health. The nurse's health is in his or her best interest as well as that of the nursing profession, the health care community, and the patients cared for.

EXPLORE 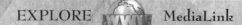 MediaLink

Critical thinking questions, essay questions, key terms, web links, activities, NCLEX review questions, and more interactive resources can be found on the Companion Website at www.prenhall.com/haynes. Click on Chapter 21 to select activities for this chapter.

REFERENCES

American Nurses Association. (1987, March). Impaired nursing practice. *ANA News*. Kansas City: Author.

Barnet, D. (2001, May 28). For stress, this job wins hands down. *The Dallas Morning News*, p. 27a.

Cannon, W. B. (1932). *The wisdom of the body*. New York: Norton.

Charnley, E. (1999). Occupational stress in newly qualified staff nurses. *Nursing Standard, 13*(29), 33–36.

Chopra, D. (1995). *Boundless energy*. New York: Harmony Books.

Covey, S. R. (1989). *The seven habits of highly effective people: Restoring the character ethic*. New York: Simon & Schuster.

Davidhizar, R., & Shearer, R. (1999). The super nurse syndrome. *Seminars for Nurse Managers, 7*(2), 59–62.

Dossey, B. (1995). Introduction. In B. Dossey, L. Keegan, C. Guzzetta, & L. Kolkmier (Eds.), *Holistic nursing: A handbook for practice*. Gaithersburg, MD: Aspen.

Elder, B. M. (2002, April). Measuring physical fitness of adults in the primary care setting. *American Journal for Nurse Practitioners*, 9–22.

Friend, J., & Guralnik, D. B. (Eds.). (1958). *Webster's new world dictionary: College edition*. New York: World Publishing.

Goliszek, A. (1992). *Sixty-six second stress management: The quickest way to relax and ease anxiety*. Far Hills, NJ: New Horizon.

Hack, M., & Hughs, T. (Eds.). (1989). *Addiction in the nursing profession*. New York: Springer.

Huber, D. (2000). *Leadership and nursing care management*. Philadelphia, PA: W. B. Saunders.

Malakh-Pines, A., & Aronson E. (1988). *Career burnout: Causes and cures*. New York: The Free Press.

McGee-Cooper, A. (1983). *Time management for unmanageable people*. Dallas, TX: Cooper Enterprises.

Merritt, S. L. (2000). Putting sleep disorders to rest. *RN, 63*(7), 26–30.

Narasi, B. (1994). A tool for living through stress. *Nursing Management, 25*(9), 73–75.

Nies, M. A., & McEwen, M. (2001). *Community health nursing: Promoting the health of populations* (3rd ed.). Philadelphia, PA: W. B. Saunders.

Nightingale, F. (1860). *Notes on nursing: What it is and what it is not*. Stamford, CT: Appleton & Lange.

Peck, M. S. (1978). *The road less traveled: A new psychology of love, traditional values and spiritual growth*. New York: Simon & Schuster.

Pender, N. (1996). *Health promotion in nursing practice* (3rd ed.). Stamford, CT: Appleton & Lange.

Pender, N., Murdaugh, C., & Parsons, M. A. (2002). *Health promotion in nursing practice* (4th ed.). Upper Saddle River, NJ: Prentice Hall.

Rossi, E. (1991). *The 20-minute break*. Los Angeles: J. P. Tarcher.

Selye, H. (1956). *The stress of life*. New York: McGraw-Hill.

Tappen, R. M., Weiss, S. A., & Whitehead, D. K. (1998). *Essentials of nursing leadership and management*. Philadelphia, PA: F. A. Davis.

Taylor, S. E., Klein, L. C., Lewis, B. P., Gruenewald, T. L., Gurung, R. A. R., & Updegraff, J. A. (2000). Biobehavioral responses to stress in females: Tend-and-befriend, not flight-or-fight. *Psychological Review, 107*(3), 411–429.

Trinkoff, A. M., & Storr, C. L. (1998). Substance use among nurses: Differences between specialties. *American Journal of Public Health, 88*(4), 581–585.

Trinkoff, A., Zhou, Q., Storr, C., & Soeken, K. (March/April 2000). Workplace access, negative prescriptions, job strain, and substance use in registered nurses. *Nursing Research, 49*(2), 83–90.

U.S. Department of Health and Human Services. (1996). *President's council on fitness and sports: Physical activity and health: A report to the surgeon general*. Washington, DC: U.S. Government Printing Office.

Winick, C. (1974). Drug dependence among nurses. In C. Winick (Ed.), *Sociological aspects of drug dependence*. Cleveland, OH: CRC Press.

SUGGESTED READINGS

DeCarlo, T. (2002). Where are the nurses? *Good Housekeeping, 243*(3), 110–113.

Lazarus, R. S. (1998). *Fifty years of the research and theory of R. S. Lazarus: An analysis of the historical and perennial issues*. London: Lawrence Erlbaum.

Lazarus, R. S. (2000). Evolution of a model of stress, coping, and discrete emotions. In V. H. Rice (Ed.), *Handbook of stress, coping, and health: Implications for nursing research, theory, and practice* (pp. 195–222). Thousand Oaks, CA: Sage.

Lazarus, R. S., & Folkman, S. (1984). *Stress, appraisal, and coping*. New York: Springer.

Phillips, K. (2001). One nurse's story. *RN, 64*(3), 47–48.

Schwam, K. (1998). The phenomenon of compassion fatigue in perioperative nursing. *AORN Journal, 68*(4), 642–648.

Sloan, A., & Vernarec, E. (2001). Impaired nurses: Reclaiming careers. *RN, 64*(2), 58–63.

Welsh, D. J. (1999). Care for the caregiver: Strategies for avoiding: "Compassion fatigue." *Clinical Journal of Oncology Nursing, 3*(4), 183–184.

22

Advanced Practice Nursing: Lessons of the Past, Challenges of the Future

DEBRA WOODARD LENERS

I have an earache:
2000 B.C. Here, eat this root.
1000 A.D. That root is heathen. Say this prayer.
1850 A.D. That prayer is superstition. Drink this potion.
1940 A.D. That potion is snake oil. Swallow this pill.
1985 A.D. That pill is ineffective. Take this antibiotic.
2000 A.D. That antibiotic is artificial. Eat this root.

Author Unknown

LEARNING OBJECTIVES

AT THE COMPLETION OF THIS CHAPTER, THE READER WILL BE ABLE TO:

➤ Discuss the evolution of advanced practice nursing and the historical context of each APN role.

➤ Analyze the influence of outcomes research and governmental task force findings.

➤ Delineate issues that will influence the future of APN practice.

➤ Synthesize information concerning licensure and regulation of APN practice.

➤ Identify various challenges facing the APN role in the twenty-first century.

MediaLink   www.prenhall.com/haynes

Additional online resources including NCLEX review questions, critical thinking questions, and real-world activities for this chapter can be found on the Companion Website at www.prenhall.com/haynes.

*A*dvanced practice nurse is a title used to describe a registered nurse who has met advanced educational and clinical practice requirements beyond basic nursing education. The American Nurses Association (ANA) recognizes four groups of APNs—certified registered nurse anesthetists (CRNAs), certified nurse midwives (CNMs), clinical nurse specialists (CNSs), and nurse practitioners (NPs). The common goals of all advanced practice roles include improved access to care, increased collaboration between various health care providers, expanded knowledge base for clinical decision-making, and increased professional autonomy.

Conceptually, the title, "advanced practice nursing/nurse" (APN), includes but is not necessarily synonymous with "advanced nursing practice." Advanced practice nursing is theoretically inclusive of but not limited to advanced nursing practice. "If one envisions advanced practice nursing as a pyramid, at the base are foundational or support factors; at the apex is advanced nursing practice" (Styles & Lewis, 2000, p. 35). Brown (1998) detailed a framework that differentiates advanced practice nursing as the broader concept subsuming advanced nursing practice. The term advanced nursing practice denotes advanced clinical practice, while APN incorporates advanced practice beyond a direct clinical focus. Unfortunately, legal titling and licensure definitions of APN identify the role as advanced clinical practice only. Therefore, nurse educators or researchers with advanced education and experience in the discipline of nursing may be unable to legally claim the title of advanced practice nurse.

The American health care system is based on a medical model of care with physicians as the gatekeepers to most services. As medical specialization has grown, there has been a tremendous focus on medical technology and treatment to the exclusion of basic primary health care services. Economics is a fundamental force driving change in the U.S. health care system. Traditional models of health care have concentrated exclusively on quantity of life which has led to a costly health care system. Today's health care system must be restructured to focus on quality of life, disease prevention, and health promotion as opposed to a sole reliance on expensive high-tech procedures and cure of disease. APNs are highly capable of providing the needed primary health care that can help transform/reform today's inefficient and costly health care system.

Specific competencies the APN must have to practice in the emerging health care system have been detailed by the work of the Pew Health Professions Commission's Taskforce on Health Care Workforce Regulation. The Commission's report directs health professions, including nursing, to meet specific health care challenges of the twenty-first century (Finocchio, Dower, Blick, Gragnola, & Task Force on Health Care Workforce Regulations, 1998). Regulation of the health care workforce is key to protecting the public's health and safety, ensuring the quality of health care services, and providing access to care. The APN is able to provide health care to individuals, families, and/or groups in a variety of settings. Advanced practice nurses act independently to offer comprehensive health assessments aimed at health promotion and disease prevention. They also diagnose and manage common acute illness and follow patients with stable chronic conditions. Advanced practice nurses are not low-priced physician substitutes—they are nurses first, with unique licensure, advanced educational preparations, and regulatory boards in all 50 states. Advanced practice nurses meet rigorous education and certification requirements. Standards of practice are identified and monitored by professional nursing organizations. The word advanced connotes increasing expertise and graduate education within nursing. The APN is uniquely qualified to resolve unmet needs in health care by serving as a point of initial contact with the health care system.

Historical Perspectives

The evolution of American advanced practice nursing has a representative history in the nursing ideals of crusading Knights Hospitallers, Nightingale's vision for nursing education, and Lillian Wald's establishment of community and public health nursing (Donahue, 1985; Kalisch & Kalisch, 1995; Seymer, 1932). History is an important domain of professional knowledge that brings to light an awareness of nursing's heritage and the ideals and issues that have shaped the profession's struggles and triumphs (Christy, 1978; Dock & Stewart, 1920). In order to learn the lessons of the past, historians advise us to first know and understand our history: "No occupation can be quite, intelligently followed, or correctly understood unless it is . . . illumined by the light of history . . ." (Dock & Stewart, 1920, p. 1).

In the eleventh century, Pope Urban II urged Christian men to take back the Holy Land from the Turks. The numerous military expeditions known as the Crusades occurred between 1096 and 1291 A.D. The series of holy wars resulted in a need for hospitals and nurses to care for the injured, as well as those stricken by disease and famine. One response to this need was the development of male nursing orders—a brotherhood of Knights Hospitallers. These men were carefully selected for their military abilities as well as their nursing ideals. The hospitallers of the Knights of Malta were noted for their organizational structure, quality of nursing care provided, public service for food distribution to the poor, and care of orphans. The hospitallers were held in high esteem by society, and membership was sought after by the best of the military knights. High status and prestige allowed the Knights Hospitallers to control and advance their nursing order (Kalisch & Kalisch, 1995; Seymer, 1932).

The Nightingale Training School of Nurses educated hospital- and community-based nurses. Students went into private homes as well as hospitals to care for and teach patients and families how to preserve and maintain health. Two levels of students were identified—the ordinary probationers and the Lady probationers. Lady probationers received more lectures, were required to take more time for private study, and received preparation for leadership positions (Seymer, 1960). The Nightingale probationers were encouraged to become "pioneers, teachers, and regenerators in hospital management and nursing systems . . ." (Nutting & Dock, 1907, p. 183). Nightingale also established the London Training School for Midwives. Probationers were educated to be midwives in order to combat the significantly high maternal mortality rates of the nineteenth century. Nightingale's study of maternal mortality from puerperal fever is an early example of evidenced-based research (McDonald, 2001). Nightingale's midwives not only worked autonomously in the hospital setting, but delivered women in their own homes (Woodham-Smith, 1951).

Lillian Wald is regarded as the founder of public health and community health nursing. She created a nursing care system that allowed nurses to have direct access to patients without the intervention of medicine. It is interesting to note, in light of current APN reimbursement issues, Wald was one of the first to encourage some form of health insurance because of the large numbers of families who could not afford health care. She worked closely with the Metropolitan Life Insurance Company to provide a nursing service for policyholders (Christy, 1970).

These historical figures provide a glimpse into the nursing leadership and expertise that led to the development of the APN role in the United States. The four officially recognized advanced practice roles—certified registered nurse anesthetists (CRNAs), certified nurse midwives (CNMs), clinical nurse specialists (CNSs), and nurse practitioners (NPs)—each have their own story and traditions that may be explored within historical nursing research literature.

Advanced Practice Roles

A definition and description of advanced nursing practice is part of the Nursing Social Policy Statement: ". . . advanced practice is used to refer exclusively to advanced clinical practice" (ANA, 1995, p. 15). The definition does not include education or administrative nursing roles. The document distinguishes between basic expertise in nursing practice and advanced practice; advanced practice knowledge and skills must be obtained through graduate nursing education. Hallmarks of advanced clinical practice include autonomy, complex clinical decision-making, and skill in managing organizations and environments from a nursing, not a medical orientation (ANA, 1995). The ANA also defines fundamental activities of the APN: "Advanced practice registered nurses manifest a high level of expertise in the assessment, diagnosis and treatment of the complex responses of individuals, families or communities to actual or potential health problems, prevention of illness and injury, maintenance of wellness and provision of comfort . . . Advanced practice registered nurses continue to perform many of the same interventions used in basic nursing practice. The difference in this practice relates to a great depth and breadth of knowledge, a greater degree of synthesis of data, and complexity of skills and interventions" (ANA, 1996, p. 2).

Nurse Anesthesia

Nurses have been involved in the specialty of anesthesia since the mid-1800s. Medicine delegated anesthesia first to medical interns, then to nurses, keeping costs and wages at a minimum (Bankert, 1989). The high degree of acceptance of nurse anesthetists became a concern of organized medicine, and post World War I saw physicians specializing in anesthesia practice. However, World War II surgical trauma needs anchored the role of the nurse anesthetist; anesthesia was declared a clinical nursing specialty within the military. High numbers of men were (and are) attracted to the specialty due to military recruitment efforts. Unfortunately, history reflects continued interprofessional tension between nursing and medicine over the role of the nurse anesthetist.

Education of the nurse anesthetist was primarily controlled and provided by physicians. Therefore, the nurse anesthetist movement met with resistance from organized nursing. In 1931, Agatha Hodgins, a leading nurse anesthetist, initiated a formal effort for nurse anesthetist to join ANA as a specialty. However, the ANA counterproposed to accept nurse anesthetists as a subspecialty of medical–surgical nursing. When the ANA rejected the direct affiliation of the nurse anesthetists, Hodgins put her efforts into establishing (the precursor to) the American Association of Nurse Anesthetists (AANA) and led her specialty into an alliance with the American Hospital Association. The AANA initiated a certification program in 1945, marking the first APN group to require credentialing (Bankert, 1989). Unfortunately, organized nursing continued to ignore the efforts of nurse anesthesia to advance the specialty within organized nursing and nursing schools resisted the inclusion of nurse anesthesia as an academic program. The first master's degree nurse anesthesia programs were finally established in the early 1970s, and the AANA mandated a baccalaureate degree for certification in 1987. As of 1998, all accredited programs are required to be at the master's level and APNs in this specialty must meet national certification requirements in order to license (ANA, 2002; Bigbee & Amidi-Nouri, 2000).

According to the American Association of Nurse Anesthetists, certified registered nurse anesthetists (CRNA) administer more than 65% of all anesthetics in the United States and are the sole providers of anesthetics in 85% of rural settings (AANA, 2002). The AANA succeeded in obtaining legal authority to receive third-party reimbursement under Medicare in 1989. However, most state nurse practice acts designated the practice of CRNAs as dependent on physician supervision. The Health Care Financing Administration (HCFA) proposed changing this rule in December 1997, with the federal agency electing to defer to individual states on the supervision issue. Currently, nursing statutes and board of nursing rules in 29 states do not require physician supervision of nurse anesthetists (AANA, 2002).

Nurse Midwifery

The history of professional nurse midwifery is interwoven with the lay practice of midwifery. Historically, midwives perceived childbirth as a "natural" phenomenon within the female domain of natural competence, and few individuals sought formal nursing education. American medicine in the early 1900s believed that midwives were unsafe and sought control over obstetrics, criticizing midwifery for high maternal and infant mortality rates. Organized nursing was not supportive of placing midwifery in nursing academia because of a perceived need for physician supervision. Nevertheless, independent nurse midwifery schools were established and patient demand for services evidenced the continued need for nurse midwifery practice.

Mary Breckinridge, an early twentieth century nurse midwife, established the Frontier Nursing Service (FNS) in 1925, serving as a model of advanced nursing practice in the Appalachian Mountains of Kentucky. The FNS recruited many of their midwives from Great Britain until Breckinridge founded her own school of midwifery in 1938 and staffed a series of clinics to serve the women of rural Kentucky. Midwives were hired to travel on horseback, delivering women in their own homes. Acutely aware of medical scrutiny, Mary Breckenridge kept thorough outcomes evaluation data, demonstrating a maternal mortality rate of 1.2 per 1,000, significantly lower than the national average at that time (Breckinridge, 1952). High support publicity of the FNS resulted in significant public support for nurse midwifery. As a result, nurse midwifery was formalized as an extension of public health nursing after World War II. Organized medicine continued to be strongly opposed to the independent education and practice of nurse midwifery because of the belief midwifery would be an intrusion on the field of medical practice (Roberts, 1954).

As a discipline, American nurse midwives have been politically active and well organized since the early 1900s. The American Association of Nurse Midwives was founded in 1928 as an extension of the FNS and later emerged as the American College of Nurse Midwives (ACNM) in 1956. Certification was established in 1971, and as of 1999 all nurse midwifery programs require a baccalaureate degree as a minimum for ACNM accreditation. The ACNM differentiates between the certified nurse midwife and the certified midwife. A CNM is educated in the two disciplines of nursing and midwifery, and possesses evidence of certification according to the requirements of the ACNM. A certified midwife (CM) may not be a baccalaureate nurse and is subsequently defined as an individual educated in the discipline of midwifery, possessing evidence of certification according to the requirements of the ACNM. "Differences in midwifery education background have not resulted in a difference in certification test results. Analysis of certification examination results demonstrate that degrees do not enhance the clinical competence of a midwife and reflects the ability of both types of programs to prepare competent beginning midwife practitioners" (ACNM, 2002). The ACNM does encourage higher degrees to prepare educators and researchers in order to advance the profession, but the ACNM believes that mandating a master's degree could limit access to maternity and gynecological services for women and specifically opposes mandatory master's degree requirements for licensure (ACNM, 2002). Furthermore, the ACNM issued a 1971 joint statement with the American College of Obstetrics and Gynecologists and the Nurses' Association of the American College of Obstetricians and Gynecologists supporting the development and utilization of CNMs in obstetrical teams—as long as they are directed by physicians (Bigbee & Amidi-Nouri, 2000).

Clinical Nurse Specialists

The title clinical nurse specialist (CNS) originally identified nurses who had advanced clinical competence and advanced knowledge vis-à-vis graduate education. Initially, graduate nursing education focused on preparing students for administration, education, or supervisory roles. Specialty roles were encouraged after organized nursing observed successful development of the psychiatric CNS role, the oldest and most highly developed CNS specialty. Therefore, by the 1990s, clinical nurse specialists were found in a variety of health care roles. In the early 1990s CNS programs were the most numerous of all master's nursing programs. The largest area of specialization was adult health/medical–surgical. In addition, a large number of clinical nurse specialists were also prepared as nurse practitioners (Bigbee & Amidi-Nouri, 2000). In reality, the CNS/NP individual tended to practice exclusively in the NP role because of increased demands for primary care providers. The role merger created controversy for the CNS as the role became ambiguous with its adaptations to meet the needs of patients, nurses, and health care organizations (Sparacino, 2000). The National Association of Clinical Nurse Specialists (NACNS) was established in 1995 and the certification began in the 1970s through the ANA. Unfortunately, because of the large variety of CNS specialties, many areas only have certification available at the basic level rather than the advanced level, or offer no certification at all. A waiver option to use the title CNS may be obtained in some states when no certification is available in a designated specialty.

The ANA (1996) provided a definition of the **clinical nurse specialist** as an expert clinician and patient advocate in a particular specialty or subspecialty of nursing practice with identified subroles of education, research, and consultation. The NACNS (1998) offers a more detailed CNS definition: A CNS independently provides theory and research-based care, facilitates attainment of health goals, works with nurses to advance nursing practice and improve outcomes cost-effectively, and/or provides clinical expertise to affect system-wide changes in organizations to improve programs of care. The CNS is a registered professional nurse who: (a) holds a graduate degree or a post-master's certificate from a program accredited by a national nursing agency, (b) holds national certification in a designated specialty, and (c) meets all state board of nursing requirements to practice as a clinical nurse specialist (NACNS, 1998). The CNS scope of practice includes (a) direct patient care, (b) evidence-based advancement of the practice of nursing through nursing personnel, and (c) system interventions to improve cost-effective interventions. The scope is wide-ranging because care includes establishing evidence-based practice, developing multidisciplinary critical pathways, and designing/testing innovations in practice affecting patient care and the outcomes of care (Lyon, Davidson, Beecroft, Bingle, & Dayhoff, 1998).

The dimensions or subroles of the CNS role include expert clinician, consultant, change agent, leader, educator, and researcher. Core competencies of CNS role performance include direct and indirect clinical practice, consulting, expert teaching and coaching, and scholarly or scientific inquiry. Scott (1999) provides a summary of common CNS practice skills discussed in the literature. The list includes psychotherapy, family therapy, grief therapy, music therapy, crisis intervention, pain management, wound management, advanced physical assessments, writing of medical and nursing orders, and pharmacological and surgical interventions and evaluations. In addition, the CNS may work in collaborative medical practices to triage, perform advanced history and physical exams, write medical orders, document patient progress, order medications, and order/interpret diagnostic laboratory tests. Medical procedures found to be performed by clinical nurse specialists include lumbar puncture, bone marrow biopsies and harvesting, gastrostomy/jejunostomy tube insertion, removal of sutures and staples, and placement of invasive lines/catheters (Scott, 1999).

Documentation of the impact of CNS practice on patient care has been slow (Sparacino 2000). Outcome studies indicate that transitional care, discharge planning, and home follow-up given by a CNS results in high quality, cost-effective care. Specific outcomes attributed to the CNS include decreased cost of care, fewer rehospitalizations, fewer hospital days per patient, increased staff knowledge, and increased patient satisfaction. The findings of outcome studies give evidence that the CNS positively affects care of patients and improves patient care outcomes (Sparacino, 2000; Urden, 2001). The efficacy of the CNS on health care outcomes includes improved quality of care as well as cost reduction. Urden (2001) provides a comprehensive listing of CNS sensitive outcomes and examples of instruments to measure the outcomes. It is evident that the CNS role may be key to delivering high-quality, cost-effective health care in a variety of inpatient and outpatient settings.

Nurse Practitioner

The NP role developed after the CNS role and was created to meet a very specific American health care need. The driving force for NP role development was the shortage of primary care physicians in the mid-1900s. Many nursing leaders were supportive of the role because of the logical fit of nursing with primary health care. However, organized nursing as a whole was not enthusiastic about the NP role. The primary concern was that the scope of practice was not nursing oriented. The ultimate result of this disagreement among nurse leaders was the creation of a wide variety of NP certificate and master's degree programs without standard educational criterion.

Loretta Ford is identified as the originator of the NP role as she developed the first NP program with Dr. Henry Silver at the University of Colorado in 1965. Ford (1991) envisioned the NP as a nurse extender deeply rooted in the values and goals of professional nursing. The outcome evaluation data collected by Ford and Silver (1967) demonstrated a 33% increase in number of patients served in pediatric primary care; the positive impact of the NP role led to a recognition of nursings' excellent contribution to primary well child care (Ford, 1991). The data attracted attention from the National Advisory Commission on Health Manpower, which issued strong statements in support of the NP role. Consequently, federal dollars were provided as incentives to academic programs for establishing innovative educational models leading to NP certificates and degrees. By 1996, the NP role became the largest APN specialty (Bigbee & Amidi-Nouri, 2000).

According to the ANA (1996), the **nurse practitioner** is a skilled health care provider who uses critical judgment in the performance of comprehensive health assessments, differential diagnosis, and prescribing of treatments in the direct management of acute and chronic illness and disease. The NP is an advanced practice nurse prepared at the graduate level with a master's degree in nursing. Numerous NP specialties were identified in the 1970s and 1980s along with the creation of the respective NP specialty organizations. Efforts to unify all NP specialty organizations into one umbrella organization resulted in the birth of four entities: the Primary Health Care Nurse Practitioner Council within the ANA, the American Academy of Nurse Practitioners (AANP), the National Organization of Nurse Practitioner Faculties (NONPF), and the American College of Nurse Practitioners (ACNP). Significant changes in the NP role occurred in the latter half of the twentieth century with the influence of the previously mentioned organizations. Educational preparation has been clearly delineated for NPs through the efforts of NONPF (1995) and AACN (1996), with certification requiring a master's degree in nursing. Nurse practitioners have prescriptive privileges in all states, but the scope of the privilege varies from state to state. The AANP specified standards for practice within the NP scope of practice. NPs provide primary health care services to individuals, families, groups of patients, and communities. NP care is characterized by an emphasis on health promotion and disease prevention in the process of diagnosis and management of common acute illnesses/injuries and stable chronic diseases. In the provision of these services, NPs may order, conduct, and interpret appropriate diagnostic and laboratory tests and prescribe pharmacological agents, treatments, and therapies. Educating and counseling individuals and their families regarding healthy lifestyle behaviors are key components of NP care.

In the last 25 years, a number of studies have documented the effectiveness of NP practice in primary care. The research consistently demonstrates that the quality of health care provided by NPs is equivalent or superior to that of physicians. NPs consistently demonstrate better outcomes in the areas of cost effectiveness, communication, and preventive care (ANA, 1993; Brown & Grimes, 1995; Crosby, Ventura, & Feldman, 1987; Mundinger et al., 2000; Office of Technology Assessment [OTA], 1986). The NP role was originally conceived to enhance access to cost-effective health care, and it appears the vision succeeded. NPs will most likely continue to assume a significant role in the primary care workforce of the American health care system.

Health care delivery systems in the United States have shifted focus from acute care in institutional settings to community-based and outpatient settings. To meet the primary care needs of increasing numbers of patients in community-based settings, greater numbers of nonphysician clinicians will be needed. These clinicians may include not only advanced practices nurses but also physician assistants and practitioners from alternative disciplines (e.g., chiropractic, acupuncture, and naturopathy). Greater understanding of the role of each of these clinicians along with evidence-based support for the efficacy of their practice should be gathered.

To this end, Mundinger et al. (2000) sought to investigate care outcomes of patients randomly assigned to nurse practitioners and physicians. While past studies have suggested that the quality of care provided by nurse practitioners is equal to that of physicians, no study had measured patient outcomes when clinicians (physician and nurse practitioner) had the same degree of clinical independence. In this study nurse practitioners provided care to a randomized patient population that was consistent with the population cared for by physicians. Nurse practitioners had the same authority, responsibility, productivity, and administrative responsibility as physicians included in the study.

Study results supported the original hypothesis, which predicted similar patient outcomes. In this study of 1981 patients, 1,181 (59.6%) were assigned to a nurse practitioner clinic while 800 (40.4%) were assigned to physician clinics. The final population enrolled in the study (1,316 patients) was from those who kept their initial appointment. No statistical difference was found based on service utilization that could account for initial or long-term patient attrition. Satisfaction interviews were completed during the studies. Of variable studies related to satisfaction, the only one found to be of statistical significance related to the provider's technical skill, personal manner, and time spent with the patient. In this case physicians rated higher. Regarding overall self-reported health status, all groups reported improved health. No statistical differences were noted between patients receiving care from nurse practitioners versus physicians. On physiological measures (including peak flow, blood pressure, and glycosylated hemoglobin), for patients reporting one chronic illness at the time of interview, there was only one statistically significant difference (mean diastolic blood pressure 82 mm Hg in patient cared for by ANP as opposed to 85 mm Hg in patients cared for by physicians, $p = .04$). In a final measure, utilization of services was also not significantly different between patients assigned to either ANPs or physicians.

While there are many pressures on the U.S. health care system to focus care on health promotion and provide community-based services, it is important to remember that evidence-based support of patient outcomes is needed. Nurses in advanced practice roles are obligated to support the efficacy of services offered, thus ensuring positive patient outcomes.

Advanced Practice Credentials

Educational Preparation

Advanced practice nursing education includes graduate education, certification, and direct practice experience. APNs achieve a graduate degree with concentration in a specialty area. The graduate level focus provides grounding in the nursing discipline through study of theory and research findings relevant to advanced practice. Historically, levels of educational preparation for the NP, CNM, and CRNA roles varied from RN continuing education certificates to master's degrees or postmaster's certificate. The CNS role has been consistently grounded in the master's degree and many programs offer postmaster's education to obtain NP, CNM, or CRNA certificates. There is general consensus today that the master's degree is the minimum level of preparation for the APN.

The AACN (1996) has developed consensus statements in the *Essentials* document for master's education in nursing. This effort established a common curriculum for APN education. The core elements of APN curriculum include (a) graduate core, basic to all master's nursing education; (b) advanced practice core, common to all advanced practice nursing roles; and (c) specialty role core, explicit to each APN role. Core content, generic to all graduate nursing programs, includes research, evidenced-based outcomes, health policy, nursing and health-related theory, organizational/leadership theory, environmental health, ethical/legal issues, multicultural care, economics and business theory, community partnerships, managed care, and health care delivery systems. Direct clinical practice is the defined area of skill performance within APN education. In addition to direct clinical practice, core competencies common to all APN roles are coaching and guidance, consultation, research, clinical and professional leadership, collaboration, and ethical decision-making skills (AACN, 1996). Delineation of curriculum for specialty content in APN programs is guided by the specialty associations' identification of unique standards of practice and competency statements for each APN role. APN educators must maintain current knowledge and skill in their advanced practice fields—achieved primarily through faculty practice arrangements.

Credentialing

Credentialing is a term that refers to regulatory mechanisms applied to individuals, programs, or organizations (Styles, 1998). From an organizational standpoint, the Commission on Collegiate Nursing Education or the National League for Nursing Accreditation Center accredits graduate nursing programs. The ACNM and the AANA oversee and review CNM and CRNA education standards, while the National Organization of Nurse Practitioner Faculties and the National Certification Board of Pediatric Nurse Practitioners and Nurses, as well as other NP specialty groups, consult on curriculum guidelines/standards. The CNS role is working to clarify curriculum structure and progression toward specialty designations in order to assure compliance with credentialing and APN regulation. Credentialing of the discipline creates a way to monitor and regulate APN practice, protect the public by ensuring compliance with standards, and ensure attention to quality.

Credentialing may be mandatory or voluntary. The first credential that advanced practice nurses must obtain is completion of an accredited APN nursing program. The master's degree is required to receive state APN titling or licensure. The second credential advanced practice nurses need to achieve is certification. **Certification** is a process by which a nongovernmental agency or association confirms that an individual has met standards specified by a professional area. In many states, APN certification is required for third-party reimbursement, prescriptive authority, or liability insurance. Confusing the issue are the multiple organizations that provide a certification credential, with a

---

Box 22–1   Major APN Accreditation, Regulatory, and Certifying Organizations

Educational Accrediting Organizations
American Association of Colleges of Nurses (AACN)
Commission on Collegiate Nursing Education (CCNE)
National League for Nursing (NLN)
National League for Nursing Accreditation Corporation (NLNAC)

Regulatory Organizations
State Boards of Nursing
National Council of State Boards of Nursing (NCSBN)

Certifying Organizations
American Academy of Nurse Practitioners (AANP)
American Association of Nurse Anesthetists (AANA)
American College of Nurse-Midwives (ACNM)
American Nurses Credentialing Center (ANCC)
National Certification Board of Pediatric Nurse Practitioners and Nurses (CNBPNP/N)
National Certification Corporation for Obstetrical, Gynecologic and Neonatal Nursing Specialties (NCC)

corresponding variety of certification requirements. Basic RN certification is granted for recognition of excellence or validation of competence; however, certification for APNs has been required for entry into practice. Most APN certifying bodies require the master's degree, and those that currently do not will require a master's by 2007 (Buppert, 1999). Box 22–1 lists major APN accreditation, regulatory, and certifying organizations.

Professional certification within a specialty area determines whether nurses meet standards for practice, and requires APNs to take a certification examination. Each certifying body determines the type of credential that it awards. For example, the American Academy of Nurse Practitioners (AANP) offers the initials "NP-C" to indicate successful certification status for a nurse practitioner that successfully completes certification requirements. The National Association of Pediatric Nurse Associates and Practitioners confer "CPNP" on their certified NPs. The AANP also allows reciprocity without examination for NPs certified by the American Nurses Credentialing Center (a subsidiary of the ANA) prior to January 1, 1995 (AANP, 2002). The ANCC has certification options in five specialty areas: gerontology, medical–surgical, pediatrics, perinatal, and psychiatric and mental health nursing. Some states may specify certification bodies they will allow for APN licensure (Illinois Department of Professional Regulation, 2002).

Because multiple entities initially began to certify APNs, the American Board of Nursing Specialties (ABNS) was established in 1991 to provide standardization and unity for the certification process. The ABNS requires APN certifying organizations to mandate a minimum of the master's degree; however, not all APN certifying organizations are members of the ABNS. The ANCC and the Council on Certification of Nurse Anesthetists are ABNS members (ABNS, 1997). NP certification has developed in a variety of specialty options for both primary and acute care. CNS certification examinations have been slower to develop in a variety of specialties. Some APN specialty areas do not have certification options at the advanced practice level. In this case, advanced practice nurses may apply for certification waivers for state or national certification requirements. The ANCC provides certification options for CNSs and NPs in several areas. A minimum of 500 hours of supervised clinical practice in the APN master's curriculum is required to take the advanced practice certification exam. The initials "APRN, BC" (advanced practice registered nurse, board certified) are used to credential nurse practitioners or clinical nurse specialtists who certify through the ANCC (2002). Box 22–2 lists ANCC options for APN certification.

Nurse anesthetists certify through the Council on Certification/Recertification of Nurse Anesthetists, a subsidiary of the American Association of Nurse Anesthetists. The American College of Nurse Midwives Certification Council, Inc., is the national certifying body for nurse midwives. Most APN specialties have mandatory practice requirements for recertification to assure that APNs are maintaining current practice competence by way of practice experience. Advanced prac-

---

Box 22–2   American Nursing Credentialing Center Certification Options for APNs

Clinical Specialist in Community Health Nursing
Clinical Specialist in Gerontological Nursing
Clinical Specialist in Home Health Nursing
Clinical Specialist in Medical–Surgical Nursing
Clinical Specialist in Pediatric Nursing
Clinical Specialist in Adult and/or Child and Adolescent
Psychiatric and Mental Health Nursing
Acute Care Nurse Practitioner
Adult Nurse Practitioner
Family Nurse Practitioner
Gerontological Nurse Practitioner
Pediatric Nurse Practitioner
Psychiatric and Mental Health—Family or Adult Nurse Practitioner

tice nurses who do not meet stipulated continuing education expectations and practice requirements must retake the national certifying exam to continue to practice. The variability of requirements for NP and CNS certification promotes confusion within the profession, the health care system and the general public. Standardization in the APN certification process has been identified as important for the future. The Pew Health Care Professions Commission Report (1995) called for consistency in how health professionals are prepared for practice, how practice is regulated, and how educational programs and certifying organizations credential students.

Institutional Credentialing and Privileging

Credentialing and privileging mechanisms initially developed for physician groups are being revised to include advanced practice nurses. The intent of **institutional credentialing** is to review qualifications and competence with periodic review of performance measures designed to ensure the quality of services being provided. **Privileging** outlines the patient care services an APN can provide in an organization. The need for hospital privileges varies for the APN depending on their practice role. Health care agency bylaws may not allow membership for nonphysicians, and Joint Commission on Accreditation of Healthcare Organizations (JCAHO) standards place the responsibility for credentialing and privileging of nonphysician practitioners with the medical staff. In addition, only medical staff may admit or discharge patients from hospitals by JCAHO standards. However, clinical privileges may be granted through APN membership in the medical staff or through other alternative privileging routes. The JCAHO has recently revised its medical staff standards to allow hospitals to extend clinical privileges to nonphysician practitioners (Kamajian, Mitchell, & Fruth, 1999). Hanson (2000) recommends that advanced practice nurses desiring agency privileges seek out nurse administrators for information on the credentialing process and what

support there may be for nonphysician providers. An application for temporary privileges should be sought when the application for institutional credentialing is requested. This would potentially allow the APN to practice while the credentialing process is in progress.

Licensure

Licensure is the regulatory method most appropriate when professional activities are complex and require specialized knowledge and skill, independent decision-making, and autonomy (Buppert, 1999). Prior to the emergence of advanced practice nursing, the legal scope of practice for nurses excluded diagnosis and treatment of medical problems. Nurse practice acts were amended to include nursing diagnoses and allow advanced practice nurses to fill gaps in the health care system. Legislation governing advanced practice nursing currently exists in every state. Title protection, scope of practice, collaborative relationships or supervision requirements, and education and certification expectations all regulate professional advanced practice nursing through individual state nurse practice act statutes. An annual overview of APN legislation in each state is published in the January issues of *Nurse Practitioner: The American Journal of Primary Health Care*.

State law oversees APN practice in two ways: statues as defined by individual state legislature through the nurse practice act, and regulations put forth by individual state agencies under the jurisdiction of the executive branch of state government (Buppert, 1999). Licensure is the authority delegated to individual states by the U.S. Constitution to provide standards to assure basic levels of public safety. In most states the board of nursing has sole authority over APN practice; however, there are some states where joint authority with the board of medicine is mandated (Buppert, 1999).

State boards of nursing are typically responsible for (a) interpreting and enforcing the scope of nursing practice; (b) adopting regulations to implement a practice act, which defines scope of practice for advanced

---

Requirements for RN licensure
Requirements for APN titling or licensure
Scope of practice; limitations to practice services
Prescriptive authority
Requirements for collaboration or supervision
Basis for license suspension, revocation, or nonrenewal
Reimbursement under Medicaid/Medicare
Reimbursement by indemnity insurers
Requirements of educational programs
Requirements for continuing education
Requirements for certification and recertification
Standards of practice

practice nurses; (c) developing and enforcing standards for all levels of nursing practice; (d) investigating complaints; (e) conducting hearings; (f) invoking disciplinary action; (g) issuing advisory opinions on nursing practice; and (h) offering examination, licensure, and renewal of licenses for qualified applicants (Buppert, 1999). The National Council of State Boards of Nursing (NCSBN) is the organization through which all state boards of nursing work together on matters of common interest. APN licensure is obtained according to the rules and regulations found in individual state nurse practice acts. Specific practice issues that fall under state regulation are listed in Box 22–3.

All states recognize APN (or APRN; advanced practice registered nurse) role, and all require licensure first as a registered nurse (RN). While variations in guidelines exists to establish APN status; the majority of states require master's degrees and advanced certification. Specifics on prescriptive authority and the degree of APN autonomy vary state by state. The term **midlevel practitioner** is used by physician groups and some regulatory agencies to identify APNs. The Drug Enforcement Administration (DEA) defines a midlevel practitioner as a provider other than a physician, dentist, veterinarian, or podiatrist. A novel approach to simplifying licensure complexity is described as mutual recognition. **Mutual recognition** refers to the use of a system similar to that used for driver's licenses: States share jurisdiction, discipline, and information to regulate practice based on an interstate pact (NCSBN, 1998). An APN could be licensed in a home state, but other states also recognize the licensure. The mutual recognition model holds the APN accountable for laws and regulations in all states where the APN practices but relies on licensure from the home state. In 1997, the NCSBN voted unanimously to endorse the mutual recognition model and authorize the development of strategies for implementation.

Advanced Practice Management

Legal Issues

The explicit goal of professional regulation is to establish standards that protect the public from incompetent health care providers. Unfortunately, these same standards protect economic privileges of some professionals by establishing barriers to practice activities for other professionals. Practice acts are often a source of conflict among health professions with territory battles over scope of practice, reimbursement, and prescriptive authority. The result has been significant variation in APN practice regulation across the nation. The Pew Taskforce on Health Care Workforce Regulation issued recommendations in 1998 calling for change in national regulatory mechanisms to reduce barriers to APN practice. The taskforce encouraged national uniformity in APN education, credentialing, and scope of practice statements (Finocchio et al., 1998). Variations in titles and roles for the APN are confusing to policy makers and regulators. It is especially problematic when authoritative agencies like the HCFA attempt to set standards for reimbursement but discrepancies among states make standard policy for advanced practice nurses extremely difficult (Hanson, 2000).

Malpractice is the failure of a professional to exercise the degree of skill commonly applied by the prudent practitioner. Negligence is the legal process for malpractice liability. Negligence includes any failure to follow up, disclose information to a patient, or give necessary care (Buppert, 1999). APNs are held to the standard of the prudent APN, not the prudent physician; however, in some cases the standards of care may be identical. Electronic data banks have the capability to monitor and screen provider competency based on successful malpractice litigation. The National Practitioner Data Bank (NPDB) was established in 1990 as a federal storehouse for information related to professional competence and conduct of physicians and nonphysicians who are granted clinical privileges. NPDB data collection prevents health care providers from simply changing locations to avoid discovery of incompetence or misconduct. Medical malpractice payments, licensure disciplinary actions, adverse clinical privilege actions taken by a health care agency, and adverse actions affecting professional society membership are all required to be reported to the NPDB. It is also mandatory for hospitals to screen all new practitioners through the NPDB and every 2 years following the date of hire (U.S. Public Health Service, 1996). A review of NPDB data suggests that APNs are at low risk for lawsuits (Birkholz, 1995).

Standards for which APNs are held accountable usually come from expert testimony and practice ideals established by the profession. Specialty organizations also publish guidelines and standards of practice, which can be admitted as evidence during litigation. Some states require advanced practice nurses to establish practice protocols or guidelines with or without physician input. Other states require protocols for prescribing drugs but not for other clinical practice decisions (Buppert, 1999). Protocols are written tools that guide the APN in **decision-making** about patient care. In states where physician involvement is required, protocols are mutually agreed-upon guidelines that define responsibilities and practice decisions of the APN and the physician. Protocols only govern aspects of APN care that require medical authorization, not independent nursing care decisions or intervention. A written protocol is considered a standard of care document because it provides a guideline for minimum level of safe practice (Buppert, 1999). Safriet (1992) criticized the restriction of mandatory physician collaboration imposed on NP practice by protocols because research demonstrates APN patient care outcomes are equivalent or superior to that of physicians.

Inasmuch as practice protocols cannot cover all possible individual clinical decision-making required, it is advisable to write them to reflect minimum, basic standards of practice. Legal authorities warn that detailed protocols may leave the APN vulnerable to litigation (Buppert, 1999; Moniz, 1992). In addition, practice protocols must be regularly updated to reflect current literature and best practice recommendations. Old protocols need to be clearly dated and archived for the time period mandated by individual state's statute of limitations. This process allows for documentation of best practice over time and allows for temporal case review in the event of a lawsuit. Buppert (1999) and Hanson (2000) recommend guidelines for protocols used by APNs in practice (Box 22–4).

Collaborative practice agreements (CPA) are legal documents that define the joint practice of a physician and APN in a collaborative and complementary working relationship (Buppert, 1999; Sebas, 1994). The contract may list all professional licensure, certification, and prescriptive authority requirements as well as

---

Box 22–4 Recommendations for APN Protocol Documents

Few details
Generalized guidelines for common, everyday practice experiences
Reference a wide source of literature and references
Include a bibliography of resources
Consider inclusions of published guidelines by organizations and agencies
Identify any common/regular alternative practices or deviations from protocols
Date all protocols
Signature of all providers on all protocols
Update on a regular basis (annually or more frequently)
Archive all old protocols by date of use

specify the manner in which the APN and employer will cooperate, consult, and control care delivery. Categories of patient diagnoses, treatment procedures, and productivity expectations on the part of the APN may also be a part of a CPA. Obligations of the employer and collaborating physicians should be specifically described, including any provision of facilities, equipment, supplies, and support personnel. The CPA should hold all parties in legal compliance with the terms of the document. Additional aspects of a CPA may include compensation decisions, noncompete clauses, termination arrangements, and support services or benefits to be provided to either party (Buppert, 1999). Most nurses are well prepared for clinical practice but, unfortunately, completely uneducated for the business aspects of practice (Porter-O'Grady, 1996).

The term collaboration is used extensively in the professional literature, but may have various contextual meanings. Hanson, Spross, and Carr (2000) recognize collaboration as a "dynamic, interpersonal process in which two or more individuals make a commitment to each other to interact authentically and constructively to solve problems and to learn from each other in order to accomplish identified goals, purposes or outcomes" (p. 318). Research suggests that advanced practice nurses and physicians view collaboration very differently. Significantly more physicians perceive that they have final authority in decision-making within a collaborative relationship compared to their NP counterparts (Moser & Armer, 1999). Mundinger (1994) indicates that collaborative practice by advanced practice nurses and physicians is more comprehensive and effective than independent practice on the part of either professional.

Ethical Practice Management

APNs today are confronted with increasingly complex ethical dilemmas given the nature of the health/illness care system, the advancement of technology focusing on quality of life and the tremendous emphasis on medical cure. An ethical dilemma is a situation involving conflict about the right thing to do. Two major perspectives are apparent in ethical discussions. The first is the perspective of justice, which seems to dominate traditional medical ethics and focuses on abstract reasoning and rationality. Some justice theories address right consequences (consequentialism) and some address right action (deontology) (Cameron & Schaffer, 1992). Caring, as an alternative perspective, involves looking at a problem in context,

taking into account personal values. Caring is defined as experiencing and understanding, as nearly as possible, what the one cared-for is feeling and acting on that person's behalf. The focus is on intuition, relationship building, and empathy rather than rationality (Noddings, 1984). The integration of both perspectives produces a more comprehensive ethical process (Cameron & Schaffer, 1992). Growing ethical pressure has been placed on APNs to control health care costs. This produces a tension between deciding on what might be best practice versus what is most cost effective, given the circumstances of the situation. No consensus exists about what constitutes a just method of balancing the desires of the individual against the diverse needs of a society.

Outcome Management

Quality of care has become a major ethical issue for the nation with concerns being voiced by consumers, payers, and governmental authorities. Outcomes of health care services have traditionally been measured by assessing health status indicators such as morbidity and mortality statistics, levels of function, comfort and well-being, and patient satisfaction survey data (U.S. Department of Health and Human Services [DHHS], 2000). Employers, insurers, and other purchasers of health care services collect data to profile the practice habits of providers. **Profiling** is defined as measuring the quality, utilization, and cost of health care resources (American Medical Association [AMA], 1995). Clinical profiles may include a providers style of practice in terms of treatment modalities, utilization of services, and outcomes of care. Economic profiling examines the financial dimensions of treatment choices, case mix, and demographic factors. Profiling has been identified as having three primary applications—quality improvement, utilization review, and assessment of provider performance (Emmons, Wozniak, Otten, & Baker, 1993).

Organizations have developed in the last decade to collect data to profile health care practice. The Agency for Healthcare Research and Quality (AHRQ) promotes research in quality measurement and provides clinical practice guidelines that define standards of best practice approach (Buppert, 1999). Performance measures also include those developed by the Foundation for Accountability and the National Committee for Quality Assurance (NCQA) to identify whether or not the needs of patient are being adequately met. NCQA collects data on quality health indicators on behalf of

HCFA. The data is identified as the Health Plan Employer Data and Information Set (HEDIS). The NCQA evaluates outcomes through the HEDIS indicators; data are used to evaluate national health care performance standards.

The Institute of Medicine (IOM) has defined **quality of care** as the degree to which health services increase the likelihood of desired health outcomes and are consistent with current professional knowledge (IOM, 1990). A nurse-sensitive patient outcome is defined as a patient state, behavior, or perception that is responsive to a nursing intervention (McCloskey & Bulechek, 2000). APN clinical decision-making must be based on the best evidence available while linking care interventions to desired outcomes. This quality process is labeled **evidence-based practice** (EBP). EBP is an approach to practice that promotes the collection, interpretation, and integration of research-based approaches to care. EBP is a way to solve clinical problems by integrating best research evidence in concert with all other sources of knowledge (Sackett, Rosenburg, Gray, Hayes, & Richardson, 1996). To integrate EBP more fully, the APN needs to ethically reflect on why they manage particular conditions as they do, identify unanswered questions, and critique current research to appraise its validity for practice application. Ethical practice management includes these steps as well as following patient care outcomes as

a measure of whether care was of high quality. EBP has been criticized for being at odds with critical thinking because of the potential for using guidelines as a "cookbook" for care. Clinical guidelines that follow EBP frameworks are not absolutes, and need to be used with other knowledge bases to reduce quality variation within typical practice problem solving (Glanville, Schirm, & Wineman, 2000). AHRQ is a primary source for guidelines on a variety of clinical conditions; professional specialty organizations are also an excellent source for practice guidelines.

The focus on reducing health care costs as an ethical practice issue has increased opportunities for the APN to demonstrate their worth to American health care policy makers and payers. At the same time, shrinking health care resources have increased the competition between physician and APN care practice. In the process, the need to demonstrate ethical, cost-conscious, best-practice approaches with positive patient care outcomes is imperative. As consumers and governmental agencies scrutinize health care practice and quality of provider services, the APN must be able to document evidence of high-quality contributions to health care. Categories of patient care outcomes are specified by Urden (1999) as clinical, psychosocial, functional, fiscal, and satisfaction. Examples of each are provided in Box 22–5. Urden (1999) also details examples of instrumentation for measuring patient care outcomes sensitive to nursing

---

Box 22–5 *Patient Care Outcomes to Measure APN Quality of Care*

Clinical Outcomes
Mortality
Morbidity
Physiological responses (e.g., BP, vital signs)
Symptom control measures (e.g., pain, nausea)

Psychosocial Outcomes
Stress management
Role functioning (e.g., return to work)
Level of anxiety
Knowledge of treatment (e.g., medications, diet)

Functional Outcomes
Quality of life
Mobility
Social interaction

Fiscal Outcomes
Length of stay
Readmission to hospital
Home care needs
ER visits
Resource utilization

Satisfaction
Consumer satisfaction with care/services provided
Payer satisfaction
Provider satisfaction

intervention. The measurement of outcomes has become a necessary element for evaluating health care. Measuring outcomes is critical to establish the effectiveness of advanced practice nursing care.

A variety of studies have been conducted exploring the effectiveness of care provided by advanced practice nurses. Early studies of APNs found that care was equivalent to that provided by physicians, and patients were highly satisfied (Brown & Grimes, 1995; OTA, 1986). Compared to physicians, APNs are more likely to talk with patients and adapt medical regimens to a patient's preferences, family situation, and environment (Brown & Grimes, 1995). Advanced practice nurses are also more likely to provide disease-prevention counseling and health promotion education to the patient (Brown & Grimes, 1995; Mundinger et al., 2000; OTA, 1986). Mundinger et al. (2000) found when nurse practitioners had the same authority, responsibility, and accountability as physicians, the quality of primary care delivered was equal to that of physicians. Safriet (1992) emphasizes the implication of outcomes research demonstrating APN care to be equivalent to physician care; advanced practice nurses are the American health system's best buy for quality care. However, even though the value of the APN has been demonstrated, health care agencies are under continued political and financial pressure and need ongoing evidence that the APN are cost effective and deliver ethical, quality outcomes.

Marketing Practice

The significant changes that have marked health care in the last half of the twentieth century brought tremendous challenges as well as opportunities for the APN. The changes have created an environment in which advanced practice nurses must take control of their careers and futures. Nursing dependence on others to define their future for them is a phenomenon of the past. Career planning and development is a continuous process requiring advanced practice nurses to understand the environment in which they live and practice; assess strengths, limitations, and what unique niche they may contribute; and market themselves to the public. **Marketing** involves articulating professional and personal qualities, attributes, and expertise to effectively communicate what APNs have to offer and why they are the best person to deliver the service. Doughty and Keller (2000) identify marketing as "anything and everything APNs do to promote their practice" (p. 656). Marketing has become a serious consideration of every aspect of health care as the competition for customers slowly intensifies. Providers can no

longer decide what is best for patients, then force it on them. APNs must discover what the "customer" wants and then develop strategic plans to provide it to the market. Key to any marketing strategy is defining the customer—be it the patient, groups of patients (business/corporations), the physician, the payer, or health care organizations or agencies.

Marketing strategy also requires understanding the goods/services the APN has to offer. Unfortunately, in the U.S. health care system, there has been an assumption that health care is equivalent to medical cure of disease. The participation of nursing in this paradigm is perceived to be that of "helper" to the ultimate goal of cure. No attention is given to illness prevention, health promotion, health education, and consumer-directed self-care—all unique health care niches for the APN. "Patients who will do especially well under the care of an APN include those who want to be educated about appropriate partnerships in their care, those with chronic disease, those who have identified risk where prevention counts, those wanting a higher level of health, or those whose frailty requires extensive support" (Mundinger, 1999, p. 9). Clearly marking "APN turf" and strategizing how to market to the customer is the work of the twenty-first-century APN.

The **professional portfolio** is a useful marketing strategy, which the APN can use to promote practice and visibility in the health care system. Graphic artists, journalists, business executives, and architects use portfolios very successfully to market themselves. Professional portfolios showcase the APN to potential employers or customers. It is a comprehensive document that details the current state of practice, background, skills, expertise, and professional growth. Portfolios are more comprehensive than resumes or vitae in that examples of one's expertise and past successes are exhibited. The professional portfolio packages APN products for display purposes. The portfolio may also be used as a data bank to collect information about APN career experiences, skills, expertise, honors, and successes to draw from when marketing to specific employers or patients. Pamphlets and brochures with profiles and images of the APN in practice may also be included in the portfolio. Professional organizations distribute fact sheets and generic brochures about APNs that explain in lay terms the advantages of choosing an APN as a health care provider.

One powerful marketing approach is the use of advertising. Advertising begins with the APN themselves. Advanced practice nurses should at all times carry business cards and brochures outlining services offered and take every subtle opportunity to educate others of

Some communities have not historically used APNs. How might you introduce an APN to a patient looking for a primary health care provider? As a staff nurse, how can you use an advanced practice nurse to improve health care outcomes for your patients?

their practice. Waiting in line at the grocery store, before PTA meetings start, and informal parent gatherings for high school sports activities are all examples of impromptu forums to offer information about APN practice. Word-of-mouth advertising can be the most effective form of advertising. Patients may be given several business cards and brochures to distribute to friends and neighbors. Advertising does not have to be expensive to be effective. Business cards and brochures can be tacked up on bulletin boards at local coffee shops, restaurants, schools, churches, and grocery stores. Direct mailings to target groups such as small businesses or larger corporations may also be considered. Advertising in telephone book yellow pages, newspapers, local magazines, radio, and television is also an option, albeit more expensive. Volunteering to speak for local service clubs is an excellent way to network and advertise what services the APN can provide—"samples" of care (e.g., blood pressure screening/health education information) may also be provided at the service club meeting. Marketing to other professionals is also a crucial source of advertising. APNs who specialize in pediatrics should market themselves to midwives and obstetric colleagues. In addition, specialists that are APN referral sources are an excellent target for developing professional relationships and marketing practice capabilities.

Marketing APNs' services is critical to promote individual practice as well as the discipline itself. As the business metaphor transforms the health care system, patients will become more sophisticated about what they want and how to find it. Educating the public about APN practice will ensure that patients will request APN services, recognizing the significant value of their care.

Advanced Practice Issues

Blending the Role of the CNS and the NP

In 1986, the ANA Council of Primary Health Care Nurse Practitioners and the Council of Clinical Specialists released a joint statement regarding the CNS and the NP role; the councils agreed that the roles were more similar than different. Historically, the major differences between the CNS and NP were the setting and focus of practice. In an early study by Elder and Bullough (1990), findings showed that the major differences in the two roles were that CNSs were more likely to become administrators or educators, while NPs were more involved in direct clinical management of acute and chronic illness. Another study of the two roles led the authors to conclude that the CNS and NP roles were distinct (Williams & Valdivieso, 1994). Lincoln (2000) repeated the Williams and Valdivieso (1994) study, finding that CNSs' and NPs' daily work activities differed significantly in 22 out of 25 categories.

The CNS has been viewed as a specialist in nursing care that provides educational development and advanced nursing care for a specific patient population, within secondary and tertiary inpatient care settings. In contrast, NPs have been identified as generalists who provide primary and preventative care and treat acute illness for a broad patient population in outpatient settings. The CNS and NP roles have been blurred with the variety of practice arenas and practice-based responsibilities taken on by both. The blended-role APN is defined as an individual who has both CNS and NP preparation. The blended-role APN is eligible for certification as a CNS specialist as well as an NP. The blended role combines the strengths of the two roles—providing patient-based care in a variety of settings to ensure continuity of health care to a specialty-based population. Skalla and Hamric (2000) assert that blending of the CNS and NP has occurred spontaneously and coexists with the traditional CNS and NP roles.

Various models of the relationship between the CNS and NP have been posited by Williams and Valdivieso (1994). These authors have conceptualized five different possible models: the additive model, the dual pathways model, overlapping roles, roles subsuming each other, and the blended role. The additive model makes the assumption that one role may be added to the other. Educationally, this would be the operative model if a practicing CNS returned to school for preparation as an NP. The dual pathways model focuses on the similarities of the CNS and the NP recognizing that ultimately they are both APNs and may function in a variety of ways. The overlapping roles model demonstrates the shared as well as unique aspects of each role. One role subsuming the other indicates that the roles are blended but one role is dominant, and the blended-role model depicts the two roles becoming so merged that the distinctions between them are not evident. Conceptual frameworks such as this confirm Skalla and Hamric (2000) in their contention that the blended role may coexist with other CNS/NP role mixes; blended role does not have to be an either–or proposition.

Many issues need to be addressed before the CNS and NP roles can be officially merged (e.g., legal and educational issues, reimbursement, and titling concerns). While boundaries between the two roles have become less distinct, the challenges of health care in the twenty-first century may require a unique, novel approach to practice roles. Some kind of blending of the two roles may meet the challenges ahead, or the distinct differences may ultimately determine how each contributes a significant need.

Prescriptive Authority

Historically, the right to prescribe medications has been the exclusive domain of the physician. However, as the twenty-first century begins, APNs have some form of prescriptive authority in all 50 states. Licensure for prescriptive privileges is under the authority of each individual state with the degree of physician collaboration required and the types of drugs allowed being the main areas of discrepancy. State nurse practice acts identify the rules and regulations for obtaining and retaining prescriptive authority for APNs. There is consistency among states regarding some requirements for obtaining prescriptive authority. Master's degree, APN licensure or state titling, national certification as an APN, and documentation of advanced pharmacology credit hours are all standard mandates.

The federal government oversees APN prescribing of controlled substances through the Drug Enforcement Administration (DEA). DEA numbers are necessary for prescription of scheduled or controlled substances, but have also become a convenient way to track prescribing practices of health care providers for nonscheduled medications. Often, the DEA number is used by pharmacies to identify health care providers; DEA numbers could become a barrier to insurance payment for prescription medications if the APN has not obtained a number. A DEA number is available to APNs in states where law allows prescriptive authority for controlled substances—the privilege is not transferable from state to state. Eligible APNs submit an application with the current fee to the DEA. If approved, the APN receives DEA registration number renewable every 3 years.

A prescription is a legal document and the prescriber is responsible for its accuracy and completeness. Although APN prescriptive authority is allowed in all 50 states, authority to prescribe may be restricted in a variety of ways. The range of drugs permitted to be prescribed by APNs may be limited to a formulary or to drugs common to a specialty area. The degree of physician involvement in APN prescribing practices may vary from use of collaborative practice protocols to significant on-site physician supervision. The lack of standardization among individual state mandates for APN prescriptive authority causes confusion among health care providers and consumers, yet the ability to prescribe drugs and therapeutic agents is considered a requisite for comprehensive primary care. The pharmaceutical industry is beginning to recognize APNs as a future market for their products. According to Scott-Levin (2000), a leading pharmaceutical consulting firm, 10% of all pharmaceutical sales calls are currently with nonphysicians, including nurse practitioners. NPs and physician assistants receive 16% of the pharmaceutical industry's educational sales calls. Pfizer, Bristol-Meyers Squibb, and Johnson & Johnson were noted to be among the top companies calling on NPs. APNs have made significant progress related to prescriptive authority in the last decade, along with other nonphysician professionals who also seek autonomy relative to prescriptive authority (e.g., psychologists, pharmacists, physician assistants). As APNs pursue the right to offer their services to the public, legal rights and responsibilities will no doubt expand beyond current physician-only barriers.

Reimbursement

Reimbursement refers to the monetary compensation for services provided to patients. Documentation of patient encounters is critical to reimbursement procedure. The discipline of nursing has developed classification systems to document care provided through the use of nursing diagnoses, nursing interventions classification (NIC), and nursing outcomes classification

(NOC). Unfortunately, there is no current economic recognition of the nursing classification systems in legal billing processes. The federal Health Care Financing Administration (HCFA) governs and guides the reimbursement process based on traditional medical systems of documenting patient encounters (AMA, 2001).

Whether an APN is employed by an agency or self-employed, the encounter between provider and patient has a third-party involved—the payer. Box 22–6 lists major categories of third party payers. Each payer has its own reimbursement policies and fee schedules and each operates under a separate set of laws. Fee-for-service is one type of payment schedule in which specific health care services are identified with an attached cost. All care services are coded using Current Procedural Terminology (CPT), and the International Classification of Diseases, 9th revision (ICD-9). Reimbursable services have CPT codes developed by the American Medical Association for use in claim submission and all medical diagnoses have a six-digit ICD-9 code. CPT codes are leveled according to evaluation and management (E&M) service codes, which represent the extent and complexity of service provided. Required information on the HCFA form includes patient identification, provider identification, ICD-9 codes, CPT codes, and E&M codes. A "superbill" lists all possible codes and is the standard documentation record for each patient encounter. HCFA determines the relative economic value for each procedural code and has developed guidelines for how to code and submit billing (HCFA, 1997).

The federal programs of Medicare and Medicaid are directed and funded nationally by HCFA, but administered through state agencies. Medicare covers enrolled patients who are 65 years and older as well as disabled individuals who qualify for Social Security disability payments and benefits. Medicaid is a federal program for families and children who qualify on the basis of poverty and for adults of poverty who are temporarily disabled (one year or less). Medicare reimburses on a fee-for-service basis unless the patient has enrolled in a managed-care health plan. In this case, Medicare pays the managed care health plan on a capitated basis (one lump sum per month per patient regardless of care provided), and the health care plan pays providers on a fee-for-service basis. Medicaid also has managed care health plans as well as fee-for-service schedules.

Under Medicare, advanced practice nurses may be directly reimbursed at 85% of the physician fee schedule. If an APN wishes to provide care to a Medicare patient, the individual applies to be a Medicare provider. (As of January 2003, a master's degree with certification is required). Once the APN has been assigned provider number, a standard billing form is filled out and submitted to the local Medicare agency for reimbursement on each visit and/or procedure. To receive Medicaid reimbursement, the APN must apply for a provider number and be admitted to the provider panel of the Medicaid managed health care plan (master's degree and certification required). Individual state law determines the degree of reimbursement to the APN (80% to 100%) but services are covered whether or not the APN is employed by or supervised by a physician.

When advanced practice nurses provide services "under direct personal supervision" of a physician, APN care can be reimbursed at 100% of the physician fee schedule. To qualify, the APN must be an employee of a physician or physician group, and provider services must be those provided during a course of treatment in which a physician is somehow involved in the patient's care. "Direct personal supervision" does not mean that a physician must be in the same room, however (Buppert, 1999). This type of reimbursement is labeled "incident to a physician's professional service." "Incident to" is Medicare language meaning services furnished as integral, but incidental to physician care in the course of diagnosis or treatment of injury/illness.

Indemnity insurers are insurance companies that pay for medical care of the insured patient on a per-visit, per-procedure basis. Indemnity insurers have fee schedules based on "usual and customary" charges,

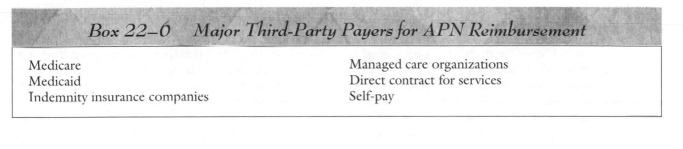

Box 22–6   *Major Third-Party Payers for APN Reimbursement*

Medicare	Managed care organizations
Medicaid	Direct contract for services
Indemnity insurance companies	Self-pay

Historically, nursing services have not been billed separately from overall patient charges. How can all nurses, including staff nurses, assure reimbursement for APN services?

meaning costs that are "typical" when compared to charges for similar conditions in the county of the policyholder. Each indemnity insurer sets its own rate of payment. If the provider charges more than what an insurer considers to be "usual and customary," the patient is usually responsible for the difference between what the provider charges and what the insurer pays.

A **managed care organization** (MCO) provides health care services as well as payment for the services. Managed care organizations include health maintenance organizations (HMOs), provider-sponsored organizations (PSOs), or physician–hospital organizations (PHOs). A health maintenance organization is a prepaid, comprehensive system of health benefits that combines financing and delivery of health service to subscribers. PSOs are groups of providers that organize to take on managed care contracts. A physician–hospital organization is an organization that bonds hospitals and medical staff in order to take on managed care contracts. In order to receive reimbursement from an MCO, the provider must obtain "primary care provider" (PCP) status through admission to the MCO provider panel. Managed care organizations reimburse primary care providers on a fee-for-service basis, a capitated basis, or a combination of both, depending on the contract negotiated. Capitation is a set fee paid by an HMO to a health care provider. Under the capitated system of reimbursement, APNs and physicians are paid a set fee per patient per month for all services agreed to by contract. Therefore, if the APN contracts to provide all primary care services for a patient, the APN must provide an unlimited number of primary care visits. However, even if the patient does not receive care, the APN receives payment. Primary care providers are almost exclusively physicians; few managed care organizations recognize APNs as PCPs. If APNs are granted PCP status, the MCO will negotiate a contract with the provider. In addition, site visits will be made to monitor and assess contract compliance as well as quality of care provided.

There are no legal barriers to advanced practice nurses who wish to contract directly with businesses, organizations, or individuals for health care services. Advanced practice nurses have successfully negotiated contracts to provide health services to a wide range of groups, such as college faculty, staff and students, occupational health care to corporations, and public organizations such as schools. Billing is achieved by filing standard forms provided by HCFA. APNs of the new millennium must be knowledgeable of state laws related to insurance practices. By learning the language of third-party payment, APNs will be in a better position to navigate the issues of reimbursement in twenty-first-century health care economics. Unfortunately, unnecessary restrictions on the APN scope of practice, prescriptive authority, and eligibility for third-party reimbursement are formidable barriers to advanced practice nursing (Safriet, 1992).

The Future of Advanced Practice Nursing

The rapid movement to managed care, along with advances in medical science, technological advances, and professional education, has caused a significant change in the scope of practice of various health care professionals. These changes have also proclaimed issues over jurisdiction of states to license and regulate health care practice. Regulation plays a crucial role in consumer protection and safeguards economic remuneration for all health care professionals. For advanced practice nursing to continue to grow, the public must be assured of competent, safe practice by APNs.

The Pew Commission was established in 1989 by the Pew Charitable Trusts and charged with the work of assisting health care professionals, workforce policy makers, and educational institutions to promote workforce reforms in response to regulatory and market pressures. The Task Force on Health Care Workforce was organized in 1994 to examine the effects of health care regulation on the consumer. Subsequent publications from the Pew Commission identified priority targets for reform: regulatory boards and governance structures, scope of practice authority, and methods of assessing and ensuring the competence of health care professionals throughout their careers (Finocchio et al., 1998). In addressing regulatory boards and governance structures, the Pew Commission identified a lack of coordination among regulatory boards and state laws resulting in underutilization of certain professionals while encouraging competition for scopes of practice, leading to decreased access to health care. APN scope of practice documents vary from state to state, yet are intimately tied to reimbursement potential. Practice acts are constantly a target of lobbying efforts to control some aspect of the health care market. The ensuing political battles are costly, bog down the legislative process, and foster competitive tension among health professionals. In this kind of process, decisions about who can competently deliver quality, cost-effective health care may be sacrificed by political partiality (Finocchio et al., 1998).

National standards of regulation, education, and credentialing of health care professionals would standardize scopes of practice throughout the country. Continued assurance of professional competence has not yet been an area for widespread regulatory control. Professional associations and credentialing organizations currently establish quality standards and evaluation procedures. The Pew Commission has recommended making decisions about practice authority based on comprehensive evidence of outcomes covering care accessibility, quality, and cost effectiveness. Safriet (1998) has expressed the need for increased APN leadership in national and state health policy reform activities. Outcomes research is demonstrating the value of the APN to the U.S. health care system, and there is evidence that the APN can provide the components of primary care just as efficiently as physicians—in some cases more efficiently (Mundinger et al., 2000). Continued leadership efforts are imperative to demonstrate the value-added contribution of APNs to the health care system.

With the complexity of advances in health care knowledge and technology, the difficulty of meeting total patient care needs has become increasingly apparent. Excellence in health care is requiring a reliance on the combined efforts of professionals who collaborate to deliver high-quality care. Future success for primary care providers will certainly be associated with the ability to share expertise with a team of health care professionals. Collegial collaboration promotes equal authority among team members with shared decision-making responsibilities. Professional collaboration in the twenty-first century will demand that advanced practice nurses and physicians work together as genuine colleagues demonstrating high levels of interpersonal skills (Mundinger, 1994; Norsen, Opladen, & Quinn, 1995). Mundinger (1994) envisions collaborative prac-

tice as merging shared expertise from the APN and physician to provide patient care. The APN makes decisions about patient care without the permission of the physician, and both professionals bring their expertise to bear on a patient care issues. The physician's strengths lie within the realm of complex diagnostic and treatment problems involving unstable and critically ill patients, while the APN takes the lead for prevention, access to community-based resources, health education, and counseling. Increases in quality of care, access to care, efficiency of care delivery and decrease in costs are all demonstrated benefits of mutual, collegial collaboration between advanced practice nurses and physicians (Norsen et al., 1995; Sebas, 1994). Mundinger (1994) asserts that this type of collaboration is more comprehensive, more cost effective, and more beneficial in terms of delivering comprehensive quality patient care. Crucial elements to collegial collaboration in the future will include establishing the right to APN autonomy and a willingness to jointly participate in a team-based approach to quality patient care.

Public visibility and professional recognition for the APN is greater now than at any other time in history. Advanced practice nurses are becoming integral to the American health system and need to become even more so to anchor their future as essential contributors to quality health care. Advanced practice nurses need to take every opportunity to describe to patients, insurers, legislators, and the media who they are and what they do. Clarification of role is crucial during patient encounters, explaining the nature of APN nursing experience, expertise, and advanced education. APNs need to be particularly clear about how they differ from physicians in philosophy, scope of practice, and authority. Research-based approaches must also be stressed, demonstrating that advanced practice nurses are well educated, knowledgeable of current evidenced-based practice guidelines, network closely with peer professionals, and have unique expertise to contribute to health care. Finally, advanced practice nurses must become involved. The greatest barriers to successful assimilation of advanced practice nurses into the health care system are indifference and ignorance about the profession. Influential people need to be educated about advanced practice nursing; assumptions can no longer be made that politicians and prominent media sources understand who advanced practice nurses are and what they do. Nurses have always been a significant part of the health care team, but in the twenty-first century the advanced practice nurses will seek, as never before, to make their contribution visible and desirable to customers of the American health care system.

TRANSITION INTO PRACTICE

Graduate nursing programs with the APN option provide a foundation for career paths to future leadership in nursing. The goal of graduate education is to develop lifelong learners who demonstrate advanced knowledge, critical thinking skills, and flexibility in problem solving. Graduate programs in nursing vary with respect to admission requirements, curriculum organization, length of program, and tuition expenses. Admission to APN programs usually requires RN licensure, graduation from an accredited baccalaureate program, an above-average grade-point average, and nursing experience.

Choosing to begin APN graduate education is an important decision, which requires careful consideration of (a) specialty or role focus, (b) clinical experience, and (c) program selection. Regarding specialization, the APN can focus on a clinical arena (e.g., pediatrics, geriatrics, adult health), the care delivery (e.g., traditional primary care, long-term care, or acute care), or the functional role (e.g., education and research).

Determining when to pursue graduate education is dependent on a number of factors including: (a) financial and travel considerations, (b) family stress issues, (c) degree of social support needed, (d) ability to work while completing educational requirements, and (e) confidence in one's nursing expertise. Graduate education provides a wealth of opportunities to explore personal interest areas; however, expertise takes time to develop. Formal graduate education cannot make experts or teach nurses to be confident in their experiential knowledge base—that process takes time. If a nurse lacks experience or expertise but desires graduate education, returning to school part time while continuing to work could lend itself to continued development of expertise. Depending on the pool of applicants, most graduate schools prefer candidates with at least 2 to 3 years of clinical experience. However, as candidate pools shrink, admission requirements are more flexible to keep classes and programs "alive" in the academic world.

Finally, with the current options of online education and Web site access, potential APN students need to do the homework of assessing graduate programs in nursing. Faculty qualifications and expertise, clinical resources and facilities, options for financial support, accreditation status, national ratings, and program requirements are all criteria for consideration by potential students. Each graduate nursing program will have unique programs of study, philosophical ideas about nursing, and conceptual frameworks that provide insightful overviews of what they believe about advanced practice nursing. Potential students need to assess which APN program most clearly articulate with career goals, personal needs, and educational expectations.

Although long- and short-term goals will be revised as life events alter the journey of a career, professional goals guide decision-making more effectively. In today's world of "change as the order of the day," career goals need to be flexible with identification of alternatives. Exploring a variety of possible choices is judicious as one can always say no to an opportunity, but being available to future options leaves the career door open for all possibilities.

KEY POINTS

1. Advanced practice nursing is a term used to describe a registered nurse who has met advanced educational and clinical practice requirements beyond basic nursing education.

2. The American Nursing Association (ANA) recognizes four groups of APNs: certified registered nurse anesthetists (CRNAs), certified nurse midwives (CNMs), clinical nurse specialists (CNSs), and nurse practitioners (NPs). The common goals of all advanced practice roles include improved access to care, increased collaboration between various health care providers, expanded knowledge base for clinical decision-making, and increased professional autonomy.

3. Advanced practice nurses are not low-priced physician substitutes—they are nurses first, with unique licensure, advanced educational preparation, and regulatory boards in all 50 states.

4. Hallmarks of advanced clinical practice include autonomy, complex clinical decision-making, and skill in managing organizations and environments from a nursing, not a medical, orientation (ANA, 1995).

5. Advanced practice nurse education include graduate education, certification, and direct practice experience.

6. Credentialing is a term that refers to regulatory mechanisms applied to individuals, programs, or organizations (Styles, 1998). From an organizational standpoint, the Commission on Collegiate Nursing Education or the National League for Nursing Accreditation Center accredits graduate nursing programs. The American College of Nurse-Midwives and the American Association of Nurse Anesthetists oversee and review CNM and CRNA education standards, while the National Organization of Nurse Practitioner Faculties and the National Certification Board of Pediatric Nurse Practitioners and Nurses, as well as other NP specialty groups, consult on curriculum guidelines/ standards.

7. Credentialing and privileging mechanisms initially developed for physician groups are being revised to include APNs. The intent of institutional credentialing is to review qualifications and competence with periodic review of performance measures designed to ensure the quality of services being provided.

8. Prior to the emergence of advance practice nurses, the legal scope of practice for nurses excluded diagnosis and treatment of medical problems. Nurse practice acts were amended to include nursing diagnoses and allow APNs to fill gaps in the health system.

9. Legislation governing advanced practice nursing currently exists in every state. Title protection, scope of practice, collaborative relationships or supervision requirements, education, and certification expectations all regulate professional advanced practice nursing through individual state nurse practice act statutes.

10. Advanced practice nurses are held to the standard of the prudent APN, not the prudent physician; however, in some cases the standards of care may be identical.

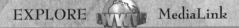

EXPLORE MediaLink

Critical thinking questions, essay questions, key terms, web links, activities, NCLEX review questions, and more interactive resources can be found on the Companion Website at www.prenhall.com/haynes. Click on Chapter 22 to select activities for this chapter.

REFERENCES

American Association of Colleges of Nursing. (1996). *The essentials of master's education for advanced practice nursing.* Washington, DC: Author.

American Association of Nurse Anesthetists. (2002, January 25). *All about the HCFA supervision issue.* Parkridge, IL: Author.

American Academy of Nurse Practitioners. (2002, February 2). *Certification program description.* Austin, TX: Author.

American Board of Nursing Specialties. (1997). *Applications for approval: Standards, rationale, criteria, required documentation.* Washington, DC: Author.

American College of Nurse-Midwives. (2002, January 15). *Mandatory degree requirements for midwives.* Washington, DC: Author.

American Medical Association. (1995). *Physician profiling and the release of physician-specific health care data: Department of Medical Review.* Chicago: Author.

American Medical Association. (2001). *Current procedural terminology.* Chicago: Author.

American Nurses Association. (1993). *Executive summary: A meta-analysis of process of care, clinical outcomes and cost effectiveness of nurses in primary care roles: Nurse practitioners and nurse-midwives.* Washington, DC: Author.

American Nurses Association. (1995). *Nursing's social policy statement.* Washington, DC: Author.

American Nurses Association. (1996). *The scope and standards of advanced practice registered nursing.* Washington, DC: Author.

American Nursing Association. (2002, January 25). *Nursing facts.* Washington, DC: Author.

American Nursing Credentialing Center. (2002, February 2). *Change of credentialing form.* Washington, DC: Author.

Bankert, M. (1989). *Watchful care: A history of America's nurse anesthetists.* New York: Continuum.

Bigbee, J., & Amidi-Nouri, A. (2000). History and evolution of advanced nursing practice. In A. Hamric, J. Spross, & C. Hanson (Eds.), *Advanced nursing practice: An integrative approach* (2nd ed.). Philadelphia, PA: W. B. Saunders.

Birkholz, G. (1995). Malpractice data from the national practitioner data bank. *Nurse Practitioner, 20*(3), 32–35.

Breckinridge, M. (1952). *Wide neighborhoods: A study of the frontier nursing service.* New York: Harper.

Brown, S. A., & Grimes, D. E. (1995). A meta-analysis of nurse practitioners and nurse midwives in primary care. *Nursing Research, 44*(6), 332–339.

Brown, S. J. (1998). A framework for advanced practice nursing. *Journal of Professional Nursing, 14,* 157–164.

Buppert, C. (1999). *Nurse practitioner's business practice and legal guide.* Gaithersburg, MD: Aspen.

Cameron, M., & Schaffer, M. (1992). Tell me the right answer: A model for teaching nursing ethics. *Journal of Nursing Education, 31*(8), 377–380.

Christy, T. E. (1970). Portrait of a leader: Lillian D. Wald. *Nursing Outlook, 18*(3), 50–54.

Christy, T. E. (1978). The hope of history. In M. L. Fitzpatrick (Ed.), *Historical studies in nursing.* New York: Teachers College Press.

Crosby, F., Ventura, M. R., & Feldman, M. J. (1987). Future research recommendations for establishing NP effectiveness. *Nurse Practitioner, 12,* 75–79.

Dock, L., & Stewart, I. (1920). *A short history of nursing.* New York: G. P. Putnam's Sons.

Donahue, M. P. (1985). *Nursing, the finest art.* St. Louis, MO: Mosby.

Doughty, S., & Keller, J. (2000). Marketing and contracting considerations. In A. Hamric, J. Sporss, & C. Hanson (Eds.), *Advanced nursing practice: An integrative approach* (2nd ed.). Philadelphia, PA: W. B. Saunders.

Elder, R., & Bullough, B. (1990). Nurse practitioners and clinical nurse specialists: Are the roles merging? *Clinical Nurse Specialist, 4,* 78–84.

Emmons, D., Wozniak, G., Otten, R., & Baker, N. (1993). Data on employee physician profiling. *Journal of Health & Hospital Law, 26,* 73–82.

Finocchio, L., Dower, C., Blick, N., Gragnola, C., & Task Force on Health Care Workforce Regulations. (1998). *Strengthening consumer protection: Priorities for health-care workforce regulation.* San Francisco: Pew Health Professions Commission.

Ford, L. (1991). Advanced nursing practice: Future of the nurse practitioner. In L. H. Aiken & C. M. Fagin (Eds.), *Charting nursing's future: Agenda for the 1990s* (pp. 287–299). New York: J. B. Lippincott.

Ford, L., & Silver, H. (1967). The expanded role of the nurse in childcare. *Nursing Outlook, 15*(8), 43–45.

Glanville, I., Schirm, V., & Wineman, N. M. (2000). Using evidence-based practice for managing clinical outcomes in advanced practice nursing. *Journal of Nursing Care Quality, 15*(1), 1–11.

Hanson, C. (2000). Understanding the regulatory and credentialing requirements for advanced practice nursing. In A. Hamric, J. Spross, & C. Hanson (Eds.), *Advanced nursing practice: An integrative approach* (2nd ed.) (pp. 679–700). Philadelphia, PA: W. B. Saunders.

Hanson, C., Spross, J., & Carr, D. (2000). Collaboration. In A. Hamric, J. Spross, & C. Hanson (Eds.), *Advanced nursing practice: An integrative approach* (2nd ed.) (pp. 315–347). Philadelphia, PA: W. B. Saunders.

Health Care Financing Administration. (1997). *1997 Documentation guidelines for evaluation and management services.* Washington, DC: Author.

Illinois Department of Professional Regulation. (2002). *Rules for the administration of the nursing and advanced practice nursing act.* Springfield, IL: Author.

Institute of Medicine. (1990). *Medicare: A strategy for quality assurance* (Vol. 1). Washington, DC: Author.

Johnson, M., Maas, M. (2000). *Nursing outcomes classification (NOC).* St. Louis, MO: Mosby.

Kalisch, P., & Kalisch, B. (1995). *The advance of American nursing* (3rd ed.). Philadelphia, PA: J. B. Lippincott.

Kamajian, M., Mitchell, S., & Fruth, R. (1999). Credentialing and privileging of advanced practice nurses. *American Association of Colleges of Nursing Clinical Issues, 10*(3), 316–336.

Lincoln, P. (2000). Comparing CNS and NP role activities: A replication. *Clinical Nurse Specialist, 14*(6), 269–277.

Lyon, B., Davidson, S., Beecroft, P., Bingle, J., & Dayhoff, N. (1998). *National Association of Clinical Nurse Specialists statement on clinical nurse specialists practice and education.* Glenview, IL: NACNS.

McDonald, L. (2001). Florence Nightingale and the early origins of evidence-based nursing. *Evidenced Based Nursing, 4,* 68–69.

Moniz, D. (1992). The legal danger of written protocols and standards of practice. *Nurse Practitioner, 17,* 58–60.

Moser, S., & Armer, J. (1999). An inside view: NP/MD perceptions of collaborative practice. *Nursing and Health Care Perspectives, 21*(1), 29–33.

Mundinger, M. (1994). Advanced practice nursing: Good medicine for physicians? *New England Journal of Medicine, 330*(4), 211–214.

Mundinger, M. (1999). Can advanced practice nurses succeed in the primary care market? *Nursing Economics, 17*(1), 7–14.

Mundinger, M., Kane, R., Lenz, E., Totlen, A., Tsai, W., Cleary, P., et al. (2000). Primary care outcomes in patients treated by nurse practitioner or physicians: A randomized trial. *Journal of the American Medical Association, 283*(1), 59–68.

National Association of Clinical Nurse Specialists. (1998). *Statement on clinical nurse specialist practice and education.* Glenview, IL: Author.

National Council of State Board of Nursing. (1998). *Advanced practice nursing: Nurse practitioner curriculum guidelines and program standards.* Washington, DC: Author.

National Organization of Nurse Practitioner Faculties. (1995). *Advanced practice nursing: Nurse practitioner curriculum guidelines and program standards.* Washington, DC: Author.

Noddings, N. (1984). *Caring: A feminine approach to ethics and moral education.* Los Angeles: University of California Press.

Norsen, L., Opladen, J., & Quinn, J. (1995). Practice model: Collaborative practice. *Critical Care Nursing Clinics of North America, 7,* 43.

Nutting, M. A., & Dock, L. (1907). *A history of nursing* (Vol. 2). New York: G. P. Putnam's Sons.

Office of Technology Assessment. (1986). *Nurse practitioners, physician assistants and certified nurse-midwives: A policy analysis* (OTA-HCS-37). Washington, DC: U.S. Government Printing Office.

Pew Health Professions Commission. (1995). *Critical challenges: Revitalizing the health professions for the twenty-first century.* San Francisco: University of California, Center for Health Professions.

Porter-O'Grady, T. (1996). Consider this—the business of partnership. *Advanced Practice Nursing Quarterly, 2,* 81–82.

Roberts, M. (1954). *American nursing, history and interpretation.* New York: MacMillan.

Sackett, D., Rosenburg, W., Gray, J., Hayes, R., & Richardson, W. (1996). Evidenced-based medicine: What it is and what it isn't. *British Medical Journal, 312,* 71–72.

Safriet, B. (1992). Health care dollars and regulatory sense: The role of advanced practice nursing. *Yale Journal on Regulation, 9*(2), 417–489.

Safriet, B. (1998). Still spending dollars, still searching for sense: advanced practice nursing in an era of regulatory and economic turmoil. *Advanced Practice Nursing Quarterly, 4*(3), 24–33.

Scott, R. A. (1999). A description of the roles, activities, and skills of clinical nurse specialists in the United States. *Clinical Nurse Specialist, 13*(4), 183–189.

Scott-Levin (2000). *Scott-Levin's nurse practitioner/physician assistant promotional audit [Online].* Available: http://www.quintiles.com/products and services/informatics/scott_levin/ (6-16-2000). Press release by Nancy Robertone, Newtown, PA.

Sebas, M. (1994). Developing a collaborative practice agreement for the primary care setting. *Nurse Practitioner, 19,* 49–51.

Seymer, L. R. (1932). *A general history of nursing.* London: Faber & Faber Ltd.

Seymer, L. R. (1960). *Florence Nightingale's nurses: The Nightingale training school 1860–1960.* London: Pitman Medical Publishing Co.

Skalla, K., & Hamric, A. (2000). The blended role of the clinical nurse specialist and the nurse practitioner. In A. Hamric, J. Spross, & C. Hanson (Eds.), *Advanced nursing practice: An integrative approach* (2nd ed.) (pp. 459–490). Philadelphia, PA: W. B. Saunders.

Sparacino, P. (2000). The clinical nurse specialist. In A. Hamric, J. Spross, & C. Hanson (Eds.), *Advanced nursing practice: An integrative approach* (2nd ed.) (pp. 381–406). Philadelphia: W. B. Saunders.

Styles, M. (1998). An international perspective: APN credentialing. *Advanced Practice Nursing Quarterly, 4*(3), 1–5.

Styles, M., & Lewis, C. (2000). Conceptualizations of advanced nursing practice. In A. Hamric, J. Spross, & C. Hanson (Eds.), *Advanced nursing practice: An integrative approach* (2nd ed.) (pp. 33–52). Philadelphia, PA: W. B. Saunders.

Urden, L. (1999). Outcome evaluation: An essential component for CNS practice. *Clinical Nurse Specialist, 13,* 39–46.

Urden, L. (2001). Outcome evaluation: An essential component for CNS practice. *Clinical Nurse Specialist, 15,* 639–616.

U.S. Public Health Service. (1996) *National practitioner data bank guidebook.* Rockville, MD: Department of Health and Human Services.

U.S. Department of Health and Human Services, Public Health Service. (2000). *Healthy people 2010.* Washington, DC: U.S. Government Printing Office.

Williams, C., & Valdivieso G. (1994). Advanced practice models: A comparison of clinical nurse specialist and nurse practitioner activities. *Clinical Nurse Specialist, 8,* 311–318.

Woodham-Smith, C. (1951). *Florence Nightingale.* New York: McGraw-Hill.

SUGGESTED READINGS

Buppert, C. (2000). Measuring outcomes in primary care practice. *Nurse Practitioner, 25*(1), 88–98.

Hamric, A. B. (1998). Using research to influence the regulatory process. *Advanced Practice Nursing Quarterly, 4*(3), 44–50.

Lyon, B. L. (2002). Legislative and regulatory update. What to look for when analyzing clinical nurse specialist statutes and regulations. *Clinical Nurse Specialist, 16*(1), 33–34.

Mundinger, M. O. (2001). Evaluating quality in nurse practitioner primary care: Comparing NP and MD primary care outcomes: Two-year follow-up. 34th Annual Communicating Nursing Research Conference/15th Annual WIN Assembly, "Health Care Challenges Beyond 2001: Mapping the Journey for Research and Practice," held April 19–21, 2001, in Seattle Washington. *Communicating Nursing Research, 34*(9), 116.

Mundinger, M. O., Cook, S. S., Lenz, E. R., Placentini, K., Auerhahn, C., & Smith, J. (2000). Assuring quality and access in advanced practice nursing: A challenge to nurse educators. *Journal of Professional Nursing, 16*(6), 322–329.

Pruitt, R. H., Wetsel, M. A., Smith, K. J., & Spitler, H. (2002). How do we pass NP autonomy legislation? *Nurse Practitioner, 27*(3), 56, 61–65.

Tingle, J. (2002). The legal implications of extending nurses' roles. *Practice Nursing, 13*(4), 148–152.

Unit 6

Challege of Management

23

Collaboration in Health Care

JENNIE ECHOLS

"Great discoveries and improvements invariably involve the cooperation of many minds.
Alexander Graham Bell (1847–1922) (as cited in Asimov & Shulmon, 1988)"

LEARNING OBJECTIVES

AT THE COMPLETION OF THIS CHAPTER, THE READER WILL BE ABLE TO:

➤ Explain the importance of collaboration in professional practice.

➤ Name the essential elements of collaboration.

➤ Identify examples of situations where collaboration is used in nursing.

➤ Discuss skills and resources necessary for successful collaboration in professional practice.

➤ Discuss the concepts of team building, negotiation, conflict resolution, and empowerment as processes critical to collaboration.

➤ Explore the benefits of collaboration for the future of nursing.

MediaLink www.prenhall.com/haynes

Additional online resources including NCLEX review questions, critical thinking questions, and real-world activities for this chapter can be found on the Companion Website at www.prenhall.com/haynes.

*C*ollaboration in *Merriam-Webster's Ninth New Collegiate Dictionary* (1987) is defined as working in partnership and involving close cooperation between participants. There are actually many definitions of collaboration found in the literature; all are similar in some respect, but different with regard to perspective and situational context. This chapter explores the meaning collaboration holds for the nurse and why it is important to be an effective collaborator. Also, the chapter provides strategies for becoming an effective collaborator in the interdisciplinary health care environment. Finally, the chapter will conclude with a summary of trends and possibilities for nurses collaborating in the future.

The Meaning of Collaboration

Peterson and Schaffer (1999) said, "individual nurse–patient relationships are only one of the relationships nurses must master" (p. 209). It is critical that nurses learn to work with each other as well as work with members of other disciplines through collaborative relationships to meet the needs of patients, provide quality care, and be cost-effective (Connolly & Novak, 2000). Patient care has become fragmented as physicians and nurses have specialized, and other disciplines have emerged as important members of the health care delivery system (McEwen, 1994). Collaboration is the link that connects the various health care disciplines to implement patient focused care.

Why Collaborate

Many researchers have found that collaboration leads to better health care outcomes and increased work satisfaction for the health care provider. This finding makes collaboration extremely important. Limited resources in today's health care environment require nurses to find ways to implement cost-effective care while maintaining positive outcomes. As collaboration promotes improved outcomes, nurses must understand collaboration and learn ways to collaborate in an effective manner.

The nurse encounters situations daily in which collaboration is required. Familiar and frequent examples include:

- Discharge planning wherein the nurse must work with the family, social workers, physician, and other providers who will follow-up with the patient after discharge.

- Treatment team meetings on the psychiatric unit or in the nursing home.
- Nursing or hospital departments such as the emergency room that call to admit a patient to the unit already at capacity.
- Utilization review with the managed care organization that will authorize admission and continued stay for the patient.
- Quality improvement studies in which the nurse is asked to join other nurses and/or other health care professionals to work to improve a particular operational or clinical process on the unit or in the hospital (e.g., reducing patient falls, or reducing medication errors, etc.).

Collaboration is a leadership quality important for nurses. Kerfoot (1994) reminds us "the nurse manager of the future will be valued for cooperation, the ability to coordinate, collaborate and synergize and to work across many different entities" (p. 100). The nursing leader of the future will need to collaborate to integrate clinical practice, education, and research. This is necessary for the development and survival of the discipline of nursing, and in a circular fashion will strengthen the ability of nurses to collaborate with other disciplines that have clearly defined roles (e.g., physicians, dietitians, respiratory therapist).

Definition of Collaboration

The term collaboration, refers to various combinations of relationships that involve communication. But collaboration is different from occasional informal or formal conversation in the workplace. Hoffman (1998) defines **collaboration** as "the highest level of partnership" (p. 194). Both partnership and collaboration require good communication, a common purpose, and acknowledgement of complementary skills and expertise (Shannon, 1998).

Collaboration is often referred to as a communication, relationship, or management style. Terms often confused with collaboration along with communication are partnership and conflict resolution. Coeling and Wilcox (1994) suggest that collaboration is more than just communication since there is an exchange of ideas among people who are committed and invested in a common goal. Collaboration requires a sharing of ownership in the problem, decision-making, and the goal along with a shared responsibility in the implementation and outcome (Ashcroft, 1996; Wells, Johnson, & Salyer, 1998). Collaboration is more than communication since the result of collaboration is the creation of a product with value. Moreover, collaboration occurs as a result of an investment in the process and outcome. According to Shannon (1998), partnership and collaboration exist at different points on the relationship continuum. Both require a common purpose; however, in a partnership a more formal agreement is usually negotiated. There are agreed-upon terms in a partnership that delineate how power is distributed and decisions are made. Kanter (1994) identified criteria for true partnerships that change the balance of power from "I" to "We." Partnerships suggest individual excellence, as well as interdependence and formal investment (Kanter, 1994). In contrast, collaboration, while requiring individual excellence and interdependence, does not require the formality, institutionalization, and interest in the individual advantages that result from the relationship.

Alpert, Goldman, Kilroy, and Pike (1992) remind us that the word collaboration comes from the Latin word meaning "with" or "together" and "to work." In the middle nineteenth century, the word collaboration suggested a process of working with another on literary, artistic, or scientific endeavors. In the more recent past, the definition of collaboration has been associated with a negative connotation of associating or cooperating with the enemy. During World War II, French citizens who sided with the Nazis were called collaborateurs. There is some element of this definition that exists today as elements of collaboration such as negotiation are used to interact with extreme enemies on an international political scale.

Collaboration focuses on trying to reach agreement among divergent opinions to accomplish mutual goals. It is the process of "joint decision-making among interdependent parties involving joint ownership of decision-making and collective responsibility for outcome" (Disch, 2001, p. 275).

Wonsetler (1987) defined collaboration as the most positive way to resolve conflict with the attributes of a high degree of assertiveness and cooperation. Key factors in collaboration include communication, negotiation, conflict resolution, and coordination (Flaherty, 1998). While each of these key factors must be present for effective collaboration, they do not in themselves define collaboration. It has been proposed that negotiation, conflict resolution, and coordination are collaborative skills, which can be learned to enhance the process of collaboration.

Both the interpersonal and intrapersonal qualities of the individual play a role in the effectiveness of the collaborative interaction. Jones (1994) and Dechairo-Marino, Jordan-Marsh, Traiger, and Saulo (2001) indicate that assertiveness and cooperation foster collaboration. Baggs (1994) describes a model of collaboration as a combination of co-cooperativeness (concern for others) with a high level of assertiveness (concern for one's own interests). Successful collaborators possess the ability to share their views without intimidation and accept criticism of their views from other. The ability to seek to understand the other person's view and position is critical to the collaboration process.

Henneman, Lee, and Cohen (1995) point out that collaboration is nonhierarchal in nature and can exist between two parties with an unequal formal power base. The power in a collaborative relationship is based on knowledge or expertise as opposed to power based on role or function. An example is the mutual power that can exist in nurse–physician interactions. The nurse and the physician, who both value and perceive equal opportunities to participate in treatment decisions, share this type of mutual power (Jones, 1994). Collaboration usually involves fewer formal behaviors related to organizational status or position, and more often relates to the individual's personal values and mission (Corser, 1998).

Definitions of collaboration vary; however, the consistent characteristics present in most definitions are presented in Box 23–1.

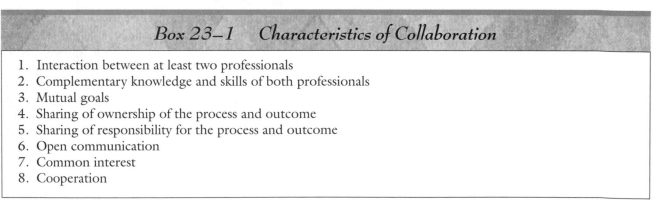

Box 23–1   Characteristics of Collaboration

1. Interaction between at least two professionals
2. Complementary knowledge and skills of both professionals
3. Mutual goals
4. Sharing of ownership of the process and outcome
5. Sharing of responsibility for the process and outcome
6. Open communication
7. Common interest
8. Cooperation

Sources: Corser (1998); Flaherty (1998); Baggs (1994); Dechairo-Marino, et. al. (2001); and Jones (1994).

Corser (1998) developed a context specific model to describe nurse–physician collaboration. The model features the complementary management of pertinent organizational/professional and personal/interpersonal influences experienced by the nurse and physician. The model also addresses other required elements, including mutual respect for each other's professional roles, abilities, and respective patient care contributions. The occurrence of a collaborative interaction requires both the nurse and physician to maintain an actual and perceived equal power base relative to one another, a circumstance that may be enhanced or impaired by any number of influences described in Corser's model, which is further detailed in Figure 23–1.

Hayward, DeMarco, and Lynch (2000) describe a model of collaboration that provides a comprehensive view of the process of collaboration. The seven-stage "interprofessional alliance" model presents a more detailed explanation of the interpersonal factors that occur among a team, along with a description of the collaborative process. Phase one includes an individual needs assessment. Phase two includes a comparison of individual and group needs. Phase three is the development of a culture of collaboration and establishing relationships. Phase four is examination and reflection. Phase five is formulating a pact to collaborate. Phase six is implementation of the project. Finally, phase seven is evaluation of the project success.

Figure 23–1   Collaborative Nurse–Physician Interaction Model

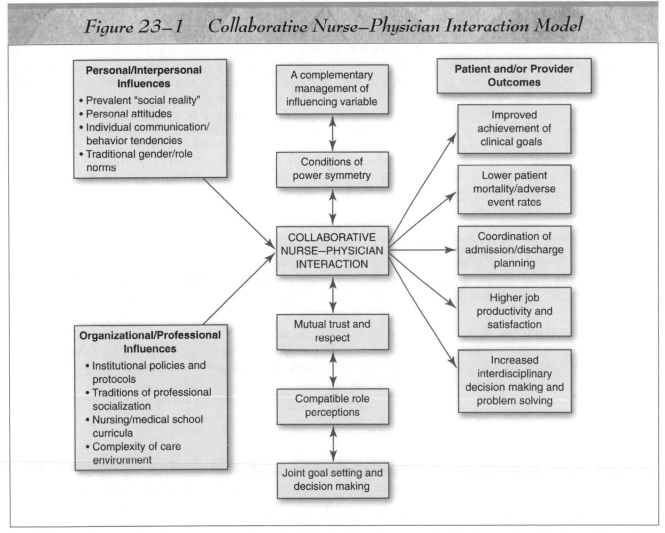

Used by permission: Corser, W. D. (1998). A conceptual model of collaborative nurse–physician interactions: The management of traditional influences and personal tendencies. *Scholarly Inquiry for Nursing Practice, 12*(14), 335. © Springer Publishing Company, Inc., New York, NY 10012.

Several instruments have been developed to measure collaboration. Baggs (1994) developed the most widely used instrument to measure nurse–physician collaboration. She based the tool on a model describing collaboration as combining a high level of co-operating and a high level of assertion. The Collaboration and Satisfaction About Care Decisions (CSACD) instrument developed by Baggs (1994) contains six collaboration questions and three satisfaction questions. Each question is scored on a Likert-type seven-point scale. The questions are displayed in Box 23–2.

Essential Elements of Collaboration

Gray (1989) suggests that collaboration is not a single-factor concept but rather behavior, which consists of several essential elements including commitment to content issues, relationships, willingness to recognize each other's ideas, and commitment to spend time talking together. The central theme to collaboration is communication. While fundamental to collaboration, effective and open communication is not sufficient for the collaborative process (Wells et al., 1998). An affirmation style of communication is required for collaboration where messages are acknowledged and recognized in a relaxed and friendly manner. This also includes active listening and an awareness of each other's communication styles (Coeling & Wilcox, 1994). Communication is defined by Jones (1997) as

"being verbal or written and involving two-channel or multichannel pathways" (p. 11). Communication can be either formal or informal and direct or indirect. Most authorities on communication agree that the majority of communication is nonverbal. Gestures, facial expressions, and tone of voice are examples of nonverbal behavior that accompanies the words exchanged in communication.

Senge (1990) explains successful communication in team building as dialogue and discussion. The word dialogue comes from a Greek phrase meaning "to pass meaning through words." "The purpose of a dialogue is to go beyond any one individual's understanding . . . to gain insights that simply could not be achieved individually" (Senge, 1990, p. 241). For dialogue to occur, individuals must suspend their own assumptions, but still communicate their assumptions regarding the issue to others as colleagues. The energy created in the group through dialogue contributes to a free flow of meaning and information among the participants. It is obvious in the process that once individuals decide "their view is the way it is," the flow of dialogue is obstructed. The key is to view "adversaries" as "colleagues" with different views. Other essential elements of collaboration are listed in Table 23–1.

In summary, a **collaborative interaction** consists of: (a) the complementary management of the pertinent organizational/professional and person/interpersonal

---

Box 23–2   The Collaboration and Satisfaction About Care Decisions (CSACD) Instrument

Collaboration
1. Nurses and physicians planned together to make the decision about care for this patient.
2. Open communication between physicians and nurses took place as this decision was made for this patient.
3. Decision-making responsibilities for this patient were shared between nurses and physicians.
4. Physicians and nurses cooperated in making this decision.
5. As this decision was considered, nurses and physicians each actively represented their professional perspectives about this patient's needs.
6. Decision-making for this patient was coordinated between physicians and nurses.

Satisfaction
1. How much collaboration between nurses and physicians occurred in making this decision for this patient?
2. How satisfied were you with the way this decision was made for the patient, that is, with the decision-making process, not necessarily with the decision itself?
3. How satisfied were you with the decision made for this patient?

Reprinted with permission from Baggs, J. G. (1994). Development of an instrument to measure collaboration and satisfaction about care decisions. *Journal of Advanced Nursing, 20*, 176–182. Blackwell Publishing, Osney Mead, Oxford, UK.

Table 23–1   Essential Elements of Collaboration

Relationship	The first element essential for collaboration is that there must be two or more parties with some degree of agreement that there is a need to work together.
Frequent communication	Baggs (1994) emphasizes the need for frequent communication as essential to facilitating collaboration. The lack of opportunity to meet face to face and develop relationships is a major barrier to effective collaboration.
Commitment	Each participant in the collaborative interaction must have a commitment to the process and the outcome. This commitment includes the ability to prioritize the time to engage in the interpersonal and intrapersonal work required for the collaborative process (Henry, Schmitz, Reif, & Rudie, 1992).
Mutual respect	Mutual respect for each other's skills and expertise and a firm belief that all participants are both inherently good and trying to provide the best care we can to our patients is absolutely critical to collaboration (Alpert, Goldman, Kilroy, & Pike, 1992). Collaboration requires that each party believes that each other is needed to achieve the goal (Ashcroft, 1996; Miccolo & Spanier, 1993; Sullivan, 1998).
Distinct body of knowledge	Wells, Johnson, and Salyer (1998) say we need a distinct body of knowledge as well as competence in our knowledge and area of clinical practice.
	Collaboration requires clear roles of each discipline that can only be accomplished through a distinct body of knowledge for each complementary member of the relationship (Jones, 1997).
Knowledge of other party's discipline	In addition to having a distinct body of knowledge, the nurse must understand what the other party's discipline is about (Coeling & Wilcox, 1994). Wells et al. (1998) also remind us that respect and acknowledgement of the expertise of others is also an essential element of collaboration.
Assertiveness	Collaboration requires that the nurse interact with others in an assertive manner. The ability to voice concerns and state problems in behavioral terms and focus on the issue in a self-assured way is necessary for collaborative interactions (Henry et al., 1992; Jones, 1994).
	Assertiveness also includes learning how to present ideas, have ideas criticized, and respond to criticism in a nondefensive, theoretically sound manner (Corser, 1998; Nugent & Lambert, 1996).
Trust	Trust is essential to most any effective communication and required for collaboration. Not only must each participant in the interaction trust that each other has the interest of the patient as the ultimate goal, but there must be trust in each other's commitment to the process (Alpert et al., 1992; Corser, 1998; Sullivan, 1998).
Coordination	Flaherty (1998) emphasizes coordination in addition to communication as an essential element in collaboration. Coordination can include such simple tasks as scheduling meeting times to complicated project management required for implementing joint solutions.
Cooperation and sharing	Collaboration requires that each person participating in the process share their concern and knowledge in a cooperative way (Baggs & Schmitt, 1988; Corser, 1998; Wells et al., 1998). All parties in the collaborative process must be willing to devote equal time and energy to collaborative endeavors as well as share ideas and concerns openly.
Collegiality	Collegiality has often been considered a precursor to collaboration. Collaborative interactions usually involve few formal behaviors and hierarchial relationships are not emphasized. Instead, relationships are more often related to the individual's personal values and presenting situation (Corser, 1998).
Openness and receptivity	Baggs (1997) emphasizes being open and receptive in the collaboration.
Interdependence	Interdependence refers to the mature relationship between individuals that are mutually dependent on the skills and expertise of each other. Corser (1998) and Baggs and Schmitt (1988) emphasize the need to increase interdependence between nurses and physicians.
Mutual goal setting	Mutual goal setting is an essential element of collaboration identified by most all of the literature on collaboration.
Consensus	Henry et al. (1992) describe that consensus is an essential element of collaboration in order to obtain agreement on the goal and implementation plan.

Why is it important to cooperate and collaborate with other health care professionals? What makes collaboration different than the normal conversation that takes place at work? What might be the effect of believing you are right and the other person is wrong in collaborating about a treatment decision?

influences that are experienced by the nurse and physician, and (b) a mutual respect for each other's professional roles, abilities, and respective patient care contributions (Corser, 1998, p. 334).

Collaboration Skills and Resources

Collaboration is a process that is learned and subject to improvement with the appropriate application of skills and resources. Important skills and resources for effective collaboration include—team building, negotiation, conflict resolution skills, and empowerment.

Team Building

Jones (1997) defines **teamwork** as health care professionals, families, and patients (with clearly defined roles) working together in partnerships. Teams are an important part of nursing that nurses need to develop. The nurse needs to know how to build teams, and be a facilitator and leader of groups that will solve problems and achieve goals.

Team-building interventions include interpersonal processes, goal setting, role definition, and problem solving. A clear focus on the task or goal is needed for effective team building. Sundstrom, DeMeuse, and Futrell (1990) also point out that with a team, the services that the group delivers or the products it makes should meet or exceed the performance standards of the people who receive it, use it, or review it. The processes and structures used by a team to carry out their work should maintain or enhance the capability of members to work together on group tasks. The characteristics that contribute to effective teams are identified in Box 23–3.

Rutan and Stone (1984) define three stages of development for groups. Stage 1 is group formation. Issues of trust and safety are important in this stage, and there is a focus on joining and finding commonalities. Stage 2 is the reactive phase. Members are focused on their reactions to belonging in the group. Emotional outbursts and unevenness of commitment

to the group often characterize this phase. Members often arrive late or not at all and may consider resigning from the group. Stage 3 is the mature phase. This is a performing, working, effective group. In this phase a flexible structure and collegial relationships develop with the leader and members. Members develop confidence in their ability to examine problems together, and there is increasing understanding of one another's strengths and weaknesses, and goals are achieved. Forsyth (1999) emphasizes the interdependence among members in a group as the group progresses through each stage. General rules for effective groups are presented in Box 23–4.

Negotiation

Fisher and Ury (1991) define **negotiation** as getting the other party in your interaction to say "yes." In negotiating, taking a position is a common natural response that serves some useful purposes since it informs another person of what you want and produces terms of an acceptable agreement. These purposes can also be served in other ways when positioning and bargaining fail to meet the basic criteria to produce an acceptable agreement. The more effective method for negotiation is negotiation based on the merits of a situation. Negotiation on the merits requires one to:

- Separate the people from the problems. Be soft on the people and hard on the problem while proceeding independent of trust. Understand from the other person's point of view by putting yourself in his shoes. Do not deduce his intentions from your own fears and do not blame him for your problem.
- Discuss each other's perception of the problem and look for opportunities to clarify misperceptions.
- Give the other party a stake in the outcome by making sure he participates in the process.
- Recognize and understand emotions, his and yours. Make emotions explicit and acknowledge them as legitimate. Allow the other side to let off steam. Do not react to emotional outbursts. Use symbolic gestures such as nodding your head in agreement of affirmative hand gestures.

Box 23–3 *Characteristics Contributing to Effective Teams*

A clear mission and shared vision and goals

Mutual trust

Supportive and effective culture with group experiences that satisfy rather than frustrate the personal needs of group members

Clearly defined roles

Motivating task

Unambiguous and constructive criticism

Innovation and improvisation

Ability to solve problems directly

Spirit of cooperation rather than competition

Realistic expectations

Just the right amount of tension to stimulate a need for change

Involvement of informal leaders

Maximum freedom of self-expression and open communication in a warm and friendly atmosphere

Inclusion and acceptance among members

Constructive feedback among members

Rewards consistent with objectives

A sense of fairness and justice prevails

Uniform standards regarding behavior and communication in the group (group norms)

Appropriate membership with distinct and unique contributions

Physical environment that balances coordination and privacy

Available technological and material resources and sufficient time

Adapted from Hackman (1987); Sundstrom, DeMeuse, and Futrell (1990); and Dyer (1994).

- Listen actively and acknowledge what is being said. Speak to be understood.
- Focus on interests, not positions. Explore interests and avoid having a bottom line. Interests define the problem. Behind opposed positions lie shared and compatible interests, as well as conflicting ones. Identify interest by asking. The most powerful interests are basic human needs like security, economic well-being, and recognition. Make interests come alive and acknowledge as part of the problem.
- Put the problem, interest, and reasoning first and your conclusions and proposals later.
- Be concrete but flexible.
- Generate a variety of possibilities before deciding what to do. Invent options with mutual gain. Develop options to choose from but decide later. Four obstacles that inhibit an abundance of options are: (a) premature judgment; (b) searching for a single answer; (c) the assumption of a fixed pie; and (d) thinking that solving their problems is their

problems. Separate inventing the options from deciding. Try brainstorming.
- Look through the eyes of different experts. Look for mutual gains and dovetail differing interests. Make their decision easy.
- Insist that the result be based on some objective standard.
- Reason and be open to reason.
- Yield to principle, not pressure.

Dealing with a more powerful person or persons requires additional strategies for the negotiation. The strategies in this case include tactics designed to protect yourself from making an agreement you should reject. In addition, you should make the most of the assets you do have so that any agreement you reach will satisfy your interests as well as possible.

A barrier to negotiation occurs when the other party "won't play." If the other party in the interaction announces a firm position, rejecting their position only

Box 23–4   General Rules for Effective Groups

1. Test assumptions and inferences.
2. Share all relevant information.
3. Focus on interests, not positions.
4. Be specific—use examples.
5. Agree on what important words mean.
6. Explain the reasons behind one's statement, questions, and actions.
7. Disagree openly with any member of the group.
8. Make statement, then invite questions and comments.
9. Jointly design ways to test disagreements and solutions.
10. Discuss undiscussable issues.
11. Keep the discussion focused.
12. Do not take cheap shots or otherwise distract the group.
13. All members are expected to participate in all phases of the process.
14. Exchange relevant information with non–group members.
15. Make decision by consensus.
16. Do self-evaluations.

From Schwarz, R. M. *The skilled facilitator: Practical wisdom for developing effective groups.* Copyright 1994 by Jossey-Bass Publishers. This material is used by permission of John Wiley & Sons, Inc.

locks the opposing party in their position. Defending the nurse's position sidetracks the negotiation. The strategy is to not (a) push back when the other party asserts their positions, or (b) reject their ideas. Channel the energy and emotion of the exchange into exploring interests, inventing options, and searching for solutions. Reframe an attack as an attack on the problem. Another tactic used by many is hard bargaining that sometimes include "dirty tricks." Common examples of these tactics are found in Table 23–2.

Dealing with someone with more power is an obstacle to anyone new to negotiation. You can negotiate with someone with more power, but how you negotiate makes a big difference. Begin by not asking who is more powerful. There are many sources of negotiation power. There is power in developing a good working relationship between the people negotiating. There is power in understanding interests and in inventing an elegant option. There is also power in making a mutual commitment. The nurse should make

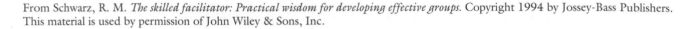

Table 23–2   Negotiation Strategies for Hard Bargaining

Hard Bargaining Tactic	Effective Strategy
Deliberate deception with phony facts and ambiguous authority; less than full disclosure	Do not trust to begin with. Never enter a negotiation with full naiveté about facts.
Psychological warfare—inducing stressful situations by personal attacks. Good guy–bad guy routine	Do not take it personally.
Refusal to negotiate with extreme demands, escalating demands, hardheaded partner, or calculated delay	Ignore threats at first; keep talking as if you didn't hear the demand or change the subject; perhaps by offering another option, let them know what they have to lose if no agreement is met.

Source: Fisher, R., & Ury, W. (1991). *Getting to yes: Negotiation agreement without giving.* New York: Penguin Books.

the most of his or her potential power in any negotiation.

Mastering the art of negotiation will help the nurse sustain productive relationships with management, peers, representatives of other disciplines, and patients. When negotiation skills are practiced and viewed as a natural process, success is assured when win–win situations are sought.

Conflict Resolution

Conflict resolution is often confused with collaboration. Accepting that conflict resolution and collaboration are synonymous assumes that collaboration always begins with conflict. Collaboration focuses on trying to reach agreement among divergent opinions to accomplish mutual goals (Dechairo-Marino et al., 2001). Weiss (1983) suggests that conflicts between nurses and physicians are due to the overlapping nature of their domains and the lack of clarification between roles. Adding to the difficulty of achieving agreement, doctors tend to bargain or negotiate while nurses avoid, accommodate, or compete.

Conflict arises from four sources: (a) differences in values; (b) dissimilar goals; (c) poor communication; and (d) personalizing issues (Kennedy, 1998). Strom-Gottfried (1998) says that conflict stems from inconsistencies in data, relationship issues, value conflicts, structural or resource problems, and different interests. It is possible to make conflict productive rather than disruptive if a solution is produced that is acceptable to everyone. The resolution of a conflict is often the route to progress or the way in which major change takes place. This requires three steps, according to Kennedy (1998): (a) value differences must be addressed; (b) communication styles must be established; and (c) everyone must commit to a satisfactory resolution of the issues.

Conflict can be healthy when it brings about new ideas and deepens relationships. For this to occur, the basis of dealing with the conflict must be win–win. Conflict is unhealthy when it leads to distrust, anger, and withdrawal. These results usually mean that conflict has been approached on a win–lose basis.

Conflict is defined as a collision or disagreement; to be at variance with or in opposition to another party; controversy, quarreling; and opposition between interests and/or principles (*Random House College Dictionary*, 1999). Methods of dealing with conflict include avoiding, accommodating, compromising, competing, and collaborating (Thomas & Kilmann,

1974). Umbreit (1995) noted that each style has advantages and disadvantages, and depending on the conflict, each style has an appropriate use.

Conflicts are so threatening to some people that they deny existence of the problem. They do not think about the problem except to deny it. They pretend that everything is all right by avoiding the conflict altogether (Bolton, 1979). The result of avoiding conflict is that neither party gets what they want, and they part with negative feelings. This is an unassertive and uncooperative encounter. The individual does not immediately pursue his or her own concerns or those of the other person. The involved parties do not address the conflict. This style is used when: (a) an issue is trivial and of only passing importance or when other more important issues are pressing; (b) you perceive no chance of satisfying your concern or when you perceive you have less power or you are frustrated by something that would be very difficult to change; (c) the potential damage of confronting a conflict outweighs the benefits of its resolution; (d) it is preferable to let people cool down to reduce tensions to a productive level and to regain perspective and composure; (e) gathering more information outweighs the advantages of an immediate decision; and (f) others can resolve the conflict more effectively.

In the competing style (win–lose) of conflict resolution, one party wins and the other person gets nothing. This is an assertive and uncooperative style of interaction. One individual pursues his or her own concerns at the other person's expense. This is a power-oriented mode, in which one uses whatever power seems appropriate to win one's own position. Competing might mean standing up for your right by defending a position, which you believe is correct. This style is used when: (a) quick, decisive action is vital; (b) important issues wherein unpopular courses of action, like cost cutting, need to be implemented; (c) issues are vital to company welfare and you know your position is right; and (d) there is a need to protect yourself against people who take advantage of noncompetitive behavior (Bolton, 1979).

Accommodation or capitulation represents a lose–win scenario. This type of behavior occurs when one person wins and the other person gets nothing. This is an unassertive and cooperative style of interaction and the opposite of competing. The individual neglects his or her own concerns to satisfy the concern of the other person. There is an element of self-sacrifice in this mode. Accommodating might take the form of selfless generosity or charity, obeying another person's order when one would prefer not to, or yielding to another's point of view. This mode is used when: (a) you realize that you are wrong—to allow a better position to be heard, to learn from others, and to show that you are reasonable; (b) the issue is much more important to the other person than to you and there is a need to satisfy others as a goodwill gesture to help maintain a cooperative relationship; (c) building up social credits for later issues that are important to you; (d) continued competition would only damage your cause; (e) you are outmatched or losing; (f) preserving harmony and avoiding disruption are especially important; and (g) aiding in the managerial development of subordinates by allowing them to experiment and learn from their own mistakes (Bolton, 1979).

Compromising, as a style of conflict resolution, results in both parties adjusting their position (fair–fair) so that the person gets part of his or her want list. This is intermediate in both assertiveness and cooperativeness. The objective is to find some expedient, mutually acceptable solution that partially satisfies both parties. It falls on a middle ground between competing and accommodating. Compromising gives up more them competing but less than accommodating. Likewise, it addresses an issue more directly than avoiding, but doesn't explore it in as much depth as collaborating. Compromising might mean splitting the difference, exchanging concessions, or seeking a quick middle-ground position. This conflict resolution mode is used when: (a) goals are moderately important but not worth the effort of potential disruption of more assertive modes; (b) two opponents with equal power are strongly committed to mutually exclusive goals—as in labor–management bargaining; (c) achieving temporary settlements to complex issues; (d) arriving at expedient solutions under time pressure; and (e) needed as a backup mode when collaboration fails to be successful (Bolton, 1979).

Collaborating is an assertive and cooperative mode of interaction that is directly opposite of avoiding and representing a win–win scenario. Collaborating involves an attempt to work with the other person to find some solution that fully satisfies the concerns of both persons. Collaboration means digging into an issue to identify the underlying concerns of the two individuals and to find an alternative, which meets both sets of concerns. Collaborating between two persons might take the form of exploring and disagreement to learn from each other's insights, concluding to resolve some condition that would otherwise have them competing for resources. Collaborative interactions are used when: (a) finding an innovative solution when both sets of concerns are too important to be compromised; (b) your objective is to learn from others and understand the views of others before acting; (c) merging insights from people with difference perspectives on a problem; (d) gaining commitment by incorporating the other's concern into a consensual decision; and (e) working through hard feelings that have been interfering with the progress of the relationship (Bolton, 1979; Coeling & Wilcox, 1994; Corser, 1998; Hoffman, 1998).

Gill (1995) suggests that there are three primary components in conflict: emotions, verbal content, and procedure. Emotions are present in every conflict. At times, the emotions can escalate to anger and rage. A typical initial emotional response to conflict is expressed in the negative (e.g., ". . . but that's not my job").

Verbal content is the primary component that is perhaps the most amenable to improvement with practice. Assertive statements may be used to clarify and defuse passive and aggressive behavior. Assertive skills convey both the substantive concerns and accurate emotions associated with the concerns, which helps keep the communication clear of overwhelming emotion or inaccurate assumptions. Assertive problem solving is a learned skill. Helpful phrases may include gentle inquiries or statements, such as "If I understand correctly, your concerns are . . ."; "I feel like I am missing something, Can you help clarify?"; or "Help me understand your point of view about. . . ."

It is critical to understand the underlying philosophy, principles, and guidelines any given solution will address in the conflict. Any misunderstanding with how or when the solution is implemented may result in further escalation of the conflict.

Though it is impossible to totally eradicate conflict, implementing conflict prevention control methods can avert frustration. To prevent conflict, treat the other person with respect; use reflective listening, assertion skills, and awareness; dump tension without creating more tension; increase emotional support; and heighten tolerance and acceptance of others (Bolton, 1979).

Empowerment

Empowerment is a resource that enables collaboration or can result from collaboration. Katz (1984), Rappaport (1984), and Rodwell (1996) indicate that empowerment facilitates desired and needed change, and is a significant process in society. Nurses and other health care professionals, especially when combining resources, are in a position to assist patients in their quest for health and satisfying health care experiences. Jones and Meleis (1993) posit that nurses need to develop skills that facilitate empowerment and create situations in which change toward healthy behaviors and outcomes are nurtured. The empowerment process can provide resources, skills, and opportunities for collaboration to occur. In addition to knowing about the process of empowerment, it is important to know what factors hinder or foster the adoption of empowered behavior by people. If empowerment contributes to increased satisfaction and eventual achievement of patient defined health goals, then it provides the same results as collaboration.

Empowerment is a process that begins with awareness of powerlessness or a need. When the person can envision a desired goal or choice, and interact synergistically with the environment, the person is enabled to make changes necessary to meet their need and achieve their goal (Echols-Hurst, 2000). Empowerment is a transactional concept, requiring mutual support tools, resources, and environment to build, develop, and increase the ability and effectiveness of others to set and reach defined goals (Gibson, 1991). Zimmerman (1995) suggests that empowerment is dynamic and involves processes and structures between individuals in partnerships, groups, or communities to enhance people's skills and provide them with the mutual support necessary to effect change in their lives. Vander Henst (1997) emphasized that the dynamic interactive nature of empowerment proposed by the distribution of power between the two parties involved must be balanced for empowerment to occur.

Freire (1973) warned that educators and other helping professionals make situations oppressive rather than empowering for humans by fostering dependency instead of creating empowering conditions. He emphasized the difference between people as subjects and people as objects; he proposed that objects are known and acted upon, whereas subjects know and act. Freire described an empowering problem-solving approach with stages that foster empowerment. The first stage is a magical period in which people do not recognize their situations as oppressive and thus conform. Individuals who blame themselves or others for the problems characterize the next stage. As a consequence of blaming himself or herself, the individual or group tries to change themselves or change each other. In the third stage, critical transformation, the individual or group is able to analyze the problem with critical think-

ing skills. They are able to assess their role in the problem and act to transform aspects of the system within their sphere of influence. This is the point where the process of collaboration begins. The action necessary to achieve successful progress through these stages starts with listening to people to find their views, longings, beliefs, hopes, and impetus to participate. Freire (1973) was very emphatic about the importance of dialogue in establishing empowerment. Dialogue requires the presence of six attitudes: love, humility, faith, trust, hope, and critical thinking.

Vogt and Murrell (1990) provide another source on the topic of empowerment cited in the management literature. In their model, empowerment is viewed as a synergistic interactive process with two or more people and the emphasis is on developing others rather than controlling others. The process involves others in goal-setting and decision-making processes. Six categories of empowering methods were proposed: educating, leading, mentoring/supporting, providing, structuring, and actualizing. Education is the sharing of information as well as helping others learn to use new information. Leading involves facilitating decision-making. Mentoring/supporting is the process of support and guidance or helping others realize their goals. With providing, resources for success are fostered and supplied. Structuring includes promoting organizational arrangements that allow or limit activities. Finally, actualizing builds on previous methods and activities as the person completes goals and performs at his or her highest level.

Empowerment is a process that parallels collaboration. The opportunity for participation in change is a critical aspect in collaboration that is achieved through the empowerment process. Likewise, successful collaboration encounters will empower nurses in the future.

Other Strategies

Disch (2001) identified several other important steps for nurses to take to foster collaboration with other disciplines. These strategies include:

- To model collaboration for students so that future nurses will know what collaboration is and what it looks and feels like through actual experience
- To offer interdisciplinary coursework at the undergraduate level with medical students and at the graduate level with residents and fellows
- To provide content on nursing in the curriculum of other disciplines and invite other health care professionals to participate in planning and conducting nursing coursework

Action research is an example of collaboration. Dechairo-Marino et al. (2001) propose that action research is an alternative to the rigorous paradigm that is prevalent in academia yet somewhat unfeasible in the practice setting. With action research, the focus is on changing knowledge, attitudes, beliefs, and behaviors rather than distant outcomes. A major aspect of action research is that it involves a collaborative, participatory process.

Pillar and Solem (1999) describe the Akron-Canton Clinical Nursing Research network as an example of collaborative research. The research network is a loosely structured, collaborative group of nurses in clinical and management practice from a variety of institutions and practice settings. The group meets quarterly to share ideas, solve problems, identify potential resources, and generally encourage the efforts of all. Sixteen organizations are involved in the network. Beginning activities of the network included sharing research articles and building a resource file of useful data, data collection instruments, and study examples. Meetings were intended to be interesting and educational and included speakers and discussions on common issues and problems. In the second year the first collaboration study was initiated within the network. The objective was to assess empathy in clinical nurses through quantitative and qualitative survey methods. The study took about one year to complete. Over 350 nurses in four hospitals participated in the study. Findings revealed that despite the diversity of settings, educational preparedness, age, and clinical specialty, there were no significant differences in empathy among the groups.

- To develop a relationship with physician colleagues with whom nurses need to consult and collaborate for improved patient outcomes
- To speak up in committees and organizations to represent nursing

Collaboration in Practice

Transdisciplinary is a term that refers to multiple disciplines that converge to implement designated tasks in a project. The specific project for the nurse and other health care professional is no simple project, but instead concerns the most complex living entity known to human kind. Disciplines working in isolation of each other cannot address the complexity of the human being. Therefore, transdisciplinary collaboration becomes a critical goal in health care delivery. While the examples of transdisciplinary collaboration in the education setting are increasing, examples in practice settings are fewer. It is hoped that through the educational process, future nurses will facilitate more active collaborative practice experiences that are detailed in the literature.

Collaborative and Service Education

Peterson and Schaffer (1999) describe service learning as reciprocal relationships between students and communities in which both parties engage in service and

What makes a team different from an ordinary work group? What are the strategies the nurse might use to initiate a collaborative relationship with another health care team member? Can you have a collaborative relationship with your supervisor or someone in a higher level of authority (e.g., nursing instructor)? If yes, what qualities and characteristics will facilitate collaboration? How do you handle conflict? What is your dominant conflict resolution style?

learning. The student and the community agency are both considered to be teachers and learners. Students reflect on the meaning of the experience in terms of their course objectives and the impact on them as an individual and on the community. Service and learning are balanced. The educators and services committees share planning for the project. It is used to help students meet learning goals in critical thinking, group work, and community relationships. There is also a research component that can be introduced. Preplanning and collaboration between faculty and the agency are required.

Connolly and Novak (2000) described another collaborative education project. The San Jose project in transdisciplinary collaboration included the disciplines of nursing, speech pathology, therapeutic recreation, occupational therapy, and social work in a collaborative educational model. Key components of the project included: weekly transdisciplinary seminars, required attendance by students from each discipline at community Alliance for the Mentally Ill (AMI) meetings, caring and sharing meetings, supervisory groups, reflective logs, and case studies. The results of the transdisciplinary collaboration were improved relationships and learning experiences for students and educators in all five disciplines.

Heath Care Alliances

Hayward, DeMarco, and Lynch (2000) define an interprofessional alliance as one or more professionals forming a relationship for the purpose of meeting a common goal. The model suggested by Hayward et al. (2000) includes five stages of collaboration. The recursive model describes the process experienced by research or education teams that work collaboratively and involve exchange, negotiation, and building an environment characterized by trust. Stage 1 involves assessment and goal setting—including assessment of individual personal goals that are identified and shared as possible research or educational opportunities. Stage

2 is determining collaborative fit and building relationships. Through the sharing and exchange of ideas, the participant must evaluate his or her personal goals and commitment, and then development of roles and trust can be initiated. Stage 3 involves resource identification and reflection. During this period of reflection, the individual examines whether he or she can work with the collaborative group and evaluates the potential benefits of the relationship. Stage 4 involves implementation of the project and is also the time when colleagues meet to negotiate results. This stage is also characterized by identification of project procedures, possible role adjustment, and assignments. Stage 5 entails the evaluation of the project outcomes and determining future goals.

Advanced Practice Collaboration

An example of professional collaboration at a national level can be found in the dance of legislation required to favorably impact the advanced nurse practitioner practice laws. During the 1960s, nurses revisited the issue of collaboration with the evolution of advanced nursing practice. Although the advanced practice nurses (APNs) were being trained to practice independently and to diagnose and prescribe drugs and therapies, few nurse practice acts created an independent scope of nursing practice. In states where the nurse practice act did create an independent scope of nursing practice, regulators were fearful of moving too far. Language in the medical practice acts was used to limit the evolution of nursing practice. Boards of Medicine suggested that nurses might be practicing medicine. Instead of directly challenging this interpretation of regulatory policy, nurses chose to emphasize the expansion of the nursing role and responsibility of the nurse in professional settings. They emphasized the collaborative role with physicians and service to rural areas. To a large extent, this strategy reflected a compromise that emerged in the face of organized physician opposition to the expansion of nursing practice.

Critical Thinking and Reflection

How would you discover the differences and similarities in goals shared with other team members? How would you build a relationship with other team members? What are your alternatives if you do not believe you can work collaboratively with the group? What model of collaboration best suits your personal style and goals?

Leaders of the American Medical Association (AMA) and American Nurses Association (ANA) met in 1993 and 1994 in an effort to reach agreement on the dimensions of nurse–physician professional relationships. After lengthy discussion and negotiation, a joint AMA–ANA task force arrived at the following definition: "Collaboration is the process whereby physicians and nurses plan and practice together as colleagues, working interdependently within the boundaries of their scope of practice with shared valued and mutual acknowledgment and respect for each other's contribution to care for individuals, their families, and their communities" (Nursing World, 2001).

Case Management

The Commission for Case Manager Certification (2000) states that "**case management** is a collaborative process that assesses, plans, implements, coordinates, and evaluates the options and services required to meet an individual's health needs, using communication and available resources to promote quality, cost-effective outcomes" (p. 1). The end goal for Case management is to achieve patient wellness and self-mastery for the patient through advocacy, communication, education, and identification of resources. "The case manager helps identify appropriate providers and facilities throughout the continuum of services, while ensuring that available resources are being used in a timely and cost-effective manner in order to obtain optimum value for both the patient and the reimbursement source" (Commission for Case Manager Certification, 2000, p. 1).

Case management is used in facilities, integrated delivery systems, public health, and managed care organizations. In most case management models, the targeted patients are those who most frequently access the system at the inpatient level of care and consume the greatest amount of resources during these episodes of care. The case management program methodology used by many managed care organizations is telephonic. Other public-funded agencies will often use a combination of face-to-face and the telephonic model. Patients are usually identified through a utilization analysis such as readmission reports. The identified patient is assigned to a designated case manager, who will assume case management responsibilities for an assigned caseload. The **case manager** works directly with the patient, family, and health care provider to prevent significant decompensation in these patients and therefore avoid unnecessary hospitalizations. The case manager then develops a care plan to address the needs of the patient, focusing on early identification of triggers to relapse, developing an action plan with necessary resources to address the patient's triggers, and having the patient access the care manager first in situations of potential decompensation.

The primary functions of the case manager are to assess the barriers to the patient's treatment progress and collaboratively develop interventions with the patient's network of therapists and doctors that address each barrier. Creativity to develop interventions that work for each individual patient is a necessary quality for the case manager. This creativity and all case management activities are practiced within the scope of practice appropriate for the case manager.

Interventions used within the case management program include such activities as calling the patient at specified intervals to support and follow-up, arranging transportation, calling the patient ahead of appointments to clear barriers and assure compliance, having the patient count pills over the phone, and reminding the patient of medication schedules. Other activities include educating families, calling the patient after appointments to determine that they were kept, setting up home interventions, home-based injections, and arranging for provider visits to the patient while still in the hospital to assist in discharge planning if an admission does occur. Coordination of care and services for the patient is extremely important as lack of communication between providers and lack of understanding of the patient's unique characteristics by multiple providers is often at the root of repeated decompensations.

The success of the case management programs can be measured in several different ways:

- Reduction of admissions in a postimplementation time frame
- Improvement in community tenure (percentage of time the patient is not in a hospital setting)
- Patient satisfaction with case management services

Quality Improvement Activities

Many health care organizations and businesses identify and prioritize quality improvement activities to pursue as an annual goal of the business. The quality improvement activity selected in a health care delivery system usually represents a relevant clinical issue that affects patients or members of a specific defined population. The process required for the successful quality improvement activity includes collaboration among the team or committee members to whom the improvement activity is assigned.

A **quality improvement team** (QIT) or committee responsible for a prioritized quality improvement activity is always formed to address complex issues and opportunities that cross several functional areas. The QIT or committee should include staff at all levels in the organization that have direct or indirect impact on the processes that are involved in the opportunity for improvement. The QIT or committee performs a barrier or root cause analysis, prioritizes causes or barriers, and identifies and implements specific interventions that address each prioritized barrier or cause. Input from members, providers, and relevant medical delivery system representatives are obtained as appropriate.

The team or committee is responsible for evaluating and monitoring all interventions at the appropriate level and frequency to determine if they resulted in an improvement. The process continues until resolution of the improvement opportunity occurs and there is evidence to demonstrate that the improvement occurred as a result of the intervention (McKeith, 2001).

Critical Paths

Critical paths are standard interdisciplinary plans of care developed for a specific type of case (e.g., diabetes, depression, etc.). The plan of care is outcome focused, identifying intermediate and long-term goals. "Therapies, diagnostic tests, medical management, and nursing management are commonly included on the critical paths with measurable outcomes and a time line" (Wells et al., 1998, p. 162). Initial development of critical paths requires communication, negotiation, and coordination among all disciplines of health care providers. Once developed, the critical path continues to provide a means of communication and coordination of patient care (Wells et al., 1998).

Future Trends and Possibilities

ANA Recommendations

The ANA, in *Nursing: A Social Policy Statement*, describes collaboration as a partnership in which the power of both sides is valued by both, with recognition and acceptance of separate and combined spheres of activity and responsibility, mutual safeguarding of the legitimate interest of each party, and a commonality of goals that is recognized by both parties (ANA, 1995). The ANA has proposed that collaboration is critical to the future of the nursing discipline.

Tri-Council Recommendations

The Nursing Agenda for Health Care Reform is a collaborative proposal of the Tri-Council of Nursing and supported by more than 60 nursing and health care organizations. The Agenda outlines plausible, constructive, and sometimes dramatic changes for the U.S. health care system. One suggestion included in the Agenda is the development of multidisciplinary clinical practice guidelines (Tri-Council for Nursing, 1991). Implicit in this goal is the need for the various health care providers to collaborate to promote cost-effective care and better patient outcomes (McEwen, 1994).

The Tri-Council testified before the House Appropriations Committee on Labor, Health and Human Services, Education and Related Agencies on fiscal year 2001 Appropriations for Nursing Education and Research. The Tri-Council collectively represents nurses in every sector of the nursing profession, including representatives from the American Association of Colleges of Nursing, American Nurses Association, American Organization of Nurse Executives, and the National League of Nursing (NLN). The Tri-Council

---

Critical Thinking and Reflection

What examples in practice can you think of that call for collaboration? You have just admitted a patient to your unit. You feel strongly that he needs nursing and medical care on an inpatient unit in preparation for surgery tomorrow, but the managed care company disagrees with your conclusion and has recommended outpatient surgery. What do you do? What opportunities for collaboration can you envision as a future nurse?

recommended increases in funding due to the impending nurse shortage and the emerging unmet health care needs that will increase the burden of the already overextended nursing workforce. In today's health care delivery system, nursing is being asked to expand its functions but also to develop innovations in care delivery. Another area of importance to nursing is the technological advances that engender innovation to provide both patient care and education for nurses (NLN, 2001).

Pew Health Professions Commission

The Pew Health Professional Commission (1998) addressed four prioritized health care challenges in the following ways:

- Health care workplace is demanding new skills and new configurations of staffing.
- There is a need to restructure the ways in which the health care professionals are regulated in order to promote responsive independence and ensure that professional credentials fit with the goals of the emerging structure.
- The number of health care professionals should be sufficient to meet the needs of the public, yet not oversupplied in a way that produces excess costs or wastes scarce resources.
- Professional schools must lead the effort to realign training and education to be more consistent with the changing need of the health care delivery system.

In their report on U.S. Health Professional Schools, the Pew Health Professions Commissions proposed a number of changes in education to prepare practitioners for 2005. They proposed that appropriate resources must be brought together to deal with a health threat and to develop solutions. The Pew document states that "due to historical, traditional, and educational determinant, the boundaries for health professionals have limited interprofessional contacts and concludes that the care delivery system would benefit from professionals who are capable of relating to other professionals through team efforts" (McEwen, 1994, p. 15). Another of the recommendations of the Pew Commission for the future by year 2005 is that practitioners be willing and able to function in new health care settings and interdisciplinary team arrangements designed to meet the primary health care needs of the public. They predict that future health care delivery will

be more integrated and coordinated with many types of providers and less reliant on physicians as the primary caregiver.

The Pew Commission supports revision of curricula to include "health care teamwork" in which the educational and care delivery arrangements of schools model integration and collaboration for health care providers. The task at hand is to promote this teamwork and collaboration. The Pew Commission recommendations for all health professional groups, advanced practice nursing, and nursing can be found in Box 23–5.

The NBNA Collaboration Model

The National Black Nurses Association (NBNA) developed its Healthy America Report based on findings from the Division of Nursing, U.S. Department of Health and Human Services in 1991. The NBNA Community Collaboration Model (1998) is based on Becker's Health Belief Model that suggests that individuals are more likely to accept preventive health strategies if they receive support from family, community, and health professionals. The NBNA Community Collaboration Model provided a mechanism for nurses in collaboration with physicians, communities, and organization partners to influence individual and communities preventive health actions. "We believe that the provision of education, supportive, and advocacy services in collaboration with community partners is an important motivating and social support strategy" (Bolton, Georges, Hunter, Long, & Wray, 1998, p. 9). The NBNA model suggests that health care professionals in partnership with other community leaders can influence health care. The decreasing availability of public dollars for health care requires additional community collaboration. The NBNA model includes the following steps to developing collaborative initiatives: (a) community assessment; (b) health professional assessment, including awareness and knowledge of health providers within the community; (c) public and private human and service agency assessment; (d) establishing community partners; and (e) implementing local initiatives like the "Great Beginnings for Black Babies" community-based program in Los Angeles, California. This program began after reviewing data from the LA County Department of Health Services that revealed an infant mortality rate of 21.1/1000 live births for African-American infants compared to a rate of 9.6/1000 live births for the overall population in the

Box 23–5   Pew Commission Recommendations (1998)

Pew Commission Recommendations for all health professional groups that will require collaboration include:

1. Change professional training to meet the demands of the new health care system. Most educational programs have not assimilated the new values, techniques, and skill sets required to pursue a satisfying and thriving practice in the managed care world. Curricula for doctors, nurses, and allied health professionals must redirect their efforts to ensure that their graduates will be successful in the type of professional practice environments and organizations that are emerging.
2. Ensure that the heath profession workforce reflects the diversity of the nation's population. By knowing the language and culture of the population they serve, they offer a more complete and effective kind of care.
3. Require interdisciplinary competence in all health professionals. Care delivery systems should work with local educational programs to describe and demonstrate how interdisciplinary skills are being incorporated into practice.
4. Continue to move education into ambulatory practice. The health care system has traditionally trained doctors in hospital settings, while the health care system is moving health care out of the hospital. Students need to be exposed to ambulatory settings early in their training.
5. Encourage public service of all health professionals students and graduates.

Pew Commission Recommendations for advanced practice nursing include:

1. Reorient advanced practice nursing education programs to prepare APNs for the changing situations and settings in which they are likely to practice.
2. Regardless of payer source, federal funding for graduate medical education should be made available to support the training of advanced practice nurses and other nonphysician providers in clinical settings.
3. Develop standard guidelines for advanced nursing practice and reinforce them with curriculum guidelines, examination requirements, and accreditation regulations.
4. Emphasize the practice styles that are a critical part of advanced practice nursing, including the emphasis on preventive and health-promoting interventions and attention to psychosocial and environmental resource factors.

Pew Commission Recommendations for nursing include:

1. Adjust education programs to produce the numbers and type of nurses appropriate to local and regional demand, rather than institutional and political needs.
2. Delineate the knowledge and outcome competencies appropriate for each level of nursing education in order to maximize efficiency, improve coordination and articulation of programs, and reduce professional conflict and public confrontation. This includes downsizing or merging diploma programs with colleges and universities.
3. Radically revamp the content and learning experiences in the nursing curriculum to produce graduates with the competencies needed for differentiated practice, including ambulatory and long-term care and community-based programs.
4. Integrate teaching, and practice enterprises of nursing education programs in order to further nursing's professional and practical goal.

Adapted from Pew Health Professions Commission. (1998). *Recreating health professions practice for a new century: The fourth report of the Pew Health Professions.* San Francisco: USCF Center for Health Professions.

county. The Los Angeles chapter of the NBNA and Chi Eta Phi Nursing Sorority, assisted by physicians, public health officials, and media experts, launched "Great Beginnings." They facilitated early entry into prenatal care through outreach education and case management and created public awareness and media campaigns to inform the community of the consequences of late prenatal care. After four years of collaboration, the infant mortality rate declined to 14.5/1000 live births. Nurses and physicians must collaborate as health professionals, citizens, and community leaders to improve the community's health (Bolton et al., 1998).

The Future

The Center for the Health Professionals (2001), University of California, San Francisco, says there is an attempt to manage care delivered to enrolled populations in such a manner as to achieve some combination of cost reduction, enhanced patient and consumer satisfaction, and improvement of health care outcomes.

Within another decade 80% to 90% of the insured population of the United States will receive its care through some type of insurance with a managed care component. The impact will be closure of as many as half of the nation's hospitals; expansion of primary care in ambulatory and community settings; consolidation of many health professional roles; and changes required for the health professional schools and the structures needed for education, research, and patient care. The future is here.

The future for nursing requires the development of partnerships and alliances—partnerships with managed care, training, clinical research, improved technology, and communications systems. New models of care and education are needed that will integrate education and the highly managed and integrated system of care. We must provide nurses with appropriate training and clinical practice opportunities that are patient-focused and encourage continual improvement and innovation through collaboration (Center for the Health Professions, 1998).

TRANSITION INTO PRACTICE

Collaborative practice is a term used to describe a type of interdisciplinary practice relationship. The leader for a case in collaborative practice is determined by the nature of the needs expressed by the patient (Connolly & Novak, 2000). The nurse transitioning to practice will become a leader in collaborative relationships with other nurses, other health care professionals, and the patient/family.

A more specific example of collaboration that the nurse might experience is with the development of best practices and policies. Wells et al. (1998) described the development of critical paths in the hospital as a type of collaborative practice. Their study showed that when perceived physician involvement played a role in collaborative development of critical paths, interdisciplinary team members are more satisfied and patient outcome

is improved. The perception of involvement is even more important than the actual method used for implementing the collaborative practice.

Collaborative practice relationships have most often been described in the health care literature as satisfying interpersonal relationships that develop over time (Corser, 1998). The collaborative practice model is a preferred model for mature organizations with nurses and physicians who are prepared and committed to mutual goals of improved patient care.

Devereux (1981) concretely describes the elements of a collaborative practice model to include: (a) primary nursing (all RN staff); (b) integrated patient record; (c) encouraging nurses in decision-making; (d) joint practice committee; and (e) joint record review.

KEY POINTS

1. Nurses must master relationships to meet the needs of patients.
2. Collaboration is the link that connects the various health care disciplines to implement patient-focused case that results in better outcomes.
3. Collaboration requires mutual goals and sharing ownership and responsibility of the problem.
4. Collaboration requires open communication through dialogue and exchange of ideas.

5. Collaboration requires complementary knowledge and skills of both/all professionals to influence health care goals.
6. Mutual respect of each other's professional discipline, knowledge, skills, role, and unique contribution is a critical requirement for collaboration.
7. Each participant in the collaborative process must contribute to the decision-making, planning, implementation, and outcomes of the interaction.
8. All participants in collaboration must invest necessary time and energy.
9. Processes necessary for collaboration include teambuilding, negotiation, conflict resolution, and empowerment. Assertive communication is a key element in each of these processes.
10. Value conflicts, relationship issues, role ambiguity, scarce resources, and different interests or goals can cause conflict. Conflict can foster problem solving and deepen relationships if managed effectively.
11. Seek to understand the other person's view.
12. Do not blame the other person for the problem.
13. Case management, advanced practice nursing, collaborative research, and service education are all examples of collaboration in practice.
14. The nurse should look for opportunities for collaboration.

EXPLORE MediaLink

Critical thinking questions, essay questions, key terms, web links, activities, NCLEX review questions, and more interactive resources can be found on the Companion Website at www.prenhall.com/haynes. Click on Chapter 23 to select activities for this chapter.

REFERENCES

Alpert, H. B., Goldman, L. D., Kilroy, C. M., & Pike, A. W. (1992). 7 Gryzmish: Toward an understanding of collaboration. *Nursing Clinics of North American, 27*(1), 47–59.

American Nurses Association. (1995). *Nursing: A social policy statement.* Washington, DC: Author.

Ashcroft, B. L. (1996). Collaboration: More than a buzz word of the 90's. *Clinical Nurse Specialist, 10*(2), 94.

Asimov, I., & Shulmon, J. (Eds.). (1988). *Issac Asimov's book of science and nature quotations.* New York: Weidenfeld and Nicholson.

Baggs, J. G. (1994). Development of an instrument to measure collaboration and satisfaction about care decisions. *Journal of Advanced Nursing, 20,* 176–182.

Baggs, J. G. (1997). Collaboration between nurses and physicians: What is it? Does it exist? Why does it matter? In J. C. McCloskey & H. K. Grace (Eds.), *Current issues in nursing* (pp. 519–524). St. Louis, MO: Mosby.

Baggs, J. G., & Schmitt, M. H. (1988). Collaboration between nurses and physicians. *Image, 20,* 145–149.

Bolton, R. (1979). *People skills: How to assert yourself, listen to others, and resolve conflicts.* Englewood Cliffs, NJ: Prentice Hall.

Bolton, L. B., Georges, C. A., Hunter, V., Long, O., & Wray, R. (1998). Community health collaboration models for the 21st century. *Nursing Administration Quarterly, 22*(3), 6–17.

Center for the Health Professions. (1998). Recreating health professional practice for a new century. The 4th report of the Pew Health Professions Commission. University of California, San Francisco: Author.

Center for the Health Professions. (2001). Critical challenges: Revitalizing the health professions for the twenty-first century. University of California, San Francisco. (*www.futurehealth.ucsf.edu/summaries/challenges*).

Coeling, H. V., & Wilcox, J. R. (1994). Steps to collaboration. *Nursing Administration Quarterly, 18*(4), 44–55.

Commission for Case Manager Certification. (2000). *CCM certification guide: Certified case manager.* Rolling Meadows, IL: Author.

Connolly, P. M., & Novak, J. M. (2000). Teaching collaboration: A demonstration model. *Journal of the American Psychiatric Nurses Association, 6*(6), 183–190.

Corser, W. D. (1998). A conceptual model of collaborative nurse-physician interactions: The management of traditional influences and personal tendencies. *Scholarly Inquiry for Nursing Practice, 12*(4), 325–341.

Dechairo-Marino, A. E., Jordan-Marsh, M., Traiger, G., & Saulo, M. (2001). Nurse/physician collaboration action research and the lessons learned. *Journal of Nursing Administration, 31*(5), 223–232.

Devereux, P. M. (1981). Essential elements of nurse-physician collaboration. *Journal of Nursing Administration, 11*(5), 19–23.

Disch, J. (2001). Strengthening nursing and interdisciplinary collaboration. *Journal of Professional Nursing, 17*(6), 275.

Dyer, W. G. (1994). *Team building: Issues and alternatives* (3rd ed.). Reading, MA: Addison-Wesley.

Echols-Hurst, J. (2000). *Examination of a structural model of empowerment and patient satisfaction.* Unpublished doctoral dissertation, The University of Alabama at Birmingham, Birmingham, Alabama.

Flaherty, M. J. (1998). Collaboration: Clinical nurse specialists can lead the way. *Clinical Nurse Specialist, 12*(4), 161–168.

Fisher, R., & Ury, W. (1991). *Getting to yes: Negotiating agreement without giving in.* New York: Penguin Books.

Forsyth, D. R. (1999). *Group dynamics* (3rd ed.). Pacific Grove, CA: Brooks/Cole.

Freire, P. (1973). *Education for critical consciousness.* New York: Seabury Press.

Gibson, C. H. (1991). A concept analysis of empowerment. *Journal of Advanced Nursing, 16*, 354–361.

Gill, S. L. (1995). Resolving conflicts: Principles and practice. *Physician Executive, 21*(4), 11–16.

Gray, B. (1989). *Collaborating.* San Francisco: Josey-Bass.

Hackman, J. R. (1987). The design of work teams. In J. Lorsch (Ed.), *Handbook of organizational behavior.* Englewood Cliffs, NJ: Prentice Hall.

Hayward, L. M., DeMarco, R., & Lynch, M. M. (2000). Interpersonal collaborative alliances: Health care educators sharing and learning from each other. *Journal of Allied Health, 29*(4), 270–276.

Henneman, E. A., Lee, J. L., & Cohen, J. I. (1995). Collaboration: A concept analysis. *Journal of Advanced Nursing, 21*, 103–109.

Henry, V., Schmitz, K., Reif, L., & Rudie, P. (1992). Collaboration: Integrating practice and research in public health nursing. *Public Health Nursing, 9*(4), 218–222.

Hoffman, S. (1998). The three new C's for nursing—collaboration, cooperation, and coalition. *Journal of Professional Nursing, 14*(4), 194.

Jones, P. S., & Meleis, A. I. (1993). Health is empowerment. *Advances in Nursing Science, 15*(3), 1–14.

Jones, R. A. P. (1994). Conceptual development of nurse–physician collaboration. *Holistic Nurse Practice, 8*(3), 1–11.

Jones, R. A. P. (1997). Multidisciplinary collaboration: Conceptual development as a foundation for patient-focused care. *Holistic Nursing Practice, 11*(3), 8–16.

Kanter, R. M. (1994, July–August). Collaborative advantage. *Harvard Business Review,* 96–108.

Katz, R. (1984). Empowerment and synergy: Expanding the community's healing resources. In J. Rappaport & R. Hess (Eds.), *Studies in empowerment: Steps toward understanding and action* (pp. 201–226). New York: The Haworth Press.

Kennedy, M. M. (1998). A crash course in conflict resolution. *Physician Executive, 24*(4), 60–61.

Kerfoot, K. (1994). The theory of cooperation and the nurse manager's challenge. *Nursing Economics, 12*(2), 100.

McEwen, M. (1994). Promoting interdisciplinary collaboration. *Nursing and Healthcare, 15*(6), 304–307.

McKeith, J. J. (2001). Establishing a CQI Program. *EMedicine Journal, 2*(3), *www.emedicine.com/emerg/topic668.*

Merriam-Webster's Ninth New Collegiate Dictionary (9th ed.). (1987). Markham, ON: Thomas Allen & Son Limited.

Miccolo, M. A., & Spanier, A. H. (1993). Critical care management in the 1990s: Making collaborative practice work. *Critical Care Clinics, 9*(3), 443–453.

NLN (2001). *http://www.nln.org/aboutnln/news_congress.htm.*

Nugent, K. E., & Lambert, V. A. (1996). The advanced practice nurse in collaborative practice. *Nursing Connections, 9*, 5–16.

Nursing World. (2001). *Collaboration and independent practice: Ongoing issues for nursing. http://www.nursingworld.org/readroom/nti/9805nti.htm.*

Peterson, S. J., & Schaffer, M. J. (1999). Service learning: A strategy to develop group collaboration and research skills. *Journal of Nursing Education, 38*(5), 208–214.

Pew Health Professions Commission. (1998). *Recreating health professions practice for a new century: The fourth report of the Pew Health Professions.* San Francisco: UCSF Center for Health Professions.

Pillar, B., & Solem, G. (1999). Cooperation and collaboration for clinical nursing research. *Orthopedic Nursing, 18*(2), 54–57.

Random House College Dictionary (2nd ed.). (1999). New York: Random House.

Rappaport, J. (1984). Studies in empowerment: Introduction to the issue. In J. Rappaport & R. Hess (Eds.), *Studies in empowerment: Steps toward understanding and action* (pp. 1–8). New York: The Haworth Press.

Rodwell, C. M. (1996). An analysis of the concept of empowerment. *Journal of Advanced Nursing, 23*, 305–313.

Rutan, J. S., & Stone, W. N. (1984). *Psychodynamic group psychotherapy.* New York: Macmillan.

Schwarz, R. M. (1994). *The skilled facilitator: Practical wisdom for developing effective groups.* San Francisco: Jossey-Bass.

Senge, P. M. (1990). *The fifth discipline: The art and practice of the learning organization.* New York: Doubleday.

Shannon, V. J. (1998). Partnerships: The foundation for future success. *Canadian Journal of Nursing Administration, 11*(3), 61–76.

Strom-Gottfried, K. (1998). Applying conflict resolution framework to disputes in managed care. *Social Work, 43*(5), 393–341.

Sullivan, T. (1998). Collaboration. *A health care imperative.* New York: McGraw-Hill.

Sundstrom, E., DeMeuse, K. P., & Futrell, D. (1990). Work teams: Applications and effectiveness. *American Psychologist, 43*, 120–133.

Thomas, K. W., & Kilmann, R. H. (1974). *Thomas-Kilmann conflict mode instrument.* Tuxedo, NY: Xicom.

Tri-Council for Nursing. (1991). *Nursing's agenda for health care reform.* Kansas City, MO: American Nurses Association.

Umbreit, M. S. (1995). *Mediating interpersonal conflicts: A pathway to peace.* West Concord, MN: CPI Publishing.

Vander Henst, J. A. (1997). Client empowerment: A nursing challenge. *Clinical Nurse Specialist, 11*(3), 96–99.

Vogt, J. F., & Murrell, K. L. (1990). *Empowerment in organizations: How to spark exceptional performance.* San Diego, CA: Pfeiffer.

Weiss, S. J. (1983). Role differentiation between nurse and physician: Implications for nursing. *Nursing Research, 32,* 133–139.

Wells, N., Johnson, R., & Salyer, S. (1998). Interdisciplinary collaboration. *Clinical Nurse Specialist, 12*(4), 161–168.

Wonsetler, L. (1987). *Perceptions of nurse–physician collaboration in an emergency department setting.* Thesis. Medical College of Ohio, Toledo, OH.

Zimmerman, M. A. (1995). Psychological empowerment: Issues and illustrations. *American Journal of Community Psychology, 23*(5), 581–598.

SUGGESTED READINGS

Bagg, J. G., Schmitt, M. H., Mushlin, A. I., Elregde, D. H., Oakes, D., & Hutson, A. D. (1997). Nurse–physician collaboration and satisfaction with the decision-making process in three critical care units. *American Journal of Critical Care, 6*(5), 393–399.

Bion, W. R. (1960). *Experiences in groups.* New York: Basic Books.

Dyer, W. G. (1994). *Team building: Issues and alternatives* (3rd ed.). Reading, MA: Addison-Wesley.

Fagin, C. M. (1992). Collaboration between nurses and physicians: No longer a choice. *Nursing and Health Care, 13*(7), 354–363.

Gill, S., & Meighan, S. (1988). Five roadblocks to effective partnerships in a competitive health care environment. *Hospital and Health Services Administration, 33*(4), 505–520.

Gladstein, D. (1984). Groups in context: A model of task group effectiveness. *Administrative Science Quarterly, 29,* 499–517.

Larson, C. E., & LaFasto, F. M. J. (1989). *Teamwork.* Newbury Park, CA: Sage.

Liedtka, J. M., & Whitten, E. (1998). Enhancing care delivery through cross-disciplinary collaboration: A case study. *Journal of Healthcare Management, 43,* 186.

Long, K. A. (2001). A reality-oriented approach to interdisciplinary work. *Journal of Professional Nursing, 17*(6), 278–282.

Miller, M. (1999). Instilling a mediation-based conflict resolution culture. *Physician Executive, 25*(4), 45–51.

Rushmer, R. (1997). What happens to the team during team-building? Examining the change process that helps to build a team. *Journal of Management Development, 16*(5–6), 316–328.

Sevel, F. (1996). Eight team-building tips that work. *Physician's Management, 36*(4), 80–87.

Strutton, D., & Pelton, L. E. (1997). Negotiation: Bringing more to the table than demands. *Marketing Health Services, 17*(1), 52–59.

Sundin-Huard, D. (2001). Subject position theory—its application to understanding collaboration (and confrontation) in critical care. *Journal of Advanced Nursing, 34*(3), 367–382.

Umiker, W. (1996). Negotiating skill for health care professionals. *Health Care Supervisor, 14*(3), 27–34.

Weiss, S. J. (1983). Role differentiation between nurse and physician: Implications for nursing. *Nursing Research, 32*(3), 133–139.

Yalom, I. D. (1985). *The theory and practice of group psychotherapy* (3rd ed.). New York: Basic Books.

24

The Baccalaureate Nurse as a Leader in Health Care Delivery

DEBORAH R. GARRISON

MERRY J. McBRYDE-FOSTER

> *Leadership is*
> *'the ability to envision a path or direction;*
> *to motivate others to follow; to join with others to reach a common goal;*
> *to work alone when solo action is called for; to withstand trouble and failure; and*
> *to refuse to be crushed by either.'*
>
> *Harriet Forman in the first volume of* Nursing Leadership,
> *as reprinted in Forman, 2001*

LEARNING OBJECTIVES

AT THE COMPLETION OF THIS CHAPTER, THE READER WILL BE ABLE TO:

- ➤ Discuss leadership and management from a historical perspective.
- ➤ Analyze the role of the new baccalaureate registered nurse as a leader.
- ➤ Differentiate leadership from management.
- ➤ Discuss a variety of theories related to leadership and management.

- ➤ Synthesize the formal and informal roles of the nurse as a manager and leader.
- ➤ Discuss the concepts of power and empowerment.
- ➤ Evaluate the concept of followership as applied to leadership and management.
- ➤ Identify strategies for the novice leader to gain recognition as an emerging leader.

MediaLink   www.prenhall.com/haynes

Additional online resources including NCLEX review questions, critical thinking questions, and real-world activities for this chapter can be found on the Companion Website at www.prenhall.com/haynes.

The graduate professional nurse of today is exposed to various leadership principles and management theory. Curriculum experiences may have provided introduction to a variety of management theories including Weber's classical bureaucracy theory (1947), McGregor's neoclassical Theory Y (1960), and Argyris's (1964, 1971) focus on employee participation. Leadership theory discussions often begin with Chapin's technical definition (1924), then progress to a discussion of Lewin's (1951) change theory, the situational leadership model of Hersey and Blanchard (1977), and Burns's (1978) transactional and transformational leader types. With this knowledge, many new professional nurses are filled with zeal, hope, and excitement at the possibilities of a rewarding professional life.

Just as the new graduate is beginning a transition into professional practice, the nursing profession itself continues its transformation from a religious vocation into a complex and often challenging profession. The constant uncertainty and change in the nursing profession is never as obvious as when facing one's first staff–nurse position. New peers and a new subordinate–superior relationship amplify feelings of being on stage. The graduate begins to wonder what nursing course prepared him or her for work as a real nurse. With the comfortable faculty–student relationships dissolved, the lack of skills and knowledge of appropriate leadership and followership behaviors leave the graduate nurse feeling powerless.

This chapter focuses on the development of leadership and management theory, change theory, and roles of the nurse leader/manager, as well as providing ideas for novice leaders to use in the development of their management skills. Followership is also defined and discussed. Influences of power, empowerment, and authority are presented as intertwining variables in professional role transition to leadership and management. Finally, suggestions will be offered for the preparation of a proactive professional development plan.

▓ The Novice Leader

A position of leadership is typically the last thought on the minds of a students preparing to complete the requirements for their degrees. Their thoughts are more often consumed with passing the NCLEX licensure exam and beginning to receive compensation for their years of hard work in the educational setting. However, upon graduation, new nurses will typically be providing leadership to a portion of the health care team on a unit within a matter of months. The nursing shortage existing presently and projected to continue into the future places demands on new nurses that are heretofore unprecedented. Many new graduates are able to move into internship positions with preceptors for a period of 1 to 3 months, which will offer them the opportunity to model their nursing practice after a more experienced nurse. Once the internship is over, nurses can expect to become involved in leadership in some way. At the very least, a new RN is expected to lead a team of individuals in providing care for a portion of the patients on the unit. Within 1 year of graduation, the new nurse often becomes the charge nurse on a patient care unit, a position that requires the coordination of patient care delivery for the entire unit; this is a challenging responsibility! The leadership characteristics that will make nurses successful in these positions can and should be the foundation on which the remainder of their nursing careers will be built. After all, it is no small feat to lead nurses, nursing assistants, and unit clerks in providing excellent patient care for a period of 8 or 12 hours under conditions that require resourcefulness, effective communication, response to crisis situations, and teamwork.

Application of Forman's definition of leadership can be applied to the role of the leader of a patient care team that encompasses other RNs, LVNs/LPNs, nursing assistants, student nurses, and unit secretaries. For the work of the team to be accomplished well, the nurse must envision the care that is to be delivered to the team's patients, identify the contributions that each individual is to make, determine what tasks may be legally and safely delegated, collaborate with others outside the team, negotiate and advocate on behalf of the patients, deal with patient crises effectively, maintain a personal balance that sustains the RN and the team throughout the day, and return for the next shift ready to do it all again. Having the skills to accomplish these tasks requires the same areas of expertise that nurse leader positions (e.g., nurse manager, director of nursing, vice president of patient care) or a leader of a professional organization such as the local nursing association must use on a daily basis. Mastery of these skills while at the bedside will form a foundation for future leadership positions at the organizational and professional level.

Nursing is in a position today that is both exciting in its possibilities and frightening in its vulnerabilities. As Forman aptly states,

In today's world, effective, visionary leadership in nursing is needed perhaps more than ever before. We are at a crossroads. Take one path and nursing will remain a vital part of health care delivery under a reformed system. Take another avenue and we might well cease to exist, at least as we know ourselves to be today (Forman, 2001, p. 4).

The desired path is quite evident; it is equally evident that all nurses have a role to play in leading our profession through the rapids of change created by the forces at play in our society and the health care delivery system. The profession cannot afford the time for new nurses to learn their leadership skills after graduation through observation and trial and error; instead, it is important to develop and nurture these emergent leaders during the final year of the baccalaureate program.

Identifying an Effective Leader

Leadership is the art and science of bringing a group of individuals together to accomplish a mission or to establish and reach mutually satisfying goals. Conflict arises in the work setting as a natural result of the lack of congruity among the priorities of the individuals who are working together. It is the leader's job to establish an environment conducive to collegial work and to bring together a team that will work collectively to achieve the goals of the organization.

One can intuit the presence of an outstanding leader when a group of individuals clearly articulates the mission and goals of their work, believes they are accomplishing their goals, and exhibits a sense of enthusiasm for the work. Inherent in this group would be the ability to manage conflict effectively and to articulate their ideas and opinions assertively rather than aggressively or, potentially more destructive than aggression, not articulating them at all except as passive–aggressive verbal attacks toward other group members or the leader.

Descriptions of leadership focus on styles, functions, and roles. There is much overlapping content among the three perspectives. A continuum of authority is an organizing theme within leadership styles, functions, and roles. Although there is much knowledge regarding leader effectiveness, no solid relationship has been demonstrated between leader effectiveness and differing styles, behaviors, or roles. In fact, research shows that styles, behaviors, and roles have varied from leader to leader and from time to time by the same leader.

Nursing's early descriptions of leadership focused on **styles** of leadership. Table 24–1 lists the major historical descriptions of leadership **styles** ranging from autocratic to laissez-faire. It is useful to think of these styles on a continuum with low and high leader authority as the two extremes. High authority rests with the autocratic leader and low authority is the hallmark of the laissez-faire style. The characteristics of each style are compared in the table.

Since concrete descriptions of functions are more conducive to research on leadership, they have become the focus of the study of leadership rather than styles. Leader behaviors can be classified using two categories: (a) task orientation and (b) interpersonal orientation. These two categories, as identified in the Ohio State University studies reference and adapted by Hersey and Blanchard (1977), align on a two-dimensional grid and create four quadrants of leader behavior: (a) low task–low interpersonal relations, (b) low task–high interpersonal relations, (c) high task–high interpersonal relations, and (d) high task–low interpersonal relations. The associated leader behaviors are (a) delegating, (b) participating, (c) selling, and (d) telling. Rowland and Rowland (1997) list additional functions of a leader to include (a) team building, (b) negotiation, (c) goal setting, (d) evaluation, (e) recruitment and retention of staff/team members, (f) marketing, (g) strategy planning, (h) role-modeling, (i) decision-making, (j) creating, (k) envisioning, (l) risk taking, (m) empowering others, (n) charismatic communication, (o) values clarification, and (p) justification. A third way to view leadership is to examine the **roles** exercised by leaders. A partial list of these roles is presented in Table 24–2.

In the nearly 100 years since Taylor's (1911) scientific definition of **management**, much research has been done to define and explore management as a concept. Today, management means many things. Rowland and Rowland (1997) define management as a five-step process: (a) planning, (b) organizing, (c) directing, (d) coordinating, and (e) controlling. The manager is employed by an organization and given the responsibility over specific resources and work designs in order to accomplish specified goals for the organization. Management "implies a dynamic and proactive approach to running operations" (p. 12). Managers are expected to teach workers the best way to perform the job; match the employee to the job; provide motivational incentives to workers; see that time, energy, and

Table 24–1 The Characteristics of Major Leadership Styles

Characteristic	Leadership Style		
	Autocratic	**Democratic**	**Laissez-faire**
Decision-making	Done by leader	Done jointly	Done by follower
Climate	Controlling	Give and take	Permissive
Outcomes	Short-lived productivity increase	Variable productivity	Variable, but usually high productivity
Major concern	Task	Task and people	People
Expectation of followers	Follow orders	Participate in problem solving	Be the leader
Follower satisfaction	Low	High	High
Management theory	X	Y	Z
Communication	One-way: Down	Two-way	One-way: Up
Rules	Many rules	Necessary rules; some are flexible	No rules, values are prime
Staff maturity	Low	Medium	High
Basic assumption	Followers are lazy and need direction	Adults will be adults if treated like adults	Professionals need little or no direction

materials are efficiently used; and ensure that outcomes are reached.

Management involves more than supervision of the workflow. Staffing and decision-making are functions currently being added to the concept of management by contemporary writers. Managers seek to (a) enhance efficiency, (b) develop resources required to reach the goals of the organization's strategic plan, and (c) manage across boundaries in the organization. It is predicted that management in nursing will draw from nursing's caretaker role, as the manager faces an increasing need to care for those "being managed" (Huber, 2000).

Management and Leadership Compared

To understand management and leadership, the reader must understand what differentiates leadership from management. **Management** is most frequently associated with the control of resources required to accomplish the organizational goals, including budgeting and staffing, with the emphasis on maintaining the functions of the organization while simultaneously balancing fiduciary responsibility for the resources of the

Table 24–2 Nursing Leader Roles

Teacher	Visionary	Information giver	Counselor
Listener	Communicator	Mediator	Decision maker
Advocate	Organizer	Forecaster	Evaluator
Mentor	Coach	Risk taker	Influencer
Caregiver	Diplomat	Role model	Problem solver
Provider	Server	Caretaker	Idealist

organization. There is no doubt that this function is an important part of any leadership position. However, there is a great deal more that is encompassed within the term leadership. **Effective leadership** calls to mind the ideas of vision, "thinking outside the box," use of power in positive ways, challenging others to join with the team to accomplish the vision or mission, and creation of a synergistic environment.

In his book *On Becoming a Leader*, Warren Bennis contrasts the concepts of management and leadership in this way:

- The manager administers; the leader innovates.
- The manager is a copy; the leader is an original.
- The manager maintains; the leader develops.
- The manager focuses on systems and structure; the leader focuses on people.
- The manager relies on control; the leader inspires trust.
- The manager has a short-range view; the leader has a long-range perspective.
- The manager asks how and when; the leader asks what and why.
- The manager has his [sic] eye always on the bottom line; the leader has his [sic] eye on the horizon.
- The manager imitates; the leader originates.
- The manager accepts the status quo; the leader challenges it.
- The manager is the classic good soldier; the leader is his own person.
- The manager does things right; the leader does the right thing (Bennis, 1994, p. 45).

The current state of health care delivery in the United States clearly calls for leaders who are innovative and able to develop superior, original solutions that challenge the status quo. The nursing shortage points out the need for a leader to focus on people and develop a collegial environment. Nurses are in such great demand that no nurse will remain in a clinical situation where the climate is charged with negativity and

a lack of trust so, in a very real sense, the climate created by the nurse manager often determines whether the unit is staffed sufficiently or not.

A Historical Perspective on Leadership and Management Theory

Drucker (2001) makes the following comment about leadership versus management in the twenty-first century: "One does not 'manage' people. The task is to lead people. The goal is to make productive the specific strengths and knowledge of each individual" (p. 81). He believes that this approach is necessary to creating a climate that supports the productivity of the "knowledge worker." Rather than being "subordinates," knowledge workers are "associates"; for the organization to work effectively, knowledge workers must actually know more about their jobs than their boss. The relationship is more like that of an orchestra leader and the musicians than the traditional concept of the superior—subordinate dyad. In his book *The Essential Drucker* (Drucker, 2001), he contrasts his current opinion of management with that in his 1954 book *The Practice of Management*. The assumption he held at that time was "There is one right way to manage people—or at least there should be" (p. 77), which he now believes is totally at odds with reality and productivity. How is it possible that one of the most respected management theorists has changed his view so drastically? This question is best answered by examining the change that has occurred in management theory from a historical perspective.

Traditional Management Methods

There are three types of traditional management: bureaucratic management, scientific management, and administrative management. These strategies were developed during the industrial revolution and dominated management at the turn of the twentieth century. The individuals who are credited with the development of each of these types of management are: (a) Max Weber, a German social historian in the early 1900s, who is considered to have established the philosophy of bureaucratic management; (b) Frederick W. Taylor, a machinist in late-nineteenth-century Philadelphia, who is considered to be the father of scientific management; and (c) Henri Fayol, a French industrialist in the early 1900s, who is the pioneer of administrative techniques. These three types of management emphasize the formal aspects of the organization. Division of labor, hierarchical arrangements of position, and rules and regulations were the chief ingredients of these models.

During the early twentieth century when Webber, Taylor, and Fayol developed these approaches to management, the world view was based on seventeenth-century science. Classical physics was established as Newton synthesized the work of Copernicus, Galileo, and Kepler. Newton's laws of motion and universal gravitation, along with the development of calculus to compute planetary orbits set the stage for a framework of cause and effect and a reliance on prediction through formulae (Whittemore, 1999). It was this perspective from which the early management theorists developed their management strategies for the Industrial Age. The ideal organization was visualized to be parallel to the physics of the time; stability and control were viewed as readily achievable if the right techniques were put into play. The emphasis of management was to master the world of work through the science and world view at the time.

Bureaucratic Management

Bureaucratic management is characterized by rules and regulations, impersonality, division of labor, hierarchical structure, lifelong career commitment, authority, and rationality. Weber believed that the more impersonal, rational, and regulated the work environment, the more likely the employees were to be treated fairly, and the more likely the organization was to reach its objectives. Within health care organizations today, one sees the continuing influence of Weber in the policy and procedure manuals; job descriptions that outline the responsibilities of each person, thereby dividing the labor; and organizational charts that depict the hierarchical structure and the areas of authority for particular positions.

The Scientific Management Movement

The Industrial Revolution gave rise to large factories and created the need to organize the efforts of the supervisors and workers in the factories. Management theory was developed to organize and teach work process in a scientific manner, fulfilling the all-important desire for profit (Taylor, 1911). Taylor's scientific management principles were based on managing time, materials, and work specialization. He developed the concept of the time and motion study with the idea that wasted time and effort could be eliminated. He implemented analyses of work flow and created an inventory of stored materials. Taylor felt that individuals should be highly specialized. To achieve this level of specialization, he implemented the concept of functional foremanship, in which each worker would have a foreman for each area of specialization. He initiated the concept of money as a motivator. He believed that the organization would be well advised to compensate employees for production over and above the basic expectations.

In organizations today these principles are still in use. Job descriptions emphasize the functions to be associated with each job, and one of the functions of the manager is to avoid overlap between positions and to clearly delineate the functions expected. And any employee today expects to be compensated fairly. Money is used as a motivator for productivity, with those employees who have performed exceptionally typically receiving greater pay increases than marginal employees.

Administrative Management

Fayol (1925) initiated the functions that have been traditionally attributed to management, including planning, organizing, leading, and controlling. In addition, he identified 14 management principles that he believed to be crucial to managerial success, including division of labor, authority, discipline, unity of command, unity of direction, subordination of individual interest to the common good, fair remuneration, centralization, scalar chain (line of authority through the hierarchy of the organization), order, equity and fairness, stability and tenure of staff, initiative for subordinates, and team spirit. These principles served to further entrench the bureaucracy of the workplace, but introduced some very forward-thinking ideas. Of course, the modern hospital personnel department has a pay scale that strives to provide fair remuneration, based on educational preparation and years of experience. Every organization strives to retain its staff because the cost of replacing an employee is great, including the cost of recruitment, training, and orientation. The development of *esprit de corps*, or team spirit, continues to be desired in today's workplace.

In conclusion, traditional management styles had advantages and disadvantages. The prime advantage was that the organization and efficiency of industry were enhanced. Many of these structures and guidelines continue to be used in today's workplace. The disadvantages of traditional management included rigid rules, slow decision-making, and authoritarianism. Thus, at the end of the 1920s, the stage was set for the era of behavioral management. The pendulum would swing from an emphasis on the structure and organization of management to a focus on the people who work in the organization.

The Behavioral Management Movement

The recognized beginning of the behavioral movement was the study which lent its name to the Hawthorne effect and which is cited in many research texts. Elton Mayo (1953), a clinical psychologist working at the Harvard Business School, conducted studies at the Hawthorne plant of the Western Electric Company from 1927 to 1932. Regardless of intervention applied to the experimental group, productivity and group pride increased in both the experimental and control groups. It was from this study that Mayo concluded that management must be concerned with preserving the dignity of the workers, demonstrating appreciation for their accomplishments and, in general, recognizing man as a social being with social needs.

Another well-known behavioral theorist, Douglas McGregor (1960), developed Theory X and Theory Y, in which Theory X represented the traditional viewpoints of management, which holds management responsible for organizing money, materials, equipment, and people as well as for directing worker's efforts, motivating them, controlling their actions, and modifying their behavior to fit the needs of the organization. Theory X suggests that, without active intervention by management, workers would be passive in their roles in the organization. Theory Y held a contrasting view of workers, which assumes that the desire to work is just as natural as the desire to play or rest, that external control and threat or punishment are not required to achieve organizational objectives because workers are self-motivated, and that the capacity to work creatively to solve problems is widely distributed in the workforce.

Lewin's Contribution of Change Theory

Lewin's (1951) Force Field Analysis Theory described the change process. This theory has been used for the past half-century as leaders have thought about change in their organizations. Lewin theorized that the likelihood of change occurring was based on assessment of driving and opposing forces, where the driving forces were those factors that favored the change and opposing forces were the barriers to change. If the driving forces were greater than the opposing forces, then change would occur more easily. He also identified a three-phase process that occurs as change is implemented, including the phases of unfreezing, moving, and refreezing. One can imagine what happens when a container of water freezes on a cold winter night, melts during the day, is poured into another shape container while liquid, and then refreezes the next night into its new shape. Unfreezing occurs as the change process is initiated; moving represents the implementation of the change; and refreezing locks the change into place. This theory has given us conceptual ways to think about change and to illustrate the fact that change takes time, has forces that act for and against the change, and that once refreezing has occurred, making another change invokes repetition of the process.

An application of this theory can be found in the hospital setting when new equipment is substituted for existing equipment. For example, the leadership may replace brand X intravenous infusion pumps with brand Y pumps for a variety of reasons. It may be that the old ones were malfunctioning; it may be that the a new model uses more cost-effective tubing; or it may be that the new equipment offers more safeguards against malfunction and negative patient outcomes. Whatever the reason, the outcome for the nurses on the unit will be that they are working with equipment that, while achieving the same purpose as the old units, functions somewhat differently. The operation of the new IV pumps will be less intuitive than the operation of the existing ones was.

The work of unfreezing will take place over the time period in which the nurses know about the change. In an optimal environment, the nurses will have been involved in making the decision about the IV pumps, and will have helped identify the driving and restraining forces associated with the change. Moving will occur once the new pumps arrive on the unit, and the nurses begin having to actually use them in patient care. There will most likely be an inservice on the new pumps and written instructions for their operation. During this period, nurses will be comparing the old and new units and will be discussing the merits and problems associated with them. Ultimately, after several months, the nurses will have acclimated to the new pumps and, should there be a need to change models in the future, the entire change process would begin again.

Twenty-First-Century Nursing Leadership

Leadership theory continues to evolve as more is learned about the best strategies for achieving the work of organizations. Theories about leadership range from transactional and transformational leadership to strategies based on chaos theory and quantum physics of science. The greatest assets of any organization are the people who carry out the roles, functions, and responsibilities within the hospital or business. It is, therefore, appropriate that much research and reflection pertains to leadership. Poor leadership decreases the productivity of the organization, creates poor morale, leads to attrition, and in the final analysis contributes to poor patient care. The mission and goals of the organization cannot be met when leadership is less than optimal.

Transactional and Transformational Leadership

Vance and Larson (2002) posit that "leadership is without meaning except as it serves the function of facilitating group performance, organizational change, and subsequent goal achievement" (p. 166). Their meta-analysis of leadership research found that over the past two decades transactional and transformational leadership styles had been the basis for much of the research.

Transactional leadership theory holds that there is an exchange, or transaction, between the leader and the employee in which the leader provides rewards and benefits to the subordinates as they contribute to the achievement of the organizational goals. The transactional leader is a hands-on leadership approach, in which the leader is involved with employees through active management-by-exception (MBEA), passive management-by-exception (MBEP), and contingent reward. MBEA involves continuous monitoring of follower's performance so that mistakes can be corrected as soon as possible or, optimally, prevented altogether. MBEP is characterized by passive monitoring and correction of mistakes and critique occurring in retrospect (Stordeur, D'hoore, & Vandenberghe, 2001).

The MBEA approach seems is an excellent philosophy for any leader who is responsible for new nurses or unlicensed assistants who are new to health care. New employees do not know how to maneuver around in the system, they don't know who the resource people are, and they are not familiar with the organization of their unit. The benefits to taking an active approach to monitoring performance at this time include maximizing the new person's success and minimizing or preventing any errors that might negatively impact patient care. MBEA is also an excellent strategy for ensuring the smooth integration of a team member who has been transferred for a single shift from another unit in the hospital. These individuals may be very competent on their own unit, but when transferred to another unit become a novice on that floor. The leader responsible for patient care in these situations may find that focusing on the exceptions in performance is the best approach to assuring quality patient care.

Transformational leadership holds that there is a relationship or interaction between the leader and the follower that results in a change, or transformation, of attitudes, beliefs, or behaviors. The leader is viewed as a change agent. Leaders who exhibits transformational leadership are concerned with a long-term sense of mission, manifests faith and respect in their followers, encourages innovative solutions to problems, transmits a sense of ethics and values, and communicates an inspiring sense of the future (Vance & Larson, 2002).

A transformational leader seeks to foster greater cohesion and teamwork and, according to Rippon and Monaghan (2001), must help to steer employees "towards new, more fluid systems which reflect the function of the team and organization, leading clinicians to deliver systems of care rather than maintain traditional organizational form" (p. 9). Transformational leadership recognizes the need to interact with different team players in a variety of ways and to consider their experience, interests, and expertise. Each person is unique and will make unique contributions to the health care team. Wise transformational leaders will seek to tailor their interactions to maximize each person's contribution to reaching the mission and goals of the unit or organization as a whole.

Chaos Theory, Quantum Theory, and Nursing Leadership

Wheatley (1994) recognizes developments in mathematics and physics as having application to leadership and wrote a very thought-provoking book entitled *Leadership and the New Science*. In this book, she recognizes the opportunity presented for application of quantum theory, founded by Neils Bohr and Werner Heisenberg, to the leadership of organizations. Just as systems in nature use periods of disequilibrium to make changes that, ultimately, maintain their order and stability, organizations can welcome change. In the quantum age, "order and change, autonomy and control were not the great opposites that we had thought them to be. It was a world where change and constant creation signaled new ways of maintaining order and structure" (Wheatley, 1994, p. 2). Wheatley believes that there is a "simpler way to lead organizations, one that requires less effort and produces less stress than the current practices" (Wheatley, 1994, p. 3). Quantum and chaos theory recognize the path between disorder and order as "order out of chaos or order through fluctuation" (Prigogine, as cited in Wheatley, 1994, p. 20).

In their review of the research pertaining to leadership, Vance and Larson (2002) found that quantum physics, chaos theory, and complexity science are appearing in the literature on leadership. The inclusion of these approaches to management is related to the changes in the environment of health care. Valadez and Sportsman (1999) state that "turmoil, multiple relationships, and new ways of 'doing business' characterize today's health care system" (p. 209). This environment is much more complex than the environment that existed 30 years ago, so it is expected that more complex, less linear approaches to leadership will be required.

Wilson and Porter-O'Grady (1999), in the second edition of their book *Leading the Revolution in Health Care*, conjecture that in a tumultuous environment a leader cannot rely on long-term vision and therefore must seek a "template, a set of principles that elucidate the relationship between what they are undertaking and the underlying values guiding their activities" (p. 26). They perceive the beginning of the twenty-first century as being a part of the unfolding of a new age, replete with unprecedented changes. The new age is emerging and four basic principles appear to be determining the way organizations will function, including partnership, accountability, equity, and ownership.

Partnership pertains to actions at the global, national, state, local, and organizational levels. Inherent in the formation of partnerships is the decreasing emphasis on old hierarchical structure present in organizations since the 1900s. "Self-directed work teams, integrative work arrangements, and transdisciplinary models of organization all demonstrate the value of partnership" (Wilson & Porter-O'Grady,

1999, p. 28). The demands made to achieve the best possible patient outcomes are envisioned to demand a fluid, flexible environment and workforce in which learning is continuous. Empowerment will become an increasingly important part, as the rigid, command and control systems become ever more outmoded.

Accountability, the second principle, is the corollary for responsibility. In the past, leaders have often been heard to say that they need the "authority to go with their responsibility." Now the emphasis will be on accountability to go with the responsibility that stems from the new partnerships that characterize the new age. In the old "industrial model," managers or supervisors were responsible for the work of the employees they supervised. In the future, "performance, outcome, and consumer satisfaction data are becoming increasingly available, which means that assessment of work and workers will be less and less dependent on personal judgment" (Wilson & Porter-O'Grady, 1999, p. 29). Instead, the team members will become self-evaluative, relying on the outcomes of care to provide direction to their interventions. In this model, if the patient outcomes are good, the nurse will know his or her role was carried out effectively. These authors differentiate responsibility and accountability as follows: "Responsibility relates to processes. Accountability is all about outcomes" (Wilson & Porter-O'Grady, 1999, p. 30). Accountability is related to the emerging partnerships and will require clear communication, reciprocal dialogue, and a mutual understanding of the mission, goals, and expected outcomes of the organization. Care must be taken to carefully differentiate roles of the various providers of care; ambiguity will cause confusion and impede the performance of the team. Ambiguity will be prevented through dialogue among members of the team so that each member can interact effectively with other team members.

Equity, the third principle, is derived from the contribution of each role to the accomplishment of the outcomes of the organization. Wilson and Porter-O'Grady (1999) predict that the industrially based hierarchical organizations are nearing the end of their usefulness. They see health care delivery as being organized around the point of delivery in the future, in which case there is no need for a hierarchy to supervise the professional knowledge workers who are the providers of care. Further, they predict that "we are watching the end of the age of the job. Now work will be reflected in role relationships and characterized by flexibility of content" (p. 34). An organization's commitment to equity will, in the future, be evidenced by the degree to which decisions are made at the point of service delivery, rather than being handed down through a hierarchical structure.

Ownership, the fourth and final principle of the new age, is seen as requisite to the new paradigm. The professional health care provider "must express ownership of that part of the work that is his or hers" (Wilson & Porter-O'Grady, 1999, p. 35). Ownership is seen as embodying empowerment, decision-making at the point of care delivery, effective methods of decision-making, partnership at every level of the organization, and work activities directed toward the accomplishment of the mission of the organization.

In this new organizational paradigm there is a need for significant shifts in accepted management practices such as:

- Continuous acknowledgement of their own and others' inner wisdom is the hallmark of successful leaders. Leaders will develop participative, relational competencies in their newly conceptualized roles.
- Leaders must recognize and act on their recognition of the interconnectedness of everyone to everything. Inherent in this realization is the fact that problems and issues can be solved only through cognitive competencies that stimulate systems thinking.
- The clockwork view of the world must be rejected. Top-down directives and the notion that people are replaceable components are old views in a rigid system when, in fact, flexibility, fluidity, innovation, and risk taking are the attributes desired in the new paradigm. Transformative leadership is required rather than transactional leadership (Wilson & Porter-O'Grady, 1999, pp. 47–48).

The paradox that disorder can be a source of order is particularly encouraging to nursing and to health care in general. Health care is in chaos. Instability is caused by many interrelated variables, including managed care and shifting demographics, age, gender, and ethnicity. According to Valadez and Sportsman (1999), three principles can be drawn from quantum theory to help leaders in nursing manage the environment, including "a) the world is unpredictable, b) the world is not independent of the observer; rather, the intent of the observer influences what is seen; and c) the relationships among things are what counts, not the things themselves" (p. 210). They emphasize that strategic planning is important, but that the plan cannot remain static; it must change, take into account new data,

examine the relationships inherent in the system, and allow for the exploration of differences of multiple perspectives of stakeholders in the organization.

Power and Empowerment

Empowerment has become one of the euphemisms of the past decade. It remains an important concept for leaders who wish to maximize the contributions of their team members. Perhaps the reason it has been viewed with skepticism in the past is that the structures within which empowerment has been attempted have been the industrial model, rigid, top-down bureaucracies. These models have not provided a good environment for empowerment. As the changes observed and predicted by Wilson and Porter-O'Grady (1999) become more prevalent in health care, nurses and other health care providers will become empowered.

Power

Before empowerment can be discussed, power itself needs to be discussed. Power has been perceived negatively in the nursing profession, primarily because it has been viewed in light of the hierarchical structures that have dominated health care organizations in the past (Kuokkanen & Leino-Kilpi, 2000). Nurses must realize that there is no power in numbers; rather, it is derived from the cohesiveness of the group (i.e., the combined common values or goals of a group). The combining of power from a variety of sources leads to synergic power, a type of power that will be needed to promote health care reform and preserve quality outcomes. In nursing, the main source of power regardless of purpose comes from the caring heart of nursing.

According to Davidhizar and Shearer (2002), power is the resource that allows nursing leaders to "gain both commitment and compliance from others." In order to facilitate the use of power, the administrator must exhibit interpersonal skills, group communication skills, negotiation skills, assertiveness, and conflict resolution" (p. 34). These authors advocate letting go of power, which allows the leaders to avoid micromanagement and let their associates make decisions on their own; it is through this letting go that the leader can facilitate and mentor decision-making. Some leaders, particularly insecure or novice leaders, may be unwilling to let go or to trust their employees with decisions. When this is the case, employees may feel that they are not trusted and may feel hurt or angry. Avoiding the urge to rush in is important, except in a true crisis. Allowing others to work through difficult situations increases their confidence, self-esteem, and future decision-making ability.

Within groups, several types of power are important. These include the connective power associated with networking, information power based on the possession of knowledge that is useful to others, and group decision-making power that is created as a group works together to solve a problem. Individual sources of power include personal power, or the ability to accomplish goals through personal effort; professional power, including the ability to make a meaningful contribution to the organization and profession; and perceived power, associated with the amount of power the group attributes to the leader (Davidhizar & Shearer, 2002).

Empowerment

The relationship of power and empowerment, according to McNay (as cited in Kuokkanen & Leino-Kilpi, 2000), is that power and the exercise thereof cannot be seen to merge within empowerment. "Empowerment is not merely the outcome of power and its exercise. Employees cannot be empowered simply by means of delegation. They all have their own personal qualities which tend to drive them to seek knowledge and to act in appropriate meaningful ways" (Kuokkanen & Leino-Kilpi, 2000, p. 239).

Davidhizar and Shearer (2002) talk about empowerment as a part of their strategy of "letting go." They define empowerment as "giving others the authority, responsibility, and freedom to act on what they know" (p. 35). By empowering the professional members of the health care team, leaders expand the sphere of influence and increase the sense of ownership. They outline the following strategies for leaders who wish to "take charge by letting go," thereby empowering their associates to:

- Avoid rushing in to solve a problem. When possible, the individuals involved should be consulted and allowed to "own" the issue.
- Not respond prematurely. Allow time for data collection and discussion with responsible individuals.
- Not say everything they know. This strategy allows time for more data collection and interpretation by group members.
- Support the authority of subordinates. Positive leadership includes empowering subordinates to accomplish group goals. Refer employees of a subordinate supervisor back to that supervisor for resolution of issues.

- Promote the self-esteem of subordinates. Place subordinates in a positive light and build up their esteem in front of others.
- Foster teamwork. Encourage members of the health care team to work together to solve problems. The administrator must trust the creative forces and energy that are created when a team successfully addresses an issue. Teamwork can decrease resistance to change, also.
- Practice active listening. Listening is one of a leader's most important actions. Active listening involves giving one's undivided attention, complete with eye contact (pp. 35–37).

A common problem in the health care setting involves disagreements among nurses on particular shifts regarding the responsibilities of each shift. A manager who uses these strategies would listen carefully to the situation, express confidence in the team to resolve the problem, avoid calling in individuals or groups to provide a "quick fix," and avoid sharing his or her own solution to the problem. These approaches support the team's ability to solve its own problems, thereby empowering the group and increasing the likelihood that the problem will be resolved positively and in a way that is satisfactory to the group.

Palmier (1998) states that "leaders must be secure professionals who do not see empowering staff as an erosion of their own power or their responsibility" (p. 17). This comment calls into question the difference between authoritative power and generative power. Authoritative power, or "power over," is seen to be a function of the organizational chart. This view of power suggests there is a limited supply of power and that it must be conserved to preserve the position of the manager. Generative power, or "power to" or "power with" sees power as occurring everywhere that there are people who are acting to accomplish the mission of the organization. From this point of view, power is unlimited and actually increases as more people are empowered to do their work to their fullest ability. The former view is more consistent with the management strategies explored under the traditional management theorists, while the latter is more consistent with the view of leadership through the lens of quantum and chaos theories.

This discussion of power and empowerment is important to the new nurse leader who is working to develop a positive organizational culture in which growth, change, and excellent patient care can flourish. Quantum theory supports the use of empowerment in the workplace. Wheatley (1994) emphasizes the contri-

Inspired by the need to evaluate creative work environments, Laschinger and Wong (1999) conducted a cross-sectional, correlational survey study to measure the relationship of selected factors to empowerment. Using a model expanding on Kanter's (1977) theory of organizational empowerment, the authors tested the associations between staff nurse perceptions of empowerment and accountability. Kanter states that access to structures of empowerment (information, support, resources, and opportunity to learn and grow) have more impact on empowerment than the characteristics of individual nurses.

For the study, empowerment was described as nurses using professional knowledge and skills for patient care decisions while being accountable for productivity and work effectiveness. A questionnaire of six established tools was administered to a random sample of 672 staff nurses in a large Canadian medical center. The data from the 477 respondents indicated that nurses perceived they:

- Were moderately empowered by their work settings
- Were mostly empowered by work opportunity
- Were least empowered by information access
- Had moderate informal power
- Had low formal power
- Had moderate accountability to one another for practice outcomes
- Contributed at a moderate level to productivity
- Were overall highly effective in their work

The presence of significant links between Kanter's theory—access to empowerment structures—and formal and informal power of staff nurses were demonstrated. In addition, well-developed alliances in the organization were linked to accountability and further to work-effectiveness. The strongest association was revealed between informal power and total empowerment.

These findings suggest that if productivity is an expectation, managers must provide the staff nurse with information, support, and resources necessary to provide quality care. The relationships among the variables in the study indicate that empowerment structures without the staff nurse control over patient-to-patient practice decisions, makes nurses shun accountability for care outcomes and decreases staff satisfaction.

The graduate must understand that empowerment, as a concept, is complex. Examining the substance rather than the physical structure of a care model must be done to evaluate the level of empowerment afforded the staff. During interviews, managers should be asked what traditional control over care decisions in the setting is relinquished to the staff nurse level. Careful examination beyond labels and marketing language will yield a truer picture of the practice expectations of the facility and the true degree to which empowerment exists in their structure.

butions made by inviting conflicts and contradictions to emerge, by processing information, and looking for ways to increase employee contribution and involvement. She expresses her confidence in participative management as a way to provide a way for human beings to meet their "strong desires for recognition and connectedness. The more they (we) feel part of the organization, the more work gets done" (p. 144).

One way that new leaders can develop the ability to use their power positively and empower their employees is through a relationship with a mentor. According to Rippon (2001), mentorship "should become a part of the everyday career experience" (p. 15). Mentorship allows the sharing of insights by the mentor, as well as providing an opportunity to see the world of work through fresh perspectives from the protégé. This partnership provides a rich learning experience for both parties.

Roles of the Leader/Manager Nurse

The nurse leader has many varied formal and informal roles. Effective leadership involves team building, decision-making, communication, negotiation, delegation, and mentorship. Whether managing a group of patients or function in the role of charge nurse, clinical manager, director of nursing, vice president of patient care, or president of the local chapter of the American Nurses Association, Sigma Theta Tau, or other professional organizations these skills are used by successful nurses who lead and manage.

Team Builder

The delivery of health care is a team activity, involving professionals from a variety of disciplines and unlicensed personnel whose contribution to patient care is vital. Until recently, group work has not been emphasized in nursing curricula. Individuals in the workplace are more likely to place credence on performing well individually as opposed to identifying how to integrate their own actions into those of the team. In the complex world of health care delivery, each individual's participation as a team member is a requirement; to do otherwise is likely to create fragmentation of care for the patient.

Leaders who desire to create a team will communicate to all team members their belief in the ability of the team to work well together. When members of the team indicate their unwillingness to participate or their lack of faith in the team members, the leader must listen carefully, avoid saying too much, help the concerned individuals to assess their own contributions to the team and their expectations of other team members, and communicate their belief in the contribution of the team to the goals of the organization. This conversation serves the purpose of empowering the team member to fully contribute to the work that is to be accomplished. However, the leader needs to gather more information about the function of the team. Perhaps there is reason for concern and, if so, the leader must take action. Often, the conversation with the team member who stepped forward is enough. Chaos theory supports the notion that small inputs may create change that is not in proportion to the original action. Sometimes more action is needed and the leader may call a team meeting or meet with others individually.

The mission and goals of the organization are the unifying principles and they don't have to be complex. A mission of "providing excellent care to the patients on the ABC unit" is a good starting point. Through reiteration of the purpose of work and the importance of teamwork, the leader can help the team refocus and move beyond personal issues.

Decision Maker

The leader is well served to recall Drucker's (2001) comments about the knowledge worker of the twenty-first century. The individual who does the work of the organization is the one who knows the most about it. Participative and transformational leaders enter into relationships with the professionals in their organizations. They share information, discuss values, and collaborate on decisions. The self-esteem of team members is related to the respect demonstrated by involvement with decision-making.

Sometimes decisions need to be made quickly, but even in those circumstances the leader is ill-advised to make the decision without gaining input from those who will be affected by the decision. If the decision will involve the need for change, the greater the number of people who believe their views have been taken into consideration, the greater will be the support for the change. A paradox that exists within organizations is that frequently there is an artificial time constraint placed on decision-making, supposedly to move the organization along more rapidly, although a decision made quickly without adequate consideration and input often results in an excessive amount of time being required to respond to the problems associated with rapid, uninformed change. A wise leader negotiates for the time to make a well-informed decision and thus avoids the frustration and time associated with outcomes of hasty decision-making.

Communicator

Information is power! Current leadership literature recognizes the importance of keeping the members of an organization informed about issues with which they are involved. Many health care organizations function around the clock, which can make the role of communicator more complex. However, the effort made to give people accurate information is worth the price. Personal face-to-face communication is optimal, and leaders must make every effort to stagger their hours in the organization to allow this communication on a regular basis.

In the past, communication books were used as a way to enhance "asynchronous" communication among various shifts of workers and the leader. Today's computer technology supports communication through listservs, e-mail, video conferencing, and discussion boards. If an organization is not taking advantage of the technology that is available, the leader should investigate the availability of that technology.

An important aspect of communication is that it must be a "two-way street." In bureaucratic organizations, information often flows only downward and there is a propensity for the information to fail to propagate to the unit lever. This type of communication is a sure recipe for disaster. The knowledge workers on the unit are lacking important information about their environment and their contributions are not being heard. A leader who identifies this approach to communication in the organization will need to create a new communication paradigm, and it may take a longer-than-expected period of time for people to trust the new system. This leader is encouraged to remember Lewin's change theory, and allow adequate time for unfreezing and moving. In time, the new communication pattern will refreeze as the expected model of communication.

Optimal communication involves a dialogue in which the ideas of all team members are viewed as meritorious. Chaos theory encourages the leader to invite divergent points of view. This author conceptualizes the organizational mission and goals to be the "strange attractor" that keeps the team focused, similar to the newly discovered attractors that operate in physics to create order out of chaos (Wheatley, 1994).

Negotiator

The leader must exhibit excellent negotiation skills. These skills are important in helping a team arrive at decisions, gaining organizational support for a new plan, gaining the cooperation of another department or organization, and in many other facets of the leader's role. New leaders are encouraged to read current literature on negotiation to hone their expertise.

The first rule of negotiation is to understand the positions of the stakeholders. Communication is an important part of negotiation, and one of the vital attributes of a negotiator is to encourage discussion among the group. Many times negotiation surrounds a decision in which it is perceived that there will be "winners" and "losers." Negotiation centers around understanding who the perceived winners and losers are; the best negotiations result in win–win solutions. Although this is not always possible, one of the questions this author advocates is "Under what circumstances do you think this goal can be accomplished?" This frequently moves participants from defending their positions to one of creativity and possibility thinking. It is a more hypothetical situation that encourages free thought. Another freeing type of question is, "If we had no con-straints, how could we make this work?" The follow-up question is, of course, "This sounds like a great suggestion. Now, how can we make it work here?"

Delegator

Every manager delegates—it is the excellent leader who enters into delegation in a way that empowers people in the organization. Additionally, the excellent leader also knows the difference between delegating accountability and abdicating responsibility. The knowledge workers of the twenty-first century hold vast stores of information about the work for which they are responsible (Drucker, 2001). Creating a sense of partnership, accountability, equity, and ownership are the hallmarks of organizations. The leader must create an environment that supports the notion of associates being partners in the delivery of health care, holding accountability for evaluating the outcomes of their interventions, having the equity in the organization to make point-of-service delivery decisions, and feeling a sense of ownership in the organization. Delegation is no longer a "top-down" activity. Instead, the leader will recognize the wisdom of his or her team members, support the interconnectedness of team members in the health care delivery system, and embrace a more fluid, innovative system (Wilson & Porter-O'Grady, 1999).

Mentor

It is often said that effective leaders are always in the business of replacing themselves so their professional development and advancement can continue. Mentorship is the process through which this can most readily be accomplished. The identification of potential protégés can occur through a variety of methods. Team members who express an interest in leadership, individuals who have recently taken on new leadership roles, or professionals who show promise in the area of leadership through their interactions with others are all likely candidates. Mentoring relationships can be formal (assigned through an organization) or can be informal (simply a handshake agreement between a seasoned leader and an aspiring one). Sigma Theta Tau International, the nursing honor society, is an example of an organization that seeks to foster formal mentoring relationships, as does the American Association of Colleges of Nursing (AACN).

Whether a mentoring relationship is formal or informal, there are a few guidelines for success. The mentoring relationship must be mutually rewarding, it must involve the opportunity for real work and stimulating challenges, there must be agreement on ownership of any projects created through the partnership, and the relationship must remain on professional grounds at all times. The mentor has the responsibility to create opportunities for professional growth and involvement, while the protégé is responsible for responding to these opportunities. The mentor has the responsibility to provide opportunities for the protégé to gain recognition for the work accomplished; the protégé is accountable for being responsible and reliable with the work he or she has accepted. The mentor empowers, encourages, and challenges the protégé.

All nurses have a professional responsibility to mentor new members of the profession. Leaders have an expectation of mentorship into leadership positions. Mutual respect, goal setting, accountability to each other, and open dialogue are hallmarks of an effective mentoring relationship. An important note here is that either party can cancel the mentorship agreement at any time. If the relationship is not working, there is little point in continuing the façade of mentorship.

In conclusion, the case can be made that there are many other roles inherent in the work of the nursing leader. However, if these roles can be assumed effectively, the work of the organization can be accomplished in a way that achieves the mission and goals, while creating an empowered workforce. The idea that fun should be involved is very important. Lewis Thomas (as quoted in Wheatley, 1994) says, "Whenever you can hear laughter and somebody saying, 'But that's preposterous!'—you can tell that things are going well and that something probably worth looking at has begun to happen in the lab" (p. 142).

Followership: The Path from Novice Nurse to Nurse Leader

All graduates should initially expect to be followers, submitting to the state of being managed in a place of employment. However, the condition of followership is taken for granted, until difficulties in the work setting arise. While vast amount of research has focused on the concept of leadership, the subject of followership has gained little attention. One barrier to recognizing the value of followership may be the misconception that followers only follow orders and cannot think

(DiRienzo, 1994). In reality, **followership** is the thoughtful and skillful use of interpersonal behavior acted in response to the leadership efforts of another.

Theoretical Development of Followership as a Concept

Followership is given scant consideration in recent nursing literature. According to Kelley (1991), followership is both an art and a craft. In writing about working relationships, Guidera and Gilmore (1988) felt that followership had to be defended as a critical element. Campbell and Kinion (1993) advised the explicit teaching of followership along with leadership in graduate education, and DiRienzo (1994) challenged nursing to not only develop leaders, but followers as well, hinting that the lack of followership ability is suspect as part of the cause of the new graduate's insecurity. Gunn (1996) described followership as courageous. Brown (1990, 1991) has twice issued a plea to professional nurses to consider followership important in their practice.

Just as leadership styles have been expressed in the literature, categories of followers have also been labeled. Kelley (1988) classified followers into five categories of engagement in the follower process: (a) sheep, (b) "yes" people, (c) alienated people, (d) survivors, and (e) effective followers. Sheep are unable to think critically and unable to take responsibility or show initiative. "Yes" people are unable to resist persuasion by others and lack initiative. Some followers are capable and can think critically, but appear passive and demonstrate resistance; these are termed alienated. Survivors never take risks but endure the change without much input. Effective followers are described as having initiative and critical thinking skills. They show responsibility and are self-managed in their ability to follow-through with solutions. Murphy (1990) applied these categories to nursing as followership styles. Table 24–3 illustrates these categories using the analogy of sheep on a cliff.

Every nursing student brings a dominant follower style to nursing education. During this educational period, followership is molded in response to relationships with nursing faculty and student peers. After graduation there is a new superior (e.g., supervisor, manager, boss) in the work setting who may have a very different leadership and/or management style than that to which the graduate has previously been exposed. New peers (co-workers) will role model differing followership styles. The new supervisor and co-workers will have a measurable effect on the development of fol-

Table 24–3	Kelley's Categories of Followers Illustrated as Sheep on a Cliff
Sheep	"Which cliff?" (Then they jump.)
"Yes" people	"I'll jump if you do."
The alienated	"You jump first."
Survivors	Look for the ambulance at the bottom of the cliff, and then jump.
Effective followers	Build a fence at the top of the cliff.

lowership behaviors in the new graduate; therefore, the development of followership as a concept demands attention and has implications for nursing education.

Precursor to Effective Leadership and Management

Although little is written about the developmental relationship of followership to leadership in nursing, Corona (1979) termed followership an important accompaniment to leadership. Bennis (1994) described three things that followers need from leaders: (a) direction, (b) trust, and (c) hope. These three things parallel the characteristics of successful leaders: (a) value systems, (b) confidence in subordinates, (c) interaction with subordinates, and (d) leader self-confidence (Tannenbaum & Schmidt, 1958). The idea that leadership and followership are related in some way is important to understanding followership (Pagonis, 1992). Followership, as "an interpersonal process of participation by following," [compliments] "the relationship between the leader and the follower [which in turn] defines leadership" (Huber, 2000, p. 66). Further exploration of followership as a concept is needed before any relationship with leadership can be credibly suggested.

Barriers to Developing Good Followership

According to Rowland and Rowland (1997) "commands in health care enterprises will be followed only if they are accepted as legitimate and reasonable by those expected to respond" (p. 4). Followers are knowledgeable in health care. But they are still liable to become "sapped" by the personality or tone of the management or by co-workers. Byham (1988) in his book, *Zapp! The Lightning of Empowerment*, cites the reasons employees (followers) get sapped (disillusioned and turned off):

- Confusion
- Lack of trust
- Not being listened to
- No time to solve problems
- Bureaucratic office politics
- Someone solving problems for you
- No time to work on bigger issues
- Not knowing whether you are succeeding
- Across-the-board rules and regulations
- A boss taking credit for others' ideas
- Not enough resources to do the job well
- Believing that you can't make a difference
- A job simplified to the point that it has no meaning
- People treated exactly the same, like interchangeable parts (p. 51)

Although followers in health care know legal and ethical boundaries, ineffective leadership, either by default or poor skills in the leader, can create an environment where being "sapped" becomes the norm. The new graduate may also find being managed a painful experience if the designated manager is ineffective and the graduate's followership skills are weak. In these situations, the development of good followership behaviors is essential.

Critical Thinking and Reflection

Is followership a precursor of leadership? How is followership learned? How should a follower respond to poor leaders and managers?

Applied Followership: Styles, Behaviors, and Rules

Examination of appropriate follower style or behaviors in relation to the experience of being led and being managed is an important activity for new nurses. There is overlap in followership behaviors and behaviors in response to being managed just as there is overlap in leadership and management behaviors. Table 24–4 contains a list of behaviors in the two categories.

In addition, there are some very important rules the new nurse follower needs to know. These rules will not be reviewed in the orientation sessions or written in the policy and procedure manuals. These rules are written on the wall behind the door to some secret room on the nursing unit. These rules, in essence, exist informally, but they are rules. These rules include, but are not limited to:

- Be a good follower, leaders need good followers if they are to be good leaders.
- No surprises, leaders don't like surprises. Keep the leader informed.
- Pick your battles. Everything is not worth fighting for.
- Don't give or take gossip. There is information you are not supposed to know. If you don't listen to it, you won't repeat it.
- Get to know the whole team, one member at a time. Show interest in them as individuals. Everyone is important to your success.
- Prompt, factual, one-on-one feedback in private surroundings is best. It's also a two-way process.
- Even when you may not need it, ask for help. Others feel complimented when you turn to them for assistance.
- Praise others. They will soon give it back to you.
- Self-evaluation is the best kind. It is less painful than when done by others. Practice it frequently and document your findings.
- Know the rules. Follow the rules. When documented rules become out-dated, seek correction (Brakey, 1991).

Table 24–4   Followership and Being Managed Behaviors

Followership Behaviors	Being Managed Behaviors
Validation	Planning
Problem identification	Organizing
Critical thinking	Conserving
Seed planting	Following through
Positive behavioring	Self-evaluation
Praising others	Taking orders
Communication	Accepting criticism
Peer evaluation	Complying
Turn taking	Reporting
Reporting	Task analysis
Team playing	Open-mindedness
Negotiating	Discovering
Valuing	Problem solving
Role modeling	Communicating
Creating	Consulting
Laughing	Attentiveness
Information gathering	
Confidence keeping	
Encouragement giver	
Facilitating	
Joining	

Leadership, management, and followership have been discussed fully in this chapter. Reflect back on the nurse's role as leader, manager, and follower.

How can leaders and managers share power with followers and find the synergy needed for the growth of professional nursing in the twenty-first century?

The Transition from Followership to Leadership

After some time and experience in nursing, baccalaureate-prepared nurses may be ready to move along the path to expand their leadership roles and responsibilities. There is a need for individuals who enjoy each of the roles discussed in this chapter. Each role requires nurses to further develop their expertise and gain additional credentials. Nurses are needed who are willing to move into central leadership positions in hospitals, public health settings, other health care organizations, professional organizations, and schools of nursing. Nurses preparing for graduation may believe that it is too early to be thinking of career planning that involves leadership and it is true that they may not know if a leadership role is one they would enjoy until later. However, here are 20 tips for preparing oneself for a future of leadership:

1. Develop a network of colleagues outside the nursing unit, including other disciplines as well as other nursing units. This will give you an appreciation of the bigger picture, exposure to other ways of thinking and new ideas, and will position you as someone who values collaboration outside the immediate work group.
2. Seek committee assignments that will involve other areas in the organization. You will learn more about your workplace and find other areas where you can make contributions that will be satisfying to you and move your career forward.
3. Learn to present your point of view in an assertive manner that is respectful of other persons while, at the same time, presenting your ideas effectively. Effective communication is vital to the emerging leader.
4. Become involved in one or more professional organizations. These may include your local chapter of the American Nurses Association, your specialty organization, or your local chapter of Sigma Theta Tau.
5. Hone your public speaking skills through self-study, participation in Toastmasters International, and by accepting opportunities to present information to small groups. Nurses who can speak effectively to groups can accomplish a great deal for both themselves and their profession. You can practice on groups such as the local parent–teacher organization, health classes, or even in such arenas as CPR instruction!
6. Learn to use a presentation software package such as PowerPoint. The ability to illustrate your presentation through audiovisual media is a vital addition. The good news is that these software packages are becoming more and more easy to master as technology becomes more and more powerful.
7. Become recognized as a person who is "part of the solution" when you approach your leader. Use your critical thinking skills to identify changes that can solve problems within your organization. A question you can ask yourself to unlock your creativity is "Under what circumstances could this problem be resolved?"
8. When you are in the leadership position, help your team solve problems through asking the following three questions: (a) What is the problem? (b) Why is it a problem? (c) What are some solutions? If solutions are not forthcoming from the team, this response may help generate solutions, "Here are some solutions I see . . . what do you think? How else could we solve the problem?"
9. Think of yourself as a person who can make a difference. Others' belief in you often begins with your belief in yourself.
10. Create your image as you want others to see you. A professional appearance, positive affect, and enthusiasm for your work are all vitally important if you would like to be perceived as the leader you are.
11. Be self-aware, recognizing both your areas of strength as well as your areas for growth—and don't beat up on yourself. You are, and always will be, in the process of evolving and becoming. Readily acknowledge your growth areas and seek assistance with your professional development.
12. "Work hard to understand the big picture and become involved in decision-making on your unit . . . read everything you can about health care reform, reengineering, and how today's business environment is affecting hospitals" (Thomas, 1995, p. 72).

13. Recognize and celebrate the specific contributions and successes of your colleagues. A focus on the real contributions of others serves many purposes, not the least of which is creating a positive work environment and improved morale.
14. Balance your life and practice self-renewal. As Dr. Patsy Keyser, a professor of nursing, once said, "You can't pour any more lemonade for others if your pitcher is empty!"
15. Find out what you love to do, and keep doing it!
16. Have business cards made. They are a small investment of around $15 to $30 at any print shop, and they will facilitate networking, create a positive image, and make you feel very professional.
17. Identify a nurse who currently practices in the role you would like to pursue and seek to establish a formal or informal mentoring relationship.
18. Investigate graduate school. Many nursing programs offer master's degrees in nursing administration. These programs are typically 36 to 50 semester credit hours in length. The admission requirements vary, but typically one can expect to take the GRE or another standardized test, submit original transcripts, provide letters of recommendation, and participate in an interview. The expense varies, depending on whether the university is public or private. Often, programs offer distance learning initiatives that will provide greater flexibility in the actual hours of course attendance on campus.
19. Take a few minutes of quiet time and keep a journal that records your professional growth. This time spent focusing on your career will pay dividends far into the future.
20. Best wishes in your quest to become a leader!

TRANSITION INTO PRACTICE

The initial task facing the graduate nurse is transition from the role of learner to that of follower. The nursing process provides a familiar critical thinking tool that can serve the new graduate in this transition as well as the staff nurse in future transitions involving leadership and management. In addition, when constructed as a two-dimensional blue print, adding the revolutionary personal–motivational–organizational format developed for future leader transition by Wilson and Porter-O'Grady (1999), the nurse can generate a matrix of ideas.

A thumbnail followership development plan is presented in Table 24–5 that demonstrates a process graduates can use to attain followership, leadership, and management skills. For example, the new nurse assesses personal toleration of chaos while observing the degree of chaos in the work environment. Judgments regarding both personal and organizational differences are made and can be compared and contrasted. While plans are made to increase motivation through spending daily planning time, the graduate can proactively plan projects and seek opportunities in decision-making within the organization. During implementation, the nurse can practice these new skills performing the job with the guidance of a mentor, maintaining positive motivation by asking for help and using the grapevine to establish unity. Keeping a personal journal helps to track accomplishments.

Table 24–5 Development Plan

Focus Process	Personal	Motivational	Organizational
Assessment	Character trait introspection	Energy levels	Territory:
	Skills inventory:	Failures	People
	Courage	Feelings	Environment
	Communication	Level of hope	Processes
	Risk taking	Degree of synergy	Problems
	Chaos toleration		Organizational goals
	Discovery		Mentor availability

Table 24–5   (continued)

Focus Process	Personal	Motivational	Organizational
	Networking Self care Power sources		Organizational personality Empowerment structure Quality of management
Diagnosis	List deficiencies	Balance of positive and negative feelings Personal dissonance	Is this a learning organization? Disparity between stated values and behavior Staff retention program
Action plan	Start a journal Write your short-term and long-term goals and general strategies for each Write your own orientation plan	Verbalize feelings Spend daily planning time Set routines Celebrate progress	Plan projects Involve others Seek opportunities in decision-making Participate in the organiza- tion's conversation
Implementation	Do your job Personal journal Find a mentor Use affirmations Read, read, read Discover, discover, discover Humor Exercise Stress management Test what you have learned	Personal journal Acknowledge failures Ask for help Use self-help resources Read current literature	Personal journal Find creative opportunities Be proactive Use the grapevine to establish unity Keep your supervisor informed
Evaluation	Personal journal Read your journal Repeat process	Personal journal Read your journal Repeat process	Personal journal Read your journal Repeat process

KEY POINTS

1. Leadership is the art and science of bringing a group of individuals into alignment to accomplish a mission or to establish and reach mutually satisfying goals.

2. Leadership is "the ability to envision a path or direction; to motivate others to follow; to join with others to reach a common goal; to work alone when solo action is called for; to withstand trouble and failure; and to refuse to be crushed by either" (Forman, 2001, p. 4).

3. The skills used by the nurse leader of a patient care team are the same skills used by nurse leaders in other leadership positions. These nurses must (a) envision team needs; (b) identify the contributions that each individual is to make; (c) determine what tasks may be legally and safely delegated; (d) collaborate with others outside the team; (e) negotiate and advocate on behalf of the organization, nurses/nursing, team members, and patients; (f) deal with crises effectively; (g) maintain a personal

balance that sustains the RN and the team throughout the day; and (h) return the day ready to begin again.

4. Mastery of leadership skills at the bedside will form a foundation for future leadership positions.

5. It is the leader's job to establish an environment conducive to collegial work and to bring together a team that will work together efficiently to accomplish the work of the organization.

6. Management is most frequently associated with the control of resources required to accomplish the organizational goals, including budgeting and staffing, with the emphasis on maintaining the functions of the organization while simultaneously balancing fiduciary responsibility for the resources of the organization.

7. Effective leadership involves vision, "thinking outside the box," use of power in positive ways, challenging others to join with the team to accomplish the vision or mission, and creation of a synergistic environment.

8. Poor leadership decreases the productivity of the organization, creates poor morale, leads to attrition, and in the final analysis contributes to poor patient care. The mission and goals of the organization cannot be met when leadership is less than optimal.

9. Partnership, accountability, equity, and ownership will determine the way organization will function in the twenty-first century.

10. Strategic planning is important, but that the plan cannot remain static; it must change, take into account new data, examine the relationships inherent in the system, and allow for the exploration of differences of multiple perspectives of stakeholders in the organization.

11. By empowering the professional members of the health care team, leaders expand the sphere of influence and increase the sense of ownership.

12. The nurse leader's role includes team building, decision-making, communication, negotiation, delegation, and mentorship.

EXPLORE · MediaLink

Critical thinking questions, essay questions, key terms, web links, activities, NCLEX review questions, and more interactive resources can be found on the Companion Website at www.prenhall.com/haynes. Click on Chapter 24 to select activities for this chapter.

REFERENCES

Argyris, C. (1964). *Integrating the individual and the organization*. New York: John Wiley & Sons.

Argyris, C. (1971). *Management and organizational development: The path from XA to YB*. New York: McGraw-Hill.

Bennis, W. (1994). *On becoming a leader*. New York: Addison-Wesley.

Brakey, M. (1991). Are you a good follower? *Nursing '91, 21*(12), 78–81.

Brown, B. (1990). Leadership and followership. *Texas Nursing, 64*(9), 13.

Brown, B. (1991). Leadership and followership. *Pennsylvania Nurse, 46*(3), 36.

Burns, J. M. (1978). *Leadership*. New York: Harper & Row.

Byham, W. (1988). *Zapp! The lightning of empowerment*. New York: Ballantine Books.

Campbell, J., & Kinion, E. (1993). Teaching leadership/followership to RN-to-MSN students. *Journal of Nursing Education, 32*(3), 138–140.

Chapin, F. S. (1924). Socialized leadership. *Social Forces, 3*, 57–60.

Corona, D. (1979). Followership: The indispensable corollary to leadership. *Nursing Leadership, 2*, 5–8.

Davidhizar, R., & Shearer, R. (2002). Taking charge by letting go. *Health Care Manager, 20*(3), 33–38.

DiRienzo, S. (1994). A challenge to nursing: Promoting followers as well as leaders. *Holistic Nursing Practice, 9*, 26–30.

Drucker, P. F. (2001). *The essential Drucker*. New York: HarperCollins.

Fayol, H. (1925). *General and industrial management*. London: Pittman & Sons.

Forman, H. (2001). Nursing leadership with the pen: Two peas in a pod. In H. R. Feldman (Ed.), *Strategies for nursing leadership* (pp. 3–6). New York: Springer.

Guidera, M. K., & Gilmore, C. (1988). Working with people: In defense of followership. *American Journal of Nursing, 88*, 1017.

Gunn, I. (1996). Courageous followership. *Nursing Management, 27*(3), 10.

Hersey, P., & Blanchard, K. (1977). *Management of organizational behavior: Utilizing human resources* (3rd ed.). Englewood Cliffs, NJ: Prentice Hall.

Huber, D. (2000). *Leadership and nursing care management.* Philadelphia, PA: W. B. Saunders.

Kanter, R. M. (1977). *Men and women of the corporation.* New York: Basic Books.

Kelley, R. (1988). In praise of followers. *Harvard Business Review, 66*(3), 142–148.

Kelley, R. (1991). The art and craft of followership. *Health Forum Journal, 34*(10), 56–60.

Kuokkanen, L., & Leino-Kilpi, H. (2000). Power and empowerment in nursing: Three theoretical approaches. *Journal of Advanced Nursing, 31*(1), 235–241.

Laschinger, H. K., & Wong, C. (1999). Staff nurse empowerment and collective accountability: Effect on perceived productivity and self-rated work effectiveness. *Nursing Economics, 17*(6), 308–316.

Lewin, K. (1951). *Field theory in social sciences.* New York: Harper & Row.

Mayo, E. (1953). *The human problems of an industrialized civilization.* New York: Macmillan.

McGregor, D. (1960). *The human side of enterprise.* New York: McGraw-Hill.

Murphy, D. (1990). Followers for a new era. *Nursing Management, 21*(7), 68–69.

Pagonis, W. (1992). The work of the leader. *Harvard Business Review, 70*(6), 118–126.

Palmier, D. (1998). How can the bedside nurse take a leadership role to affect change for the future? *ConceRN, 27*(1), 16–17.

Rippon, S. (2001). Nurturing nursing leadership: How does your garden grow? *Nursing Management, 8*(7), 11–15.

Rippon, S., & Monaghan, A. (2001). Clinical leadership: Embracing a bold new agenda. *Nursing Management, 8*(6), 6–9.

Rowland, H. S., & Rowland, B. L. (1997). *Nursing administration handbook* (4th ed.). Gaithersburg, MD: Aspen.

Stordeur, S., D'hoore, W., & Vandenberghe, C. (2001). Leadership, organizational stress, and emotional exhaustion among hospital nursing staff. *Journal of Advanced Nursing, 35*(4), 533–542.

Strader, M. K. (1995). Role transition to the workplace. In M. K. Strader & P. J. Decker (Eds.), *Role transition to patient care management* (pp. 57–93). Norwalk, CT: Appleton & Lange.

Tannenbaum, R., & Schmidt, W. (1958). How to choose a leadership pattern. *Harvard Business Review, 51*(3), 162–180.

Taylor, F. (1911). *The principles of scientific management.* New York: Harper & Row.

Thomas, D. O. (1995). Speak up! We need good followers, too. *RN, 57*(9), 72.

Valadez, A. M., & Sportsman, S. (1999). Environmental management: Principles from quantum theory. *Journal of Professional Nursing, 15*(4), 209–213.

Vance, C., & Larson, E. (2002). Leadership research in business and health care. *Journal of Nursing Scholarship, 34*(2), 165–171.

Weber, M. (1947). *The theory of social and economic organization.* Translated by A. M. Henderson & T. Parsons. New York: Free Press.

Wheatley, M. J. (1994). *Leadership and the new science.* San Francisco: Berrett-Koehler.

Whittemore, R. (1999). Natural science and nursing science: Where do the horizons fuse? *Journal of Advanced Nursing, 30*(5), 1027–1033.

Wilson, C. K., & Porter-O'Grady, T. (1999). *Leading the revolution in health care* (2nd ed.). Gaithersburg, MD: Aspen.

SUGGESTED READINGS

Bennis, W., & Goldsmith, J. (1997). *Learning to lead: A workbook on becoming a leader.* Reading, MA: Addison-Wesley.

Blanchard, K. P., & Vincent, N. (1988). *The power of ethical management.* New York: William Morrow and Company, Inc.

Brakey, M. (1991). Are you a good follower? *Nursing '91, 21*(12), 78–81.

Campbell, J., & Kinion, E. (1993). Teaching leadership/followership to RN-to-MSN students. *Journal of Nursing Education, 32*(3), 138–140.

Corona, D. (1979). Followership: The indispensable corollary to leadership. *Nursing Leadership, 2*, 5–8.

Hatcher, S., & Laschinger, H. K. (1996). Staff nurses perceptions of power and opportunity and level of burnout: A test of Kanter's structural theory of organizational behavior. *Canadian Journal of Nursing Administration, 9*(2), 74–94.

Laschinger, H. K. (2001). Promoting nurses' health: Effect of empowerment on job strain and work satisfaction. *Nursing Economics, 19*(2), 42–53.

Laschinger, H. K., & Wong, C. (1999). Staff nurse empowerment and collective accountability: Effect on perceived productivity and self-rated work effectiveness. *Nursing Economics, 17*(6), 308–316.

Laschinger, H. K., Wong, C., McMahon, L., & Kaufmann, C. (1999). Leader behavior impact on staff nurse empowerment, job tension and work effectiveness. *Journal of Nursing Administration, 29*(5), 28–30.

Puccio, G. J., & Chimento, M. D. (2001). Implicit theories of creativity: Lay persons' perceptions of the creativity of adaptors and innovators. *Perceptual & Motor Skills, 92*(3 Pt 1), 675–681.

25

Legal Issues for the Nurse Manager

GINNY WACKER GUIDO

"An employer is directly liable for torts caused by his employees against others. The employer could have prevented these torts by reasonable care in hiring, supervising, and, if necessary, firing the tortfeasor."

Hunter v. Allis-Chambers Corporation, *Engine Division, 1986, at 1419*

LEARNING OBJECTIVES

AT THE COMPLETION OF THIS CHAPTER, THE READER WILL BE ABLE TO:

➤ Discuss risk management strategies involving the nurse manager.

➤ Discuss the importance of policy and procedure development as part of risk management strategies.

➤ Apply federal safety regulations, including application of labor codes, to the health care setting.

➤ Describe measures to prevent discrimination and harassment in health care settings.

➤ Describe the impaired employee, including needed crisis management resources.

➤ Analyze employer/employee relationships, including collaborative practice issues, promoting relationships for mutual growth, working with impaired employees, and independent contractor status.

➤ Analyze compensation packages, including evaluation of compensation proposals.

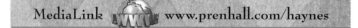

MediaLink www.prenhall.com/haynes

Additional online resources including NCLEX review questions, critical thinking questions, and real-world activities for this chapter can be found on the Companion Website at www.prenhall.com/haynes.

As the chapter opening quote aptly states, the nurse manager is concerned not only with his or her individual competencies, but also with the competencies of health care employees. Employees become the employer's representatives and, because of that special legal status, can impose liability to the employer. As nurses become more independent, serving as independent contractors and entrepreneurs, aspects of legal liability are altered. This chapter addresses risk management strategies and legal concepts vital for nurse managers to understand and apply in health care settings.

Risk Management Strategies

Risk management programs identify, evaluate, and take corrective action against potential risks that could lead to the injury of patients, staff, and/or visitors. Historically, risk management programs have focused on unsafe health care by members of the health care team, informed consent issues, and a person's right to refuse recommended health care options. Thus, risk management programs are problem focused and seek to prevent potential untoward outcomes.

Risk management strategies in health care approximate product liability prevention in industry. Goals of the program are to identify, analyze, and evaluate the potential for risk and then develop a plan to reduce the frequency and severity of these risks. Involving all departments of an organization, risk management is a continuous daily program of detection, intervention, and education. All levels of the health care team are involved in risk management, from the director of nursing to nurse managers and nursing staff members. Box 25–1 outlines the steps of an effective risk management program.

In establishing a risk management program, administration assigns the needed resources to achieve success, a process in which the nursing department plays an integral role. Nurse managers are vital at this level because their participation and commitment ensures daily implementation of the program.

Areas that nurse managers monitor most frequently in risk management programs include: medication administration; complications from procedures; patient falls; patient and/or family dissatisfaction with care, both nursing and medical; and patient refusal of recommended therapy or treatment. Though medical staff may have the primary accountability in some of these areas (e.g., refusal for treatments and procedures and the ordering of needed medications), the nursing staff is often at the front line for implementing risk management interventions. The nurse manager's role in the success of any risk management program is key. He or she continuously evaluates the effectiveness of the current program, educating nursing personnel about the benefits and worth of the program and assuring that all incidents, complaints, and instances of less than competent care are investigated and resolved.

Incident reports are often the starting point for risk management programs. **Incident reports,** sometimes called unusual occurrence reports or variance reports, document unplanned or unexpected occurrences that could potentially affect a patient, family member, or health care provider. Accurate and complete incident reports are essential in protecting the organization and caregiver from potential liability. Synthesizing and analyzing these reports as a group rather than merely looking at individual reports, is often the backbone of an effective risk management program. Once an incident report or verbal complaint is received, the nurse manager should take the following steps:

- Recognize the incident or complaint as important.
- Investigate the incident or complaint in a calm and prompt manner.
- Involve others as needed to fully investigate the occurrence, including relevant staff members and supervisory or mid-level management personnel.
- Follow up with appropriate action. Enact measures to prevent future occurrences.

Prompt care and attention by the nurse manager protects the patients and may actually prevent the filing of a future liability claim. The vast majority of patient and staff concerns can be effectively managed at the nurse manager level and communication is the best tool for resolving those concerns.

A case example illustrating the need to closely monitor occurrences is *Gess v. United States* (1996). In that case, a medical technician, who was in a position to care for infants in the newborn nursery had a history of psychiatric hospitalizations and reports of domestic violence, was tried for injecting newborn infants with lidocaine.

The court in *Gess v. United States* held that an obvious pattern of adverse patient care incidents should have alerted the risk manager that the incidents were neither random nor isolated. The court also held that if the institution had designated a single person to read all incident reports the fact that Gess was the only common denominator would have come to light more quickly. The court emphasized the health care institu-

Box 25–1   Steps in an Effective Risk Management Program

1. Identify potential risks for injury, accidents, or financial loss, using formal and informal lines of communications.
2. Review all sources of organizational-wide monitoring systems, including incident reports, patient and/or family complaints, patient satisfaction surveys, committee minutes, and staff complaints. Determine if additional means of monitoring for risk management are needed and implement such systems as needed.
3. Analyze data collected through monitoring the above reports and oral communications. Look for patterns that may exist and begin to devise means of preventing their future occurrence.
4. Continuously review safety and risk aspects of patient care procedures and treatments, eliminating or reducing risks as much as possible.
5. Monitor pertinent case law and federal codes relating to patient safety, care, and consent issues. Include in this review of pertinent legal issues federal codes concerning the safety of health care workers and ensure that such codes are fully implemented in the agency.
6. Analyze the work of other committees, such as infection control, medical, nursing, and pharmacy audit, and safety/security committees, to determine how their work complements the risk management program being implemented and to ensure that no obvious potential hazards are being overlooked.
7. Identify needs for continuing education regarding risk management and implement such an educational program if needed. Educational program should entail programs designed to include all levels of persons in the agency including patient and family members; auxiliary personnel; nursing and medical staff members; and administrative personnel.
8. Evaluate the effectiveness of the risk management program and provide periodic reports to the appropriate level of administration, including staff nurses.

tion's responsibility to discover and eliminate the cause of such incidents before significant damage had been done. Through careful analysis of incident reports, risk management can become one mechanism that institutions use to alert personnel about suspicious patterns and/or persons causing adverse patient care situations.

Though most incidents may not rise to this level of liability, an institution may discover a pattern of patient falls while evaluating a new type of patient slipper, or an increase in medication errors when a new IV pump is introduced. Reviewing all reports of the same type of incident could show an evolving trend and quickly unveil an unsafe piece of equipment or new patient care garment. Additionally, all incident reports from multiple nursing units should be reviewed, since a pattern may not emerge unless reports from different units are compared.

Vital to the success of any risk management program is having institutional policies and procedures well defined. Written policies and procedures, a requirement set by the Joint Commission on Accreditation of Healthcare Organizations (JCAHO),

set standards of care for the institution, which serve to direct practice. Policies and procedures must be clearly stated, well delineated, and based on current, evidence-based practice. Nurse managers should periodically review the written policies and procedures to ensure their relevancy, currency, and compliance. If policies are outdated or absent, the nurse manager should request that the appropriate committee or risk manager update or initiate a new policy and procedure.

Development of policies and procedures is often based on current research concerning evidence-based practice and standards set by state nurse practice acts and national organizations. For example, individual state nurse practice acts define the functions of licensed nurses and give direction concerning the scope of a nurse's practice. Policies and procedures would then be written to incorporate the scope of the nurse's practice, without requiring nurses to exceed their legal authority. The American Nurses Association issues standards for basic nursing care, as well as care specific standards for given specialty areas. Organizations such as the American Association for Critical Care Nurses and the

Review the policies and procedures of the institution where you work or have educational experiences. How current are they? Are they inclusive of recent changes in the institution or are there unwritten policies and procedures nurses are expected to implement? Are there contradictions between the policies and procedures as written and the actual implementation of the same policies and procedures within the nursing units?

How would you begin to change the current policies and procedures? Do you know the person or committee responsible for the currency and correctness of the policies and procedures?

Emergency Nurses Association publish standards specific to care of patients within those clinical settings and the Oncology Nursing Society and the Association of Neuroscience Nurses publish standards specific to care of patients with those diagnoses.

Federal Safety Regulations

Federal and individual state governments have enacted laws regarding employment. To be legally effective, nurse managers must be familiar with these laws and how the laws affect agency and labor relations. Box 25–2 gives examples of selected federal labor legislation.

By understanding and correctly applying employment laws, nurse managers reduce their potential liability.

Collective Bargaining

Collective bargaining, sometimes referred to as **labor relations,** is the joining together of employees for the purpose of increasing their ability to influence the employer and improve working conditions. Typically, the employer is referred to as management and employees as labor (or more commonly the labor union or union). Persons involved in the hiring, firing, scheduling, disciplining, and evaluating of employees are considered management and may not be part of a collective

---

Box 25–2   Selected Federal Labor Laws

1. Wagner Act or the National Labor Relations Act (1935) established the National Labor Relations Board and unionization in the United States.
2. Taft-Hartley Act or the Labor Management Relations Act (1947) served to equal the balance of power between unions and management and addressed unfair union labor practices.
3. Labor management Reporting and Disclosure Act (1959) enacted further protection for union members and the public against arbitrary action by union officials.
4. Executive Order 10988 (1962) allowed employees of the executive branch to unionize.
5. Civil Rights Act (1964) protected against discrimination due to race and color.
6. Age Discrimination Act (1967) protected against discrimination due to age.
7. Occupational Safety and Health Act (1970) established safe and healthy working conditions.
8. Wagner Amendments (1974) allowed unionization for nonprofit organizations.
9. Americans with Disabilities Act (1990) barred discrimination against disabled workers.
10. Civil Right Act (1991) addressed sexual harassment in the workplace.
11. Family and Medical Leave Act (1993) allowed leaves based on family and medical needs.
12. Ergonomics Program Standard (1999) addressed the issue of work-related musculoskeletal injuries and disorders.
13. Ergonomics Program Standard Repealed (2000).

bargaining unit. Nurse managers may or may not be part of management; if they have hiring and firing authority, then they are considered part of management.

Collective bargaining is defined and protected by the National Labor Relations Act (NLRA) and its multiple amendments. The National Labor Relations Board (NLRB) oversees and enforces the NLRA. The Board ensures that employees are able to choose freely whether they want to be represented by a particular bargaining unit and it serves to prevent or remedy any violation of the labor laws.

While collective bargaining is relatively new to nursing, the American Nurses Association (ANA) has continually supported the right for nurses to bargain collectively. There are two main reasons for this support: (a) collective bargaining allows for achieving the basic elements of professional status and (b) collective bargaining allows a mechanism for nurses to resolve conflicts within the workplace setting, thus enhancing the quality of patient care. Other areas in which collective bargaining can be influential include: basic economic issues such as salary, overtime pay, shift differentials, and benefits; unfair or arbitrary scheduling, staffing, seniority rights, and posting of job openings; and maintenance and promotion of professional practice, including standards of care and adequate staffing ratios.

Those nurse managers confronted with union activity should be aware that there are five categories of unfair labor practices described by the NLRB. These unfair labor practices concern both the organizing phase as well as the actual collective bargaining contract. All are to be avoided. These unfair labor practices include: (a) interference with the employees' right to organize; (b) domination of issues by promising rewards to employees if the union is defeated or threatening pay cuts and demotions if the union is successful; (c) encouraging or discouraging union membership; (d) discharging an employee for giving testimony or filing a grievance with the NLRB; and (e) refusal to bargain collectively. Once the contract has been ratified, there are some issues that nurse managers should know. A thorough understanding and following of the contract provisions can prevent most employee grievances from being filed. Second, treating all persons being supervised with respect and consideration, whether union members or nonmembers, will avoid charges of discrimination and promote morale. Should an issue arise, the nurse manager should act professionally, avoid being defensive, and not succumb to pressure.

The nurse manager should also admit wrong statements or decisions and work collectively toward a better solution, while maintaining institution goals. Assistance from upper-level management should be sought as needed, especially if a conflict cannot readily be resolved. As always the manager should continue to learn more about management principles through formal education or continuing education.

Equal Employment Opportunity Laws

Federal laws have been enacted to ensure equal employment opportunities by prohibiting discrimination based on gender, age, race, religion, disability, national origin, and pregnancy. The Equal Employment Opportunity Commission (EEOC) enforces these laws. Some states have also enacted laws to compliment these federal laws with their own state agencies to enforce them and nurse managers should consider all applicable laws when hiring, firing, disciplining, and assigning staff members.

Perhaps the most significant legislation affecting equal employment opportunities is the Civil Rights Act of 1964, and its amendments (also known as "Title VII"). This act prevents discrimination with respect to compensation, terms, conditions, or privileges of employment because of the individual's race, color, religion, gender, or national origin. Title VII applies to private institutions with 15 or more employees, to state and local governments, labor unions, and employment agencies.

Title VII also protects employees against sexual harassment in the workplace. **Sexual harassment** is unwelcome sexual conduct. It can be requests for sexual favors directly linked to job benefits or opportunities. It can be physical or verbal behavior. It can involve supervisors or co-workers. It can also involve harassment by members of the same sex. Sexual harassment involves any conduct that creates an intimidating, hostile, or offensive environment that interferes with an employee's ability to work (a **"hostile work environment"**). The United States Supreme Court's decisions in *Burlington Industries, Inc. v. Ellerth* (1998) and *Faragher v. City of Boca Raton* (1998) identified two categories of harassment. The first category involves a "tangible employment action," while the second category arises from a hostile environment but does not result in any **"tangible employment action."** Tangible employment actions normally involve financial loss to an employee or a significant change in workload or work assignment. Most episodes of sexual harassment in health care settings typically concern hostile work environment sexual harassment.

A case that shows how nurse managers should respond to complaints of sexual harassment is *Grodzdanich v. Leisure Hills Health Center, Inc.* (1998). In that case, a female staff member brought a charge of hostile work environment sexual harassment against her employer after a male charge nurse had fondled her. While the court agreed that such actions did create a hostile work environment sexual harassment cause of action, there was no liability found against the nursing home. Following notification by the staff nurse that she had been sexually harassed, the nurse manager at the nursing home followed an already disseminated policy on harassment. Within minutes of the complaint, the manager talked with witnesses whom the nurse had identified. The nurse was immediately given the choice to work in another unit, away from the perpetrator, once witnesses had collaborated the nurse's charges. Then, the perpetrator was fired after all charges against him were validated.

The court in this case stressed the need for the employer to take seriously the victim's complaint and act swiftly for the victim's sake as well as avoiding or minimizing potential liability. Such a ruling contrasts with the holding in *Smith v. St. Louis University* (1997) in which the employer took 4 months to speak with the alleged perpetrator. Four months, said the court, did not meet the employer's legal responsibility of prompt remedial action reasonably calculated to end the harassment.

Courts have not mandated the firing of the perpetrator, but have allowed other remedial actions, such as a transfer of the offender to other units or disciplinary warnings. What is important is that some action must be taken and taken promptly.

Nurse managers have an important role in preventing sexual harassment in the workplace. A widely publicized harassment policy is the first important step toward preventing harassment in the workplace and avoiding legal liability. The policy should clearly identify and explain prohibited conduct, indicate there is a "zero tolerance" for such activity, and warn that perpetrators will be severely disciplined or fired. It is also critical that the policy include a confidential complaint procedure, which allows an employee to complain to more than one person. The policy should be posted on a bulletin board or placed on the institution's Internet site so as to be available 24 hours a day. Just as important, nurse managers should ensure that the policy is disseminated to all employees. Managers and supervisors need to know the policy exists and understand the procedure to be followed in dealing with complaints. All complaints should be taken seriously, even if the behavior or comments alleged would not offend all in the workplace. For example, some individuals take offense at the hanging of a Playboy calendar in the lunch area, while other staff members see the same calendar as funny or ridiculous. When one employee considers the calendar display to be offensive, the perception of a hostile work environment is present.

Once a complaint has been voiced, investigate the matter thoroughly and promptly. Ask the person voicing the complaint for witnesses to the event and privately question them about the comment or behavior. If the complaint appears valid, question the perpetrator and initiate appropriate action. Such action could include transferring the perpetrator to another unit or shift or beginning disciplinary measures. If these remedies are beyond the scope of the nurse manager, seek assistance from upper-level management or the appropriate department in the agency.

Harassment and possible legal liability may be avoided if the nurse manager stops any potential offensive behavior or comments the first time he or she becomes aware of it. For example, when the nurse manager overhears staff members telling sexually explicit jokes, that is the time to remind staff that such behaviors and comments are not allowed in the workplace. One of the most effective and proactive ways to prevent sexual harassment is to teach employees about what conduct is prohibited and how to complain if they are subjected to such conduct. In addition, the nurse manager can devise educational sessions, conduct informal staff meetings, or request that the education coordinator plan such a program to teach all staff about sexual harassment in the workplace.

Americans with Disabilities Act of 1990

The Americans with Disabilities Act (ADA) provides protection to persons with disabilities. The purposes of the ADA are to provide a clear and comprehensive national mandate for the elimination of discrimination against disabled persons and to provide a strong, consistent, and enforceable standard addressing discrimination in the workplace. The ADA is closely related to the Civil Rights Act of 1964 and incorporates the antidiscrimination principles established in that act.

The ADA has five sections or titles. The pertinent concerns of each are shown in Table 25–1. Title 1 is the section of the ADA that most concerns workers in the health care industry. This section eliminates discrimina-

Table 25–1	Americans with Disabilities Act of 1990
Title	**Provisions of the Title**
I	Defines the purpose of the act, who is qualified under the act, and employment issues.
II	Concerns services, programs, and activities of public entities as well as public transportation.
III	Addresses public accommodations and services operated by private entities; prohibits discrimination against the disabled in the areas of public accommodations, commercial facilities, and public transportation services.
IV	Attempts to make telephone services accessible to individuals with hearing or speech impediments.
V	Addresses multiple miscellaneous provisions, including certain insurance matters and incorporated this act with other federal and state laws.

Adapted from *42 USC*, 12101 et. seq., 1990.

tion against disabled persons in employment by enforcing equal access to jobs and accommodations. The ADA seeks to assure that no employer, public or private, who employs 15 or more workers, discriminates against a qualified worker who has a disability merely because of the disability. Thus, the ADA attempts to equalize job opportunities for disabled and nondisabled workers, without placing undue hardship on employers.

Disability is defined broadly in the ADA. With respect to an individual, a disability is defined by:

- A physical or mental impairment that substantially limits one or more of the major life activities of the individual

- A record of such impairment (e.g., a diagnosed impairment)
- Being regarded as having such impairment (e.g., viewed by others as disabled)

The overall effect of the law is that persons with disabilities will not be excluded from employment opportunities or adversely affected in any aspect of employment unless they are not qualified or are otherwise unable to perform the essential functions of their job. The ADA protects qualified disabled individuals with regard to job applications, hiring, compensation, advancement, and all other aspects of employment. It applies not only to job applicants, but also to employ-

Research Application

Hernandez, Keys, and Balcazar (2000) reviewed 37 research studies that were published from 1987 to 1999. The authors found that employers, representing a diverse group of American workplaces, continue to express positive global attitudes toward workers with disabilities and that it has become socially appropriate for employers to espouse such attitudes toward the disabled worker. Workers were viewed as dependable, productive, and able to interact with others. These positive views were evident for workers with different types of disabilities, including physical disabilities, epilepsy, and mental and emotional disabili-

ties. Employers of larger companies reported more positive attitudes and hired proportionately more disabled workers than employers of smaller companies.

Although the employers were supportive of ADA as a whole, the employment provision evoked some concern. When appropriate supports are provided, employers continue to have positive attitudes toward workers with intellectual and psychiatric disabilities. Workers with physical disabilities, though, are viewed more positively than those with intellectual or psychiatric disabilities. Employers expressed willingness to hire applicants with disabilities, though this exceeds their actual hiring of disabled workers.

The authors concluded that these positive attitudes and support for the ADA are a significant change from similar studies conducted in the early 1980s. It was unclear, though, if these more positive attitudes stem from personal experiences, lack of information, or from global myths and stereotypes. If the latter is true, then educational programs are needed to assist employers in understanding disabled workers and their potential value to the company. Second, though the gap between those employers with positive attitudes toward this worker and the actual numbers of disabled workers they employ is narrowing, it again speaks to the fact that additional educational programs are needed. The study supports the inclusion of people with disabilities in the workforce as fully as possible. Additional workers could erode these attitudinal barriers and ultimately increase employment opportunities for people with disabilities.

Though not written from the perspective of a health care facility, the research article has implications for health care agencies. Nurse managers are at a pivotal point to begin to assess their own attitudes and those of staff members about disabled workers, developing informational programs to more fully assist staff in understanding the capabilities and assets of workers with disabilities. They are also in a position to ensure that capable, qualified disabled workers are given employment opportunities, thus furthering more positive attitudes about workers with disabilities.

ees who develop a disability during their tenure of employment.

Though the intention of the ADA is straightforward, the difficulties posed by its practical day-to-day application in the workplace is depicted by the sheer number of court cases filed just in the first 10 years since the law was enacted (Guido, 2001). Determining which categories of physical and mental impairment are covered or not covered under the ADA has been the basis of many lawsuits. For example, conditions that some courts have found not to constitute a disability include:

- Lifting disabilities (*Thompson v. Holy Family Hospital,* 1997)
- Depression and anxiety (*Cody v. Cigna Healthcare of St. Louis, Inc.,* 1998)
- Migraine headaches and latex allergies (*Howard v. North Mississippi Medical Center,* 1996)
- Pregnancy (*Jessie v. Carter Health Care Center, Inc.,* 1996)

It is generally held today that physical handicaps as well as diseases affecting the physical condition of the person are covered, including AIDS and HIV infections. Communication and learning disabilities are covered, as are vision impairments. Mental retardation, organic brain syndrome, and emotional and mental illnesses are also covered conditions. The ADA specifically excludes from the definition of who is disabled homosexuality and bisexuality, sexual behavioral disorders, gambling, kleptomania, pyromania, and current use of illegal drugs. Those persons who are still abusing drugs or drinking are not protected under the ADA; recovering alcoholics and drug abusers who are currently enrolled in or have successfully completed a supervised rehabilitation program are protected. Nevertheless, under the ADA, employers can still hold alcoholics to the same employment qualifications and job performance standards as other employees, even if their unsatisfactory behavior or performance is related to the alcoholism [42 USC sec. 12211(a) and (b) and sec. 12114(c)(4)].

While an employee may have a disability covered by the ADA, the employee must still be able to perform the essential functions of his or her particular job in order to be protected under the ADA. The essential functions of a job are defined by the ADA as those job functions that the person must be able to perform in order to be qualified for that employment position. If the disabled person is not able to perform the essential functions of the position, he or she is not qualified (i.e., protected) under the ADA. What constitutes the essential functions of a job is also the subject of many lawsuits. For example, in *Jones v. Kerrville State Hospital* (1998), the court found that an essential function for psychiatric nurses was the ability to restrain patients and in *Laurin v. Providence Hospital and Massachusetts Nurses Association* (1998), the court held that the ability to work rotating shifts was an essential job function of nursing staff members.

The ADA also requires an employer provide reasonable accommodations for a disabled employee so that they may fulfill the requirements of employment. The law does not mandate that the disabled individual be hired before fully qualified, nondisabled persons; rather, it mandates that the disabled not be disqualified merely because of a disability that can be reasonably be accommodated. Reasonable accommodations may include: a leave of absence with or without pay; allowing the employee to work from home for a period of time; providing devices, such as a special telephone for a hearing impaired worker; and assigning other members of the staff to work with the disabled worker as part of a team. Lawsuits regarding what constitutes "reasonable accommodations" are almost as frequent as litigation regarding what constitutes a disability.

As the courts continue to further interpret the ADA, nurse managers are reminded that each day brings additional knowledge of what constitutes a disability, what constitutes the essential job functions of selected nursing positions, and what are reasonable accommodations. Thus, nurse managers are encouraged to stay current in this area of the law and to seek outside advice about the ADA and how it applies in their work environment.

Occupational Safety and Health Act

The Occupational Safety and Health Act (OSHA) was established to ensure a safe and healthy work environment for employees and to preserve human resources. OSHA standards are sets of rules designed to minimize selected on-the-job risks for employees. Those with particular application to nursing and the health care industry include rules that require isolation procedures, protecting areas for containing ionizing radiation,

proper grounding of electrical equipment, protective storage of flammable and combustible liquids, and the gloving of all personnel handling bodily fluids. Under OSHA guidelines, if no federal standards have been established, then state law standards prevail. Three administrative bodies are established under OSHA to enforce its provisions:

1. Occupational Safety and Health Administration, which oversees the creation and enforcement of standards and procedures to enhance employee safety and health
2. National Institute of Occupational Safety and Health, which oversees safety research and makes recommendations to the Occupational Safety and Health Administration
3. Occupational Safety and Health Review Committee, which reviews contested actions by employers cited for noncompliance with OSHA rules

With the increased awareness of HIV/AIDS and the dangers of hepatitis B and now C, OSHA began publishing regulations in 1991 designed to reduce workplace risks of infection from exposure to bloodborne pathogens. Steps required by OSHA include:

- Developing an exposure control plan to minimize or eliminate risks from exposure
- Making hepatitis B vaccine available to all at risk employees
- Ensuring that employees are tested and provided with follow-up treatment and counseling after exposure
- Implementing engineering and work practice control to minimize or eliminate risks in the workplace
- Storing or maintaining sharps or contaminated materials in the way prescribed by regulation

Critical Thinking and Reflection

What are the essential job functions for the staff nurses and nurse managers in area health care institutions? Write a list of the essential job functions for a nurse manager within a selected health care setting, giving rationale for each of the essential job functions.

What accommodations could disabled nurses reasonably expect when applying for a nurse manager position? Is it essential that a nurse manager

position be fully mobile or could a wheelchair bound individual serve in the role of nurse manager?

How do you think the members within the health care setting you are familiar with would respond to a disabled worker or student? How would you change this attitude so that a disabled worker or student would be accepted in the workplace, if the answer to the first part of this question would be negative?

- Affixing biohazard labels to containers to warn employees and the public that the contents are contaminated wastes
- Providing educational programs to all new employees and on a yearly basis thereafter
- Maintaining accurate and confidential records relating to employee education, immunization, and management of exposures (White, 1992)

A newer area in OSHA standards, the *Ergonomics Program Standard*, initially became law on January 16, 2001. That standard was created to address work-related musculoskeletal disorders (MSDs) that result from mismatch between a worker's physical capacity and the physical demands of the workplace. Ergonomics, defined as the science of fitting the job to the worker, is seen as one way to prevent this mismatch.

The new OSHA standard required the employer provide its employees with certain basic information:

- Common MSDs, their signs and symptoms
- The importance of reporting MSDs as soon as possible
- How to report MSDs in the workplace
- Risk factors, job and work activities associated with MSD hazards
- A brief description of OSHA's ergonomics standard (*CFR 29*, Standard 1910.900, 2000)

However, with a projected cost to employers in excess of $4.5 billion annually, that standard was soon repealed (March 6 and 7, 2001), with future plans to develop a more cost-effective approach. While that OSHA standard is no longer in effect, the 2-month window when the standard was law illustrates how nurse managers should be aware of laws that affect the workplace.

Family and Medical Leave Act of 1993

The Family and Medical Leave Act (FMLA) is designed to balance the demands of the workplace with the demands of the family. This act allows employed individuals to take unpaid leaves of absence from work for their own serious health problems; for the care of a spouse, child, or parent who has serious health problems; or for the birth or adoption of a child. This federal law was initially passed because of the ever-increasing numbers of single parent and two-parent households with parents working full time, thus placing parenting needs and job security at odds. Additionally, the law also helps with some of the demands placed on working adults by their aging parents. The law is gender neutral and allows both men and women the same leave provisions.

However, the law applies only to employers with 50 or more employees. Additionally, to be eligible, the employee must have worked for at least 12 months and for at least 1,250 hours during the preceding 12-month period. The eligible employee may take up to 12 weeks of unpaid leave, after exhausting all or part of any paid vacation time, personal leave, or sick leave the employer may provide. Equally important, the employer must continue the employee's health insurance benefits during the leave, and guarantee employment in the same job or comparable job when the employee returns to work. Employees must give their employer 30 days' notice or whatever shorter notice as is practical in emergency cases. Nurse managers should be familiar with the FMLA and offer assistance to employees who might qualify for such a leave of absence, since employers are expected to know whether or not an employee's request or situation qualifies for family medical leave or not.

Employment-at-Will and Wrongful Discharge

Historically, employment relationships have been considered a "free-will" relationship. Basically, the **"employment-at-will"** concept has meant that an employee was free to quit a job at any time and an employer was free to hire or fire employees for any reason. Over time, exceptions to this employment-at-will doctrine evolved, most notably through collective bargaining agreements by labor unions and also specific exceptions under some federal and state laws.

One area of exceptions are those based on public policy. These exceptions involve cases in which an employee's firing directly conflicts with a state's public policy, such as firing an employee for serving on a jury, for reporting an employer's illegal actions (sometimes called "whistle-blower"), or for filing a worker's compensation claim (Pozgar, 1999). A second area of exceptions involves situations in which courts have "implied" that a contract exists between an employer and employee, even though no specific written contract has been signed. Contracts limit an employer's right to fire an employee. Courts in some states treat employee handbooks, company policies, and oral statements made at the time a person was hired as "implied" contracts. A third area is referred to as "good faith and fair dealing" exceptions, which prevents unfair or malicious terminations, but are not favored by the courts. In *Fortune v. National Cash Register Company* (1997), an employee was discharged just before a contract was signed between his employer and another company, which would have entitled the employee to a large commission. The court in that case held the employer had discharged the employee in bad faith, solely to avoid payment of the employee's commission.

Nurse managers should familiarize themselves with state and federal laws concerning employment-at-will and wrongful discharge. Nurse managers should review the employer's internal policies, especially employee handbooks and employee recruiting brochures for statements implying job security or other unintentional promises and bring these to the attention of upper level management. Interactions with job applicants should not imply job security or unintentionally promise job benefits to potential employees. To prevent successful lawsuits by employees for wrongful discharge or retaliation, nurse managers must carefully monitor the treatment of any employee who has filed a job-related complaint, to ensure that his or her performance evaluations are accurate (and not biased), performed according to policy, and placed in the appropriate files.

Independent Contractor

An **independent contractor** performs services for another person or entity, but that other person or entity does not have the right to control the details of how the independent contractor performs his or her job. In health care settings, independent contractor status usually applies to private-duty nurses, selected advance practice roles, and selected physicians. For example, many institutions employ emergency care nurse practitioners or physicians to staff emergency centers, especially at night or on weekends. From a liability standpoint, the key issue is control or the right to control. In other words, can the actions (or misdeeds) of an independent contractor be imputed to the agency because the health care agency had the right to control the work setting and thus the worker?

As with all roles in nursing or medicine, individuals are responsible and accountable for their own actions. If an independent contractor is negligent in providing care and that patient successfully sues for malpractice, the independent contractor will be liable for damages to the patient. But the health care agency employing that negligent independent contractor may also be liable to the patient, under what is known as the doctrine of "apparent agency." Courts employ four criteria to determine if the doctrine of apparent agency applies. The first criterion is subjective and looks at whether outsiders or third parties see the person as an employee of the institution. In the case of the emergency care nurse practitioner, the court might look to whether or not the patient or the patient's family member saw (or assumed) that nurse was a hospital employee.

The second criterion centers on whether or not the independent contractor is furthering the "primary function" of the employer. For example, nurse practitioners employed as independent contractors to staff an emergency center are normally and easily viewed as furthering the primary function of the institution (i.e., patient care).

The third criterion, "reliance," involves the faith that a patient places in the institution's judgment. If an institution contracts with an emergency care nurse practitioner to perform certain services, the patient and family members assume the agency has investigated the nurse practitioner's credentials and skills and the nurse practitioner is fully competent to perform the role of an emergency care provider.

Finally, control is the fourth criterion in determining whether or not an independent contractor is the apparent agent of an institution. To determine who had the greater control, courts look at the following factors:

- The extent to which the employer determines the details of the work and work settings
- Whether the work is supervised by the employer or the independent contractor is free to perform the work in whatever manner he or she deems appropriate
- Who supplies the instruments, equipment, and materials needed to perform the work
- The actual workplace
- Benefits given the independent contractor, if any
- The method of payment

The more control an institution has over these factors, the more likely it is that a court will hold the institution liable for injuries or damages caused by the independent contractor.

In theory, a nurse who is an independent contractor is solely liable for his or her actions, which relieves the institution from any liability. However, in reality, courts frequently find institutions liable for the negligence or intentional misconduct of independent contractors working there. In *Hansen v. Caring Professionals, Inc.* (1997), the court determined that a nurse was an independent contractor because she paid her own employment taxes, received a Form 1099 rather than a W-2 form, and paid for her own worker's compensation insurance. However, since the hospital where she worked controlled the patients who were assigned to her care and directly supervised the nurse's performance, the hospital was also found to be liable for the patient's injury caused by the nurse.

Given the potential for liability, nurse managers are urged to ensure that any independent contractors in the workplace know the institution's policies and procedures have the same requirements for in-service and other educational offerings that staff members have, and that their work is appropriately supervised. Additionally, assigning a resource person to serve as a mentor to an independent contractor may also prevent problems caused by the independent contractor's lack of knowledge about policies and procedures. When the nurse manager has reason to suspect that the quality of care given by the independent contractor is substandard or likely to cause patient injury, the nurse manager must intervene to protect the patient.

◾ Impaired Employee: Crisis Management Resources

Substance abuse by health care members places both patients and organizations at risk. A chemically dependent staff member affects morale, jeopardizes patient care, and increases his or her employer's potential liability. Early recognition of substance abuse, including alcohol and drug dependency, followed by prompt referral for treatment are responsibilities of nurse managers. The nurse manager is cautioned to know his or her employer's expectations since institution policy may vary greatly concerning who first speaks with the employee suspected of abusing alcohol or drugs and who makes referrals.

One of the first steps is recognizing the signs and symptoms of substance abuse. Typically, the initial reaction of an impaired employee is to deny having a problem. Since an employee without a substance abuse problem would react the same way, identifying the person requiring assistance may not be readily apparent.

Once a nurse with a substance abuse problem has been identified, careful documentation is essential. Documentation supporting the existence of substance abuse could include (a) records of absenteeism and tardiness, especially if these are recent problems and escalating in occurrence; (b) records of patient complaints regarding ineffective medications or poor quality nursing care; (c) records of controlled substance usage; (d) complaints by other staff members regarding patient care delivered by this individual nurse; and (e) any signs and symptoms that the nurse manager may have noted. Dates, times, and behaviors should be well documented, since it is the pattern of behavior, not the isolated incident, that identifies whether a problem exists.

Before intervening, the nurse manager should carefully review the institution's policy and procedure manual for guidance, since state laws vary in what must be reported, to whom it is reported, and the existence of peer (or employee) assistance programs. Such peer assistance programs, also called diversion programs, offer referral, assistance, and monitoring, rather than disciplinary actions.

Prompt and appropriate assistance increases the chance to assist the recovery of the chemically dependent nurse. Appropriate resources to assist the chemically dependent nurse should be identified. These include an employee assistance program (if one exists within the institution), assistance from other nurses recovering from alcohol or drug abuse who have offered to help, and the names and phone numbers of treatment centers or support groups that exist in the community, such as Alcoholics Anonymous or Narcotics Anonymous. It is essential that several sources be provided so that the chemically dependent nurse can receive support from someone the individual is comfortable working with and who knows what the nurse is experiencing.

Moreover, the nurse manager's own attitude is also important throughout this process. Often, nurse managers can be frustrated, have little patience, or be downright hostile toward a nurse with a substance abuse problem, especially where there have been problems on the job over a long period of time. Managers can best help this person and the staff understand that chemical abuse is an illness, and that the person can be helped to full recovery. Allowing the staff to vent their feelings about the situation as well as educating them about treatment for substance abuse may provide a supportive setting for the recovered individual's return to work on the same unit.

Collaborative Practice Issues: Promoting Relationships for Mutual Growth

The continuous advancement of technology and the ever-increasing complexity of health care settings provide health care practitioners with more opportunities for developing collaborative practices. Collaborative practice opportunities occur between medical and nursing members of the health care team, among nurses who work together in clinical practice settings, and also among nurses and nursing management. One type of collaborative practice employs team building or team development. Team building promotes productivity and effectiveness of individuals, and in so doing, assists the overall delivery of competent, high-level health care.

Nurse managers play vital roles in developing effective collaborative work relationships, so all members of the health care team work at the highest level of performance. To foster collaboration the nurse manager promotes (a) open, clear, and effective communication; (b) well-defined and attainable goals; and (c) trust and collegiality (Antai-Otong, 1997). Attainment and maintenance of these qualities allows for mutual growth of all team members and delivery of quality health care in all clinical settings.

Case management enhances collaborative practice. As the health care system becomes more interdependent, with shared planning, goal setting, decision-making, interventions, and problem solving, case management plays a larger role (Sullivan, 1998). "Case management is a collaborative process that assesses, plans, implements, coordinates, monitors, and evaluates options and services to meet an individual's health needs through communication and available resources to promote quality cost-effective outcomes" (Case Management Society of America, 1995, p. 1). Box 25–3 presents some of the varied goals of case management.

Nursing case management organizes patient care by major diagnoses and focuses on attaining predetermined patient outcomes within specific time frames, using specific resources (Zander, 1992). One of the more important concepts within this approach is the promotion of professional growth, among both nurses and the interdisciplinary health care team members. Using this approach, all members of the health care delivery team are equal, and all members agree on the development of critical pathways, take ownership of patient outcomes, and accept responsibility and accountability for patient interventions. The nursing care manager directs and coordinates the case management process.

A third approach to collaborative practice involves the practice partnership model. In this model, professional and nonprofessional nursing members become partners, working the same schedules and caring for a single group of patients. The professional nurse directs the work of the junior partner within the limits of the

---

Box 25–3   Selected Goals of Case Management

1. Ensure, through early assessment, that services are initiated in a timely manner.
2. Assist patients to achieve an optimal level of wellness by facilitating timely and appropriate health care delivery.
3. Assist patients to be decision makers to the degree that is possible.
4. Enhance employee productivity, satisfaction, and retention.
5. Promote competent, quality health care, focusing on holistic care of patients.
6. Achieve expected or standardized patient outcomes, using critical pathways to achieve these goals in a timely and cost-effective manner.
7. Promote collaborative practice and mutual growth.
8. Promote professional development and satisfaction among members of the interdisciplinary team.
9. Promote patient and family satisfaction with health care delivery.
10. Assist patients to be more cognizant of their role in improving and maintaining their health status.

What collaborative practice models might be employed in health care organizations in your area? How are these models superior to what is currently in use? How would you begin to implement a new collaborative practice model?

What types of collaborative practice models are in place in health care settings where you practice? Are they being utilized to promote the individual growth of staff members or merely as a means to ensure more efficient patient care?

state nurse practice act (Manthey, 1989). This model encourages the mutual growth of the partners while increasing the continuity of care and accountability for patient care.

None of these approaches are ideal. Moreover new methods for competent and effective delivery of health care will develop in the future. It is likely all models will include collaborative practice as a primary mode of health care delivery. Well-prepared nurse managers will be aware of current developments in collaborative practice, understanding the benefits of this type of system, as well as the advantages of one approach holds over another, so it can be adapted to the unique qualities of an individual institution. Nurse managers provide the leadership and mentorship skills needed to ensure the success of collaborative practice methodologies.

Compensation Packages

As nursing has expanded into multiple health care settings, the idea of a "traditional" nurse employed by one institution, working a 40-hour week is no longer the norm. Flexibility and creativity are now the watch words that best describe today's employment options.

Before exploring different options, nurses should understand what an employment contract is and how it is made. A contract is a legally binding agreement made between two or more persons to do or refrain from doing certain actions. For contracts to be enforceable, they must have four essential features:

1. Promises or agreements to perform a certain action or restraint from doing certain actions
2. Mutual understanding of the terms and meanings of the contract
3. Compensation in the form of something valuable in exchange for a person's action
4. Fulfill a lawful purpose

Aside from how much a nurse would be paid, provisions in an employment contract of particular concern to nurses might include:

- Working schedules
- Provisions for paid time off
- Holidays, float policies
- Philosophy of nursing and style of nursing care delivered (e.g., primary or team nursing)
- Collective bargaining agreements
- Leave of absence for medical leave or jury duty
- Seniority within the institution
- Grievance procedures

This is certainly not a complete list. Nurses may also negotiate for mileage allowance if they work in community settings, paid continuing education hours if the state has mandatory continuing education as part of the licensing process, or paid educational leave. Nurses may also negotiate for on-site child care services and paid professional liability insurance. Whatever the parties agree to, once an agreement has been formed these provisions become binding on the nurse and the employer.

Traditionally, the compensation package offered to nurses in health care settings included a set salary (usually calculated per hour of work), a fixed number of paid holidays per year, overtime pay at either the set salary rate or time and-a-half, and personal time (including sick time and paid vacation time—based on a fixed amount of hours per pay period). For example, nurses might earn 4 hours of paid personal time per pay period. Most institutions included insurance benefits in their basic package, with additional insurance and retirement options. There was little to evaluate using this system, as there was no negotiation (essentially a "take it or leave it" proposition) and everyone had the same basic package.

With the advent of a widespread nursing shortage and more nurses desiring less fixed packages, institutions began offering more part-time and less restrictive options. For example, nurses began to negotiate for "per diem" work, an option that allowed nurses to work when they wanted to work, usually for a salary at a higher hourly rate but without the benefits of accrued paid personal time or sick leave options. This option did not guarantee the nurse a certain amount of work per pay period, but was seen by many nurses as the perfect means to supplement their income or allow them more time with their family. Since this was often the choice of a "working wife" whose husband had full insurance coverage, many opted for "per diem" work. This arrangement also allowed individual nurses to set their own schedules, including prolonged vacations or time away from work for other reasons.

Some institutions, desperate to fill weekend shifts, also began to offer weekend work options. In these options, the nurse typically worked less than 40 hours per week (e.g., either 32 or 24 hours per weekend), but was eligible for full employment benefits. While salary was commensurate with the actual number of hours worked, the nurse still received all benefits (such as health insurance) of a full-time employee. Of course, the main drawback of this system was the nurse's commitment to work every weekend. Many evaluated this option as ideal for students working on further degrees in nursing or other fields or for those nurses who had other obligations during the week. Health care institutions saw this as a "win–win" solution; staffing improved dramatically, and full-time weekday nurses no longer complained about working weekends. As the numbers of advanced practice nurses also increased, some contracts began to be negotiated with pay based on a percentage of profit. Essentially, this model offers to the advanced nurse practitioner or nurse anesthetist the ability to share in the profits of the corporation or partnership. A nurse's salary under this model is often determined by taking the total monies received by the business, subtracting the total cost of overhead and outside consultation, and multiplying the difference by the particular percentage negotiated in the nurse's contract. This model works well for nurses who have been in practice for some time and do not depend on a fixed salary per pay period, since payments received will fluctuate from month to month depending on the earnings and outside consultation costs required for complex patients. This model usually establishes no set benefits, rather the individual nurse pays their own health insurance costs and any additional expenditures, such as workers compensation insurance premiums, and continuing education costs.

Some advanced practice nurses negotiate for a fixed (base) salary, plus a percentage of profit. This hybrid model not only assures the nurse a certain fixed monthly income, but also provides additional compensation should the nurse's work generate income to the employer in excess of a predetermined amount. Sometimes benefits are part of this model, but it depends on what the parties are willing to negotiate before the nurse is hired. Nurses willing to work under this arrangement require a predetermined amount of salary per pay period but who also want to have their labors rewarded by sharing in their employer's profits.

Compensation packages will continue to be as creative as the nurses who desire more flexibility and options. Nurse managers should remember that while the nurse and his or her employer are free to negotiate the terms to suit their needs, once the terms of the contract are agreed to by both parties, those contract terms can be enforced in a court of law.

TRANSITION INTO PRACTICE

Comprehending that the role of the nurse manager is threefold, incorporating leader, manager, and follower characteristics, is the beginning of becoming an effective manager. Role transition into nursing manager positions involves understanding that the leading role creates an interface which allows for supporting innovation, discussing concerns, solving problems, and dreaming about new possibilities (Porter-O'Grady, 1997). The nurse who assumes the role of manager must have a good understanding of the persons being led, including their individual capabilities, strengths, and expectations. The new manager must also understand these same characteristics about his or her new peer group, determining how their strengths and expectations compliment one's own qualities and expectation.

In the role of leader, the nurse manager learns to be an expert listener, understanding not only what is being discussed, but also what is not being discussed. The nurse manager becomes an encourager, a motivator, and a developer, thus encouraging staff and peers to excel in their productivity and expectations. The nurse manager is a supporter and a problem solver, assisting personnel in striving for excellence while using the most expeditious means of attaining that excellence. "People skills" are essential to this part of the role. The nurse manager should spend some time in assessing these skills, improving on those where improvement is needed and using all the skills to the best advantage of patient care and staff development.

The role of manager involves linking the team or nursing unit to the larger organization. The nurse manager interfaces with persons being supervised, peers, administrators, and to some extent, regulating agencies. This part of the nurse manager role involves using organizational skills such as budgeting, hiring, evaluating, reporting, and communication competence. It also involves knowing current aspects of labor law and codes and ensuring that all comply with the current laws. The nurse manager is both an expert listener and informer since much of management entails effective communications.

The nurse manager is also a follower, working with supervisors and peers. This portion of the role involves contributing to the effectiveness of the whole institution, implementing effective interventions, and seeing that assignments are completed. Respect for others' authority and working within the system to attain organizational outcomes are essential. The recognition of accountability and responsibility that nurse managers have to those in higher organizational positions is vital to the success of the nurse manager.

Continuously striving to improve as leader, manager, and follower is essential for one to become an effective nurse manager. The nurse manager must be able to recognize that any one of these parts of the role may be more important at different times, but that one must excel in all in order to be successful as a manager.

KEY POINTS

1. Risk management programs identify, evaluate, and take corrective action against potential risks that could lead to the injury of patients, staff, and/or visitors.

2. Accurate and complete incident reports are essential to protect the institution and care giver from potential liability. The group synthesis and analysis of these reports provide the backbone of an effective risk management program.

3. Vital to the success of a risk management program are written policies and procedures, which set the standards of care for the institution and serve to direct practice.

4. Nurse managers must be familiar with federal and state employment laws, including how the laws affect agency and labor relations in order to ensure corporate and personal liability.

5. The most significant legislation affecting equal employment opportunities is Title VII of the Civil Rights Act of 1964, as amended, which prevents discrimination with respect to compensation, terms, conditions, or privileges of employment because of the individual's race, color, religion, gender, or national origin.

6. The Americans with Disabilities Act provides a clear and national mandate for the elimination of discrimination against disabled persons and provides a strong, consistent, and enforceable standard addressing discrimination in the workplace.

7. The Occupational Safety and Health Act was established to ensure a safe and healthy work environment for employees and to preserve human resources.

8. The Family and Medical Leave Act of 1993 attempts to balance the demands of the workplace and the demands of the family, allowing employees to take unpaid leaves of absence for medical reasons, for themselves or for the care of a spouse, child, or parent who has serious health problems or for the birth or adoption of a child.

9. Substance abuse by health care workers affects staff morale, jeopardizes patient care, and increases the employer's potential liability for the mistakes and actions of the chemically dependent worker.

10. Compensation packages offer nurses the ability to be more flexible and creative in their discipline and afford nurses the opportunity to negotiate for work schedules, benefits, and scheduled hours.

Critical thinking questions, essay questions, key terms, web links, activities, NCLEX review questions, and more interactive resources can be found on the Companion Website at www.prenhall.com/haynes. Click on Chapter 25 to select activities for this chapter.

REFERENCES

Antai-Otong, D. (1997). Team building in a health care setting. *American Journal of Nursing, 97*(7), 48–51.

Burlington Industries Inc. v. Ellerth, 118 S. Ct. 2257, 1998.

Case Management Society of America. (1995). *Standards of practice for case management.* Little Rock, AR: Author.

CFR 29, Standard 1910.900 (2000).

Cody v. Cigna Healthcare of St. Louis, Inc., 139 F.3d 595 (8th Cir., 1998).

Faragher v. City of Boca Raton, 118 S. Ct. 2275, 1998.

Fortune v. National Cash Register Company, 272 Mass. 96, 264 N.E. 2d 1251 (1997). 42 USC 12101 et. seq., 12211 (a) and (b), and 12114(c)(4), (1990).

Gess v. United States, 952 F.Supp. 1529 (M.D. Ala., 1996).

Grodzdanich v. Leisure Hills Health Center, Inc., 25 F.Supp. 2d 953 (D. Minn., 1998).

Guido, G. W. (2001). *Legal and ethical issues in nursing* (3rd ed.). Upper Saddle River, NJ: Prentice Hall Health.

Hansen v. Caring Professional, Inc., 676 N.E. 2d 1349 (Ill. App., 1997).

Hernandez, B., Keys, C., & Balcazar, F. (2000). Employer attitudes toward workers with disabilities and their ADA employment rights: A literature review. *Journal of Rehabilitation, 66*(4), 4–16.

Howard v. North Mississippi Medical Center, 393 F.Supp. 505 (N.D. Miss., 1996).

Hunter v. Allis-Chambers Corporation, Engine Division, 797 F.2d 1417 (Cir. App. 7, 1986).

Jessie v. Carter Health Care Center, Inc., 926 F.Supp. 613 (E.D. Ky., 1996).

Jones v. Kerrville State Hospital, 142 F.3d 263 (5th Cir., 1998).

Laurin v. Providence Hospital and Massachusetts Nurses Association, 150 F.3d 52 (1st Cir., 1998).

Manthey, M. (1989). Practice partnership: The newest concept in care delivery. *Journal of Nursing Administration, 19*(2), 33–35.

Pozqar, G. D. (1999). *Legal aspects of health care administration* (7th ed.). Gaithersburg, MD: Aspen.

Porter-O'Grady, T. (1997). Quantum mechanics and the future of health care leadership. *Journal of Nursing Administration, 27*(1), 15–20.

Smith v. St. Louis University, 109 F.3d 1261 (8th Cir., 1997).

Sullivan, T. (1998). Concept analysis, Part 1. In Collaboration: A health care imperative (pp. 1–42). New York: McGraw-Hill.

Thompson v. Holy Family Hospital, 122 F.3d 537 (9th Cir., 1997).

White, L. C. (1992). Protecting workers from pathogens. *Health Progress, 4*, 38–42.

Zander, K. (1992). Focusing on patient outcome: Case management in the 90s. *Dimensions of Critical Care Nursing, 11*(3), 127–129.

SUGGESTED READINGS

Benda, C., & Rozovsky, F. (1998). *Liability and risk management in managed care.* Gaithersburg, MD: Aspen.

Guido, G. W. (2001). *Legal and ethical issues in nursing* (3rd ed.). Upper Saddle River, NJ: Prentice Hall Health.

Hughes, T. L. (1995). Chief nurse executives responses to chemically dependent nurses. *Nursing Management, 26*(3), 37–40.

Iversen, J. K. (1997). Combined incident and quality management report. *Home Health Care Management and Practice, 9*(6), 57–78.

Lundy, M. C. (1997). How nurses can organize for the purposes of collective bargaining. *Revolution, 7*(4), 38.

Ponte, P. R., Fay, M. S., Brown, P., Doyle, M., Peron, J., Lizzi, L., & Barrett, C. (1998). Factors leading to a strike vote and strategies for reestablishing relationships. *Journal of Nursing Administration, 28*(2), 35–43.

Epilogue: Toward the Future

Daniel J. Pesut PhD RN CS FAAN

To create a preferred future, nursing needs nurse leaders with foresight. The profession needs nurses who are lifetime learners, attuned to emerging trends. Resilient, curious, creative, and courageous nurses are needed. Nursing also needs clinical scholars who act on values that support their visions. Nursing needs individuals who commit time, energy, and talents to looking ahead and are willing to see the future as full of opportunity rather than full of threats, danger, and anxiety (Bower, 2000). To be an effective leader, one needs to learn about and appreciate the role that future study plays in one's professional commitments and career development (Chaska, 2001; Sullivan, 1999). One also needs to do the inner work required to support personal and professional transformation that enhances the commitment to professional ideals, aspirations, and service (Pesut, 2001).

In order to have vision one needs to use one's values and beliefs as a guide to contrast the present reality with a desired future. The juxtaposition of both the probable and preferred future creates tension and opportunities that are mediated and resolved through thoughtful analysis and action. A preferable future is what nurses want to have happen by creating it. In order to do this it is useful to connect with those in the futurist community and to learn how to think like a futurist (Pesut, 2001, 2000, 1999a, 1999b, 1997a, 1997b, 1997c). Future thinking has consequences for education, practice, research and personal and professional development (Sullivan, 1999; Sullivan & Pesut, 1999).

Responding to the Future

Responding to the future is a matter of awareness, choice, and action. To what degree do individuals create the future they desire? Much of what happens depends on one's responses to emerging trends. Using trend-based information to develop personal and professional plans supports proactive individuals who can take advantage of opportunities that are evolving. Nurses who consider future trends as decision variables that demand engagement, choice, and action are in a position to positively influence the future of the profession. An individual's response to the future can be reactive or proactive. The essential tension between the present and a desired future creates the energy, commitment, and momentum for change and work excitement. Responding to the future is a matter of learning and engaging in strategic conversations that stimulate and enhance professional learning. Scenarios about the future support the initiation of strategic conversations and learning about the future (Van der Heijden, 1996). Future trends will have consequences on professional nursing (Porter-O'Grady, 2001). Consider how thinking about and responding to the following scenarios stimulates ideas and conversations about the future of the nursing profession.

Nursing 2020: Scenarios and Strategic Conversations

Canadian nurse-futurist Martha Rogers (1997) was commissioned to develop five scenarios about Canadian nursing in the year 2020. These scenarios used emerging trends to paint different pictures and stories about possible nursing futures in Canada. The stories that Rogers developed can easily be applied to nursing in the United States. Consider each of these scenarios and a professional nursing response to each. What kind of strategic conversation does each story suggest?

The title of the first 2020 scenario is *Technology Eclipses Care*. In this story, health care and health management are technology driven. Hospitals are high-tech

543

centers. Sensors, monitors, and voice-activated equipment and smart machines monitor and adjust care parameters. Genetic engineering decreases or eliminates disease development. For example, enzymes dissolve organs like the appendix and gallbladder. A cast of health supporters that include massage therapists, palliative care assistants, elder care assistants, health communication specialists, and child development specialists emerge and support health initiatives. Nursing disappears. Analysis reveals that the reason for the nursing profession demise was rooted in the fact that nurses defined practice as a set of skills and tasks rather than a profession supported and sustained in knowledge-based service, care, and evidence.

Consider a second 2020 scenario entitled *Control, Manage, and Measure*. In this scenario, because of debt, social programs are eliminated. The business of health care is organized around programs of managed care. Health activities are centralized. Genetic fingerprints result in predicted illness patterns. People are given personalized care maps based on genetic analysis. Compliance is monitored via a personal health record, called a "smart card." People who do not follow the care map are required to finance their own health care. Physicians are directors of medical teams and choose which individuals will be hired. Nurses on teams decrease in number because others are less expensive. A small band of nurses continue to exist believing in the power of nursing. However, most decisions are made through an economic, rather than social, values-based decision-making lens.

The title of the third 2020 scenario is *Return to Care*. Social, political, and economic stability lead to "values-based" politics. Health becomes a value. Resources are shifted from illness care to health care. Some believe nursing needs to be replaced with more cost-effective workers. However, the panacea of managed care did not realize its promise. In fact, managed care contributed to increases in morbidity, mortality, and consumer dissatisfaction. Nursing studies contributed knowledge and evidence that supported the achievement of health outcomes by nurses. Healing rooms and lay learning centers accelerate healing and maintain health. Collective political action results in nursing education reforms, and the value of health and nursing are supported because evidence and knowledge contribute to respect and appreciation of nursing's contributions to the health politics of the time.

In a fourth 2020 scenario titled *The Transformation*, society discovers caring, and spiritual development begets better health and a meaningful life. The quest for balance results in appreciation of diversity, balance in work and play, and a renewed interest in the concept of community. People conclude that not everything can be measured. The mystery of life is valued. Boundaries between health disciplines blur and are replaced by educational programs for healing and health. Healing competencies are documented on smart cards. The international exchange of ideas contributes to global health.

Of course, there is a fifth scenario, and that is the one that each nurse wants to create based on his or her understanding and professional aspirations for the future. Creating and sharing stories about what nurses want to see happen and what nurses do not want to see happen is an important professional activity and responsibility. Rogers (1997) suggests, when thinking of scenarios, the following questions guide thinking, reacting, and strategic learning conversations:

- How plausible does the scenario seem?
- What thoughts does it bring to mind?
- What feelings, if any, does it generate?
- What are the implications for society, health, health care, and nursing?
- If parts of the scenario are desirable, what actions need to be taken to increase the chances of the scenario happening?
- If parts are undesirable what actions should be taken to prevent them from happening?

Rogers (1997) writes,

> Every nurse has the capability to influence the future: to create a positive future for the profession as well as health, and health care of those we serve. To make informed decisions and choices we need to think about the future beyond tomorrow and or the next day. We need to explore the possibilities, both good and bad. We need to use our minds, hearts, and imagination to generate images of the future, use our voice, hands and feet to create our destiny. (p. vi)

Slow Death versus Deep Change

Robert Quinn (1996) notes that the major dilemma professionals face in organizational life is the issue of slow death versus deep change. Slow death is evident in an organization when people fail to anticipate and actively participate in personal, professional, and organizational renewal. A nurse recognizes slow death when he or she hears other health care providers talk about burnout or hears individuals say, "I don't want to rock the boat." Slow death exists when self-interests triumph over collective professional responsibilities. One can recognize slow death in an organization when people cope by pulling back, withdrawing, or staying busy with insignificant things. Slow death is apparent when people exhibit signs and symptoms of hopelessness and helplessness and feel trapped by their circumstances. Slow death creeps in when people do not have aspirations for a desirable future. Quinn (1996) defines three basic organizational lifestyles to which one can commit: a technical, transactional, or transformational organizational lifestyle.

If one chooses to commit to a technical organizational lifestyle, one becomes an individual contributor to the technical success of the organization. Personal survival is a key objective of a technical lifestyle commitment. Development of technical skills and competencies is a priority. Pride in technical competence is the aspiration.

If one commits to a transactional organizational lifestyle, then one values curiosity and courage. With transactional commitment, individuals aspire to management roles and become concerned about politics, interpersonal communication, and interpersonal transactions. Personal survival is still a top priority in this paradigm of organizational life. However, one is attuned to the politics of the system and becomes invested in the development of competencies and skills associated with the art and science of compromise. Such a skill set contributes to one's success and insights related to the complexity of relationships, events, and strategic goals in an organizational context. Concepts and ideas facilitate communication and influence. Some nurses believe that the technical (individual) and transactional (manager) mode of operation is the essence of aspiration. Quinn notes that there is a third alternative and possibility that one can choose in regard to an organizational lifestyle. He calls this the transformational paradigm. Transformational leadership is built on creative management of the tensions that exist between what the reality of the organization is, or its truth, and the organization's vision—that which the organization and the people in the organization aspire to be.

The Challenge of Being a Transformational Professional

Transformational leadership requires a commitment to leadership with an eye on the future. One of the main objectives in a transformational model is creating a vision and sense of community built on core values. In a transformational leadership paradigm, behavioral integrity is more valued than organizational position. Transformational leaders are self-authoring and engage in action learning. Transformational leaders engage in deep change that results in a continuous quest to create and redefine themselves based on inner work that results in outer-focused service.

Being transformational is a choice. Being transformational requires inner-driven change that is manifested in outer-focused service. What deep changes do you want to see in the nursing profession? How might you contribute to "deep change" and the future integrity and development of the profession? Quinn (2000) offers the following seed thoughts for individuals who want to make extraordinary change:

- Envision productive community.
- First look within.
- Embrace the hypocritical self.
- Transcend fear.
- Embody a vision of the common good.
- Disturb the system.
- Surrender to the emergent process.
- Entice through moral power.

As nursing moves toward the future, here are a few thoughts about strategies for change in regard to Quinn's seed thoughts.

Envision Productive Community

Communities are created when people who have a shared purpose and goal come together to find and make meaning. Communities enhance capabilities through dialogue and commitment. Building community ensures continuity, collaboration, and conscience. Productive community is characterized by clarity of purpose and high standards of performance. Productive communities are synergistic. Quinn notes, "A social movement begins when someone allows the personal to become public. When the change agent chooses to live undivided, focuses on the good of the system, and becomes a servant to the system, other people are attracted to empower themselves and the system changes" (Quinn, 2000, p. 54). The first step to changing the world is to envision a productive professional community of nursing.

First Look Within

Nurses increase the likelihood for changing the world if they look within, clarify their own values as they go, and then discipline themselves to more fully live those values. This requires what Quinn calls *soul force*. The world creates individuals, and they create the world. Profession nursing can be recreated by inner work (Pesut, 2001). Intrapersonal inner work supports personal growth that is in turn manifested in outer work of social relevance. The creation of a productive community begins when each nurse owns and manages his or her own soul force.

Embrace the Hypocritical Self

Because some nurses value control, winning and suppression of negative feelings, and the pursuit of rational objectives, some nurses find ways to discount or neutralize negative feedback about themselves. Some nurses project dark feelings on others as they blame and seldom ask how they contribute to the problems or dynamics of a situation. Once individuals accept their own hypocrisy, they get closer to their integrity gaps and can renew and recreate themselves. Embracing a hypocritical self requires acknowledgment, appreciation, and successful negotiation of an individual's shadows and dark sides. Working through shadow issues makes individuals whole.

Transcend Fear

There are two motivational forces in the world: fear and aspiration. Often, fear is based on a need to conform. "Unexamined conformity can limit our perceptions about life and its many possibilities (Quinn, 2000 p.90)" Transformational leaders have many fears and are willing to face them. They also are clear about their aspirations. They are committed to a passionate YES! "When we find a unique purpose, life takes on greater meaning. We can transcend the actual because we envision the possible" (Quinn, 2000, p. 108). What is your passionate YES? It is easier to transcend fear when one is clear and courageous about aspirations.

Embody a Vision of the Common Good

Each nurse moves along his or her own path. Task types or technical lifestyle-oriented professionals often depend on authorities to provide vision, direction, and approval. Intense achievement types want to take charge, provide direction, and overcome barriers. They have high achievement needs, are inner directed, and know what they want. Some but not all nurses take the path of responsive service. The path of responsive service supports and sustains collective fulfillment and visions of the common good. Those on the journey to responsive service are idealistic and dedicated to serve others. They are open, intuitive, and proactive. Transformational leaders value co-creating, cohesion, and trust, and are open to feedback and alternatives that support and sustain the common good.

Disturb the System

Transformational power resides at the edge of chaos. Resistance is where transcendence begins. Quinn writes, " Human collectives can never transform until someone cares enough and dares enough to deviate and disturb the system" (p. 169). He also offers this advice: The disruption must challenge and not overwhelm.

Surrender to the Emergent Process

Future thinking involves paying attention to self-organizing patterns and discerning the logical consequences of those patterns through time. Future thinking requires critical, creative, and network thinking. Transformational leadership is built on the tension that exists between truth and vision. Transformational leaders have a sense of the future. One of the main objectives in a transformational model is creating a vision and sense of community built on core values.

Entice Through Moral Power

Nurses must remind themselves that service rather than recognition is a higher standard of leadership (Nair, 1997). If responsibilities are met then rights are not an issue (Nair, 1997). At the most fundamental level all conduct is individual. When moral dimensions are brought to individual action integrity becomes an essential feature of the entire work environment (Nair, 1997). Nurses are moral agents who manage the tension between negligence and nursing on a daily basis.

Summary

Many of the authors in this text have challenged you with information, insights and aspirations. The knowledge gained from the readings in this text has equipped you with data, information, and knowledge. To what degree will nurses use this information to develop wisdom? What organization lifestyle will most nurses choose: technical, transactional, or transformational? As nurses make the transition, each must decide if he or she will be a nurse-witness to slow death or a nurse-advocate-leader of deep change? Leadership consciousness calls one to create deep change and preferred futures. The future of the profession depends on deep change and navigating the future. As Mikela and Phillip Tarlow (1999) note, a large part of navigating the future is the realization that what the future holds for each person depends on what each person contributes to the future.

REFERENCES

Bower, F. (Ed.). (2000). *Nurses taking the lead: Personal qualities of effective leadership*. Philadelphia, PA: Saunders.

Chaska, N. (Ed.). (2001). *The nursing profession: Tomorrow and beyond*. Thousand Oaks, CA: Sage.

Nair, K. (1997). *A higher standard of leadership: Lessons from the life of Gandhi*. San Francisco: Berrett Koehler.

Pesut, D. J. (2001). Healing into the future: Recreating the profession of nursing through inner work. In N. Chaska (Ed.), *The nursing profession: Tomorrow and beyond* (Chapter 70, pp. 853–867). Thousand Oaks, CA: Sage.

Pesut, D. J. (2000). Looking forward: Being and becoming a futurist. In F. Bower (Ed.), *Nurses Taking the Lead: Personal Qualities of Effective Leadership* (Chapter 3, pp. 39–65). Philadelphia, PA: Saunders.

Pesut, D. (1999). Leadership and the spirit of service. *Journal of Professional Nursing, 15*(1), 6.

Pesut, D. (1998a). Twenty-first century learning. *Nursing Outlook, 46*(1), 37.

Pesut, D. (1998b). Scenarios: Stories about the future. *Nursing Outlook, 46*(2), 55.

Pesut, D. (1997a). Facilitating futures thinking. *Nursing Outlook, 45*(4), 155.

Pesut, D. (1997b). Connecting with the futures community. *Nursing Outlook, 45*(5), 251.

Pesut, D. (1997c). The future, virtue-ethics, and sigma theta tau. *Reflections, 23*(3), 56–59.

Porter-O'Grady, T. (2001). Profound change: 21st century nursing. *Nursing Outlook, 49*(4), 182–187.

Quinn, R. (1996). *Deep change: Discovering the leader within*. San Francisco: Jossey Bass.

Quinn, R. (2000). *Changing the world: How ordinary people can achieve extraordinary results*. San Francisco: Jossey Bass.

Rogers, M. (1997). *Canadian nursing in 2020: Five scenarios*. Ottawa: Canadian Nurses Association.

Sullivan, E. (Ed.). (1999). *Creating nursing's future: Issues, opportunities, and challenges*. St. Louis, MO: Mosby.

Sullivan, E., & Pesut, D. (1999). Challenges for nursing in higher education. In E. Sullivan (Ed.). *Creating nursing's future: Issues, opportunities, and challenges* (Chapter 16, pp. 151–163). St. Louis, MO: Mosby.

Tarlow, M., & Tarlow, P. (1999). *Navigating the future*. New York: McGraw-Hill.

Van der Heijden, K. (1996). *Scenarios: The art of strategic conversation*. New York: John Wiley & Sons.

Appendix A

Nursing Organizations

Academy of Medical–Surgical Nurses
http://www.medsurgnurse.org/
East Holly Ave., Box 56
Pitman, NJ 08071-0056
Phone: 856-256-2323
Fax: 856-589-7463

Aerospace Nursing Association North Carolina Central University Dept. of Nursing
P.O. Box 19798
Durham, NC 27707
Phone: 919-560-6431

American Academy of Nurse Practitioners
http://www.aanp.org/
Capital Station,
P.O. Box 12846
Austin, TX 78711
Phone: 512-442-4262
Fax: 512-442-6469

American Academy of Nursing
http://www.nursingworld.org/aan/index.htm
600 Maryland Ave., SW, Suite 100 West
Washington, DC 20024-2571
Phone: 202-651-7238
Fax: 202-554-2641

American Assembly for Men in Nursing
http://people.delphiforums.com/brucewilson/
AAMN % NYSNA
11 Cornell Rd.
Latham, NY 12110-1499
Phone: 518-782-9400 Ext. 346

American Association for the History of Nursing
www.aahn.org
P.O. Box 175
Lanoka Harbor, NJ 08734
Phone: 609-693-7250
Fax: 609-693-1037

American Academy of Ambulatory Care Nursing
AAACN National Office, East Holly Ave., Box 56
Pitman, NJ 08071-0056
Phone: Main number 856-256-2350
Toll Free: 800-AMB-NURS
Fax: 856-589-7463

American Association of Colleges of Nursing
http://www.aacn.nche.edu
One Dupont Circle, Suite 530
Washington, DC 20036-1120
Phone: 202-463-6903
Fax: 202-785-8320

American Association of Critical Care Nurses
www.aacn.org
101 Columbia
Aliso Viejo, CA 92656
Phone: 949-362-2000
Fax: 949-362-2020

American Association of Legal Nurse Consultants
http://www.aalnc.org/
401 N. Michigan Ave.
Chicago, IL 60611
Phone: 877-402-2562
Fax: 312-673-6655

American Association of Neuroscience Nurses
http://www.aann.org
4700 W. Lake Ave.
Glenview, IL 60025
Phone: 847-375-4733
Fax: 877-734-8677

American Association of Nurse Anesthetists
www.aana.com
222 South Prospect Ave.
Park Ridge, IL 60068-4001
Phone: 847-692-7050

American Association of Nurse Attorneys
http://www.taana.org
7794 Grow Dr.
Pensacola, Fl 32514
Phone: 877-538-2262
Fax: 850-484-8762

American Association of Occupational Health Nurses
http://www.aaohn.org
Brandywine Rd., Suite 100
Atlanta, GA 30341
Phone: 770-455-7757
Fax: 770-455-7271

American Association of Spinal Cord Injury Nurses
www.aascin.org
75-20 Astoria Blvd.
Jackson Heights, NY 11370-1177
Phone: 718-803-3782
Fax: 718-803-0414

American College of Nurse Practitioners
http://www.nurse.org/acnp/
1111 19th St. NW, Suite 404
Washington DC 20036
Phone: 202-659-2190
Fax: 202-659-2191

American College of Nurse-Midwives
http://www.acnm.org
818 Connecticut Ave. NW, Suite 900
Washington, DC 20006
Phone: 202-728-9860
Fax: 202-728-9897

American Forensic Nurses
http://www.amrn.com/
255 N. El Cielo, Suite 195
Palm Springs, CA 92262
Phone: 760-322-9925
Fax: 760-322-9914

American Holistic Nurses Association
http://ahna.org
P.O. Box 2130
Flagstaff, AZ 86003-2130
Phone: 800-278-2462

American Nephrology Nurses Association
http://anna.inurse.com/
East Holly Ave., Box 56
Pitman, NJ 08071-0056
Toll Free: 888-600-ANNA (2662)
Phone: 856-256-2320
Fax: 856-589-7463

American Nurses Association
http://www.ana.org
600 Maryland Ave. SW, Suite 100 West
Washington, DC 20024-2571
Phone: 800-274-4ANA

American Nurses Credentialing Center
600 Maryland Ave. SW, 100 West
Washington, DC 20024-2571
http://www.nursingworld.org/ancc/
Email: *ancc@ana.org*

American Organization of Nurse Executives
http://www.aone.org
325 Seventh Street NW, Suite 700
Washington, DC 20004
Phone: 202-626-2240
Fax: 202-638-5499

American Psychiatric Nurse Association
www.apna.org
Colonial Place Three
1555 Wilson Blvd., Suite 515
Arlington, VA 22209
Phone: 703-243-2443
Fax: 703-243-3390

American Radiological Nurses Association
www.rsna.org/about/orgs/arna
820 Jorie Blvd.
Old Brook, IL 60523
Phone: 630-571-2670
Fax: 630-571-7837

American Society of Ophthalmic Registered Nurses
http://webeye.ophth.uiowa.edu/asorn/
P.O. Box 193030
San Francisco, CA 94119
Phone: 415-561-8513
Fax: 415-561-8575

American Society of Pain Management Nurses
http://www.aspmn.org/
7794 Grow Dr.
Pensacola, FL 32514
Phone: 888-342-7766
Fax: 850-484-8762

Commission on Graduates of Foreign Nursing Schools
www.cgfns.org
3600 Market St., Suite 400
Philadelphia, PA 19104
Phone: 215-349-8767
Fax: 215-349-0026

American Society of PeriAnesthesia Nurses
http://www.aspan.org
10 Melrose Ave., Suite 110
Cherry Hill, NJ 08003-3696
Phone: 877-737-9696
Fax: 856-616-9601

Dermatology Nurses Association
http://www.dnanurse.org
East Holly Ave., Box 56
Pitman, NJ 08071
Phone: 800-256-2330
Fax: 609-582-1915

Association of Black Nursing Faculty, Inc.
5823 Queens Cove
Lisle, IL 60532
www.abnfinc.org
Phone: 630-969-3809

Association of Nurses in AIDS Care
http://www.anacnet.org/
3538 Ridgewood Rd.
Akron, Ohio 44333
Phone: 330-670-0101 or 800-260-6780
Fax: 330-670-0109

Association of Operating Room Nurses
http://www.aorn.org
2170 South Parker Rd., Suite 300
Denver, CO 80231-5711
Phone: 303-755-6304 or 800-755-2676
Fax: 303-750-2927

Association of Pediatric Oncology Nurses
www.apon.org
4700 West Lake Ave.
Glenview, IL 60025-1485
Phone: 847-375-4724
Fax: 877-734-8755

Association of Rehabilitation Nurses
http://www.rehabnurse.org
4700 West Lake Rd.
Glenview, IL 60025-1485
Phone: 800-229-7530
Fax: 877-734-9384

Association of Women's Health, Obstetric and Neonatal Nursing
http://www.awhonn.org
2000 L Street, NW, Suite 740
Washington, DC 20036
Phone: 800-673-8499
Fax: 202-728-0575

Developmental Disabilities Nurses Association
www.ddna.org
1733 H St., Suite 330, PMB 1214
Blaine, WA 98230
Phone: 800-888-6733
Fax: 360-332-2280

Emergency Nurses Association
http://www.ena.org/
915 Lee St.
Des Plaines, IL 60016-6569
Phone: 800-900-9659
Fax: 847-460-4001

Federation of Nurses and Health Professionals
http://www.aft.org/fnhp/
555 New Jersey Ave.
Washington, DC 20001
Phone: 202-879-4491
Fax: 202-879-4597

Haitian Nurses Association
113-63 Hook Creek Blvd.
Valley Stream, NY 11580

Hospice and Palliative Nurses Association
www.hpna.org
Penn Center West One, Suite 229
Pittsburgh, PA 15276
Phone: 412-787-9301
Fax: 412-787-9305

International Council of Nurses
http://www.icn.ch/
Place Jean-Marteau
Geneva, Switzerland 1201
Phone: 41-22-908-01-00
Fax: 41-22-908-01-01

International Society of Nurses in Genetics, Inc. Foundation for Blood Research
http://www.globalreferrals.com
Phone: 603-643-5706

Intravenous Nurses Society (Therapy)
http://www.ins1.org
220 Norwood Park South
Norwood, MA 02062
Phone: 781-440-9408
Fax: 781-440-9409

National Association Directors of Nursing Administration in Long Term Care
www.nadona.org
10101 Alliance Rd., #140
Cincinnati, OH 45242
Phone: 800-222-0539
Fax: 513-791-3699

National Association of Hispanic Nurses
www.thehispanicnurses.org
1501 16th Street NW
Washington, DC 20036
Phone: 202-387-2477
Fax: 202-483-7183

National Association of Neonatal Nurses
http://www.nann.org
4700 W. Lake Ave.
Glenview, IL 60025-1485
Phone: 800-451-3795
Fax: 888-477-6266

National Association of Nurse Practitioners in Women's Health
www.npwh.org
503 Capitol Court NE, Suite 300
Washington, DC 20002
Phone: 202-543-9693
Fax: 202-543-9858

National Association of Orthopedic Nurses
http://www.orthonurse.org
401 N. Michigan Ave., Suite 2200
Chicago, IL 60611
Phone: 800-289-6266
Fax: 312-527-6658

National Association of Pediatric Nurses and Practitioners
http://www.napnap.org
20 Brace Rd., Suite 200
Cherry Hill, NJ 08034
Phone: 856-857-9700
Fax: 856-877-1600

National Association of School Nurses
www.nasn.org
P.O. Box 1300
Scarborough, ME 04070-1300
Phone: 207-883-2117 or 877-627-6476
Fax: 207-883-2683

National Black Nurses Association, Inc.
www.nbna.org
8630 Fenton St., Suite 330
Silver Spring, MD 20910-3803
Phone: 301-589-3200

National Consortium of Chemical Dependency Nurses
167 Cleveland St.
P.O. Box 2749
Eugene, OR 97402
Phone: 800-876-2236
Fax: 541-485-7372

National Council of State Boards of Nursing, Inc.
http://www.ncsbn.org
111 East Wacker Dr., Suite 2900
Chicago, IL 60601
Phone: 312-525-3600
Fax: 312-279-1032

Air and Surface Transport Nurses Association aka National Flight Nurses Association
http://www.astna.org/
9101 E. Kenyon Ave., Suite 3000
Denver, CO 80237
Phone: 800-897-NFNA (6362)
Fax: 303-770-1812

National Gerontological Nursing Association
www.ngna.org
7794 Grow Dr.
Pensacola, FL 32514
Phone: 800-723-0560
Fax: 850-484-8762

North American Nursing Diagnosis Association
www.nanda.org
1211 Locust St.
Philadelphia, PA 19107
Phone: 215-545-8105
Fax: 215-545-8107

National Institute of Nursing Research
http://www.nih.gov/ninr/index.html
NIH Building 31
Bethesda, MD 20892-2178
Phone: 301-496-0207
Fax: 301-480-4969

National League for Nursing
http://www.nln.org
61 Broadway, 33rd Floor
New York, NY 10006
Phone: 800-669-1656

National Nursing Staff Development Organization
http://www.nnsdo.org/
7794 Grow Dr.
Pensacola, FL 32514
Phone: 800-489-1995
Fax: 850-484-8762

National Organization for Associate Degree Nursing
http://www.noadn.org/
P.O. Box 3188
Dublin, OH 43016
Phone: 614-451-1515

National Student Nurses Association
http://www.nsna.org
45 Main St., Suite 606
New York, NY 11201
Phone: 718-210-0705
Fax: 718-210-0710

Navy Nurses Corps Association
www.nnca.org
P.O. Box 1229
Oak Harbor, WA 98277

Nurses Christian Fellowship
www.ncf-jcn.org
P.O. Box 7895
Madison, WI 53707-7895
Phone: 608-274-4823 Ext. 401

Nurses Organization of Veterans Affairs
www.vanurse.org
1726 M St. NW, Suite 1101
Washington, DC 20036
Phone: 202-296-0888
Fax: 202-833-1577

Oncology Nursing Society
http://www.ons.org
125 Enterprise Dr.
Pittsburgh, PA 15275-1214
Phone: 866-257-4ONS (4667)
Fax: 877-369-5497

Philippine Nurses Association of America
http://www.pnaamerica.org
151 Linda Vista Dr.
Daly City, CA 94014
Phone: 415-468-7995
Fax: 415-468-7995

Respiratory Nursing Society
www.respiratorynursingsociety.org
RNS c/o NYSNA
11 Cornell Rd
Latham, NY 12110
Phone: 518-782-9400 Ext. 286

Sigma Theta Tau International
www.nursingsociety.org
550 West North St.
Indianapolis, IN 46202
Phone: 317-634-8171
Toll Free: 888-634-7575
Fax: 317-634-8188

Society for Vascular Nursing
www.svnnet.org
7794 Grow Dr.
Pensacola, FL 32514
Phone: 888-536-4786
Fax: 850-484-8762

Society of Gastroenterology Nurses and Associates
www.sgna.org
401 North Michigan Ave.
Chicago, IL 60611-4267
Phone: 800-245-7462
Fax: 312-527-6658

Society of Gynecologic Nurse Oncologists
www.sgno.org
1411 Silverleaf
St. Louis, MO 63146
Phone: 321-434-8639

Society of Trauma Nurses
www.traumanursesoc.org
PMB 300 223 N. Guadelupe
Sante Fe, NM 87501
Phone: 505-983-4923
Fax: 505-983-5109

Transcultural Nursing Society
www.tcns.org
36600 Schoolcraft Rd.
Livonia, MI 48150
Phone: 888-432-5470
Fax: 734-432-5463

Wound, Ostomy, and Continence Nurses Society
www.wocn.org
4700 W. Lake Ave.
Glenview, IL 60025
Phone: 888-224-WOCN
Fax: 866-615-8560

Appendix B

State Boards of Nursing
(Including U.S. Territories)

Alabama State Board of Nursing
www.abn.state.al.us/
770 Washington Ave., RSA Plaza, Suite 250
Montgomery, AL 36104-3900
Phone: 334-242-4060
Fax: 334-242-4360

Alaska Board of Nursing
Department of Commerce and Economic
Development
Division of Occupational Licensing
http://www.dced.state.ak.us/occ/pnur.htm
P.O. Box 110806
Juneau, AK 99811-0806
Phone: 907-269-8161
Fax: 909-269-8196

Arizona State Board of Nursing
www.azboardofnursing.org
1651 East Morten Ave., Suite 210
Phoenix, AZ 85020
Phone: 602-331-8111
Fax: 602-906-9365

Arkansas State Board of Nursing
www.state.ar.us/nurse
University Tower Building, Suite 800
1123 South University Ave.
Little Rock, AR 72204
Phone: 501-686-2700
Fax: 501-686-2714

California Board of Registered Nursing
www.rn.ca.gov
400 R St., Suite 4030
Sacramento, CA 94244-2100
Phone: 916-322-3350
Fax: 916-327-4402

Colorado State Board of Nursing
www.dora.state.co.us/nursing
1560 Broadway, Suite 880
Denver, CO 80202
Phone: 303-894-2430
Fax: 303-894-2821

Connecticut Board of Examiners for Nursing
Dept. of Public Health
410 Capitol Ave., MS# 13PER
Hartford, CT 06134-0308
http://www.dph.state.ct.us/Licensure/licensure.htm#N
Phone: 860-509-7624
Fax: 860-509-7553

Delaware Board of Nursing
Cannon Building, Suite 203
861 Silver Lake Blvd.
Dover, DE 19904
http://www.professionallicensing.state.de.us/boards/nursing/index.shtml
Phone: 302-744-4500
Fax: 302-739-2711

District of Columbia Board of Nursing
Dept. of Public Health Board of Nursing
825 N. Capitol St. NE, 2nd Floor
Room 2224
Washington, DC 20002
http://www.nurse.org/dc-index.shtml
http://www.dchealth.dc.gov/prof_license/services/boards_main_action.asp?strAppId=11
Phone: 202-442-4776
Fax: 202-442-9431

Florida Board of Nursing
http://www.doh.state.fl.us/mqa [Dept. of Health]
4080 Woodcock Dr., Suite 202
Jacksonville, FL 32207
Phone: 904-858-6940
Fax: 904-858-6964
Nursing License
http://www.doh.state.fl.us/mqa/nursing/nur_home.html

Georgia Board of Nursing
http://www.sos.state.ga.us/plb/rn/
237 Coliseum Drive
Macon, GA 31217-3858
Phone: 478-207-1640
Fax: 478-207-1660

Hawaii Board of Nursing
Professional and Vocational Licensing Division
http://www.state.hi.us/dcca/pvl/areas_nurs.html
Box 3469
Honolulu, HI 96801
Phone: 808-586-3000
Fax: 808-586-2689

Iowa Board of Nursing
www.state.ia.us/government/nursing/
400 SW 8th Street, Suite B
Des Moines, IA 50309-4685
Phone: 515-281-3255
Fax: 515-281-4825

Kansas State Board of Nursing
www.ksbn.org
Landon State Office Building
900 SW Jackson St., Suite 551-S
Topeka, KS 66612
Phone: 785-296-4929
Fax: 785-296-3929

Kentucky Board of Nursing
www.kbn.state.ky.us
312 Whittington Parkway, Suite 300
Louisville, KY 40222
Phone: 502-329-7000 or 800-305-2042
Fax: 502-329-7011

Louisiana Board of Nursing
http://www.lsbn.state.la.us/
3510 N. Causeway Blvd., Suite 501
Metairie, LA 70002
Phone: 504-838-5791
Fax: 504-838-5279

Idaho State Board of Nursing
http://www2.state.id.us/ibn/ibnhome.htm
280 N. 8th Street, Suite 210
P.O. Box 83720
Boise, ID 83720-0061
Phone: 208-334-3110
Fax: 208-334-3262

Illinois Department of Professional Regulation
www.dpr.state.il.us/
James R Thompson Center
100 West Randolph, Suite 9-300
Chicago, IL 60601
Phone: 312-814-2715
Fax: 312-814-3145

Indiana State Board of Nursing Health Professions Bureau
http://www.state.in.us/heb/boards/isbn/
402 West Washington Street, Suite W066
Indianapolis, IN 46204
Phone: 317-234-2043
Fax: 317-233-4236

Maine State Board of Nursing
www.state.main.gov/boardofnursing
158 State House Station
Augusta, ME 04333
Phone: 207-287-1133
Fax: 207-287-1149

Maryland Board of Nursing
www.mbon.org
4140 Patterson Ave.
Baltimore, MD 21215
Phone: 410-585-1900
Fax: 410-358-3530

Massachusetts Board of Registration in Nursing
www.state.ma.us/reg/boards/rn
239 Causeway St.
Boston, MA 02114
Phone: 617-727-9961
Fax: 617-727-1630

Michigan Board of Nursing
CIS/Office of Health Services
http://www.michigan.gov/healthliscense
Ottawa Towers North
611 West Ottawa, 4th Floor
Lansing, MI 48933
Phone: 517-373-0918
Fax: 517-373-2179

Minnesota Board of Nursing
www.nursingboard.state.mn.us
2829 University Ave. SE, Suite 500
Minneapolis, MN 55414
Phone: 612-617-2270
Fax: 612-617-2190

Mississippi Board of Nursing
www.msbn.state.ms.us
1935 Lakeland Dr, Suite B
Jackson, MS 39216-5014
Phone: 601-987-4188
Fax: 601-364-2352

Missouri State Board of Nursing
www.ecodev.state.mo.us/pr/nursing/
P.O. Box 656
Jefferson City, MO 65102-0656
Phone: 573-751-0681
Fax: 573-751-0075

Montana State Board of Nursing
http://www.discoveringmontana.com/dli/bsd/license
/bsd_boards/nur_board/board_page.htm
301 South Park
Helena, MT 59620-0513
Phone: 406-841-2340
Fax: 406-841-2343

Nebraska Board of Nursing
http://www.hhs.state.ne.us/crl/nursing/nursingindex.htm
Department of Health and Human Services
Regulation and Licensure
Nursing Section
301 Centennial Mall South
Lincoln, NE 68509-4986
Phone: 402-471-4376
Fax: 402-471-1066

Nevada State Board of Nursing
www.nursingboard.state.nv.us
4330 S. Valley View #106
Las Vegas, NV 89103-4051
Phone: 702-486-5800
Fax: 702-486-5803

New Hampshire Board of Nursing
http://www.state.nh.us/nursing/
P.O. Box 45010
78 Regional Drive, Bldg. B
Concord, NH 03301
Phone: 603-271-2323
Fax: 603-271-6605

New Jersey Board of Nursing
http://www.state.nj.us/lps/ca/medical.htm
P.O. Box 45010
124 Halsey St., 6th Floor
Newark, NJ 07101
Phone: 973-504-6586
Fax: 973-648-3481

New Mexico Board of Nursing
www.state.nm.us/clients/nursing
4206 Louisiana Blvd. NE, Suite A
Albuquerque, NM 87109
Phone: 505-841-8340
Fax: 505-841-8347

New York State Education Department
http://www.op.nysed.gov/nurse.htm
89 Washington Ave. 2nd Floor, West Wing
Albany, NY 12234
Phone: 518-474-3817 Ext. 120
Fax: 518-474-3706

North Carolina Board of Nursing
www.ncbon.com
3724 National Dr. #201
Raleigh, NC 27612
Phone: 919-782-3211
Fax: 919-781-9461

North Dakota Board of Nursing
www.ndbon.org
919 South 7th St., Suite 504
Bismarck, ND 58504
Phone: 701-328-9777
Fax: 701-328-9785

Ohio Board of Nursing
http://www.state.oh.us/nur/
17 South High St., Suite 400
Columbus, OH 43215-3413
Phone: 614-466-3947
Fax: 614-466-0388

Oklahoma Board of Nursing
2915 N. Classen Blvd., Suite 524
Oklahoma City, OK 73106
http://www.youroklahoma.com/nursing/
Phone: 405-962-1800
Fax: 405-962-1821

Oregon State Board of Nursing
www.osbn.state.or.us
800 NE Oregon St., Box 25, Suite 465
Portland, OR 97232
Phone: 503-731-4745
Fax: 503-731-4755

Pennsylvania State Board of Nursing
http://www.dos.state.pa.us/bpoa/cwp/view.asp?a=1104&q=432869
P.O. Box 2649
Harrisburg, PA 17105-2649
Phone: 717-783-7142
Fax: 717-783-0822

Rhode Island Board of Nurse Registration and Nursing Education
www.health.ri.org/hsr/professions/nurses.htm
105 Cannon Building, Three Capitol Hill
Providence, RI 02908
Phone: 401-222-5700
Fax: 401-222-3352

South Carolina State Board of Nursing
www.llr.state.sc.us/pol/nursing
110 Centerview Dr., Suite 202
Columbia, SC 29210
Phone: 803-896-4550
Fax: 803-896-4525

South Dakota Board of Nursing
www.state.sd.us/dcr/nursing
4305 South Louise Ave., Suite C-1
Sioux Falls, SD 57106-3124
Phone: 605-362-2760
Fax: 605-362-2768

Tennessee State Board of Nursing
http://www.gov/health
426 Fifth Ave. North
1st Floor, Cordell Hull Building
Nashville, TN 37247
Phone: 615-532-5166
Fax: 615-741-7899

Texas Board of Nurse Examiners
www.bne.state.tx.us
333 Guadalupe, Suite 3-460
Austin, TX 78701
Phone: 512-305-7400
Fax: 512-305-7401

Utah State Board of Nursing
www.Commerce.state.ut.us/
160 East 300 South
Salt Lake City, UT 84111
Phone: 801-530-6628
Fax: 801-530-6511

Vermont State Board of Nursing
http://www.vtprofessionals.or/opr1/nurses
109 State St.
Montpelier, VT 05609-1106
Phone: 802-828-2396
Fax: 802-828-2484

Virginia Board of Nursing
www.dhp.state.va.us/
6603 West Broad St., 5th Floor
Richmond, VA 23230-1712
Phone: 804-662-9909
Fax: 804-662-9512

Washington State Nursing Quality Assurance Commission
Department of Health
http://www.doh.wa.gov/nursing/default.htm
HPQA #6
310 Israel Rd. SE
Tumwater, WA 98501-7864
Phone: 360-236-4700
Fax: 360-236-4738

West Virginia Board of Examiners for Registered Professional Nurses
www.state.wv.us/nurses/rn
101 Dee Dr.
Charleston, WV 25311
Phone: 304-558-3596
Fax: 304-558-3666

Wisconsin Department of Regulation and Licensing
www.drl.state.wi.us/
1400 E. Washington Ave.
P.O. Box 8935
Madison, WI 53708-8935
Phone: 608-266-0145
Fax: 608-261-7083

Wyoming State Board of Nursing
http://nursing.state.wy.us/
2020 Carey Ave., Suite 110
Cheyenne, WY 82002
Phone: 307-777-7601
Fax: 307-777-3519

United States Territories

American Samoa Health Services Regulatory Board
LBJ Tropical Medical Center
Pago Pago, American Samoa 96799
Phone: 684-633-1222
Fax: 684-633-1869

Guam Board of Nurse Examiners
P.O. Box 2816
Barrada, GU 96913
Phone: 671-735-7411
Fax: 671-477-4733

Northern Mariana Islands Commonwealth Board of Nurse Examiners
Public Health Center
P.O. Box 501458
Saipan, Northern Mariana Islands 96950
Phone: 011 670-664-4812
Fax: 011 670-664-4813

Commonwealth of Puerto Rico Board of Nurse Examiners
800 Roberto H. Todd Ave.
Room 202, Stop 18
Call Box 10200
Santurce, PR 00908
Phone: 787-725-7506
Fax: 787-725-7903

Virgin Islands Board of Nurse Licensure Veterans Drive Station
Veterans Drive Station
St. Thomas, VI 00803
Phone: 340-776-7397
Fax: 340-777-4003

Appendix C

State Nursing Associations

Alabama State Nurses' Association (ASNA)
http://www.alabamanurses.org
360 North Hull Street
Montgomery, Alabama 36104-3658
Phone: 334-262-8321
Fax: 334-262-8578

Alaska Nurses Association (AaNA)
www.aknurse.org
2207 East Tudor Road, Suite 34
Anchorage, Alaska 99507-1069
Phone: 907-274-0827
Fax: 907-272-0292

Arizona Nurses Association (AzNA)
http://www.aznurse.org/
1850 E. Southern Ave., Suite #1
Tempe, Arizona 85282
Phone: 480-831-0404
Fax: 480-839-4780

Arkansas Nurses Association (ArNA)
1401 W. Capitol Avenue, Suite 155
Little Rock, Arkansas 72201
Phone: 501-664-5853
Fax: 501-664-5859

ANA\California (ANA\C)
http://www.anacalifornia.org/
1121 L Street, Suite 409
Sacramento, California 95814
Phone: 916-447-0225
Fax: 916-442-4394

Colorado Nurses Association (CNA)
http://www.nurses-co.org/
5453 East Evans Place
Denver, Colorado 80222
Phone: 303-757-7483
Fax: 303-757-8833
E-mail: cna@nurses-co.org

Connecticut Nurses Association (CNA)
http://www.ctnurses.org
Meritech Business Park
377 Research Parkway, Suite 2D
Meriden, Connecticut 06450
Phone: 203-238-1207
Fax: 203-238-3437

Delaware Nurses Association (DNA)
http://www.nursingworld.org/snas/de/
2644 Capitol Trail, Suite 330
Newark, Delaware 19711
Phone: 302-368-2333
Fax: 302-366-1775

District of Columbia Nurses Association, Inc. (DCNA)
http://www.dcsna.org/
5100 Wisconsin Ave., N.W., Suite 306
Washington, D.C. 20016
Phone: 202-244-2705
Fax: 202-362-8285

Florida Nurses Association (FNA)
http://www.floridanurse.org/
P.O. Box 536985
Orlando, Florida 32853-6985
Phone: 407-896-3261
Fax: 407-896-9042

Georgia Nurses Association (GNA)
http://www.georgianurses.org/
3032 Briarcliff Road, NE
Atlanta, Georgia 30329-2655
Phone: 404-325-5536
Fax: 404-325-0407

Guam Nurses Association (GNA)
E-mail: guamnurs@ite.net
P.O. Box CG
Hagatna, Guam 96932
Tel/Fax: 671-477-6877

Hawaii Nurses Association (HNA)
http://www.hawaiinurses.org/
677 Ala Moana Boulevard, Suite 301
Honolulu, Hawaii 96813
Phone: 808-531-1628
Fax: 808-524-2760

Idaho Nurses Association (INA)
http://www.nursingworld.org/snas/id/
200 North 4th Street, Suite 20
Boise, Idaho 83702-6001
Phone: 208-345-0500
Fax: 208-385-0166

Illinois Nurses Association (INA)
http://www.illinoisnurses.com/
105 West Adams Street, Suite 2101
Chicago, Illinois 60603
Phone: 312-419-2900 Ext. 226
Fax: 312-419-2920

Indiana State Nurses Association (ISNA)
http://www.indiananurses.org/
Director
2915 North High School Road
Indianapolis, Indiana 46224
Phone: 317-299-4575
Fax: 317-297-3525

Iowa Nurses Association (INA)
http://www.iowanurses.org/
1501 42nd Street, Suite 471
West Des Moines, Iowa 50266
Phone: 515-225-0495
Fax: 515-225-2201

Kansas State Nurses Association (KSNA)
http://www.nursingworld.org/snas/ks/
1208 S.W. Tyler
Topeka, Kansas 66612-1735
Phone: 785-233-8638
Fax: 785-233-5222

Kentucky Nurses Association (KNA)
http://www.kentucky-nurses.org/
1400 South First Street
P.O. Box 2616
Louisville, Kentucky 40201-2616
Phone: 502-637-2546
Fax: 502-637-8236

Louisiana State Nurses Association (LSNA)
http://www.lsna.org/
5700 Florida Blvd., Suite 720
Baton Rouge, Louisiana 70806
Phone: 225-201-0993
Toll-Free: 800-457-6378
Fax: 225-201-0971

ANA-MAINE (ANA-ME)
http://www.nursingworld.org/snas/me/
ANA-MAINE
P.O. Box 254
Auburn, Maine 04212-0254
Phone: 207-667-0260

Maryland Nurses Association (MNA)
http://www.nursingworld.org/snas/md/
21 Governor's Court, Suite 195
Baltimore, MD 21244
Phone: 410-944-5800
Fax: 410-944-5802

Massachusetts Association of Registered Nurses (MARN)
http://www.marnonline.org/
Massachusetts Association of Registered Nurses, Inc.
P.O. Box 70668
Worcester, MA 01607-0668
Phone & Fax: 508-881-8812

Michigan Nurses Association (MNA)
http://www.minurses.org/
2310 Jolly Oak Road
Okemos, Michigan 48864-4599
Phone: 517-349-5640 Ext. 14
Fax: 517-349-5818

Minnesota Nurses Association (MNA)
http://www.mnnurses.org/
1625 Energy Park Drive
St. Paul, Minnesota 55108
Phone: 651-646-4807 Ext. 152 or 800-536-4662
Fax: 651-647-5301

Mississippi Nurses Association (MNA)
http://www.msnurses.org/
31 Woodgreen Place
Madison, Mississippi 39110
Phone: 601-898-0670
Fax: 601-898-0190

Missouri Nurses Association (MONA)
http://www.missourinurses.org/
1904 Bubba Lane, P.O. Box 105228
Jefferson City, Missouri 65110-5228
Toll-Free: 1-888-662-MONA
Phone: 573-636-4623
Fax: 573-636-9576

Montana Nurses Association (MNA)
http://www.mtnurses.org/
104 Broadway, Suite G-2
Helena, Montana 59601
Phone: 406-442-6710
Fax: 406-442-1841

Nebraska Nurses Association (NNA)
http://www.nursingworld.org/snas/ne/
715 South 14th Street
Lincoln, Nebraska 68508
Phone: 402-475-3859
Fax: 402-475-3961

Nevada Nurses Association (NNA)
http://www.nvnurses.org/
P.O. Box 34660
Reno, Nevada 89533
Phone: 775-747-2333
Fax: 775-747-1337

New Hampshire Nurses Association (NHNA)
http://www.nhnurses.org/
48 West Street
Concord, New Hampshire 03301-3595
Phone: 603-225-3783
Fax: 603-228-6672

New Jersey State Nurses Association (NJSNA)
http://www.njsna.org/
1479 Pennington Road
Trenton, New Jersey 08618-2661
Phone: 609-883-5335 Ext. 10
Fax: 609-883-5343

New Mexico Nurses Association (NMNA)
http://www.nmna.org/
P.O. Box 29658
Santa Fe, New Mexico 87592-9658
Phone: 505-471-3324
Fax: 505-471-3326

New York State Nurses Association (NYSNA)
http://www.nysna.org/
11 Cornell Road
Latham, New York 12110
Phone: 518-782-9400 Ext. 279
Fax: 518-782-9530

North Carolina Nurses Association (NCNA)
http://www.ncnurses.org/
103 Enterprise Street
Box 12025
Raleigh, North Carolina 27605
Phone: 919-821-4250
Fax: 919-829-5807

North Dakota Nurses Association (NDNA)
http://www.ndna.org/
531 Airport Road, Suite D
Bismarck, North Dakota 58504-6107
Phone: 701-223-1385
Fax: 701-223-0575

Ohio Nurses Association (ONA)
http://www.ohnurses.org/
4000 East Main Street
Columbus, Ohio 43213-2983
Phone: 614-237-5414 Ext. 1020
Fax: 614-237-6081

Oklahoma Nurses Association (ONA)
http://www.oknurses.com/
6414 North Santa Fe, Suite A
Oklahoma City, Oklahoma 73116
Phone: 405-840-3476
Fax: 405-840-3013

Oregon Nurses Association (ONA)
http://www.oregonrn.org/
18765 SW Boones Ferry Road
Tualatin, Oregon 97062
Phone: 503-293-0011
Fax: 503-293-0013

Pennsylvania State Nurses Association (PSNA)
http://www.psna.org/
2578 Interstate Drive, Suite 101
Harrisburg, PA 17110-9601
Phone: 717-657-1222 or 888-707-7762
Fax: 717-657-3796

Rhode Island State Nurses Association (RISNA)
http://www.risnarn.org/
550 S. Water Street, Unit 540B
Providence, Rhode Island 02903-4344
Phone: 401-421-9703
Fax: 401-421-6793

South Carolina Nurses Association (SCNA)
http://www.scnurses.org/
1821 Gadsden Street
Columbia, South Carolina 29201
Phone: 803-252-4781
Fax: 803-779-3870

South Dakota Nurses Association (SDNA)
http://www.nursingworld.org/snas/sd/index.htm
P.O. Box 1015
Pierre, South Dakota 57501-1015
Phone: 605-945-4265
Fax: 605-945-4266
E-mail: sdnurse@midco.net

Tennessee Nurses Association (TNA)
http://www.tnaonline.org/
545 Mainstream Drive, Suite 405
Nashville, Tennessee 37228-1201
Phone: 615-254-0350
Fax: 615-254-0303

Texas Nurses Association (TNA)
http://www.texasnurses.org/
7600 Burnet Road, Suite 440
Austin, Texas 78757-1292
Phone: 512-452-0645
Fax: 512-452-0648

Utah Nurses Association (UNA)
http://www.utahnurses.org/
4505 South Wasatch Blvd. #290
Salt Lake City, Utah 84124
Phone: 801-272-4510
Fax: 801-293-8458
E-mail: una@xmission.com

Vermont State Nurses Association (VSNA)
http://www.uvm.edu/~vsna/
100 Dorset Street, Suite 13
South Burlington, Vermont 05403-6241
Phone: 802-651-8886
Fax: 802-651-8998

Virgin Islands State Nurses Association (VISNA)
P.O. Box 583
Christiansted, St. Croix
U.S. Virgin Islands 00821-0583
Phone: 809-773-1261
E-mail: vcgvina@viaccess.net

Virginia Nurses Association (VNA)
http://www.virginianurses.com/
7113 Three Chopt Road, Suite 204
Richmond, Virginia 23226
Phone: 804-282-1808/2373
Fax: 804-282-4916

Washington State Nurses Association (WSNA)
http://www.wsna.org/
575 Andover Park West, Suite 101
Seattle, Washington 98188-3321
Phone: 206-575-7979 Ext. 3002
Fax: 206-575-1908

West Virginia Nurses Association (WVNA)
http://www.wvnurses.org/
100 Capitol Street, Suite 1009
P.O. 1946
Charleston, West Virginia 25301
Phone: 304-342-1169 or 800-400-1226
Fax: 304-346-1861

Wisconsin Nurses Association (WNA)
http://www.wisconsinnurses.org/
6117 Monona Drive
Madison, Wisconsin 53716
Phone: 608-221-0383
Fax: 608-221-2788

Wyoming Nurses Association (WNA)
http://nursing.state.wy.us/
Majestic Building, Room 305
1603 Capitol Avenue
Cheyenne, Wyoming 82001
Phone: 307-635-3955
Fax: 307-635-2173

American Nurses Association (ANA)
http://www.nursingworld.org/
600 Maryland Avenue, SW, Suite 100W
Washington, DC 20024-2571
Phone: 202-651-7000
Toll-Free: 800-274-4ANA
Fax: 202-651-7001

Appendix D

Canadian Nursing Associations

Aboriginal Nurses Association of Canada
www.anac.on.ca
ODAWA Native Friendship Centre
56 Sparks St., Suite 502
Ottawa, ON K1P 5A9
Phone: 613-724-4677
Fax: 613-724-4718

Alberta Association of Registered Nurses
www.nurses.ab.ca
11620-168 St.
Edmonton, AL T5M 4A6
Phone: 780-451-0043
Fax: 780-452-3276

Association of Registered Nurses in Newfoundland
http://www.arnn.nf.ca/
55 Military Rd., P.O. Box 6116
St. John's, Newfoundland AIC5X8
Phone: 709-753-6040
Fax: 709-753-4940

Canadian Association of Critical Care Nurses
www.caccn.ca
P.O. Box 25322
London, ON N6C 6B1
Phone: 519-652-5284
Fax: 519-649-1458

Canadian Association of University Schools of Nursing
http://www.causn.org/
99 Fifth Avenue, Suite 15/15A
Ottawa, ON KIS 5K4
Phone: 613-235-3150
Fax: 613-235-4476

Canadian Intravenous Nurses Association
http://www.cina.ca
P.O. Box 66572
685 McCowan Rd.,
Toronto, Ontario M1J 3N8
Phone: 416-696-7761
Fax: 416-696-8437

Canadian Nurses Association
http://www.cna-nurses.ca/default.htm
50 Driveway
Ottawa, ONK2P 1E2
Phone: 613-237-2133
Fax: 613-237-3520

Canadian Nurses Foundation
http://www.cna-nurses.ca/cnf/
50 Driveway
Ottawa ONK2P 1E2
Phone: 613-237-2133
Fax: 613-237-3520

The Canadian Nursing Students' Association
http://www.aeic.ca/
325-350 Albert St.
Ottawa, ONK1R 1B1
Phone: 613-563-1236
Fax: 613-563-7739

National Federation of Nurses' Unions
http://www.nursesunions.ca
2841 Riverside Dr.
Ottawa ON KlV 8X7
Phone: 613-526-4661
Fax: 613-526-1023

Registered Nurses Association of British Columbia
http://www.rnabc.bc.ca/
2855 Arbutus St.
Vancouver, BCV6J 3Y8
Phone: 604-736-7331
Fax: 604-738-2272

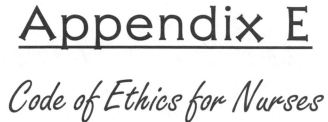

Appendix E

Code of Ethics for Nurses

1. The nurse, in all professional relationships, practices with compassion and respect for the inherent dignity, worth and uniqueness of every individual, unrestricted by considerations of social or economic status, personal attributes, or the nature of health problems.

2. The nurse's primary commitment is to the patient, whether an individual, family, group, or community.

3. The nurse promotes, advocates for, and strives to protect the health, safety, and rights of the patient.

4. The nurse is responsible and accountable for individual nursing practice and determines the appropriate delegation of tasks consistent with the nurse's obligation to provide optimum patient care.

5. The nurse owes the same duties to self as to others, including the responsibility to preserve integrity and safety, to maintain competence, and to continue personal and professional growth.

6. The nurse participates in establishing, maintaining and improving health care environments and conditions of employment conducive to the provision of quality health care and consistent with the values of the profession through individual and collective action.

7. The nurse participates in the advancement of the profession through contributions to practice, education, administration, and knowledge development.

8. The nurse collaborates with other health professionals and the public in promoting community, national, and international efforts to meet health needs.

9. The profession of nursing, as represented by associations and their members, is responsible for articulating nursing values, for maintaining the integrity of the profession and its practice, and for shaping social policy.

Reprinted with permission from American Nurses Association Code of Ethics for Nurses with Interpretive Statements, © 2001 American Nurses Publishing, American Nurses Foundation/American Nurses Association, Washington DC.

Appendix F

International Council of Nurses Code of Ethics for Nurses

▨ Preamble

- Nurses have four fundamental responsibilities: to promote health, to prevent illness, to restore health, and to alleviate suffering. The need for nursing is universal.
- Inherent to nursing is respect for human rights, including the right to life, to dignity, and to be treated with respect. Nursing care is unrestricted by consideration of age, color, creed, culture, disability or illness, gender, nationality, politics, race, or social status.
- Nurses render health services to the individual, the family, and the community and coordinate their services with those of related groups.

The *ICN Code of Ethics for Nurses* has four principle elements that outline the standards of ethical conduct.

▨ 1. Nurses and People

- The nurse's primary responsibility is to those people who require nursing care.
- In providing care, the nurse promotes an environment in which the human rights, values, customs, and spiritual beliefs of the individual, family, and community are respected.
- The nurse holds in confidence personal information and uses judgment in sharing this information.
- The nurse shares with society the responsibility for initiating and supporting action to meet the health and social needs of the public, in particular those of vulnerable populations.
- The nurse also shares responsibility to sustain and protect the natural environment from depletion, pollution, degradation, and destruction.

▨ 2. Nurses and Practice

- The nurse carries personal responsibility and accountability for nursing practice, and for maintaining competence by continual learning.
- The nurse maintains a standard of personal health such that the ability to provide care is not compromised.
- The nurse uses judgment regarding individual competence when accepting and delegating responsibilities.
- The nurse at all times maintains standards of personal conduct, which reflect credit upon the profession and enhance public confidence.
- The nurse, in providing care, ensures that use of technology and scientific advances are compatible with the safety, dignity, and rights of people.

▨ 3. Nurse and the Profession

- The nurse assumes the major role in determining and implementing acceptable standards of clinical nursing practice, management, research, and education.

- The nurse is active in developing a core of research-based professional knowledge.
- The nursing acting through the professional organization, participates in creating and maintaining equitable social and economic working conditions in nursing.

4. Nurse and Co-workers

- The nurse sustains a cooperative relationship with co-workers in nursing and other fields.
- The nurse takes appropriate action to safeguard individuals when their care is endangered by a co-worker or any other person.

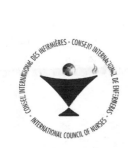

Copyright © 2000 by ICN—International Council of Nurses, 3, Place Jean-Marteau, CH-1201 Geneva (Switzerland).

Appendix G

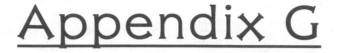

A Patient's Bill of Rights

A Patient's Bill of Rights was first adopted by the American Hospital Association in 1973
This revision was approved by the AHA Board of Trustees on October 21, 1992

Introduction

Effective health care requires collaboration between patients and physicians and other health care professionals. Open and honest communication, respect for personal and professional values, and sensitivity to differences are integral to optimal patient care. As the setting for the provision of health services, hospitals must provide a foundation for understanding and respecting the rights and responsibilities of patients, their families, physicians, and other caregivers. Hospitals must ensure a health care ethic that respects the role of patients in decision-making about treatment choices and other aspects of their care. Hospitals must be sensitive to cultural, racial, linguistic, religious, age, gender, and other differences as well as the needs of persons with disabilities.

The American Hospital Association presents A Patient's Bill of Rights with the expectation that it will contribute to more effective patient care and be supported by the hospital on behalf of the institution, its medical staff, employees, and patients. The American Hospital Association encourages health care institutions to tailor this bill of rights to their patient community by translating and/or simplifying the language of this bill of rights as may be necessary to ensure that patients and their families understand their rights and responsibilities.

Bill of Rights

These rights can be exercised on the patient's behalf by a designated surrogate or proxy decision maker if the patient lacks decision-making capacity, is legally incompetent, or is a minor.

1. The patient has the right to considerate and respectful care.
2. The patient has the right to and is encouraged to obtain from physicians and other direct caregivers relevant, current, and understandable information concerning diagnosis, treatment, and prognosis.

   Except in emergencies when the patient lacks decision-making capacity and the need for treatment is urgent, the patient is entitled to the opportunity to discuss and request information related to the specific procedures and/or treatments, the risks involved, the possible length of recuperation, and the medically reasonable alternatives and their accompanying risks and benefits.

   Patients have the right to know the identity of physicians, nurses, and others involved in their care, as well as when those involved are students, residents, or other trainees. The patient also has the right to know the immediate and long-term financial implications of treatment choices, insofar as they are known.

566

3. The patient has the right to make decisions about the plan of care prior to and during the course of treatment and to refuse a recommended treatment or plan of care to the extent permitted by law and hospital policy and to be informed of the medical consequences of this action. In case of such refusal, the patient is entitled to other appropriate care and services that the hospital provides or transfer to another hospital. The hospital should notify patients of any policy that might affect patient choice within the institution.

4. The patient has the right to have an advance directive (such as a living will, health care proxy, or durable power of attorney for health care) concerning treatment or designating a surrogate decision maker with the expectation that the hospital will honor the intent of that directive to the extent permitted by law and hospital policy.

   Health care institutions must advise patients of their rights under state law and hospital policy to make informed medical choices, ask if the patient has an advance directive, and include that information in patient records. The patient has the right to timely information about hospital policy that may limit its ability to implement fully a legally valid advance directive.

5. The patient has the right to every consideration of privacy. Case discussion, consultation, examination, and treatment should be conducted so as to protect each patient's privacy.

6. The patient has the right to expect that all communications and records pertaining to his/her care will be treated as confidential by the hospital, except in cases such as suspected abuse and public health hazards when reporting is permitted or required by law. The patient has the right to expect that the hospital will emphasize the confidentiality of this information when it releases it to any other parties entitled to review information in these records.

7. The patient has the right to review the records pertaining to his/her medical care and to have the information explained or interpreted as necessary, except when restricted by law.

8. The patient has the right to expect that, within its capacity and policies, a hospital will make reasonable response to the request of a patient for appropriate and medically indicated care and services. The hospital must provide evaluation, service, and/or referral as indicated by the urgency of the case. When medically appropriate and legally permissible, or when a patient has so requested, a patient may be transferred to another facility. The institution to which the patient is to be transferred must first have accepted the patient for transfer. The patient must also have the benefit of complete information and explanation concerning the need for risks, benefits, and alternatives to such a transfer.

9. The patient has the right to ask and be informed of the existence of business relationships among the hospital, educational institutions, other health care providers, or payers that may influence the patient's treatment and care.

10. The patient has the right to consent to or decline to participate in proposed research studies or human experimentation affecting care and treatment or requiring direct patient involvement, and to have those studies fully explained prior to consent. A patient who declines to participate in research or experimentation is entitled to the most effective care that the hospital can otherwise provide.

11. The patient has the right to expect reasonable continuity of care when appropriate and to be informed by physicians and other caregivers of available and realistic patient care options when hospital care is no longer appropriate.

12. The patient has the right to be informed of hospital policies and practices that relate to patient care, treatment, and responsibilities. The patient has the right to be informed of available resources for resolving disputes, grievances, and conflicts, such as ethics committees, patient representatives, or other mechanisms available in the institution. The patient has the right to be informed of the hospital's charges for services and available payment methods.

The collaborative nature of health care requires that patients, or their families/surrogates, participate in their care. The effectiveness of care and patient satisfaction with the course of treatment depend, in part, on the patient fulfilling certain responsibilities. Patients are responsible for providing information about past illnesses, hospitalizations, medication, and other matters related to health status. To participate effectively in decision-making, patients must be encouraged to take responsibility for requesting additional information or clarification about their health status or treatment when they do not fully understand information and instructions. Patients are also responsible for ensuring that the health care institution has a copy of their written advance directive if they have one. Patients are responsible for informing their physicians and other caregivers if they anticipate problems in following prescribed treatment.

Patients should also be aware of the hospital's obligation to be reasonable efficient and equitable in providing care to other patients and the community. The hospital's rules and regulations are designed to help the hospital meet this obligation. Patients and their families are responsible for making reasonable accommodations to the needs of the hospital, other patients, medical staff, and hospital employees. Patients are responsible for providing necessary information for insurance claims and for working with the hospital to make payment arrangements, when necessary.

A person's health depends on much more than health care services. Patients are responsible for recognizing the impact of their life-style on their personal health.

Conclusion

Hospitals have many functions to perform, including the enhancement of health status, health promotion, and the prevention and treatment of injury and disease; the immediate and ongoing care and rehabilitation of patients; the education of health professionals, patients, and the community; and research. All these activities must be conducted with an overriding concern for the values and dignity of patients.

Reprinted with permission of the American Hospital Association, copyright © 1992.

Index

Page numbers followed by f indicate figure or box; those followed by t indicate table.

American Association of Colleges of Nursing (AACN)
  on curriculum, 38, 40f
  on essential knowledge, 192, 193f, 193t
American Board of Nursing Specialists (ABNS), 464
American Holistic Nurses Association, 305–6
American Journal of Nursing, history of, 21
American Nurse's Association (ANA), political
    influence of, 340
American Nurses Association (ANA)
  Code of Ethics, 55, 123
  on essential knowledge, 195
  on ethical principles, 116–17, 118t
  history of, 9
  listing of standardized nursing languages, 167f
  Standards of Practice, 55
American Nursing Credentialing Center (ANCC), 64,
    66, 464, 464f
Americans with Disabilities Act (ADA), 531–34,
    532t
  essential functions, 533–34
  reasonable accommodation, 534
  research on, 531–33
Ancestral medicine, defined, 290t
Andrews, M., cultural assessment, 222, 222f
Anesthetist, certified registered nurse, 458–59
Antibiotic resistance education resolution, 60, 61f
"Apparent agency," independent contractor and, 536
Appleton, C., 133, 133t
Applied science, 148
Aromatherapy, 293t
Art
  caring as an, 132–35, 133t, 142
  nursing as, 4, 148, 235f
Artistic interests, 377
Assault, 359
Assertiveness, in collaboration, 487t
Assessment
  in education curriculum, 41
  in nursing process, 94
Associate degree (ADNs), 43–45, 54
  entry into baccalaureate programs, 44–45
  entry into practice and, 43–45
Autonomy, 117, 118t
  defined, 55, 117
  in nursing, 55
  as nursing value, 117, 118t, 121f

Baccalaureate degree, 54
  associate degree (ADNs) entry into, 44–45
  curriculum, 38–43, 40f
    knowledge, 39
    old habits, 42–43

practice, 40–41
  role, 38–40
Bandura, A., 404
Bar coding, 174–75
Basic science, 148
Battery, 359
Behavioral management, 510
Belonging, spirituality and, 238–39
Benchmarking, information technology in, 174
Beneficence, 112–13, 113t, 121f
Benner's stages of nursing proficiency, 190, 190f
Bennis, W., 508
Beta-carotene supplements, 295t
Bicultural socialization, 407
Biculturalism, defined, 407
Biofeedback, 293t
Biologic weapons, 203–4, 204t
Biological-based interventions, 297, 297t
Boards of nursing, state, 357
  advance practice nursing and, 465–66, 466f
Boards of Nursing Examiners (BNEs)
  current responsibilities, 418–22
    delegation, 421–22
    disciplinary action, 420–21, 428–29
    education supervision, 419, 421
    foreign students, 420
    scope of practice supervision, 419–22
  history of, 418
Boolean search, 257
Boykin, A. and Schoenhofer, S.
  conceptual framework of, 75t
  Nursing as Caring Model, 139
  writings of, 86t
Boyle, J., cultural assessment, 222, 222f
Breach of confidentiality, 359–60
Breast cancer
  risk factors for, 277
  screening guidelines, 278f, 285t
Breast self-examination, 277
Breckinridge, M., 459
Bunge, H. L., 23t
Bureaucratic management, 509
Burnout, 447–48
  defined, 447
  stages of, 448

Calcium supplements, 295t
Calling, nursing as a, 53, 234
Cancer
  breast, 277, 278f, 285t
  cervical, 278t, 286t
  colorectal, 285t

Clinical reasoning (*See also* Critical thinking)
  components of, 152
  in education curriculum, 41
  reflective (*See* Reflective clinical reasoning)
Co-insurance, defined, 327
Cochrane Collaborative, 252, 256–57
Cochrane systematic review, 257–58, 258f
Code for Academic and Clinical Professional Conduct, 58
Code of ethics, 121–23
  American Nurses Association (ANA), 55, 123
Cognitive development, Piaget's stages of, 108, 109t
Cognitive strategies for learning, 189
Collaboration, 482–501
  in advance practice nursing, 467–68, 475
  characteristics of, 483–84, 484f
  communication and, 483, 486
  defined, 468, 483
  essential elements of, 486, 487t, 488
  future trends, 497–500
    National Black Nurses Association (NBNA), 498, 500
    Pew Health Professions Commission, 498, 499f
    Tri-Council of Nursing, 497–98
  key points, 500–501
  measurement tool for, 486, 486f
  nurse-physician, 467–68, 485, 485f
  in practice, 494–97
    advance practice nursing, 495–96
    case management, 496
    critical paths, 497
    health care alliances, 495
    quality improvement teams (QIT), 496–97
    transdisciplinary, 494
  purpose of, 483
  skills for
    conflict resolution, 491–92
    empowerment, 492–93
    negotiation, 488–91, 490t
    team building, 488, 489f, 490f
  stages of, 495
  transdisciplinary, 494
  transition into practice, 500
  vs. partnership, 484
Collaboration and Satisfaction About Care Decisions (CSACD) instrument, 486, 486f
Collaborative education, 494–95
Collaborative health record, 326
Collaborative practice
  case management, 538
  interdisciplinary teams, 538
  practice partnership model, 538–39

Collaborative practice agreements (CPA), in advance practice nursing, 467–68
Collective bargaining, 529–30
Collegiality
  in collaboration, 487t
  defined, 56
Colorectal cancer, screenings recommendations for, 285t
Commission on the Graduates of Foreign Nursing Schools (CGFNS), 420
Commitment
  in caring, 137
  in collaboration, 487t
  political influence and, 338
  in time management, 445
Communication
  in collaboration, 483, 486, 487t
  defined, 486
  in education curriculum, 40–41
  electronic, 177
  leadership and, 516–17
  legal considerations, 366–67, 367f
  technology and, 30
  in time management, 445
Compassion, defined, 136
Compassion fatigue, 448–49
Compensation packages, 539–40
Competence
  in caring, 137
  clinical, 407–8
  defined, 188
  emotional, 408–10, 409t
Competency, 184–206
  continuing, 187
  continuing professional nursing, 187–88
  defined, 187
  developing, 188
  errors and, 200–202
  essential nursing, 191–92, 194–95
    American Association of Colleges of Nursing (AACN), 192, 193f, 193t
    American Nurses Association (ANA), 195
    Pew Health Professions Commission, 192, 194–95, 194f
  expectations about, 199–200
    health care team, 199–200
    institutional, 199
    patient, 200
  key points, 205
  levels of nursing, 191, 191f
    core, 191, 191f
    patient care management, 191, 191f
    specialty, 191, 191f

Medical self-care, 329–30

Medicare, advance practice nursing and, 473

Medication compliance, health care costs and, 332

Medication Errors Reporting Program (MERP), 174

MEDLINE, 256

MedMARx, 174

MedWatch, 174

Men in nursing, 26, 27t–28t, 28–29

Mentorships, 515
  leadership and, 517–18
  transition into practice and, 413–14

Merciless Master, 446

Meta-analysis, 258, 258f

Metacognition, 150

Metaparadigms, 73–76
  characteristics of, 74–75
  defined, 74, 77t
  of nursing, 75–76
    caring, 76
    environment, 76
    health, 76
    nursing, 75–76
    person, 75–76
    transition, 76
  of various nursing conceptual frameworks, 88t–93t

Midlevel practitioner, 466

Midwife, certified nurse, 459–60

Military, impact on nursing, 8, 18, 108

Mill, J. S., 120–21

Mind-body interventions, 297, 297t

Minors, legal considerations, 351, 365

Mission statement, economic considerations, 324–25

Modem, defined, 177

Moral development, 108–11
  defined, 108
  Gilligan's ethic of caring, 111, 112t
  Kohlberg's theory of, 109–11, 110t

Morbidity
  in adolescents, 275
  in children, 273
  in men, 279–81
  in older adults, 280
  in women, 276–79

Mortality, leading causes of
  in adolescents, 275
  in children, 273, 275t
  in men, 277t, 279
  in older adults, 280
  risk factors for, 268–69, 270t
  in United States, 268, 269t
  in women, 276, 277t

Motivation, 409–10, 409t

Motorized sporting vehicles, 352f

Multiculturalism, defined, 218

Multistate licensure, 429–30

Multistate privilege to practice, 430

Muslim, 236

Mutual recognition, in advance practice nursing, 466

National Advisory Council on Nurse Education and Practice (NACNEP), on information technology, 164–65

National Black Nurses Association (NBNA), collaboration model, 498, 500

National Caring Conferences, 129

National Center for Complementary and Alternative Medicine (NCCAM)
  purpose of, 299–300
  research centers, 301–2, 302t

National Committee for Quality Assurance (NCQA), 468

National Council Examination (NCLEX) (*See* NCLEX)

National Council of State Boards of Nursing (NCSBN), 422

National Leagues of Nursing (NLN), 340

National Organization for Public Health Nursing (NOPHN), 340–41

National Practitioner Data Bank, 429, 467

National Student Nurses' Association (NSNA), 57–60
  Code for Academic and Clinical Professional Conduct, 58
  leadership development, 59–60
  Leadership U, 58–59
  mission of, 57
  purpose and function of, 57, 58t
  resolutions, 59–64

NCLEX, 422–29
  application for, 423
  Computer Adaptive Testing (CAT), 422, 424
  failing, 431–32
  innovative test items, 422–23
  job analysis survey, 42
  licensure and, 427–28
  preparing for, 424–26
  purpose of, 423
  research about, 424–25
  review courses for, 426–27

Needs, self appraisal of, 379, 379t

Negligence, 358, 359t, 467

Negotiation
  in collaboration, 488–91, 490t
  defined, 488

Unfair labor practices, 530
Uninsured, economic considerations, 315–16
Union activity, 530
United American Nurses (UAN), 64, 66
United States health care, 214–17, 317–18
    demographics, 215–17
    disparities in health care, 215–17
    health insurance, 214–15
Unlicensed assistive personnel (UAP), delegation to,
        421–22
Urbanization, global demographics, 212
Utilitarianism, 120–21

Validity
    external, 257
    internal, 257
Value system, defined, 115
Values (*See also* Nursing values)
    defined, 115
    ethics and, 115–19
    in policy development, 344–45
    professional, 115
    public policy and, 337
    self appraisal of, 375–77, 377t
    spirituality and, 238
Values clarification, 116
Values conflict, 116
Veracity, 113t, 114
Violence
    in men, 280
    teen, 276, 276f, 338
    workplace, 202–3
Visual impairments, in older adults, 280–81
Vitamin A, 295t

Vitamin C, 295t
Vitamin D, 295t
Vitamin K, 295t
Vitamins
    commonly used, 295t
    supplementation of, 295t
Vocation, defined, 234

Wald, L., 9, 25t, 458
War, impact on nursing, 8, 18, 108
Watson, J.
    conceptual framework of, 75t
    holistic view of, 453
    nursing as an art, 134
    transpersonal caring-healing model, 137–39, 138t
    writings of, 86t
Web-based instruction (WBI), 179f
Web course development tools, 179f
Weber, M., 509
Welsh, D., 402, 403t
Wheatley, M. J., 511–13
White House Commission on Complementary and
        Alternative Medicine Policy, 300
Wholeness, defined, 232
Witnesses, 362
Women's movement, political influence of, 340–41
Women's work
    caring and, 128–29
    in history of nursing, 11–12, 22, 25
    subordinate sex, 25–26
Workplace violence, 202–3
World Wide Web (WWW), defined, 177

Zone therapy, 293t